Endocrinology

Endocrinology

MAC E. HADLEY

Department of Biology
University of Arizona
Tucson, Arizona

PRENTICE-HALL, INC., *Englewood Cliffs, New Jersey 07632*

Library of Congress Cataloging in Publication Data

HADLEY, MAC E.
Endocrinology.

Includes bibliographical references and index.
1. Endocrinology. I. Title. [DNLM: 1. Endocrinology.
WK 100 H131e]
QP187.H17 1984   599'.0142   83-8701
ISBN 0-13-277137-3

43,284

Editorial/production supervision and
interior design: Virginia Huebner
Cover design: Photo Plus Art, Celine Brandes
Manufacturing buyer: John Hall

Printed in the United States of America

10 9 8 7 6 5 4 3 2 1

ISBN 0-13-277137-3

Prentice-Hall International, Inc., *London*
Prentice-Hall of Australia Pty. Limited, *Sydney*
Editora Prentice-Hall do Brasil, Ltda., *Rio de Janeiro*
Prentice-Hall Canada Inc., *Toronto*
Prentice-Hall of India Private Limited, *New Delhi*
Prentice-Hall of Japan, Inc., *Tokyo*
Prentice-Hall of Southeast Asia Pte. Ltd., *Singapore*
Whitehall Books Limited, *Wellington, New Zealand*

This text is dedicated to my wife, Trudy, in appreciation
for her constant encouragement and assistance during the
preparation of this book, and to my daughter,

Martha Sharon Hadley

Contents

4 GENERAL MECHANISMS OF HORMONE ACTION

7

NEUROHYPOPHYSIAL HORMONES   140

8

THE MELANOTROPINS   160

12 GROWTH HORMONES 264

13 THYROID HORMONES 292

14 CATECHOLAMINES AND THE SYMPATHOADRENAL SYSTEM

15 ADRENAL STEROIDS   344

18 HORMONES AND FEMALE REPRODUCTIVE PHYSIOLOGY

421

21   NEUROHORMONES   488

Preface

This textbook of ENDOCRINOLOGY was written to fill the need for a modern and complete coverage of the field of neuroendocrine physiology, and to use in teaching a course in general endocrinology. The outline of this book is quite similar to the lecture schedule followed in my general endocrinology course, and also uses material from a course in comparative endocrinology that I taught for many years.

The central theme of this text is the role of chemical messengers, hormones, whether they are of endocrine or neural origin, in the control of physiological processes. Although, classically, endocrine physiology has been separated from neurophysiology, it is now amply documented that hormones may originate from either endocrine or neural tissue. Thus, has emerged the field of *neuroendrocrinology*. The awarding of Nobel prizes in Physiology or Medicine to a number of eminent endocrinologists for their monumental efforts leading to the discovery and elucidation of the chemical structure of several brain neuropeptides (neurohormones), clearly emphasizes the importance of the concept of neuroendocrine physiology. It is now also realized that the so-called "classical" hormones are produced in many sites throughout the body and may be released either directly into the blood, into neuronal synapses, or into the immediate intercellular space to affect adjacent cellular activity. A more inclusive definition of "hormone" has, therefore, been employed, as suggested by the Nobel Laureate, Roger Guillemin. The important point emphasized in this concept is that it is the method of delivery rather than the source of the hormone that is of greatest physiological significance.

In the INTRODUCTION TO ENDOCRINOLOGY a short chronology of the history of endocrine research is presented. The concept of homeostasis is then discussed with special reference given to the roles of chemical messengers in the control of homeostatic systems. The reader is then provided with a general description of THE VERTEBRATE ENDOCRINE SYSTEM wherein an initial working vocabulary is established. Included here is a discussion of: the general classes of chemical messengers and other cellular regulators (steroid and peptide hormones, neurohormones, chalones, growth factors, prostaglandins, pheromones), the cellular synthesis of chemical messengers, their secretion, delivery, and metabolism, and a general overview of the physiological roles of hormones. In consideration of the variety of methodologies utilized in present-day endocrine research, it was considered necessary to add a chapter on ENDOCRINE METHODOLOGIES early in the text. Classical surgical and histological techniques are discussed as are more recent methods including: radioimmunoassay, radioreceptor assay, radioisotope enzyme assay, autoradiography, and recombinant DNA methodology. It was also considered important to provide, early in the book, a discussion of GENERAL MECHANISMS OF HORMONE ACTION, because these concepts are a necessary component of each of the following chapters. Included within this chapter is a discussion of cellular receptors, cyclic nucleotides as second messengers, prostaglandins (and prostacyclins, thromboxanes and leukotrienes), kallikrein-kinin systems, stimulus-response coupling, calmodulin (a cellular calcium receptor) and phosphorylated proteins as physiological effectors.

The source, synthesis, chemistry and general role of the PITUITARY HORMONES in the control of endocrine physiology is discussed next because the pituitary gland is a major source of hormones regulating many other endocrine glands. More specific details of the roles and actions of these hormones are provided in subsequent chapters. Because the secretion of each of the pituitary hormones is controlled by hypophysiotropic hormones of hypothalamic origin, a chapter on the role of THE ENDOCRINE HYPOTHALAMUS is provided. The evidence supporting the neurovascular hypothesis is emphasized.

Chapter seven, NEUROHYPOPHYSIAL HORMONES, provides a complete coverage of the source, synthesis, chemistry, secretion, metabolism, biological actions and mechanisms of action of the posterior pituitary hormones, oxytocin and the vasopressins. The evolution of hormone structure is emphasized under the comparative endocrinology of neurohypophysial hormones. Chapter 8, THE MELANOTROPINS emphasizes the recent discovery that pro-opiomelanocortin is the precursor protein of α-melanotropin, adrenocorticotropin, and man's own analgesic hormones, the endorphins (opiate-like peptides). The author has done considerable research in the field of melanotropins and vertebrate pigmentation, particularly in relationship to the control of melanocyte stimulating hormone secretion and the mechanisms of action of the melanotropins. Because the secretion and actions of most all hormones involve the calcium ion, the roles of parathormone, calcitonin and vitamin D in the HORMONAL CONTROL OF CALCIUM HOMEOSTASIS are discussed early in the book.

The next six chapters are grouped together because they all relate importantly to aspects of metabolic endocrinology. The GASTROINTESTINAL HORMONES play important roles in the control of the movement of foodstuffs through the gastrointestinal tract, and their transport through the intestinal mucosa and into the general circulation. The chapter on PANCREATIC HORMONES AND META-

BOLIC ENDOCRINOLOGY discusses the roles of the endocrine pancreas in the storage and utilization of metabolic substrates. The contrasting roles of insulin and glucagon are explored as are the possible roles of the newer pancreatic hormones, somatostatin and pancreatic polypeptide. In a chapter on GROWTH HORMONES, the varied roles of the somatomedins and other peptide growth hormones, such as nerve growth factor, epidermal growth factor, erythropoietin, and the thymic growth factors, as well as growth inhibitory factors (chalones) are discussed in addition to a coverage of pituitary somatotropin.

In the THYROID HORMONES, evidence is marshalled that triiodothyronine is the physiologically relevant thyroid hormone at the cellular level. An extensive review of several models of thyroid hormone action is provided. A discussion of the integrated functional aspects of CATECHOLAMINES AND THE SYMPATHOADRENAL SYSTEM provides recent data on the developmental biology of catecholamine biosynthesis within adrenal chromaffin tissue and sympathetic neurons. The physiological roles of catecholamines as mediated through adrenergic receptors is discussed, and the pharmacology of the autonomic nervous system, particularly the sympathoadrenal system, is reviewed. The chapter on the ADRENAL STEROIDS completes the general discussion of the roles and acitons of hormones in the control of metabolic homeostasis. Steroid hormone structure and nomenclature is reviewed. The newly recognized roles of the renal kallikrein-kinin system in the actions of aldosterone, the major mineralocorticoid of the adrenal, on the kidney is summarized.

The next five chapters deal with the endocrinology of vertebrate reproductive systems, mostly mammalian systems. In the ENDOCRINOLOGY OF SEX DIF-FERENTIATION AND DEVELOPMENT, the recently recognized role of the H-Y antigen (a hormone) in the regulation of gonadal differentiation is discussed. The early organizational roles of gonadal steroids in the development of neural centers (e.g., dimorphic nucleus) within the central nervous system, and the activational roles of steroids in CNS function in the adult animal are reviewed. In HORMONES AND MALE REPRODUCTIVE PHYSIOLOGY, as in HORMONES AND FEMALE REPRODUCTIVE PHYSIOLOGY, the origin, synthesis, chemistry, secretion, metabolism, biological roles and mechanisms of actions of the male and female reproductive hormones are reviewed. A discussion of the pathophysiology of reproductive function in the human male and female provides an insight into the many genetic and congenital defects that affect normal growth and development of the human reproductive systems. In ENDOCRINOLOGY OF PREGNANCY, PAR-TURITION, AND LACTATION, the roles of hormones in the fertile period of the female are reviewed. Next is included a chapter on the ENDOCRINE ROLE OF THE PINEAL which reviews its putative role in reproduction physiology. This chapter is long overdue; the pineal gland is clearly an endocrine organ.

A final chapter devoted to NEUROHORMONES emphasizes the emerging understanding of the importance of neuropeptides to endocrine system function. For example, the discovery and physiological roles of the endorphins, the opiate-like peptides, or "analgesic hormones," are discussed. The role of other newly discovered brain peptides which include substance P, neurotensin, bombesin, and other gastrointestinal peptides, in brain function and behavior is reviewed.

An outline is provided for each chapter. Generally, each chapter is subdivided as follows: 1) INTRODUCTION, (which provides a historical perspective to the particular topic), 2) SOURCE, 3) SYNTHESIS, 4) CHEMISTRY, 5) SECRETIONS, 6) METABOLISM, 7) PHYSIOLOGICAL ROLES, 8) MECHANISM OF ACTION, 9) PATHOPHYSIOLOGY (of endocrine dysfunction), and 10) COMPARATIVE ENDOCRINOLOGY. Due to space limitations and other considerations the coverage of neuroendocrine physiology has been generally restricted to vertebrates, mainly mammals, particularly the human. Therefore, this book should be of special appeal to preprofessional students in medicine, dentistry, pharmacology, and other related medical or animal sciences. Within each chapter, however, where appropriate, is included a short coverage of comparative endocrinology.

References are provided with each chapter, but, because space limitations place a premium on those selected, those most recently available were used. These references will provide the reader with most of the important earlier studies related to a particular topic. The author, therefore acknowledges the unreferenced contributions of many investigators in the field of neuroendocrine physiology. I am particularly grateful to my past students, both in the classroom and the research laboratory, who provided me with an opportunity to develop those thoughts which are now presented in this textbook of ENDOCRINOLOGY. I am also grateful to those individuals who have critically read all or part of the manuscript. Acknowledgement of these individuals does not, however, necessarily imply that they totally endorse the content of any one chapter as it is presented to the reader. The reviewers include the following (chapter reviewed are indicated):

Dr. Earl B. Barnawell (all); Dr. Mohammed Bedzadian (12); Dr. Sue A. Binkely (20); Dr. David E. Blask (20); Dr. David W. Borst (19); Dr. Jean B. Burnett (8); Dr. Robert B. Chiasson (15, 16); Dr. Walter Chavin (many); Dr. Russell P. Davis (17, 18); Dr. James A. Edwardson (8); Dr. Milton Fingerman (many); Dr. Sally K. Frost (12); Dr. Blake A. Gosnell (6, 10, 21); Dr. Robert L. Hazelwood (11); Dr. Mark R. Haussler (9); Dr. Andre J. Van Herle (13); Dr. Henry W. Kircher (many); Dr. Victor J. Hruby (7); Dr. Sigmund Hsiao (6, 10, 21); Dr. James P. Hughes (3, 4, 15); Dr. David G. Johnson (11); Dr. Hugh E. Laird (14); Dr. Bruce Magun (12); Dr. Lynn M. Matrisian (12); Dr. Frank L. Meyskens (8); Dr. Peter K. T. Pang (9); Dr. Elizabeth K. Perryman (7, 8); Dr. Brian T. Pickering (7); Dr. Russel J. Reiter (20); Dr. Sami I. Said (10); Dr. Melvin S. Soloff (7); Dr. Richard L. Stouffer (10, 16, 17, 18, 19); Dr. David L. Vesely (4, 13); Dr. Brian Weatherhead (8, 9).

Most of the figures in the book were prepared by Mr. Paul Martin and Ms. Thelma Reinhard. A few were prepared by Ms. Ginney Childs. The author greatly appreciates the fine efforts of these three individuals.

Helpful criticisms, corrections, or other comments are most welcome and may be addressed to the author.

MAC E. HADLEY
Tucson, Arizona

Endocrinology

1

Introduction
to Endocrinology

INTRODUCTION

Development of a multicellular organism commences upon fertilization and subsequent division of the egg. Further development is then dependent on continued cell proliferation, growth, and differentiation, including histogenesis and organogenesis. The integration of these developmental events as well as the coordination of such physiological processes as metabolism, respiration, excretion, movement, and reproduction, are dependent on chemical cues—substances—synthesized and secreted by specialized cells within the animal. The role of these *chemical messengers*, *endocrines*, in the growth and regulation of cellular function in the vertebrate is the topic of this book.

Endocrinology is a subdiscipline of the broader field, physiology, and is concerned with chemical messengers or *hormones*, substances secreted by cells of endocrine glands (ductless glands) and tissues that regulate the activity of other cells in the body. Besides the obvious study of the physiological roles of hormones, endocrinologists also study the cellular source and synthesis of hormones, hormonal chemistry and storage, the factors and mechanisms controlling hormonal secretion, the cellular mechanisms of action of hormones, and the pathophysiology of endocrine system dysfunction. The comparative endocrinologist is particularly interested in the study of the endocrine systems of a number of vertebrate or invertebrate species.

HISTORICAL PERSPECTIVE

Endocrinology is a relatively infant science which began with the first recorded endocrine experiment published by Berthold (1849). No other truly significant discoveries were made until about 50 years later (1889–1902). The pace quickened after 1910, and the outlines of vertebrate and invertebrate endocrine systems were generally complete by 1950. From then on, chemistry played a most important role in the development of the science and many advances in the field were made. With the discovery of cyclic AMP in 1957 and the discovery of brain hormones more recently, the interested individual has difficulty keeping abreast of this expanding field.

An Endocrine Chronology

The history of endocrinology progressed, as one might expect, from simple observations to complex experimentation. Early medical writings described the general symptoms of many endocrine dysfunctions long before the pathophysiology of any of the now well-characterized *endocrinopathies* were at all understood. In the age of the great microscopists of the nineteenth century most tissues and organs of the vertebrate body were described in great detail, but the functional significance of what we now refer to as endocrine glands was not evident. Clinical correlations between tissue or organ abnormalities, such as atrophy or enlargement, and a change in a particular physiological state were occasionally noted. This led to the study of the possible effects of tissue or organ removal from animals and subsequent alteration in physiological function. The utilization of organ transplants or extracts to determine whether they could serve as adequate replacement therapy for the absent tissue or organ then followed. Successful replacement therapy led to the purification of these physiologically active extracts and ultimately to the identification of the hormonal substances concerned.

Berthold, in the earliest endocrinological study on record, noted that if he castrated cockerels they failed to develop their comb and wattles and they also failed to exhibit male behavior. Replacement of the testes (one or both) back into the abdominal cavity of the same or another bird resulted in normal development of the comb and wattles, and the birds exhibited male behavior, which involved an interest in hens and an aggressive action toward other males. The transplanted testes were functional and therefore not dependent on any direct nervous innervation for their activity. Berthold even observed that a transplanted single testis was larger than either testis of the host when both were present together in the bird. He thus discovered, but may not have appreciated, what is now referred to as *compensatory hypertrophy*, an increase in the size of an organ to compensate functionally for the activity of the other lost organ. His results also demonstrated that an organ from one (donor) animal could be transplanted to another (host) animal where it became functional (Fig. 1.1).

Berthold concluded that the testes secreted something that conditioned the blood, and he speculated that the blood then acted on the body of the cockerel to cause the development of male characteristics. Actually these experiments only demonstrated the need for the presence of the testes to maintain male characteristics. The testes could maintain such behavioral and physiological functions by a number of

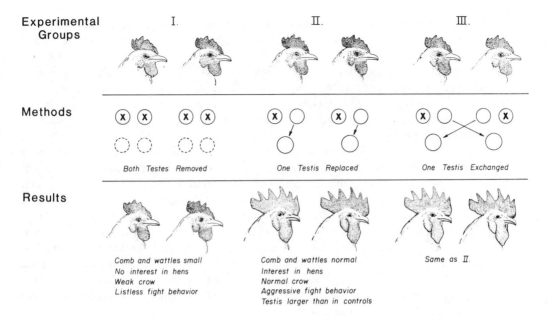

Experimental Groups

I. II. III.

Methods

Both Testes Removed   One Testis Replaced   One Testis Exchanged

Results

Comb and wattles small
No interest in hens
Weak crow
Listless fight behavior

Comb and wattles normal
Interest in hens
Normal crow
Aggressive fight behavior
Testis larger than in controls

Same as II.

Figure 1.1 Berthold experiment: the first endocrine experiment.

possible means: (1) activation or transformation of one or more constituents of the blood into active agents, hormones, (2) removal of an inhibitory substance from the blood or, as is now known, (3) release of a hormone into the circulation. That the testes produce a substance that is released into the blood to affect masculine features and behavior was not proven until many years later when it was shown that extracts of the testes could functionally replace the testes of a castrated animal. The hormone of the testes, testosterone, was finally obtained in pure crystalline form in 1935.

In 1902 the first critical experiment, the *experimentum cruces*, demonstrating the existence of a hormone was reported [2]. Bayliss and Starling, Canadian physiologists, discovered that a substance was liberated by the mucosa of the small intestine that stimulates the flow of pancreatic juice. It was known that the acid present in chyme stimulated pancreatic secretion after it entered into the small intestine from the stomach. Introduction of acid into an isolated (denervated) but vascularized section of the jejunum caused a similar flow of pancreatic juice. This observation supported the view that the control of pancreatic enzyme secretion was mediated by humoral rather than nervous stimulation. Extracts of jejunal epithelium produced similar effects on pancreatic secretion. The active substance was given the name *secretin* and was further shown to be localized only to those regions of the small intestine that could be stimulated by acid to induce pancreatic fluid flow. Starling (1905) introduced the term *hormone* (Greek: I arouse to activity or I excite) for this humoral factor [22].

In 1889 Von Mering and Minkowski showed by surgical methods that removal of the pancreas from dogs led to symptoms that are similar to those characteristic of human *diabetes mellitus*. In these dogs, as in diabetic humans, blood sugar levels were remarkably elevated; this suggested that diabetes mellitus might result from a defect of carbohydrate metabolism due to lack of pancreatic function. Banting and Best [1] concluded from other investigations that the islets of Langerhans, rather than the pancreatic acini, which make up the bulk of the pancreas, are essential in the control of carbohydrate metabolism. They suggested that the pancreatic islets regulate blood glucose levels by producing an internal secretion, rather than by modifying the blood. In 1922 they successfully obtained extracts of the pancreatic islets, and showed that these preparations caused a dramatic drop in blood glucose levels when administered to diabetic dogs. This hormone of the pancreas had been given the name insulin by Schaefer in 1912.

Although many hormones are released from cells into the general circulation to mediate their effects on distant target cells, an equally large number of chemical messengers are released from neurons into close proximity to the effector cells which they regulate. These chemical messengers of neural origin play important roles in *central nervous system* (CNS) and *autonomic nervous system* (ANS) function. Cannon was the first physiologist to stress the role of the autonomic nervous system in the "self-regulation of physiological processes" [6]. As is described in Chapter 14, the ANS regulates the activity of such so-called autonomic activities as gastrointestinal smooth muscle contraction and relaxation, gastrointestinal secretions (including hormone secretions from the stomach and gut), cardiovascular muscle contraction and relaxation, and adipose tissue metabolism.

That nerves release chemical messengers that control effector cell activity was first demonstrated in 1921 by Loewi [15]. A frog heart with its attached vagus nerve was incubated in physiological saline solution, and after residing therein for a period of time, the solution was pipetted off and used to bathe a second heart. There was no effect of the solution on the *inotropic* (amplitude of beat) or *chronotropic* (rate of beat) characteristics of the incubated heart. If, on the other hand, the vagus nerve innervating an incubated heart was stimulated a number of times and the saline solution then pipetted off into another beaker containing another frog heart, a decreased (negative) inotropic and chronotropic activity was noted. These diminished myotropic responses could be blocked by addition of the drug, atropine, which was known to be inhibitory to vagal nerve-induced relaxation of the heart. The atropinized heart preparations did, however, respond to saline solution taken from vagus nerve-stimulated hearts by an increased rate and strength of contraction. These experiments demonstrated that the vagus nerve released substances that affect the relaxation and contraction of cardiac muscle. For this work Loewi received a Nobel Prize. The "vagustuff" (vagal substance) was identified as *acetylcholine* and the accelerator substance as *norepinephrine*. These two neurohormones play very important roles in endocrine physiology (Chapter 14).

In 1953, Sanger established the amino acid sequence for the protein hormone insulin [19]. For this crucial work in the characterization of hormone structure he received a Nobel Prize. By his methods the structures of most peptide hormones have been elucidated. At the same time du Vigneaud carried out the first laboratory syntheses of peptide hormones by synthesizing oxytocin and a vasopressin. For this work he, too, received a Nobel Prize. Most interestingly, he also synthesized a related structure (analog) of oxytocin, which turned out to be a hormone found in the pituitaries of most vertebrates. He thus determined the structure of a hormone (vasotocin) before it was even discovered (Chapter 7).

The Discovery of Cyclic AMP

In 1962 Sutherland and his colleagues presented a number of papers describing the presence of adenosine 3′, 5′-monophosphate (*cyclic AMP, cAMP*) in biological materials. These papers also dealt with adenylate cyclase, the enzyme which was responsible for the cellular production of this cyclic nucleotide. Sutherland and his coworkers had previously demonstrated that hormones could stimulate broken cell membrane preparations to activate liver phosphorylase, the enzyme responsible for the normal breakdown of liver glycogen. These workers established that when hormones were incubated with a particulate (cell membrane) fraction of liver cells, a factor was produced which could in turn activate the phosphorylase enzyme present in the supernatant fraction of the tissue homogenate. This substance was identified by Sutherland as cyclic AMP (Fig. 1.2).

For this monumental discovery Sutherland received a Nobel Prize in Physiology or Medicine in 1971 [23]. Cyclic AMP, the so-called second messenger of hormone action, is now implicated in the actions of many hormones and other stimuli on cellular physiological processes. The importance of this cyclic nucleotide to biochemistry, pharmacology, physiology, and medicine is enormous. Much of this book is, in fact, a discussion of the role of cyclic AMP in hormone action and cellular function.

Neuropeptides and Nobel Prizes

Another crucial discovery was the demonstration that the pituitary gland, the so-called master gland of the body, was controlled by the brain, specifically the area known as the hypothalamus. Harris had provided data suggesting that the release of the pituitary hormones was controlled by humoral factors probably of hypothalamic origin [14]. A number of workers then showed that extracts of the hypothalamus contained substances that affected the release of pituitary hormones [16, 21, 25]. The "race to Stockholm" was then on [26]. Schally and Guillemin, working independently of each other, began purification of hypothalamic extracts from porcine and ovine sources. After the extraction of about 250,000 pig hypothalami, Schally and his group were able to provide the structure of the factor that stimulates the release of thyroid stimulating hormone (TSH) from the pituitary gland. The structure of this thyrotropin releasing

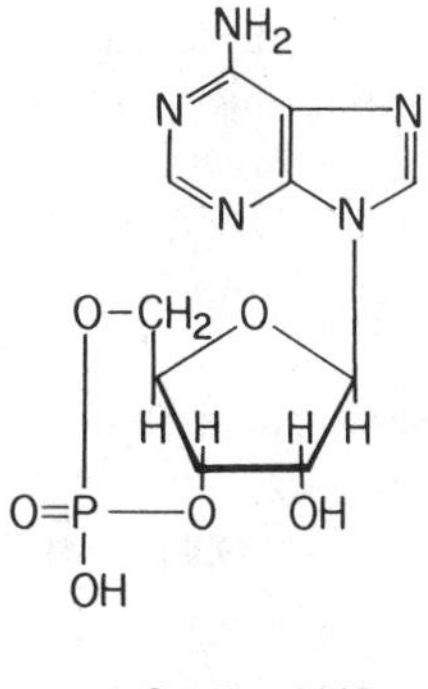

Cyclic AMP

Figure 1.2 Structure of cyclic AMP, the second messenger of hormone action.

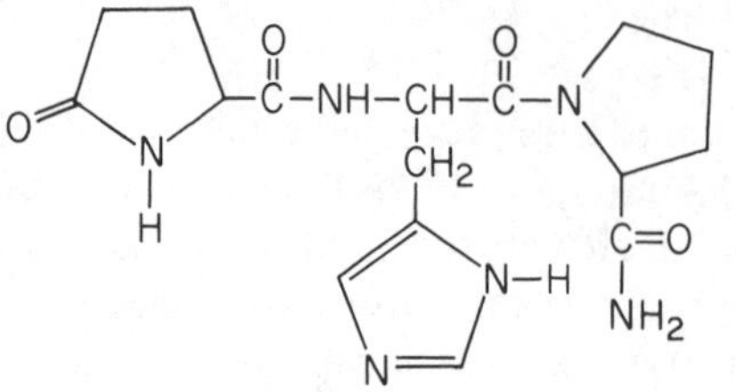

Figure 1.3 Structure of thyrotropin releasing hormone (TRH), a neurohormone.

hormone (TRH) was similar (Fig. 1.3) to that of the same factor isolated from sheep brains by Guillemin and reported at about the same time. This work was followed by the isolation and structural identification of the hypothalamic hormones which control the secretion of pituitary gonadotropins and growth hormone.

Schally and his collaborators were also able to provide the chemical structure of porcine gonadotropin releasing hormone (GnRH), which controls the release of the gonadotropins from the pituitary. Guillemin and his group then revealed that sheep GnRH was identical in structure. The potential importance of the elucidation of the structure of GnRH is immense. It may now be possible to control fertility in humans and domestic animals with synthetic GnRH. It is also possible to improve on the structure of the natural GnRH to provide analogs that enhance gonadotropin secretion from the pituitary, which may enhance the probability of conception. On the other hand, antihormone analogs may also be produced which may then be used as contraceptive agents.

Guillemin and his colleagues were the first to discover and report the structure of a peptide, somatostatin, that was inhibitory to pituitary somatotropin (growth hormone) secretion. Somatostatin, also found in other regions of the brain and in the pancreas, inhibits a number of hormone secretions including the pancreatic hormones, glucagon and insulin. The implications of this discovery for medicine may be vast. Already there is a hope that somatostatin or related analogs may be utilized in the treatment of diabetes mellitus, a major endocrine dysfunction of humans.

For their contribution to the isolation and determination of the structures of the hypothalamic regulatory peptides, Guillemin and Schally received a Nobel Prize in Physiology or Medicine in 1978 [11, 20]. Certainly the pioneering work of Harris and many others provided the great impetus for the important accomplishments of Schally and Guillemin, as they have acknowledged. Many other chemists and endocrinologists provided important discoveries that facilitated greatly the determination of the structures and roles of hypothalamic peptide hormones. The knowledge of the structures and functions of these hypothalamic regulatory hormones is of the greatest importance for the welfare of humanity. As discussed later, other hypothalamic factors are being discovered and their roles in endocrine physiology elucidated (Chapters 6 and 21).

The ability to isolate and characterize chemically the hypothalamic factors was enhanced by the development of the radioimmunoassay (RIA). By the use of RIA's it is possible to detect the presence of hormones in the blood or in tissues at very minute concentrations. Future possibilities for other uses of RIA's appear to be limitless [28]. For the development of the RIA, Yalow received a Nobel Prize in Physiology or Medicine in 1978 along with Schally and Guillemin.

Important new information in endocrine physiology is being reported at a rapid rate. Certainly knowledge of the molecular mechanisms of peptide [8] and steroid [7] hormone action are being defined in exquisite detail. One might predict that future Nobel Prizes will be awarded in this exciting field of *neuroendocrine physiology*.

THE SCIENCE OF ENDOCRINOLOGY

Endocrine glands secrete their hormones into the immediate extracellular space from where the hormones then enter the circulatory system. These ductless glands differ from *exocrine glands* (e.g., salivary glands) whose products are released into ducts that lead to the digestive tract and then to the exterior of the body. Endocrinology is therefore the study of the ductless glands or tissues and their hormonal products. Hormones were originally considered to be synthesized within specific endocrine organs and then secreted into the bloodstream to act on specific target tissues some distance away to evoke a specific physiological response. These definitions of endocrine glands and their hormones are too restrictive and must therefore be modified to be of any instructive value. For example, Bayliss and Starling clearly demonstrated that secretin is released from the small intestine, specifically the jejunum. Secretin is actually produced and secreted by individual cells distributed individually through the epithelial lining of the jejunum. The gastrointestinal tract is the source of other hormones and could well be considered the largest endocrine organ of the body [17]. Secretin travels by way of the blood to act on the pancreas to induce pancreatic secretion, but it also has many other sites of action and therefore produces a number of other effects. Secretin may also be released from nerve cells within the brain to act on adjacent or nearby neurons. In this case, the hormone secretin does not travel from its source of origin to its site of action by way of the bloodstream.

Such bloodborne hormones as secretin will be considered as one example of the numerous chemical messengers within the body that control physiological processes. As for other chemical messengers, they or their precursors are synthesized by cells, but they may travel to a distant target tissue by way of the blood or they may function as local hormones. The various classes of chemical messengers that exist are discussed in Chapter 2.

Comparative Endocrinology

Much of what is known about the endocrine physiology of humans derives from data obtained from patients manifesting signs of endocrine dysfunction. Research on other animals, particularly the rat and the mouse, has also provided a wealth of information on the endocrine system of mammals including that of humans. One should appreciate, however, the contributions that comparative endocrinology has provided for a broader evolutionary view of the endocrine system [9].

Although the chemical structures of most hormones of humans have been elucidated, this information obviously does not provide knowledge of the evolution of these hormones. Once the structures of the related hormones of other vertebrates are determined, however, it becomes possible to trace the changes in the structure of the hormones that have evolved. In comparing the amino acid sequences of similar peptide structures from primitive and more recent vertebrates one can determine the approximate rates of evolutionary change in the hormones and the time in earth history when particular chemical changes probably occurred. Knowledge of comparative hormone structure allows one to synthesize related structural analogs with possible predictions on biological activity. This is important as some hormones are not available in large enough quantities to supply the medicinal needs of humans. A lack of somatotropin (STH) results in a failure of growth in humans. If STH were commercially available, normal growth could be initiated and normal bodily stature attained, but supplies of STH are severely limited. Although primate STH might be compatible, such supplies of the hormone are limited and not feasible for such a use. With a knowledge of the comparative structure of STH it might be possible to determine the active site of the molecule. The entire structure of STH is too large to synthesize chemically, especially on a commercial basis, but it might be possible to synthesize some smaller sequence comprising the active site of the hormone. Introduction of the human STH gene into bacteria by recombination DNA techniques, may provide a means for the large-scale production of the hormone (Chapter 3). The recent discovery and chemical elucidation of the structure of a putative hypothalamic STH releasing factor may also provide a medically important tool for stimulating pituitary STH secretion [13, 18].

Knowledge of how hormones work owes much to studies on the large chromosomes from salivary glands of such dipteran flies as *Drosophila* and *Chironomus*. The action of hormones on genes can be visualized using the large chromosomes from these glands. Certain insect hormones cause so-called puffs in the chromosome structure which represent areas where DNA has become exposed and RNA synthesis is increased. One can follow completely the puffing patterns of these large chromosomes during the larval development of the insects. Knowledge of invertebrate hormone structure and mechanisms of action may provide a potent tool in the fight against the insect world. Understanding the endocrine system of other vertebrate and invertebrate species provides important information that may be essential to animal husbandry and the culture and growing of exotic species, such as shrimp and other edible crustaceans or mollusks [3].

THE CONCEPT OF HOMEOSTASIS

Claude Bernard, the nineteenth-century French physiologist, first formulated the concept of homeostasis [12]. He pointed out that an individual lives within two environments: the exterior environment that surrounds us, and, more importantly, a *milieu interieur*. This internal environment is the fluid compartment within which the cells of our body are bathed. Bernard noted that this fluid is produced and controlled by the individual organism. Organisms become more independent from changes in the outer world by maintaining constant their own internal environment. He emphasized that "it is the fixity of the milieu interieur which is the condition of free and independent life" and that "all the vital mechanisms, however varied they may be, have only one objective, that of preserving constant the conditions of life in the internal environment" [4].

This internal fluid environment bathes the cells with nutrients and inorganic and organic ions of critical importance to normal cell functioning. The blood carries important metabolites to all the cells in the body: metabolic substrates, such as sugars, fatty acids, and amino acids; cofactors, such as the vitamins which are needed for enzyme function; and electrolytes, such as calcium, sodium, and potassium, which are necessary for stability of the electrical properties of cells.

Cannon[6], however, stated that "the coordinated physiological processes which maintain most of the steady states in the organism are so complex and so peculiar to living beings—involving, as they may, the brain and nerves, the heart, lungs, kidneys and spleen, all working cooperatively that I have suggested a specific designation for these states, homeostasis." Mammals, for example, maintain a very stringent control over the concentration of glucose, calcium, sodium, and other constituents of the body fluids. Only small fluctuations in these important fluid components are tolerated or the animal will suffer rather immediate and often fatal consequences. Homeostatic settings, however, are not invariant; they depend on the time of day, time of year, stage of development, age, and reproductive status of an animal. It is the ability to maintain a constant internal environment in the face of adverse environmental conditions that has undoubtedly favored the wide distribution of mammals to all types of environmental habitats. Many poikilothermic vertebrates, on the other hand, are restricted to rather narrow environmental niches. The price that homeotherms must pay for maintenance of the homeostatic state is a need for a constant food supply. Many poikilotherms hibernate or estivate until more favorable climatic conditions occur when they become active again. They are, nevertheless, successful in their particular niches as they need not always depend on a continuous supply of metabolic substrates.

Feedback Systems

How does the body maintain such precise control over the concentrations of such fluid components as glucose, calcium, and sodium ions? Certain sensory (endocrine) cells in the body either individually or functioning as a unit seem to possess a definite set point (like a thermostat) for monitoring the concentrations of these substances. If the plasma concentration of a metabolite is diminished, for example, by loss through the urine or by perspiration, these receptive cells respond by releasing a substance, in this context, a hormone, which then acts on other cells to release their stores of the needed metabolite or to prevent its loss from the body. These responses to hormonal stimulation elevate the levels of such factors as sodium or glucose in the blood to a point where, for example, the cellular osmostat or glucostat now shuts off release of its chemical

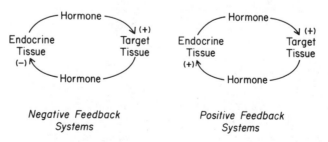

Figure 1.4 General scheme of negative and positive feedback systems.

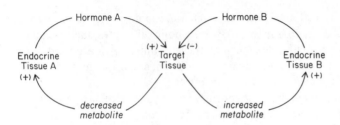

Figure 1.5 General scheme of two-hormone feedback systems.

messenger. Increased metabolite availability therefore functions as a *negative feedback* stimulus (Fig. 1.4).

Many such systems within the vertebrate body have been discovered, and there are even examples of *positive feedback* where rising concentrations of a hormone cause another gland to release a second hormone which is then stimulatory to an increased output of the first hormone (Fig. 1.4). A positive feedback system must have some mechanism of shutting off release of the first hormone or the system would increase continuously in amplitude. In the primate, estradiol, a gonadal estrogen, increases the release of pituitary hormones which, in turn, stimulate ovarian estrogen production. Consequently estrogen levels as well as gonadotropin levels increase concomitantly. The monthly demise of the ovarian follicle, the source of estradiol, results in a subsequent fall in plasma estrogen and gonadotropin levels (Chapter 18). There are only a few presently recognized examples of positive feedback.

In a number of feedback systems an increase in the plasma levels of one hormone may be stimulatory to the release of a metabolite (e.g., glucose) from a target tissue. Elevated plasma levels of the metabolite may then be stimulatory to the release of a second hormone, which has an inhibitory effect on the release of the metabolite from the target tissue. The lowered level of the metabolite would, in turn, be the stimulus to the release of the first hormone (Fig. 1.5). Some specific examples of the roles of hormones in plasma metabolite homeostasis will now be discussed.

HORMONES AND HOMEOSTASIS

Maintenance of a constant internal environment is necessary for the normal functioning of the various cellular components of tissues and organs. Nerve cells, for example, must be bathed in an extracellular fluid of a definite electrolyte composition and concentration. If the concentration of monovalent cations, such as sodium or potassium, or the divalent cation, calcium, is altered, the activity of the neurons will also be affected, which will lead to depressed or hyperactive neuronal activity. The following three examples illustrate the homeostatic control of metabolic and mineral constituents of the blood.

Glucose Homeostasis

Blood glucose in humans is maintained at a rather precise concentration. Many factors affect the circulating levels of glucose such as food intake, rate of digestion, excretion, exercise, psychological state, and reproductive state. These influences, individually or

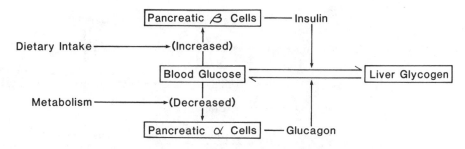

Figure 1.6 Hormonal control of glucose homeostasis.

in combination, constantly affect the physiological processes that regulate plasma glucose levels. The glucose level may drop momentarily due to muscular activity, especially if food intake is limited. The diminished level of blood glucose is in some way recognized by certain cells in the pancreas, specifically, the *alpha* (α) *cells* of the *islets of Langerhans*. These cells then release glucagon, a hormone which acts on cells of the liver to cause the release of glucose. Thus, the blood glucose level is brought back to normal. If, on the other hand, blood glucose is elevated, as occurs usually after a meal, other pancreatic islet cells, *beta* (β) *cells*, release the hormone, insulin. Insulin induces the uptake of glucose from the blood into the liver and other cells. Thus, the glucose level of the blood is lowered to the normal circulating concentration. There is greater likelihood to develop hyperglycemia than there is to develop hypoglycemia as most hormones have a hyperglycemic effect. Lack of insulin, therefore, results in a serious inability to lower blood glucose, which results in diabetes mellitus. The feedback control of blood glucose is shown schematically in Figure 1.6.

Calcium Homeostasis

Calcium is required by all cells of the body for a variety of functions. Calcium is needed for clotting of the blood and it is a requirement for cellular secretory processes. This divalent cation is also required for muscle contraction and is undoubtedly required for many other more subtle cellular functions not presently understood. In most mammals the concentration of calcium in the blood is maintained within very narrow limits. Any deviation from this set point will cause homeostatic mechanisms to bring the concentration of Ca^{2+} back to this level. If Ca^{2+} levels fall, this is in some way perceived by cells in the parathyroid glands and they secrete parathormone. This hormone then acts on bone to release the stored Ca^{2+} from that organ. In addition parathormone causes enhanced absorption of Ca^{2+} from the gut and resorption of Ca^{2+} from the urine in the kidney. All these actions tend to bring the concentration of the cation back to normal. Lack of parathormone, on the other hand, leads to a lowering of serum Ca^{2+}, which may lead to tetanic convulsions and death [24].

If serum Ca^{2+} becomes elevated, as it may after a meal, then other cells release a hormone, calcitonin, which lowers the level of circulating calcium. In mammals this hormone is released from parafollicular cells within the thyroid gland. Somehow these cells are capable of detecting elevated levels of calcium. Calcitonin causes deposition of Ca^{2+} into bone, and it may have other actions on the gut and kidney

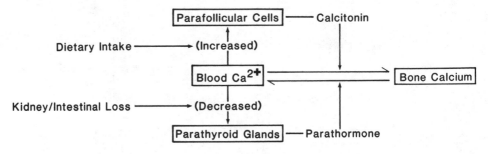

Figure 1.7 Hormonal control of calcium homeostasis.

to prevent Ca^{2+} uptake and resorption. The hormonal homeostatic mechanisms controlling serum Ca^{2+} levels are shown in Figure 1.7.

Sodium Homeostasis

Although sodium is the major electrolyte in body fluids, it is continuously being lost from the body in urine and perspiration. Specialized cells within the walls of certain blood vessels within the kidney act as *osmoreceptors* and continuously monitor the sodium concentration of the blood. If a drop in osmolarity is noted, these cells release a substance, renin, which, acting as an enzyme, is able to split a plasma protein into a smaller peptide. This peptide is then acted upon by yet another enzyme to release a still smaller peptide, angiotensin II, a hormone. Angiotensin II then stimulates certain cells of the adrenal cortex to release aldosterone, another hormone. This hormone then acts on certain collecting tubules of the kidney to cause resorption of sodium from the urine. Thus, a complex set of hormonal actions are brought into play to maintain the proper levels of blood sodium (Fig. 15.10).

NEUROENDOCRINE INTEGRATION IN HOMEOSTASIS

A variety of stimuli of both *extrinsic* (environmental) and *intrinsic* (within the body) origin affect physiological processes within an animal. The body must interpret changes in environmental temperature and day length. The recognition of odors produced by members of the opposite sex may be important in the control of reproductive behavior. Changes in fluid electrolyte levels or metabolic substrate levels must be monitored. Pain stimuli, whether of extrinsic or intrinsic origin, must be perceived. The recognition of these factors is accomplished by cellular sensory elements (receptors), which may be referred to as mechanoreceptors, chemoreceptors, osmoreceptors, or baroreceptors, depending on which modality is monitored. These sensory elements may be cellular components of glands, such as the pancreas, or they may be neural elements of the eye, nasal (olfactory) epithelium, or other tissues. These sensory cells respond to sensory cues by releasing a hormone directly into the blood or by transmitting a nerve impulse to other neurons or cellular elements which then release one or more chemical messengers. After the stomach contents (chyme) are released into the small intestine, hydrogen ions (from hydrochloric acid) interact with specific cells of the gut epithelium, which results in the release of the hormone, secretin. Secretin then enters the blood and interacts with cells of the pancreas to release a fluid secretion which neutralizes the acid within the small intestine. This is the classical example of a hormone, as first described by Bayliss and Starling [2], and a further example of a homeostatic mechanism (Fig. 10.6).

The control of release of most hormones is not as simple as the example of secretin. Sensory cues are often transmitted from one neuron to one or more other neurons, which may ultimately result in the release of a hormone. The nervous system working through the endocrine system therefore plays an important role in the homeostasis of a number of such physiological processes as water balance, temperature regulation, and even feeding behavior. The following examples of neuroendocrine integration are discussed in more detail in Chapter 21.

Control of Water Balance

If water is lost and not replaced, dehydration results. The hyperosmolality and hypovolemia are detected by *osmoreceptors* and *baroreceptors*, sensory cells which monitor changes in sodium concentration or volume (pressure), respectively, of the blood. Baroreceptor neurons, located within the carotid sinus, for example, relay information to specific sites within the brain. Integration of this information within the hypothalamus results in the release of a hormone, vasopressin, from neurons which are components of the posterior pituitary gland. This antidiuretic hormone is released into the blood and acts on certain cells of the collecting tubules of the kidney to cause water reabsorption. Vasopressin also causes contraction of certain smooth muscles of the vasculature, which results in partial restoration of blood pressure. In addition sensory neurons within the brain may also monitor fluid osmolarity, and, under dehydrating conditions, neurohormones are released to act within the brain to initiate drinking (*dipsogenic*) behavior. The complexity of this neuroendocrine control of water balance is discussed more fully in Chapters 7 and 21.

Control of Body Temperature

The temperature of the body, at least that of humans, is maintained at a precise level although it does exhibit a circadian (daily) variation. Hormones and neuronal mechanisms are crucial in temperature regulation. Alterations in body temperature are monitored by sensory neurons within the brain. These neurons release neurotransmitter substances which stimulate other neurons to initiate physiological processes that lead to warming or cooling of the body back to the normal state. Under cooling conditions where body heat is lost, neurons within the brain release one or more neurohormones which increase metabolic activity and heat production within the body. Specifically, a hormone (Fig. 1.3) released from nerves within the hypothalamus of the brain stimulates the release of a thyroid stimulating hormone (TSH) from the pituitary [25]. This hormone released into the circulation stimulates cells of the thyroid to release one or more other thyroid hormones, thyroxine and triiodothyronine, which then stimulate metabolism within various cells of the body with resulting heat production. In addition neurohormones released within the brain also activate the *sympathetic nervous system* and the adrenal gland to release hormones which also affect metabolic processes by causing the release of glucose from the liver which can then be utilized as a metabolic substrate for heat production (Chapter 21). The sympathetic nervous system will also release hormones which cause vasoconstriction, which will result in decreased heat loss from the skin. These are only a few of the neuroendocrine mechanisms involved in the complex physiological processes that maintain temperature homeostasis [27].

Control of Feeding Behavior

Blood glucose not only triggers the direct release of pancreatic hormones to restore normal blood sugar levels, but cellular *glucostats* within the brain may also monitor glucose levels and set into motion complex physiological processes to restore the normal blood glucose concentration. These glucostats are located in the basal hypothalamus (*satiety center*) of the brain. Neurons from this center apparently maintain a tonic inhibitory control over neurons in the lateral hypothalamus (*feeding center*). Under conditions of low blood glucose, satiety center neurons no longer inhibit the feeding center neurons. Neuronal pathways from the feeding center then activate other neuronal centers concerned with the sensation of hunger [10]. This leads to food intake and the restoration of blood glucose levels back to normal (Chapter 21).

REFERENCES

[1] BANTING, F. G., and C. H. BEST. 1922. The internal secretion of the pancreas. *J. Lab. Clin. Med.* 7:251–66.

[2] BAYLISS, W. M., and E. H. STARLING. 1902. Mechanisms of pancreatic secretion. *J. Physiol.* 28:325–53.

[3] BERN, H. A. 1977. Some possible contributions of comparative endocrinology to mammalian and human endocrinology. *Zool. Mag.* 86:1–9.

[4] BERNARD, C. 1965. *Introduction a l'étude de la mèdicine experimentale*. Paris: J. B. Ballière et Fils.

[5] BERTHOLD, A. A. 1849. Transplantation der Hoden. *Arch. Anat. Physiol. Wiss. Med.* 16:42–46.

[6] CANNON, W. B. 1960. *The wisdom of the body*. New York: W. W. Norton & Co., Inc.

[7] CHAN, L., and B. W. O'MALLEY. 1976. Mechanism of action of the sex steroid hormones. *New Engl. J. Med.* 294:1322–28;1372–81;1430–37.

[8] GREENGARD, P. 1979. Cyclic nucleotides, phosphorylated proteins, and the nervous system. *Fed. Proc.* 38:2208–17.

[9] GORBMAN, A., W. W. DICKHOFF, S. R. VIGNA, N. B. CLARK and C. L. RALPH. 1983. *Comparative endocrinology*. New York: John Wiley & Sons, Inc.

[10] GROSSMAN, S. P. 1977. Neuroanatomy of eating and drinking behavior. *Hosp. Prac.* May: 45–53.

[11] GUILLEMIN, R. 1978. Peptides in the brain: the new endocrinology of the neuron. *Science* 202:390–402.

[12] GUILLEMIN, R., and L. GUILLEMIN, translators. 1974. Claude Bernard. *Lectures on the phenomena of life common to animals and plants.* Springfield, Ill.: Charles Thomas, Publisher.

[13] GUILLEMIN, R., P. BRAZEAU, P. BÖHLEN, F. ESCH, N. LING and W. B. WEHRENBERG. 1982. Growth hormone-releasing factor from a human pancreatic tumor that caused acromegaly. *Science* 218:585–87.

[14] HARRIS, G. W. 1955. *Neural control of the pituitary gland.* London: Edward Arnold, Ltd.

[15] LOEWI, O. 1921. Uebertragbarkeit der Herznervenwirkung. *Pflüger's Arch. ges Physiol.* 189:239–42.

[16] MOSS, R. L. 1979. Actions of hypothalamic-hypophysiotropic hormones on the brain. *Ann. Rev. Physiol.* 41:617–32.

[17] REHFELD, J. F. 1979. Gastrointestinal hormones. *Intern. Rev. Physiol.* 19:291–321.

[18] RIVIER, J., J. SPIESS, M. THORNER and W. VALE. 1982. Characterization of a growth hormone-releasing factor from a human pancreatic islet tumour. *Nature* 300:276–78.

[19] SANGER, F. 1959. Chemistry of insulin. *Science* 129:1340–44.

[20] SCHALLY, A. V. 1978. Aspects of hypothalamic regulation of the pituitary gland. *Science* 202:18–28.

[21] SÉTÁLÓ, G., and B. FLERKÓ. 1978. Brain cells as producers of releasing and inhibiting hormones. *Intern. Rev. Cytol.* 7(Suppl.):1–50.

[22] STARLING, E. H. 1905. The chemical correlation of the functions of the body. *Lancet* 1:340–41.

[23] SUTHERLAND, E. 1972. Studies on the mechanisms of hormone action. *Science* 177:401–408.

[24] TALMAGE, R. V., and R. A. MEYER, Jr. 1976. Physiological role of parathyroid hormone. In *Handbook of physiology*, Sect. 7: Endocrinology, eds. E. B. Astwood and R. O. Greep, vol. 7, pp. 343–51. Washington, D.C.: Amer. Physiol. Soc.

[25] VALE, W., C. RIVIER, and M. BROWN. 1977. Regulatory peptides of the hypothalamus. *Ann. Rev. Physiol.* 39:473–527.

[26] WADE, N. 1978. Guillemin and Schally. *Science* 200:279–82; 411–15; 510–13.

[27] WILSON, J. A. 1979. *Principles of animal physiology.* 2nd ed. New York: Macmillan, Inc.

[28] YALOW, R. S. 1978. Radioimmunoassay: a probe for the fine structure of biologic systems. *Science* 200:1236–45.

2

The Vertebrate Endocrine System

INTRODUCTION

After fertilization of the vertebrate egg, a number of inductive processes ensue which cause the zygote to divide and develop into an embryo. The chemical messengers regulating early embryonic differentiation and development, however, are presently undetermined. The fetus will grow, develop, utilize metabolic substrates, respire, move, and excrete various waste products. The extent to which these physiological processes are regulated by hormones of fetal or maternal origin is also poorly understood. Whether the embryo will develop in a male or female direction is, however, determined by early endocrine influences (Chapter 16). The fetus will be liberated from the environment of the womb at parturition; the fetus will continue to grow and develop, and new physiological functions and morphological changes will occur during growth and development of the young animal. The adolescent will develop into an adult and the adult may bear offspring of its own. A large number of hormones are required to control and coordinate these various physiological activities. Some hormones may only function during specific developmental stages, and their physiological roles may even change in time. Growth hormone and thyroid hormones, for example, are necessary for normal bone growth in the young animal; these same hormones assume additional functions in the adult.

Some hormones cause rapid responses after being secreted, such as milk release and uterine contraction in response to oxytocin. Epinephrine, a

16

hormone of the adrenal medulla, causes an almost instantaneous change in the rate and force of the heart beat. Other hormones, such as gonadal steroids, initiate a slower response such as protein synthesis within muscle and other tissues. Testosterone or one of its metabolites affects the development of the brain at an early developmental period, but these effects may not become manifest until the animal approaches sexual maturity. In some animals this may occur many years later. Some hormones, for example, corticotropin (ACTH), may only control a few physiological functions; others like testosterone may affect physiological processes in many target tissues. A large and diverse number of hormones are required for coordinating the complex physiological events associated with reproductive processes, especially in the female. These may include differentiation of the gonads, germ cell maturation, development of secondary sexual characteristics, milk production, labor at parturition, and sexual behavior.

In this chapter the general characteristics of the vertebrate endocrine system are considered. Each of the endocrine glands or tissues and their hormones will be discussed in detail later in the text.

ENDOCRINE GLANDS AND THEIR HORMONES

Although it is reasonable to conclude that all the so-called endocrine glands of vertebrates have been discovered, new hormones are still being found in a variety of tissues, distributed diffusely throughout the gastrointestinal (GI) tract as well as in the CNS and peripheral nerves. Therefore, it is not easy to pinpoint the origin of all the documented vertebrate hormones or to characterize definitely their putative physiological roles.

Tissues are composed of one particular cell type and a number of tissues usually function together to form an organ. An endocrine gland, for example, is composed of a prominent mass of secretory cells as well as connective tissue, blood vessels and nerves. Endocrine glands (ductless glands) secrete their products directly into the bloodstream. This is in contrast to exocrine glands (e.g., salivary glands), which release their products into ducts that lead into the lumen of other organs, such as the intestine, or to the outside of the animal. The hormones of the adrenal steroidogenic tissue are synthesized within a rather compact mass of tissue, but some hormones are secreted by individual cells or groups of cells found distributed within other nonendocrine tissue. The pancreatic islets, for example, which are the source of insulin and glucagon, are found embedded within the much larger exocrine pancreas. Gastrointestinal hormones are produced by individual isolated cells, distributed diffusely throughout the endothelial lining of the stomach and gut [15]. A few endocrine glands are transient in nature. For example, hormones are produced by the placenta during pregnancy; the placenta and its endocrine tissues are lost during parturition but return, de novo, during a subsequent pregnancy. Endocrine glands usually secrete more than one hormone, but the parathyroids may be an example where an endocrine organ secretes but one hormone.

The pituitary gland is the source of a large number of hormones. The anterior lobe or pars distalis contains at least six well-characterized hormones and a number of other hormonal candidates (Chapter 5). The pars intermedia (the intermediate lobe of the pituitary) contains one or more hormones and the posterior lobe or neurohypophysis contains at least two hormones. Although the pituitary gland was once considered the master gland of the body, its function is subservient to the brain, in particular, the hypothalamus. The secretion of the pituitary principles of the pars distalis and pars intermedia is under the control of hypothalamic releasing and inhibiting hormones [16]. Some of these hypothalamic substances have not yet been chemically characterized and are only considered as candidate hormones; they are often referred to as factors rather than hormones (e.g., prolactin releasing factor, PRF). Numerous other hormones are also present within the hypothalamus and other parts of the brain; the brain is one of the richest sources of hormones. The hormones of the hypothalamus and pituitary (Table 2.1), as well as hormones from other sources (Table 2.2), are listed with a brief statement of their functions.

Hormones Defined

Bayliss and Starling [3] discovered that the small intestine is the source of a substance which is released into the bloodstream to act on cells of the exocrine pancreas to cause fluid (bicarbonate) secretion necessary to neutralize the acid present within the chyme. This substance, secretin, was subsequently referred to as a hormone. Hormones are generally considered to be chemical messengers which are released from cells into the bloodstream to exert their action on target cells some distance away. These bloodborne messengers of the endocrine system have been, until recently, distinguished from *neurotransmitters*, which are chemical messengers released from neurons into a synapse between the nerve and its *effector cells*, such as secretory cells, muscle cells, or other neurons. It was discovered that the posterior pituitary gland consisted mainly of axonal endings of neurons that stored the hormones oxytocin and vasopressin. These hormones are released upon appropriate stimulation into the bloodstream to regulate target tissues of the mammary gland, uterus, and kidney. These peptide hormones of neural origin were referred to as *neurosecretions* to distinguish them from such neurotransmitter substances as acetylcholine, norepinephrine, and serotonin [17].

It has been discovered that many peptide hormones, secretin, adrenocorticotropin (ACTH), cholecystokinin (CCK), and others, which function in the classical sense as bloodborne hormones, are also synthesized within specific neurons within the central and peripheral nervous systems. There is evidence that some of these peptide hormones may function as neurotransmitters within the nervous system. On the other hand, dopamine, which has always been considered a classic example of a neurotransmitter, is released from nerves within the brain (hypothalamus) into the bloodstream (hypophysial portal system) and carried to the pituitary gland where it functions in the control of prolactin and α-MSH secretion. Here, then, is an example of a neurotransmitter functioning as a classical hormone. One can no longer separate the

TABLE 2.1 Vertebrate Hypothalamic and Pituitary Hormones

Source of hormone			Major physiological roles[a]
Hypothalamus			
Gonadotropin releasing hormone	GnRH	↑	FSH and LH secretion
Thyrotropin releasing hormone	TRH	↑	TSH secretion
Corticotropin releasing hormone	CRH	↑	ACTH secretion
Prolactin inhibiting factor	PIF[b]	↓	Prolactin secretion
Melanocyte stimulating hormone (MSH) release inhibiting factor	MIF[b]	↓	MSH secretion
Somatostatin (somatotropin release inhibiting hormone)	SS	↓	STH secretion
Somatocrinin (somatotropin releasing factor)		↑	STH secretion
Pituitary Gland			
Posterior Lobe[c]			
Oxytocin		↑	Milk secretion; uterine contraction
Vasopressin (arginine vasopressin) (antidiuretic hormone)	AVP ADH	↑	Renal water absorption; vasoconstriction
Pars Intermedia			
Melanocyte stimulating hormone	MSH	↑	Integumental melanogenesis; melanosome movement
Pars Distalis			
Follicle stimulating hormone (follitropin)	FSH	↑	Female: ovarian follicle growth; estradiol synthesis
		↑	Male: spermatogenesis
Luteinizing hormone (lutropin)	LH	↑	Female: ovulation; ovarian estradiol and progesterone synthesis
		↑	Male: testicular androgen synthesis
Prolactin	PRL	↑	Milk synthesis; corpus luteum progesterone synthesis in some species
Thyrotropin (thyroid stimulating hormone)	TSH	↑	Thyroid hormone (T_4 and T_3) synthesis and secretion
Corticotropin (adrenal cortical stimulating hormone)	ACTH	↑	Adrenal steroidogenesis
Somatotropin (growth hormone, GH)	STH	↑	Hepatic somatomedin biosynthesis

[a]The effect of each hormone on either an increased or stimulated (↑) or a decreased or inhibited (↓) physiological response is indicated.

[b]There is some evidence for putative prolactin and MSH releasing factors (PRF and MRF, respectively).

[c]See Chapter 7 for other vertebrate neurohypophysial hormones.

endocrine and nervous system into unrelated physiological entities. The hypothalamus, for example, is the richest source of chemical messengers and should be considered the "endocrine hypothalamus" (Chapter 6).

Based simply on anatomical considerations, hormones derived from nerve cells may be called *neurohormones*, a specific subclass of hormones; they may be *neuropeptides* or nonpeptidergic in nature (e.g., dopamine). Although neurohormones may be secreted into the bloodstream, they also regulate neuronal function within the nervous system as neurotransmitters or *neuromodulators*. In contrast to the rapid actions of

TABLE 2.2 Some other Vertebrate Hormones

Source of hormone			Major physiological roles[a]
Thyroid			
Thyroxine	T_4	↑	Growth; differentiation; calorigenesis (↑ metabolic rate and oxygen consumption)
Triiodothyronine	T_3		Same as for thyroxine
Adrenal steroidogenic tissue			
Cortisol		↑	Carbohydrate metabolism; sympathetic function
Corticosterone		↑	Carbohydrate metabolism; sympathetic function
Aldosterone		↑	Sodium retention
Adrenal chromaffin tissue			
Epinephrine	E		Multiple ↑ and ↓ effects on nerves, muscles, cellular secretions, and metabolism
Norepinephrine	NE		Generally same physiological roles as epinephrine
Ovary (preluteal follicle)			
Estradiol		↑	Female sexual development and behavior
Ovary (corpus luteum)			
Progesterone		↑	Uterine and mammary gland growth; maternal behavior
Relaxin		↑	Relaxation of pubic symphysis and dilation of uterine cervix
Placenta			
Chorionic gonadotropin (choriogonadotropin)	CG	↑	Corpus luteum progesterone synthesis
Placental lactogen		↑	Possibly fetal growth and development, mammary gland development in the mother
Testes (leydig cells)			
Testosterone		↑	Male sexual development and behavior
Testes (sertoli cells)			
Inhibin		↓	Pituitary FSH secretion
Müllerian regression factor	MRF		Müllerian duct regression (atrophy)
Pineal (epiphysis)			
Melatonin		↓	Gonadal development (antigonadotropic action)
Thymus gland			
Thymic hormones		↑	Proliferation and differentiation of lymphocytes
Pancreatic islets			
Insulin		↓	Blood glucose; ↑ protein, glycogen, and fat synthesis
Glucagon		↑	Blood glucose; gluconeogenesis; glycogenolysis
Somatostatin	SS	↓	Secretion of other pancreatic islet hormones
Pancreatic polypeptide	PP	↑↓	Secretion of other pancreatic islet hormones

TABLE 2.2 *(Cont.)*

Source of hormone		Major physiological roles[a]
Gastrointestinal tract		
Gastrin		↑ HCl secretion
Secretin		↑ Pancreatic acinar cell fluid (bicarbonate) secretion
Cholecystokinin	CCK	↑ Pancreatic acinar cell enzyme secretion; gall bladder contraction
Gastric inhibitory peptide	GIP	↓ Gastric acid (HCl) secretion
Vasoactive intestinal peptide	VIP	↑ Intestinal secretion of electrolytes
Chymodenin		↑ Chymotrypsinogen secretion from the exocrine pancreas
Motilin		↑ Gastric acid secretion; villous motility
Neurotensin	NT	Enteric neurotransmitter
Substance P	SP	Enteric neurotransmitter
Gastrin releasing peptide	GRP	Increased gastrin secretion; decreased gastric acid secretion
Parathyroid glands		
Parathormone	PTH	↑ Blood calcium; ↓ blood phosphate
Thyroid parafollicular cells (or ultimobranchial glands)		
Calcitonin		↓ Blood calcium
Skin, liver, kidney		
Vitamin D		↑ Blood Ca^{2+}; bone formation, intestinal Ca^{2+} and PO_4^{3-} absorption
Plasma angiotensinogen		
Angiotensin II		↑ Vasoconstriction; aldosterone secretion; thirst (dipsogenic) behavior
Kidney		
Erythropoietin (erythrocyte stimulating factor, ESF)	EP	↑ Erythropoiesis
Most all tissues		
Prostaglandins	PGE_2	↑ Cyclic nucleotide (cAMP) formation
	$PGF_{2\alpha}$	↑ Cyclic nucleotide (cGMP) formation
Prostacyclins	PGI_2	↑ Cyclic nucleotide (cAMP) formation
Thromboxanes	TXA_2	↑ Cyclic nucleotide (cGMP ?) formation
Leukotrienes	LTE_4	↑↓ Cyclic nucleotide formation
Various tissues		
Epidermal growth factor	EGF	↑ Epidermal cell proliferation
Fibroblast growth factor	FGF	↑ Fibroblast proliferation
Nerve growth factor	NGF	↑ Neurite development
Somatomedins		↑ Cellular growth and proliferation
Endorphins		Opiatelike activity
Epithelial tissue		
Epidermal chalone		↓ Epithelial proliferation

[a]The major effect of each putative chemical messenger on either an increased or stimulated (↑) or a decreased or inhibited (↓) physiological response is indicated.

neurotransmitters, neuromodulatory substances are considered to exert slower but more sustained neurotropic actions [1, 2]. Their actions are believed to enhance or inhibit (and therefore modulate) the response of neurons to neurotransmitters. Neuromodulators and neurotransmitters are also referred to in a more general sense as *neuroregulators*. Neuromodulatory hormones may also originate from nonneuronal sources. For example, adrenocortical steroids, such as cortisol, or androgens and estrogens of gonadal origin may modulate central nervous system activity and therefore play an important role in sexual and other behavior (Chapter 16).

Some cells within the gastrointestinal epithelium and other tissues of the body apparently secrete peptide hormones and neurotransmitter substances (e.g., serotonin) locally to regulate adjacent cells. Here are possible examples of neurotransmitter substances acting nonsynaptically and hormones acting locally rather than by a bloodborne route. Epithelial growth inhibitory substances, *chalones*, are other examples of local hormones. Some chemical messengers are released to the exterior of animals where by air convection or ingestion they interact with cells of other members of the same species to evoke a response; these substances are referred to as *pheromones*.

In consideration of the multiple sources of peptide hormones, within glandular cells or within neurons, and the observation that classical neurotransmitters may function as bloodborne messengers, and that either type of chemical messenger may function as a local hormone, neurotransmitter, or neuromodulatory substance, a broader definition of a hormone is required. Guillemin has suggested that a hormone be defined as "any substance released by a cell and which acts on another cell near or far, regardless of the singularity or ubiquity of the source and regardless of the means of conveyance, blood stream, axoplasmic flow, or immediate intracellular space"[10]. In this book the term *hormone* will be used in this context, but such terms as neurotransmitter, neuromodulator, or neurohormone may be used to indicate specific examples of hormones (Table 2.3). Endocrinology is by this definition the study of hormones derived from the classical endocrine glands (e.g., pituitary, thyroid, adrenal, gonads) or from other cells or tissues such as the brain or GI tract. Some teachers and students may prefer to restrict the use of the term hormone in the classical sense and may use the more cumbersome term, chemical messenger, to include hormones, neurohormones, pheromones, and so on.

One problem which arises from the recognition of the varied distribution of hormones is that relating to the physiological roles of a hormone. If one wants to know the functional role of a specific hormone, it is necessary to inquire as to which source of the hormone is being discussed. For example, the hormone somatostatin is released from specific neurons in the brain to regulate somatotropin secretion from the pituitary gland. This peptide hormone is also present within other neurons within the CNS where it may function as a neurohormone (neurotransmitter or a neuromodulator). Somatostatin is also found within the gut epithelium and the pancreas, and it undoubtedly functions in these sites by a local mechanism to regulate gastrin, glucagon, and insulin secretion. Portal plasma levels of somatostatin are elevated after a meal; the peptide may function in this example as a bloodborne chemical messenger (hormone in the classical sense) as it does in the regulation of pituitary STH secretion. Somatostatin eventually may be shown to have as many functions as have been

TABLE 2.3 Hormone Terminology

Chemical messenger:	Any substance produced by a cell of exogenous or endogenous origin that plays a physiological role in the control of the physiological activity of another cell.
Hormone:	Any substance elaborated by one cell to regulate another cell (used here synonymously with chemical messenger). May be delivered by an endocrine, neuroendocrine, neurocrine, paracrine, autocrine, or even pheromonal route.
Neurohormone:	A hormone produced by a nerve cell.
Neuropeptide:	A peptidergic neurohormone (e.g., substance P).
Nonpeptidergic neurohormone:	Any nonpeptidergic neurohormone, such as acetylcholine, histamine, norepinephrone, serotonin, and so on.
Neurotransmitter:	A neurohormone that acts transynaptically.
Neuromodulator:	A hormone that modulates the response of a neuron to a neurotransmitter or other hormone.
Neuroregulator:	A generalized term for any neurohormone that acts as a neurotransmitter or a neuromodulator.
Pheromones:	Chemical messengers released to the exterior of one animal to stimulate a response in another member of the same species.
Chalones:	Putative cellular mitotic inhibitors.
Growth factors:	Mitogenic substances that may, in time, become established hormones.

described for the particular neurons or cells within which it is localized. Like the neurotransmitter dopamine, which is distributed widely within the brain and which subserves many functions, the localization of peptide hormones to specific neurons suggests that they too probably regulate a diverse number of functions.

GENERAL CLASSES OF CHEMICAL MESSENGERS

Although there are many vertebrate hormones, they may be conveniently categorized into a small number of groups which bear structural similarities. Generally these groupings also imply some major difference in cellular source and synthesis of the particular chemical messengers which comprise the group. Peptide hormones, thyroid hormones, and all neurotransmitters are of neuroectodermal or endodermal origin, whereas steroid hormones are of mesodermal origin [14].

Peptide Hormones

As implied by the subgroup classification, these hormones are composed of amino acids. There may be as few as three amino acids (as in thyrotropin releasing hormone, TRH, Fig. 1.3) to as many as 180 or more in the pituitary gonadotropins. Although the individual hormones could be referred to as peptide, polypeptide, or protein in nature depending on their specific chain length, for the sake of brevity they are here referred to as peptide hormones. The shorter peptides may be composed of a linear chain, as in α-MSH or angiotensin II, or the peptide may contain a ring structure due to bridge formation through disulfide bonds as in the *neurohypophysial hormones*, oxytocin and vasopressin (Fig. 7.2), or as in somatostatin (Fig. 6.6). Some of the larger protein hormones are composed of two chains as in insulin (Fig. 11.5), thyrotropin (TSH), and the gonadotropins (follicle stimulating hormone, FSH, and luteinizing hormone, LH). The dimeric structure of insulin is held together by interchain disulfide bonds. Intrachain disulfide bonds are also present in insulin and in prolactin (PRL), somatotropin (STH) and other hormones. These covalent bonds may be important for establishing the *tertiary structure* necessary for producing the active site within these peptides or, in some instances, for protecting the hormones from enzymatic degradation.

In some hormones tyrosine is sulfated (e.g., gastrin, Fig. 10.1), and the glutamic acid moiety may be cyclized into a pyrrole structure (as in TRH, Fig. 1.3). Because peptide hormones are composed of a linear sequence of amino acids, there is usually an amino (NH_2)- or N-terminal and a carboxy (COOH)- or C-terminal group present in the structure. In some peptides the C-terminal end may be amidated (to a carboxamide) and the N-terminal group may be acetylated (as in α-MSH, Fig. 8.1). Some of the larger peptides (FSH, LH, TSH, and hCG) are *glycoproteins*, that is, they are conjugated to one or more carbohydrate residues. Incorporation of carbohydrate into their structure may be necessary for establishing the *quaternary* structures of these glycoproteins.

The amino acid sequence (*primary structure*) of a hormone may differ between species (for example, ACTH and calcitonin, Figs. 5.8 and 9.4, respectively). Knowledge of such species differences in primary structure provides information on the evolution of the hormone. Single amino acid substitutions may even lead to the evolution of new hormone structures within an individual species. Although oxytocin and vasopressin are closely related structurally and presumably evolutionarily, they play entirely different physiological roles within an individual animal. Based on similarity of structure, one can group hormones into families of peptides which undoubtedly are derived from a common evolutionary precursor. The insulin family of peptides includes nerve growth factor (NGF), relaxin, and one or more of the somatomedins (Figs. 12.2 and 19.3). The melanotropin family of peptides includes ACTH, α-MSH, and possibly other melanotropins (Fig. 8.1). Invariant sequences of amino acids within the primary structure of a peptide may suggest that such sequences are components of the active site of the hormone.

Thyroid Hormones

The thyroid gland synthesizes two hormones, thyroxine (T_4) and triiodothyronine (T_3), from the precursor amino acid tyrosine (Fig. 13.1). These two iodinated hormones have a diverse number of functions within and between members of the different vertebrate classes. These hormones are unique in that an inorganic ion is incorporated into their structures.

Steroid Hormones

Steroid hormones are produced by steroidogenic tissue of adrenal or gonadal origin. The adrenal steroidogenic *tissue* produces *glucocorticoids* (e.g., cortisol, cortico-sterone, and cortisone) and *mineralocorticoids* (e.g., aldosterone). These steroids play

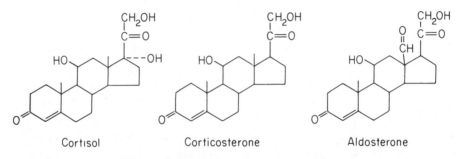

Figure 2.1   Examples of adrenal steroid hormones.

important roles in carbohydrate metabolism and electrolyte balance, respectively. The pathway of steroid biosynthesis is complex and many steroid precursors are formed in the synthesis of any particular steroid hormone (e.g., Fig. 15.3). Under abnormal conditions the production of these metabolites may increase and exert undesirable physiological effects. Figure 2.1 shows the structures of three adrenal steroid hormones.

The steroidogenic tissue of the gonads produces a number of sex (gonadal) steroids: *androgens* (masculinizing), *estrogens* (feminizing), and *progestins*. The testes produce testosterone; in the ovary estradiol and progesterone are the main steroids synthesized and secreted. During pregnancy the placenta is an additional source of estrogens and progestins. Under certain developmental conditions the adrenal steroidogenic tissue may be an important additional source of androgens and estrogens. Figure 2.2 shows the structure of three important gonadal steroid hormones.

Neurotransmitters

These neurohormones are synthesized by neurons and are usually released into a specialized structure, a synaptic cleft, adjacent to the cell to be regulated (effector or target cell). These neurotransmitters regulate another nerve cell, a muscle cell, or a secretory cell (e.g., salivary gland cell). The common neurotransmitters are acetylcholine, norepinephrine, dopamine, and serotonin (5-hydroxytryptamine, 5-HT), but there are a number of other putative neurotransmitters (Chapters 6 and 21).

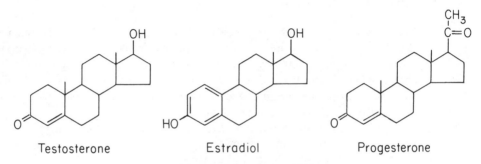

Figure 2.2   Examples of gonadal steroid hormones.

General Classes of Chemical Messengers

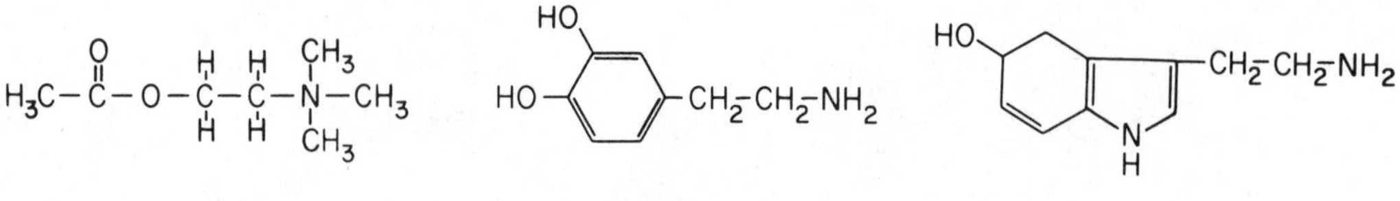

Figure 2.3 Examples of neurotransmitters.

Dopamine released from hypothalamic neurons of the brain may also function as a bloodborne hormone to regulate pituitary hormone secretion. Figure 2.3 shows the structures of three important neurotransmitters.

Neuropeptides

Many of the peptide hormones have been found in the brain where they are synthesized by specific neurons and localized to specific nerve tracts. Such a discrete localization argues strongly for a function of these neuropeptides within the nervous system. It is speculated that these hormones act as neuroregulators, either as neurotransmitters (to conduct information synaptically, between neurons) or as neuromodulators (to affect the response of a neuron to neurotransmitters released from other neurons). Some neuropeptides are distributed widely throughout the central nervous system. The *endorphins*, for example, may function as neuroregulators to act on so-called opiate receptors and, in humans at least, as analgesic hormones. Methionine enkephalin and leucine enkephalin and β-endorphin are examples of endorphins (Fig. 21.2). New peptides in the brain are being discovered and it is expected that exciting advances in neuroendocrinology will result from the discovery of the physiological roles of these hormones. These neuropeptides are discussed in Chapter 21.

OTHER CHEMICAL MESSENGERS

Besides the clearly defined hormones of animals, there exist other chemical messengers that are less well characterized (Table 2.2). In time these *candidate hormones* will undoubtedly be considered as bona fide hormones.

Chalones

Endogenous mitotic inhibitors are referred to as *chalones* [6]. These growth factors are capable of inhibiting the mitotic activity of a given cell type. This cell specificity is not, however, associated with any species specificity. The first and most carefully studied chalone system was the so-called *epidermal chalone*. Extracts of the epidermis contain a factor which affects a number of different epithelia, suggesting that this factor might better be referred to as an *epithelial chalone*.

Other so-called granulocyte, liver, fibroblast, and lymphocyte chalones have been proposed. Although most of these factors are ill defined, they might prove to be of importance in the control of cancer.

Peptide Growth-Stimulating Factors

A number of proteinaceous substances of diverse origin possessing growth-promoting activity have been identified. In some cases the structural characteristics of the molecules have been partially or fully determined. The thymus may produce one or more *thymosins* which are believed to induce maturation of white blood cells which then function in the immune response. Nerve growth factor (NGF), another putative chemical messenger, is responsible for neuron maturation in developing systems. These and other growth-stimulating peptides [8], such as erythropoietin (erythrocyte stimulating factor, ESF), epidermal growth factor (EGF), fibroblast growth factor (FGF), and the somatomedins will be discussed in Chapter 12.

Prostaglandins

Prostaglandins are a new class of chemical messengers. Although discovered relatively recently [13], they are ubiquitous and affect the activity of many physiological processes. Prostaglandins are synthesized from fatty acid substrates (e.g., arachidonic acid) within the membranes of cells. Their generic name was derived because they were first discovered within seminal fluid. They are composed of a 20-membered fatty acid carbon skeleton folded into a hairpinlike structure by incorporating a five-membered ring at the bend of the molecule. The thromboxanes, prostacyclins, and the leukotrienes are related chemical messengers that may prove to play significant roles in many physiological processes (Chapter 4). Figure 2.4 shows the structure of two important prostaglandins.

Pheromones

Most hormones act on cells within the animal in which they are produced. Chemical signals are also utilized for transmitting information between individuals. The term *pheromone* denotes a chemical substance that is liberated by one animal and which causes a relatively specific modification of the behavior of a recipient animal following its chemoreception [19]. This chemical communication is implied to function within a species. Pheromones are classified into two types, a *signaller* (or *releaser*) pheromone, which brings about a prompt behavioral reaction, and a *primer* pheromone, which causes a slower effect, such as an alteration of the endocrine and reproductive systems. These effects are produced through neuroendocrine mechanisms for which the primary stimulus is olfactory. Pheromones play important roles in insects and other invertebrates. Pheromones are generally aliphatic, thus facilitating their volatilization and subsequent transport by the wind. The structure of the vertebrate pheromone,

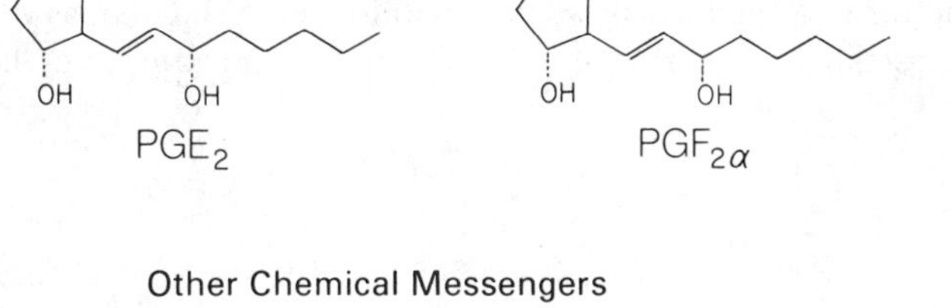

PGE_2 $PGF_{2\alpha}$

Figure 2.4 Examples of two common prostaglandins.

H–C–C–C–C=C–C=C–C–C–C–C–C–C–C–C–C–C–OH

Bombykol

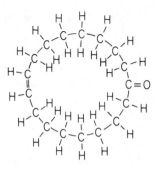

Civetone

Figure 2.5   Examples of vertebrate and invertebrate pheromones.

civetone (from the civet), and the invertebrate pheromone, bombykol (from the silk worm moth), are shown (Fig. 2.5).

Other Cellular Regulators

Besides the well-recognized classes of hormones, other substances play important roles as chemical messengers controlling cellular function. The simplest such messenger is the hydrogen (H^+) ion. The hydrochloric acid present within chyme is responsible for stimulating secretin release from cells of the duodenal epithelium. Because other acids will similarly stimulate secretin release, it can be presumed that interaction of the hydrogen ion with specific cellular receptors of secretin-producing cells elicits release of this hormone. Osmoreceptors also monitor sodium ion (Na^+) levels within the plasma. These chemoreceptor cells undoubtedly have special recognition sites for this monovalent cation. The divalent calcium (Ca^{2+}) ion is an important regulator of parathormone and calcitonin secretion from the parathyroid glands and parafollicular cells, respectively. These cells apparently have specific recognition sites for this important cation.

Glucose is a specific stimulus for insulin secretion from the *beta* cells of the pancreatic islets. Glucose is also inhibitory to glucagon secretion from the *alpha* cells of the pancreatic islets. *Glucostats* are apparently present within the hypothalamus where they may function as the receptive units of the so-called *satiety center*. These cells must have special sensory elements for recognizing this metabolic substrate [9].

Certain amino acids (e.g., arginine) may function as specific stimulants of insulin secretion from the pancreatic islets. Certain neurons within the hypothalamus also monitor the levels of certain circulating amino acids; these sensory elements may then regulate the release of pituitary somatotropin. The simplest amino acid, glycine, probably functions as a neurotransmitter within the brain. Glutamine, a derivative of glutamic acid, may also function as a chemical messenger within the CNS. Other as yet unrecognized metabolic substrates or end products may play important roles in cellular regulation.

HORMONE SYNTHESIS

Because of the diversity of hormone structures, a number of interesting synthetic processes are involved in hormone biosynthesis.

Peptide Hormones

Most vertebrate hormones are peptide in nature and are therefore composed of amino acids. Like other proteins, they are synthesized on ribosomes where their specific amino acid sequence is determined (*translated*) by a specific messenger RNA sequence (condon). The nucleotide sequences of the RNA are dictated (*transcribed*) from specific nucleotide sequences (genes) in the DNA of chromosomes. The nascent proteins are then released and transported into the cisternae of the rough endoplasmic reticulum and then to the Golgi elements where they may be altered (e.g., sulfated or combined with carbohydrate moieties). Vesicles containing the hormone and possibly other products (e.g., proteolytic enzymes) are then pinched off the terminal cisternae of the Golgi apparatus. These secretory vesicles are distributed within the cytoplasm in patterns generally characteristic of the cell type involved.

Steroid Hormones

These hormones are synthesized within elements of the smooth endoplasmic reticulum. Steroid-secreting cells are easily identified by the large amounts of smooth endoplasmic reticulum present within these cells. However, a complex multiple-enzyme system is required for the synthesis of steroids. These enzymes are present within the mitochondria as well as the cytoplasm. Steroid hormone synthesis can, therefore, be blocked by protein synthesis inhibitors. Nevertheless, the preponderance of the cellular synthesizing machinery is smooth endoplasmic reticulum.

Thyroid Hormones

These iodinated hormones are synthesized on a proteinaceous substrate (thyroglobulin) which is extracellular (intraluminal). They are then taken up by endocytosis and transported through the follicular cells of the thyroid gland where they are enzymatically released from the carrier protein prior to secretion (Chapter 13). Thyroid hormone production and secretion within the thyroid gland is a unique process which provides important clues for understanding cellular function.

Neurotransmitters

Neurotransmitters are synthesized within the axonal endings of neurons (Chapter 14). The enzymes needed for the many steps required for neurotransmitter production are, however, synthesized on ribosomes in the perikarya (cell bodies) of neurons and are subsequently transported by axoplasmic flow to the neuron terminals. The secreted neurotransmitter (e.g., norepinephrine) may then be taken back up into axon terminals for further use. Acetylcholine is inactivated by enzymatic cleavage after secretion, but the constituent moieties (acetate and choline) are then taken up for resynthesis of the hormone.

Neuropeptides

The peptide neurohormones (e.g., oxytocin and vasopressin) are synthesized in neuronal perikarya and are transported within vesicles for long distances to the axon terminals for storage. One might assume that the recently discovered neurohormones, such as the enkephalins, and other brain peptides are synthesized, packaged, and stored in a similar manner as the neurohypophysial hormones.

Prohormones

Some peptide hormones are composed of only a small number of amino acids. Oxytocin and other neurohypophysial hormones, for example, contain only nine amino acids (nonapeptides). These hormones are probably not coded directly by the DNA. Rather, sequences of about 100 amino acids and longer (e.g., neurophysins) are initially synthesized (Chapter 7). These proteins are then packaged within secretory vesicles along with proteolytic enzymes. These enzymes (endopeptidases) then cleave the protein into one or more smaller peptides, in some cases the definitive hormone. A number of cleavage events may, however, take place before the definitive hormone is produced. Thus some hormones are derived indirectly by way of a prohormone [5]. The prohormone may be derived from a preprohormone (Fig. 2.6). Some large plasma proteins also serve as prohormones for hormone production. Renin, an enzyme released from the juxtaglomerular cells of the kidneys, acts on a substrate protein, angiotensinogen produced by the liver, to convert it to a smaller fragment. This fragment, angiotensin I, is then converted by another enzyme to the active hormone, angiotensin II. Large precursor plasma proteins, the kininogens, are converted by certain serine proteases, referred to as kallikreins, to kinins, such as bradykinin, which is an important hormone in regulating blood flow in certain vascular beds (Chapter 15). Bradykinin and antiotensin II are examples of hormones even though they are

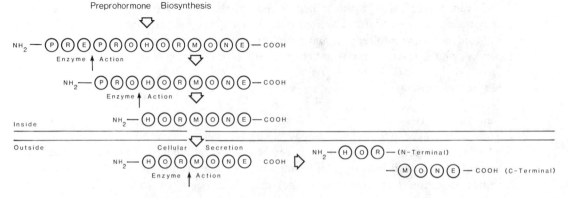

Figure 2.6 General scheme for hormone production from a prohormone.

released from cells (probably the liver) as larger prohormones to be converted into active hormonal peptides within the blood.

Certain steroids serve as prohormones in the production of other definitive steroid hormones. For example, certain cells possess the enzyme 5α-reductase which converts testosterone to dihydrotestosterone, the effector molecule for activating these cells (Fig. 16.6). Within the brain testosterone is also aromatized within certain neurons to estradiol which is the biologically active steroid structure required for activation of these cells.

CONTROL OF HORMONE SECRETION

Hormones are synthesized within cells and, except for the thyroid and steroid hormones, they are packaged within secretory vesicles until released. Stimuli of both an intrinsic (internal) or extrinsic (light, sound, smell, temperature, etc.) nature affect hormone secretion. Stimulation of the hormone-secreting cells results in vesicular fusion with the plasma membrane and *exocytosis* of the granule contents. Hormones often stimulate hormone secretion from other endocrine glands. For example, pituitary hormones, such as TSH, FSH, LH, and ACTH, stimulate target tissue cells of the thyroid, gonads, and adrenal gland, respectively, to secrete their own respective hormones: thyroxine, gonadal steroids, and adrenal glucocorticoids (Fig. 6.13). Hormone-secreting cells of the neurohypophysis, the adrenal medulla (*chromaffin tissue*), and the pineal gland are regulated by direct neural innervation. Stimulation of hormone secretion by nerves is referred to as *neuroendocrine transduction* [20]. Metabolic substrates and inorganic ions also provide a selective stimulus to hormone secretion by some cells.

Calcium levels are monitored directly by parathormone- and calcitonin-secreting cells. Thus, the hormone-secreting cells that regulate calcium levels do so by sensing the extracellular Ca^{2+} concentration, but the exact cellular mechanisms involved in such detection are not well understood. Glucose concentration is monitored by the glucagon- and insulin-secreting cells of the pancreatic islets. Thus the hormones that regulate blood glucose levels do so by determination of the circulating glucose concentration. Models describing the mechanism glucose detection suggest that products of glucose metabolism within these cells provide important intracellular cues in the control of glucagon and insulin secretion. Somatotropin stimulates tissue uptake of amino acids, and the amino acids that are present in the blood at increased levels after a meal provide cues to STH secretion.

The pituitary hormones, FSH, LH, TSH, and ACTH, stimulate hormone secretion from the gonads, thyroid and adrenal, respectively, and are controlled through negative feedback mechanisms. Target organ hormones, gonadal steroids, and thyroxine or adrenal glucocorticoids feed back to the hypothalamus and pituitary to inhibit further secretion of pituitary hormones (e.g., Fig. 6.14). Examples of positive feedback have also been described (Chapter 18). It has even been suggested that some hormones exert a negative feedback on the cells within which they were synthesized by a so-called autoinhibition.

The factors that stimulate cellular secretion, whether they are hormones or metabolites, interact with cellular receptors of the secretory cells. For example, epinephrine, a bloodborne hormone, or norepinephrine, a neurotransmitter, interacts with cell membrane adrenergic receptors (Chapter 14). Hormone interaction with some membrane receptors results in membrane *depolarization*. This stimulates the movement of calcium into the cells, which results in secretory vesicle exocytosis (so-called *stimulus-secretion coupling*). Some chemical messengers are inhibitory to cellular secretion, and their effects are mediated by cell membrane *hyperpolarization*. Changes in cellular secretion are generally correlated with changes in levels of intracellular cyclic nucleotides. Secretion is usually correlated with elevation of cyclic adenosine monophosphate (cyclic AMP) levels, whereas inhibition of secretion may be correlated with lowered cyclic AMP and elevated cyclic GMP levels. At present the precise relationship of cyclic nucleotides to membrane transmembrane potential changes is unclear.

Most hormone-secreting cells only exhibit minimal (basal) secretion in the absence of stimulatory cues. Prolactin- and MSH-secreting cells of some species are unique as hormone-secreting cells, in that they spontaneously secrete their hormones when studied in vitro or when the pituitary is transplanted to an ectopic site in the animal. These cells are normally under tonic inhibition by the brain, and they spontaneously secrete their hormones in the absence of such inhibitory input.

HORMONE DELIVERY

Chemical messengers are delivered from the cell of origin to their target cells by one of four or more routes [7, 10]: (1) *endocrine*, where the messenger substance is bloodborne (the classical definition of a hormone); (2) *neurocrine*, where a neuron contacts its target cells by axonal extensions and then releases the hormone into a synaptic cleft between the two cells; (3) *neuroendocrine*, where the hormone released by a nerve is bloodborne; and (4) *paracrine*, where the released hormone diffuses to its target tissue through the immediate extracellular space (Fig. 2.7). There is some evidence that following the release of a hormone it may feed back on the cell of origin by a so-called *autocrine* mechanism [11]. Somatostatin is a possible example of a hormone that may be delivered to its target tissue by all these routes. It is delivered to the pituitary by way of the hypophysial portal system (neuroendocrine route) to regulate somatotropin secretion. Somatostatin is localized within other specific neurons of the CNS and controls target tissue neurons by a neurocrine mechanism. Somatostatin regulates pancreatic islet function by a local paracrine mechanism, and in the gut it may also function as a local hormone and control gastrin secretion by a

Endocrine   Neuroendocrine   Paracrine   Neurocrine

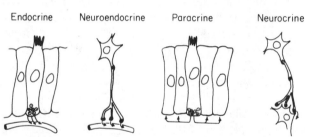

Figure 2.7 Methods of hormone delivery. (From Dockray [7], with permission.)

paracrine mechanism [12]. Portal blood somatostatin levels are increased after a meal, suggesting an additional endocrine method of delivery to undetermined target sites.

Hormones achieve selectivity of target cell activation by many ways. Neurotransmitters may be delivered (by a neurocrine mechanism) only to those target cells being regulated. Some selectivity of hormone action is achieved by delivery through specialized circulatory routes, such as the hypophysial portal system linking the hypothalamus to the pituitary. The specificity of target tissue receptors also assures that these cells will only respond to certain hormones. Under certain pathological states, overproduction of a hormone and its excessive release results in undesirable target tissue responses due to excess amounts of the hormone. Most neurons in the brain are protected from systemic endocrine influences by a so-called blood-brain barrier.

HORMONE METABOLISM

Hormones are secreted from endocrine cells to initiate immediate target tissue responses or to set in motion more long-term effects. In either case hormones must be continuously inactivated or the cellular response cannot be terminated. Both intracellular and extracellular mechanisms function in the cessation of hormone-mediated responses [4].

Peptide Hormones

Peptide hormones have rather short half-lives. The half-life of a hormone or other active agent is defined as the amount of time required for half of the molecules to become inactivated or removed from the circulation. Smaller peptides or such hormones as MSH and oxytocin have particularly short half-lives (possibly 2 to 30 minutes). The large protein hormone, TSH, is reported to have a half-life of 60 minutes, and this may be one example of a rather long half-life. Peptide and protein hormones are inactivated mainly in the liver and the kidney, and each hormone is affected differentially in these two organs. Some hormones may be enzymatically inactivated at the site of their actions (receptors). Peptide hormones have been found inside certain target tissue cells. It is unknown whether the hormone has an intracellular site of action or has become internalized to become degraded. Both suggestions may be correct.

Enzymes inactivate peptide hormones by splitting the molecule at specific peptide bonds. *Exopeptidases*, both *carboxypeptidases* and *aminopeptidases*, cleave off the C-terminal or N-terminal amino acids, respectively. Peptide hormones may also be inactivated by simple deamination at either the N- or C-terminal (if amidated) ends of the molecule. *Endopeptidases* split the molecule at other specific peptide bonds within the molecule. The sites of internal cleavage are quite specific, for example, often between repeating sequences of certain basic amino acids, such as Lys-Lys- as found in β-LPH (Fig. 8.4). The clinical use of some peptides has been limited because of their short half-lives. A knowledge of biodegradation mechanisms may facilitate the preparation of appropriate analogs with longer lasting actions.

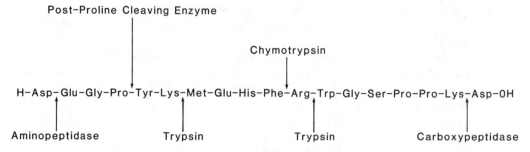

Figure 2.8 Model of peptide degradation by proteolytic enzymes.

Insulin is composed of two chains held together by a pair of disulfide bonds. The hormone is inactivated by a so-called insulinase, an enzyme complex which inactivates the hormone by reduction of the interchain disulfide bonds, thus splitting the hormone into two individual chains. A hypothetical model for the action of various proteolytic enzymes on hormone degradation is shown (Fig. 2.8).

Steroid and Thyroid Hormones

Most steroid hormones are bound to plasma proteins which are specific for each hormone. The half-life of steroid hormones is apparently enhanced by the hormones' ability to be bound to these plasma proteins. Aldosterone, a steroid which is not readily bound, has a shorter half-life than other steroid hormones that have specific carrier (transport) proteins. In the liver both adrenal and gonadal steroids are usually conjugated to glucuronic acid or they are sulfated (Fig. 2.9). This structural modification may render them inactive and more soluble so that they can be rapidly excreted in the urine. Some of the glucuronide salts are secreted with the bile salts and may be reabsorbed into the blood. Thyroxine and triiodothyronine are deaminated in many tissues. These hormones are also conjugated in the liver to form sulfates and glucuronides which enter the bile to pass into the intestine to be reabsorbed or eliminated from the bowel.

Adrenal Catecholamines and Neurotransmitters

The metabolism of circulating catecholamines occurs mainly in the liver by ortho-methylation and oxidative deamination by catechol-0-methyl transferase (COMT) and monoamine oxidase, respectively (MAO) (Fig. 14.4). Neurotransmitter action

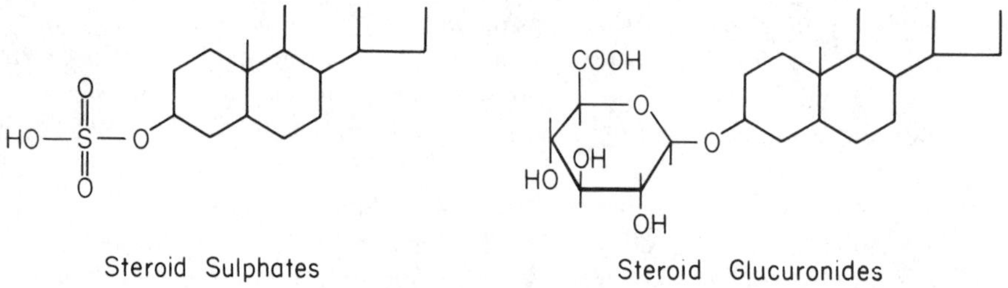

Steroid Sulphates

Steroid Glucuronides

Figure 2.9 Steroid hormone sulfation and glucuronide formation.

within synapses is terminated rapidly by a number of enzymatic or other processes. Norepinephrine and dopamine are inactivated in the synapse by COMT. These neurotransmitters are also taken back into the presynaptic axon to be utilized again or to be inactivated by MAO. Acetylcholine liberated into the synapse from cholinergic neurons is split into choline and acetate by the enzyme acetylcholinesterase. The reaction products, choline and acetate, are also taken back into the presynaptic axon to be resynthesized into acetylcholine.

PHYSIOLOGICAL ROLES OF HORMONES

Hormones control the activity of probably all cells in the body. The vast number of effects produced by hormones can, however, be reduced to a few general processes.

1. Hormones affect cellular synthesis and secretion of other hormones whether in endocrine glands or within neurons. Hormones affect the secretion of products of the digestive tract, such as enzymes, hydrochloric acid, and bile salts. They also affect epithelial mucus and milk synthesis and secretion as well as integumental sebum and sweat production and release. Hormones also affect the production and secretion of pheromones and probably other odoriferous substances.

2. Hormones affect metabolic processes, both *anabolic* and *catabolic*, in most cells. The synthesis and degradation of carbohydrates, lipids and proteins are controlled by hormones to meet the specific energy or growth needs of the individual.

3. Hormones affect contraction, relaxation and metabolism of muscle. They cause contraction and relaxation of vascular and gastrointestinal smooth muscle as well as genital tract musculature such as the uterus and oviducts. Hormones also affect cardiac and skeletal muscle contractile properties. Some steroid hormones profoundly affect anabolic and catabolic processes within muscle.

4. Hormones control reproductive processes, such as gonadal differentiation, maturation, and gametogenesis.

5. Hormones are stimulatory or inhibitory to cellular proliferation and thus they affect growth.

6. The excretion and reabsorption of inorganic cations and anions is regulated by hormones. Sodium, potassium, calcium, and phosphate ions are particularly affected.

7. Hormones have a permissive action on the effects of other hormones: The effectiveness of certain hormones is often considerably enhanced by the action of another hormone. The permissive hormone may be without any noticeable effect of its own but it is an absolute requirement for the actions of the other hormone.

8. Hormones play important roles in animal behavior. Sexual and aggressive behaviors are affected by hormones, particularly during phases of the reproductive cycle. Maternal behavior is controlled by gonadal hormones and

pituitary. Group behavior may even be affected by the release of chemical messengers (pheromones) into the environment.

Hormones may control a physiological function at one stage in life and another at a later developmental stage. Some hormones are secreted on an off and on basis to control fluctuations in serum constituents, such as glucose and calcium. Some hormones are secreted spasmodically to meet particular needs; oxytocin, for example, is generally secreted at parturition and during suckling. Adrenal catecholamines, on the other hand, are usually secreted under conditions of stress. The continuous secretion of hormones under prolonged stress may debilitate an organism [18]. Some hormones are not secreted in large amounts until a later time in development. The gonadotropic hormones, for example, increase in secretion after puberty to cause growth and development of the secondary sex characteristics.

Some hormones may come into existence once or but a few times in the life of an individual. Human chorionic gonadotropin and other peptide hormones are made by the placenta and therefore are only produced during pregnancy. Some hormones lose their function with time; after menopause, for example, FSH secretion is enhanced but the ovary no longer responds to the hormone.

GENERAL MECHANISMS OF HORMONE ACTION

The physiological processes regulated by hormones result from interaction of the hormone with specific constituents of the cell, referred to as *receptors*. All peptide hormones as well as nonpeptidergic neurotransmitters act on membrane receptors. The exact nature of these receptors is unclear, but knowledge of the structure of hormones and related analogs provides some general information.

Stimulation of membrane receptors leads to activation of cyclizing enzymes, which initiate the production of a cyclic nucleotide, either cyclic AMP or cyclic GMP. These so-called second-messengers induce one or more specific protein phosphorylation events within the cell. Addition of a phosphate group to a protein, an enzyme for example, may result in its activation. Phosphorylation of another protein might enhance its contractile activity. This is an exciting and changing field, and many aspects of hormone action will be uncovered by these studies.

Steroid hormones, unlike most other chemical messengers, interact with cytoplasmic receptors. These receptors with attached hormone migrate to the nucleus where the complex interacts with the chromatin of specific chromosomes, which initiates RNA and protein synthesis. Evidence suggests that thyroid hormones also interact with intracellular receptors to activate protein synthetic processes.

The cellular response to membrane receptor activation may be instantaneous as in nerve-nerve or nerve-muscle communication. The ultimate physiological response of cells to steroid or thyroid hormones is obviously much slower as the synthetic events require more time to be consummated. Other complex events are also associated with hormone receptor interaction and subsequent intracellular molecular processes (Chapter 4).

ENDOCRINE PATHOPHYSIOLOGY

Endocrine glands release their hormones in response to bodily needs. The released hormones exert their effects on target tissues and are rapidly degraded and excreted. Failure of a gland or tissue to secrete enough hormones can lead to fatal consequences. For example, in the absence of insulin, elevated blood glucose (hyperglycemia) adversely affects other physiological processes. Individuals with diabetes mellitus may go into coma and die, or they may ultimately succumb from destructive alterations of other physiological processes. Lack of parathormone leads to hypocalcemia and resulting tetanic convulsions and death. Failure to secrete vasopressin will result in severe water loss (*diabetes insipidus*) and dehydration.

TABLE 2.4 Some Examples of Endocrinopathies

Disease	Etiology	Symptoms
Diabetes mellitus	Lack of insulin	Hyperglycemia, glucosuria
Diabetes insipidus		
Pituitary	Lack of ADH	Water loss, hypovolemia, dehydration
Nephrogenic	Renal unresponsiveness to ADH	Water loss, hypovolemia, dehydration
Addison's disease		
Primary	Adrenal cortical destruction (lack of all adrenal steroids)	Altered carbohydrate metabolism; salt-losing syndrome
Secondary	Lack of ACTH secretion	Altered carbohydrate metabolism
Cushing's syndrome		
Primary	Adrenal tumor (excess cortisol secretion)	Protein catabolism, hyperglycemia
Secondary	Pituitary adenoma (excess ACTH secretion, excess cortisol secretion)	Protein catabolism, hyperglycemia
Cretinism (infantile hypothyroidism)	Lack of $T_4 - T_3$ secretion	Lowered BMR, decreased mentation, growth failure
Myxedema (adult hypothyroidism)	Lack of $T_4 - T_3$ secretion	Lowered BMR, decreased mentation
Hyperthyroidism (thyrotoxicosis)	Excess $T_4 - T_3$ secretion	Enhanced BMR, hyperexcitability
Hypoparathyroidism	Parathyroid gland destruction	Lowered blood Ca^{2+} levels
Hyperparathyroidism	Parathyroid gland tumor or hypertrophy (increased PTH secretion)	Elevated blood Ca^{2+} levels
Pseudohypoparathyroidism	Lack of renal response to PTH	Lowered blood Ca^{2+} levels
Testicular feminizing syndrome	No androgen receptors	Genital tract feminization in the male
Hyperaldosteronism (Conn's disease)	Adrenocortical tumor (excess aldosterone secretion)	Sodium retention (hypernatremia), hypervolemia, hypertension

Overproduction of hormone secretion, on the other hand, can also lead to pathophysiological states and possibly death. Excess cortisol secretion (*Cushing's syndrome*) can cause altered carbohydrate, fat, and protein metabolism. This usually leads to hyperglycemia and pancreatic beta cell exhaustion resulting in diabetes mellitus. Oversecretion of aldosterone (*Conn's syndrome*) may lead to severe hypertension because of the hypervolemia (increased blood volume) caused by the hypernatremia (increased blood Na^+) which is characteristic of *hyperaldosteronism*.

Many endocrinopathies of excess hormone secretion result from neoplasms where the tumor produces too much of a hormone or too much of another product. Adrenal cortical tumors may secrete tremendous amounts of cortisol (*Cushing's syndrome*). Insulinomas secrete excessive amounts of insulin, which results in lowered blood glucose levels. The resulting hypoglycemia may cause rapid coma and death as nerve cells must have a constant supply of glucose to function.

Failure to secrete enough hormone may result from destruction of the endocrine gland, as can happen to the adrenal cortex due to tuberculosis. Failure to secrete cortisol (*Addison's disease*) may result from destruction of the adrenal cortex or failure of the pituitary to secrete ACTH which is responsible for stimulation of adrenal cortisol formation. Failure to secrete ACTH can result from pituitary gland dysfunction or failure of the hypothalamus to secrete corticotropin releasing hormone (CRH). Diabetes insipidus may result from a lack of vasopressin, but also, if the kidney fails to respond to the hormone, this results in *nephrogenic diabetes insipidus*.

Endocrine disorders can result from a number of events related to hormone-target cell interaction. For example, the structure of a peptide hormone may be altered due to a mutation (nucleotide base change) in the gene coding for the hormone, as in one form of familial hyperinsulinemia. In the *testicular feminizing syndrome*, target tissues lack receptors for testosterone, and the body may differentiate along the direction of the female phenotype. In pseudohypoparathyroidism, although blood calcium levels are low, there is an excess of parathormone. The target tissue of the hormone, the kidney, apparently lacks a functional adenylate cyclase system responsible for the production of cyclic AMP and therefore the cells fail to respond to the hormone. Other examples of endocrine dysfunction are discussed in Table 2.4 and within the following chapters.

COMPARATIVE ENDOCRINOLOGY

Most information on the vertebrate endocrine system is derived from experiments on mammals, particularly the rat and the mouse. Endocrine dysfunction in humans has, of course, contributed immensely to understanding the role of hormones in normal physiological processes. Primates, the closest relatives of humans, provide important experimental model systems for understanding the roles of hormones.

Much less is known about the endocrinology of nonmammalian forms. Studies on these vertebrates have, however, provided particularly interesting insights into the specialized aspects of endocrine regulation. Thyroid hormones, for example, are required for the metamorphic change necessary for the emergence of some amphibians (e.g., frogs, toads, salamanders) from the aquatic to the terrestrial environment.

Vitamin D_3, because of its crucial role in calcium homeostasis, is of special importance to egg laying in the bird. Prolactin is necessary for successful transition of certain species of fishes from the saline (marine) to the freshwater environment. Prolactin is required for brood patch development in some birds. Melanocyte stimulating hormone plays an important role in regulating color changes of the integument of many vertebrates. Understanding the diverse roles of each of the vertebrate hormones provides interesting insights into the evolution of hormone structure and function.

REFERENCES

[1] BARCHAS, J. D., H. AKIL, G. R. ELLIOT, R. B. HOLMAN, and S. J. WATSON. 1978. Behavioral neurochemistry: neuroregulators and behavioral states. *Science* 200:964–73.

[2] BARKER, J. L. 1977. Physiological roles of peptides in the nervous system. In *Peptides in neurobiology*, ed. H. Gainer, pp. 295–341. New York: Plenum Publishing Corporation.

[3] BAYLISS, W. M. and E. H. STARLING. 1902. The mechanism of pancreatic secretion. *J. Physiol.* 28:325–53.

[4] BENNETT, H. J., and C. McMARTIN. 1979. Peptide hormones and their analogues: distribution, clearance from the circulation, and inactivation in vivo. *Pharmacol. Rev.* 30:247–92.

[5] BROWNSTEIN, M. J., J. T. RUSSELL, and H. GAINER. 1980. Synthesis, transport, and release of posterior pituitary hormones. *Science* 207:373–78.

[6] BULLOUGH, W. S. 1975. Mitotic control in adult mammalian tissue. *Biol Rev.* 50:99–127.

[7] DOCKRAY, G. J. 1979. Evolutionary relationships of the gut hormones. *Fed. Proc.* 38:2295–2301.

[8] GIORDANO, G., J. J. VAN WYK, and F. MINUTO, eds. 1979. *Somotomedins and growth.* New York: Academic Press, Inc.

[9] GROSSMAN, S. P. 1980. The neuroanatomy of eating and drinking behavior. In *Neuroendocrinology*, eds. D. T. Krieger and J. C. Hughes, pp. 131–140. Sunderland, Mass.: Sinauer Associates, Inc.

[10] GUILLEMIN, R. 1977. The expanding significance of hypothalamic peptides, or, is endocrinology a branch of neuroendocrinology. *Rec. Prog. Horm. Res.* 33:1–28.

[11] KARLSON, P. 1982. Was sind Hormone? Der Hormonbegriff in Geschichte und Gegenwart. Naturwissenschaften 69:3–14.

[12] LARSSON, L.-I, N. GOLTERMANN, L. DE MAGISTRIS, J. F. REHFELD, and T. W. SCHWARTZ. 1979. Somatostatin cell processes or pathways for paracrine secretion. *Science* 205:1393–94.

[13] NELSON, N. A., R. C. KELLY and R. A. JOHNSON. 1982. Prostaglandins and the arachidonic acid cascade. Chem. & Engin. News, Aug. 16:30–44.

[14] PEARSE, A. G. E. 1979. The endocrine division of the nervous system: a concept and its verification. In *Molecular endocrinology*, eds. I. MacIntyre and M. Szelke, pp. 3–18. New York: Elsevier North-Holland, Inc.

[15] SAID, S. I. 1980. Peptides common to the nervous system and the gastrointestinal tract. *Front. Neuroendocrinol.* 6:293–331.

[16] SCHALLY, A. V., A. J. KASTIN, and A. ARIMURA. 1977. Hypothalamic hormones: the link between brain and body. *Amer. Sci.* 65:712–19.

[17] SCHARRER, B. 1977. Peptides in neurobiology: historical introduction. In *Peptides in neurobiology*, ed. H. Gainer, pp. 1–8. New York: Plenum Publishing Corporation.

[18] SELYE, H. 1976. *The stress of life*. New York: McGraw-Hill Book Company.

[19] STODDART, D. M. 1976. *Mammalian odours and pheromones*. London: Edward Arnold Publ. Ltd.

[20] WURTMAN, R. J. 1980. The pineal as a neuroendocrine transducer. *Hosp. Prac.* Jan.: 82–92.

3

ENDOCRINE METHODOLOGIES

INTRODUCTION

Some of the methods presently used in endocrinological studies were developed for more practical purposes. In many cultures castration as a form of punishment was practiced. In the Middle and Far East castration was performed to provide servants (eunuchs) for harems; in Italy castrated young boys were trained to be adult sopranos. Castration is presently used to improve the flavor of meat from some domestic animals (e.g., in the chicken to produce a capon). These "practical" operations were the forerunners of the gonadectomies of present-day endocrinological studies.

The idea that glands contained humors or substances that could act as replacement therapy for a lost function of a gland was first entertained seriously by a French physician, Charles Brown-Séquard. He injected himself with extracts from dog, guinea pig, and rabbit testicles and proclaimed that the extracts had remarkable rejuvenating effects. Brown-Séquard even recommended that extracts be obtained from the mature calf to give to man the vigor of horses and other larger animals. It is now believed that these extracts had only a placebo effect. Nevertheless, glandular extraction, purification, and injection into animals have become important methods in elucidating the hormonal role of particular tissues and organs.

Although hormones control a large variety of physiological events, their basic function is to act at the level of the cell to stimulate cellular physiological processes inherent in the cell. Melanocytes, for example, synthesize the pigment melanin. Melanocyte stimulating hormone (MSH) enhances melanin formation by increasing the activity of the rate-limiting enzyme, tyrosinase. Cortisol is a hormone produced by adrenal steroidogenic tissue. Corticotropin (ACTH) activation of adrenocortical enzyme activity leads to elevated cortisol biosynthesis. Thus physiological effects of hormones are reflected in the physiological processes in the many cell types present within an organism. This chapter summarizes some of the methods utilized by endocrinologists to study endocrine glands and the cells and tissues which they regulate.

METHODS OF STUDY

The methods now employed to study endocrine systems are highly diverse. They include surgical manipulations, tissue extract preparation for hormone isolation and identification, immunological methods of histochemistry, and numerous assay methods. The techniques described below will be mentioned in later chapters.

Histological-Cytological Studies

The early endocrine studies were, as expected, anatomical and purely descriptive. The light microscope was used to determine the histological nature of the endocrine glands. Many early observations were made on these tissues even before their endocrine role was suspected. Much of this work was accomplished by the great German, Italian, and other European cytologists of the nineteenth century. Although light microscopic methods are still important, the electron microscope is now the tool in the investigation of cellular function at the ultrastructural level. Recently the scanning electron microscope has bridged the gap between light and electron microscopy.

Gross anatomical observations of endocrine tissue only provide general details of anatomical localization, organ size, vascularization, and innervation. Severe alterations from the normal in organ size may provide clues to an underlying pathophysiology. The thyroid gland, for example, may become enlarged or goitrous under certain conditions of hyperstimulation. At the histological level, one is able to discern the cytological characteristics of endocrine tissues. The cells may be *hypertrophic* or *atrophic* depending on whether they are hyperactive or hypoactive. Hypertrophic cells contain an abundance of endoplasmic reticulum and Golgi bodies, as these organelles function in many cellular synthetic processes. Atrophic cells, on the other hand, lack this synthetic machinery and contain a much diminished cytoplasmic mass.

Histological stains are available to provide further information on chemical components of cells. Hematoxylin and eosin are two popular dyes for staining cells for routine histological observation. Hematoxylin, a basic dye, interacts with acidic components of the cell, such as the phosphoric acid of DNA and RNA. These components are said to be *basophilic* or to exhibit basophilia. On the other hand, eosin, an acidic dye, interacts with the basic components of the cell which are then said to be *acidophilic*. Used in combination, hematoxylin and eosin usually stain the nucleus and cytoplasm blue and pink, respectively.

By the use of a battery of histological stains one can characterize each cell present in the pituitary. With hematoxylin and eosin it is only possible to separate the basophils from the acidophils. Other histological stains are needed to differentiate the basophils. Certain stains can also be used to demonstrate the presence of specific organic constituents, such as glycoproteins, in such cells as the gonadotrophs of the pituitary.

Immunocytochemistry.   In techniques using immunocytochemistry, antibodies to peptide or protein hormones are conjugated to a fluorescent dye and used to identify hormone-producing cells. After the tissue is placed on a microscope slide, a solution of the antibody-conjugate is added to the tissue, and the excess solution is then rinsed from the slide several times. Microscopic observations usually reveal that the fluorescent antibody is deposited only in those cells that produce the hormone, the antigen (Fig. 10.7). Specificity is determined by prior treatment with the nonfluorescent antibody which interacts with the cellular antigen and thus prevents (swamps out) the fluorescent antibody from binding to the antigen.

In immunoenzyme histochemistry an antibody to a hormone is conjugated to an enzyme, such as peroxidase. The antibody-enzyme conjugate is then allowed to interact with the tissue slice. When substrate for the enzyme is added, the conjugated enzyme catalyzes very localized reactions which yield a color or opaque product in the vicinity of the antigen (the hormone). By this immunoperoxidase method and use of the electron microscope, it is even possible to localize the site of the enzyme activity to the secretory vesicles of a cell, which provides strong evidence that these organelles contain the hormone under investigation [26].

Surgical Methods

The use of surgical methods involves removal of a putative endocrine gland or tissue from an animal and subsequent assessment of physiological alterations [28]. A change in functional activity of suspected target organs (i.e., atrophy) suggests an endocrine function for the extirpated tissue. One might also monitor changes in blood or urinary levels of certain metabolites or electrolytes. Removal of the adrenals, for example, would result in lowered circulating levels of adrenal steroids and catecholamines and a reduction in the plasma sodium concentration. Transplantation of an organ back into the same or different animal also provides information on the functional role of the organ. In mammals transplantation of an organ from a donor to a host is usually done in genetically related (inbred) strains of animals so that the transplant is not rejected by immunological processes. Endocrine organs can be transplanted to an *ectopic* site in the animal, usually beneath the kidney capsule or within the eye where rapid vascularization often occurs. Removal of the pituitary is referred to as a *hypophysectomy*. The pituitary target organs of "hypox" animals become atrophic due to the absence of hormonal stimulation. In a few examples endocrine tissue is normally under a tonic inhibitory control; the tissue becomes hypertrophic when transplanted to an ectopic site within the animal or when incubated in vitro.

Removal of both members of paired target organs (for example, adrenal glands or gonads) usually leads to complete loss of the dependent tissue function. If only one of the pair is removed, the remaining organ usually undergoes compensatory hypertrophy. In other words, there is an increase in cell size and number in the remaining organ to compensate functionally for the loss of hormone secretion from the ablated organ (Fig. 1.1).

Certain experimental animals can be sutured together and their vascular systems joined. Under these conditions if the endocrine (or other) organs of one *parabiosed* animal are removed, the organs of the other animal hypertrophy (Fig. 3.1). Obviously, some form of chemical communication must be transferred between the parabiotic animals to produce this compensatory hypertrophy. Removal of the gonads (castration: either orchidectomy in the male, or ovariectomy, spaying, in the female) of one of the animals would be expected, for example, to remove partially a negative feedback to the hypothalamus as the total circulating levels of gonadal steroids of both animals would be decreased compared to that of a pair of intact animals. This would result in enhanced gonadotropin secretion from the pituitary of both animals and compensatory growth of the remaining gonads of the nongonadectomized animal.

Other examples of endocrine ablations include pinealectomy (epiphysectomy), adrenalectomy, thyroidectomy, and thymectomy. The diverse nature of such endocrine tissues as the gastrointestinal hormone-secreting cells prevents such a surgical procedure. The pancreatic islets are similarly impossible to remove without removing concomitantly the exocrine tissue which comprises most of the mass of the pancreas. Islet ablation can, however, be accomplished by the use of alloxan or streptozotocin, drugs which specifically destroy the insulin-secreting cells of the islets. Cobalt chloride is similarly effective in the elimination of the glucagon-secreting cells of the pancreatic islets. How these chemicals specifically destroy either of these pancreatic hormone-secreting cells is unknown.

Immunological Neutralization Of Hormone Activity

Antibodies can be prepared against most of the peptide hormones. Injected into the intact animal these antibodies neutralize the biological activity of the endogenous hormones. This methodology may have clinical applications as such an immunological

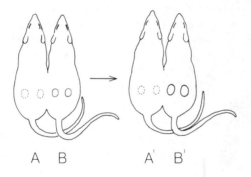

A   B   A' B'

Figure 3.1 Parabiosis accompanied by compensatory organ hypertrophy after removal of the same organs from one of the parabiotic animals.

approach may be useful for contraception in both the male and the female. Many experimental uses of this methodology can be foreseen. For example, injections of antibodies to nerve growth factor (NGF, Chapter 12), a hormone required for growth and development of the sympathetic nervous system, result in failure of this system to develop. The injected animals are effectively immunosympathectomized.

Tissue Extracts And Purification

Crude extracts of endocrine or other tissues were used by some early investigators to determine whether these materials could replace the excised endocrine tissue. With improved chemical techniques these preparations were purified with respect to the hormonal entities contained within the extracts. This led eventually to the preparation of rather pure substances that were, and still are in many cases, marketed by pharmaceutical houses for medicinal or experimental use. Replacement therapy with these preparations can lead to full restoration of target organ function or even to hypertrophy, an overshoot, if too much of the preparation is provided. Many diabetics must receive daily injections of exogenous insulin to augment insufficient quantities produced endogenously by the pancreatic islets. Until recently the only source of the protein hormones, such as insulin, that are too large to synthesize was from endocrine glands obtained from the abattoir (slaughterhouse). Generally the hormones extracted are of *bovine* (cattle), *ovine* (sheep), *porcine* (pig) or even *equine* (horse) origin. Often these foreign proteins are immunologically neutralized within the body following administration, therefore necessitating a change in the type (source) of the hormone which is utilized.

Chemical Identification And Synthesis

A purified hormone must next be chemically identified. The simplest analysis of the hormonal entity may only yield information relative to the percentage of carbon, hydrogen, oxygen, nitrogen, sulfur, or other atoms present and thus provide only an empirical formula. Further analysis, for example of a protein, may then indicate the number of amino acids present (an amino acid analysis). This may be followed by a determination of the *primary structure* (exact amino acid sequence) of the peptide or protein under study. This is not easy if a large protein hormone is being studied. Nevertheless one may obtain information on the N-terminal or C-terminal sequences of these large protein hormones. Recently primary structures of a number of large proteins have been determined by analyzing the nucleotide sequences of the DNA which codes for the molecules. Secondary (helical) and tertiary (intrachain bonding) structures may often be implied from such information as the distribution of basic or acidic amino acids or the presence of sulfhydryl (—SH) groups within the protein. Some peptide hormones, such as insulin, possess a quaternary structure, that is, the hormone is made up of two peptide chains folded together into a three-dimensional structure. A number of the larger peptide hormones, for example, FSH, LH, and TSH, are composed of two chains, the so-called α- and β-subunits of their structures.

Chemical analysis may indicate that proteins are modified through sulfation or conjugation to carbohydrate moieties. Again the pituitary hormones, FSH, LH, and

TSH are examples of *glycoproteins*. Determination of steroid or other hormone structures requires different chemical and physical methods of analysis. After determination of the putative hormone structure, it is necessary to synthesize the proposed structure and demonstrate that the natural and synthetic structures are identical with respect to chemical, physical, and biological characteristics. One can then synthesize related structural analogs of the hormone to determine the structural basis for the biological activity of the hormone [5].

Bioassays

The physiological activity of a hormone was originally determined by bioassay. Although some assays have been replaced by more modern methods, in some instances the only method available is bioassay [28]. In a bioassay the activity of a hormone is studied on living tissue or cells. Physiological responses, such as muscle contraction or glandular secretion, are monitored. The assay may be performed in vitro or in vivo (in situ) depending on the assay utilized. Usually a tissue or organ is selected that is naturally responsive to the hormone. These biological preparations are usually responsive to hormones in the nanomolar (10^{-9} M) to picomolar (10^{-12} M) range. Other hormones may also affect these tissues, but usually in pharmacological (micromolar 10^{-6} M) doses. The following are specific examples of bioassays.

The frog skin bioassay for melanophore stimulating hormone (MSH) is simple, specific, and exquisitely sensitive. Melanin granules within melanophores of frog skin disperse in response to the hormone, causing the skins to turn from light green to dark brown (Chapter 8). This change can be measured in a number of ways, but one objective method is to monitor light reflectance off the surface of the skin [18].

The toad bladder and such epithelia as frog skin and the mammalian renal nephron have been used in vitro to study the actions of vasopressin on transport of water and other components, such as sodium and urea, across these tissues. Studies of ion transport in the toad bladder have contributed detailed information of the mechanisms involved in vasopressin action (Chapter 7).

The steroid-primed uterus of the rat has been used in vitro to study the mechanisms of oxytocin-induced contraction of this organ. Mammary tissue from the lactating mouse is used in vitro to determine milk-ejecting potency of oxytocin and related analogs. Other bioassays include in vitro adrenal steroidogenesis and secretion in response to ACTH; prostate and seminal vesicle growth in vivo in response to testosterone in the castrated male rodent; measurement of iodine uptake by the thyroid after exogenous TSH injections; measurement of growth of the epiphysial (cartilage) plate in the young rat in response to somatotropin. These and other bioassays are listed in Table 3.1.

Radioisotope Studies

A number of endocrine methods utilize the radioactive isotopes of various elements (e.g., ^{125}I, ^{45}Ca, ^{35}S, ^{32}P, ^{23}Na, ^{14}C, ^{3}H) to determine physiological and biochemical responses within a cell [8]. The half-life of a hormone, for example, can be ascertained by radiolabeling the hormone and then determining its distribution, excretion rate,

TABLE 3.1 Some Examples Of Bioassays[a]

Hormone	Assay system	Responses monitored[b]
In vivo:		
Insulin	Fasted rodent	↓ Blood glucose
Follitropin	Immature or hypox rodent	↑ Weight or follicular size of ovaries
Thyrotropin	Any vertebrate	↑ Thyroid uptake of ^{131}I; release of ^{131}I-T$_4$ and ^{131}I-T$_3$ from thyroid tissue
Thyroxine	Larval amphibian	Metamorphic change
Somatotropin	Tibia test (rat)	↑ Width of epiphysial (cartilage) plate
Oxytocin	Rat uterus	Contraction
Parathormone	Parathyroidectomized rat	↑ Ca^{2+} in plasma
Estrogens	Castrated or immature rodent	Vaginal cornification
Androgens	Castrated or immature rodent	↑ Weight of prostate and seminal vesicles
Prolactin	White squab pigeon	↑ Height of crop sac epithelium
Choriogonadotropin	Female frog	Induced ovulation
	Galli–Mainini male frog test	Induced spermiation
	Ascheim–Zondek test, mature rodent or rabbit	Formation of hemorrhagic follicles and corpora lutea
In vitro:		
Melanotropins	Frog skin	↑ Darkening of skin, melanosome dispersion
	Melanoma cells	↑ Tyrosinase activity, melanin production
Corticotropin	Perfused adrenal	↑ Synthesis and release of cortisol

[a] See [28] for references to bioassays.

[b] The effect of each hormone on an increased (↑) or decreased (↓) physiological response is indicated.

and metabolism within the body of an animal. Iodide [^{125}I] is taken up by thyroid cells and incorporated into thyroid hormones (T$_4$ and T$_3$). Radiometric methods can be used to measure uptake of radioactive iodide atoms by the thyroid. Information obtained often reflects the biosynthetic activity of the thyroid gland, and this method is also used to localize hyperplastic thyroid tissues.

The radioisotope of carbon [^{14}C] can be incorporated synthetically into the structure of a molecule, such as glucose. Subsequent metabolism of glucose with the concomitant evolution of radioactive carbon dioxide [^{14}C]O$_2$ is a measure of the metabolic activity of the cell. Insulin, for example, increases release of radioactive CO$_2$ by stimulating the uptake of radiolabeled glucose into diaphragm muscle where it is metabolized. This is also a good example of a bioassay. Tritium, a radioisotope of hydrogen [^{3}H], is widely used in autoradiography and in enzyme assays. The tritium isotope is generally used as a component of some organic structures, such as an amino acid or sugar. The sodium radioisotope [^{23}Na] is most often utilized to measure Na$^+$

uptake into nerve or muscle cells during studies on transmembrane potential changes in response to chemical messengers or other stimuli. Radioactive [^{45}Ca] is often used to measure uptake of this divalent cation during muscle contraction and relaxation, nerve stimulation, or cellular secretion. Moreover, this isotope can localize Ca^{2+} sequestration within mitochondria or in the sarcoplasmic reticulum. Incorporation of sulfur [^{35}S] into the amino acid, cysteine, has been particularly productive in the study of neurohypophysial hormone synthesis because neurohypophysial peptides contain a high percentage of this amino acid. Such labeling of newly synthesized neurophysins and neurohypophysial hormones has greatly facilitated studies on the movement of these proteins by axoplasmic transport down the neuronal secretory axons.

Radioactive phosphorus [^{32}P] in the form of phosphate can be used to monitor protein phosphorylation as induced, for example, by hormonal stimulation of cells. A variety of assays utilize radioisotopes to determine the concentration of a hormone in an endocrine tissue, in the blood, or in the urine. Radioisotope assays can also be utilized to determine enzyme activation or inhibition by a hormone or other chemical messengers. In each of these assays specialized equipment capable of measuring the decay of the isotope is utilized (liquid scintillation counters or gamma counters, for example).

Radioimmunoassays.   These assays are routinely employed to determine the concentration of hormones and other molecular structures in blood or other body fluids [19]. Antibodies against the antigenic principle (e.g., hormone) are usually raised in the rabbit or other animal. The hormone or other structure is iodinated or tritiated; in peptide hormones or in other proteins the tyrosine moiety incorporates iodine. The radiolabeled ligand (e.g., hormone) can then be shown to combine with a given quantity of antibody in a dose-related manner to provide a standard curve. Unknown samples containing native (unlabeled) hormone compete with labeled hormone for the antibody, and the concentration of the hormone is then determined from a standard curve. Because the native and labeled hormones compete equally well (sometimes an assumption) with the antibody, the decreased binding of the labeled hormone to the antibody is a reflection of the amount of the native hormone bound to the antibody. Cyclic nucleotides and many other nonprotein substances are also measured by radioimmunoassay. They are, however, usually conjugated to an antigenic principle to produce antibodies for their assay.

Radioreceptor Assays.   In the radioreceptor assay target tissue plasma membranes or intact cells are carefully prepared and a dose-related binding of radiolabeled hormone to the membranes is then demonstrated [25]. Instead of an antigen-antibody reaction, the assay employs interaction between hormone and natural membrane receptors. The detailed mechanisms are, nevertheless, similar to those described for the radioimmunoassay. The specificity of the binding is determined by the ability of the cold, native hormone to compete with the radiolabeled hormone for receptor. Other cold or radiolabeled hormones or other ligands can be used to determine the specificity of the hormone for its receptor. Both ACTH as well as prostaglandins, for example, interact with adrenal cortical cell membranes to initiate steroidogenesis. Radiolabeled ACTH can be displaced from its receptor by cold ACTH but not cold prostaglandin. Cold prostaglandin, but not cold ACTH, will displace radiolabeled prostaglandin from the membrane preparation. These results demonstrate that the receptors for these active agonists are separate because each agonist can be specifically blocked while the integrity of the other receptor is uncompromised.

Enzyme Assays. Enzyme activity can also be measured by radioisotope methods [14]. Adenylate cyclase or guanylate cyclase are measured by quantitation of the conversion of an appropriately radiolabeled precursor, ATP or GTP, to radiolabeled cyclic nucleotide. This is a true measure of cyclizing activity of the membrane fractions as measurements of cyclic nucleotide levels in the cell fail to indicate how the nucleotide levels are altered. Cyclic AMP levels, for example, may be altered by a number of processes, such as increased or decreased phosphodiesterase activity, which are unrelated to cyclase activity and cyclic AMP formation. Measurement of tyrosinase activity of melanocytes is monitored by production of radiolabeled water from the appropriately labeled precursor, tyrosine (Fig. 3.2). Many other examples of enzymatic assays are used to measure a variety of cellular enzyme systems.

Autoradiography. This technique determines the cellular site of incorporation of a radiolabeled substrate [20]. A radioisotope is injected into an animal or placed in the medium within which cells are grown. A sample of tissue from the animal or the cell culture is then placed on a microscope slide and fixed as is done for routine microscopy. The slide is immersed in a photographic emulsion and placed in the dark for a certain period of time. Decay of the isotope (usually tritium) leads to reduction of the silver bromide in the overlying emulsion to silver crystals. Because the beta particles released by the tritium only travel a short distance, the silver grains directly over the emulsion are preferentially exposed as they are closest to the source of isotope decay. The tissue with emulsion is then placed in developer and stained if desired. By this method one can determine the incorporation of tritium-labeled thymidine into DNA [20]. This nucleotide is generally utilized to determine the mitotic activity of cells of a tissue. After orchidectomy, for example, there is enhanced hypothalamic activation (due to lack of negative feedback inhibition by testosterone) of pituitary gonadotrophs. This leads to increased incorporation of radiolabeled thymidine into the DNA of these cells which can be visualized by autoradiographic methods. The mechanism of action of steroid hormones involves interaction with nuclear chromatin. Autoradiography using tritium-labeled steroids provides a method for demonstrating the cellular site of action of these hormones (Fig. 3.3).

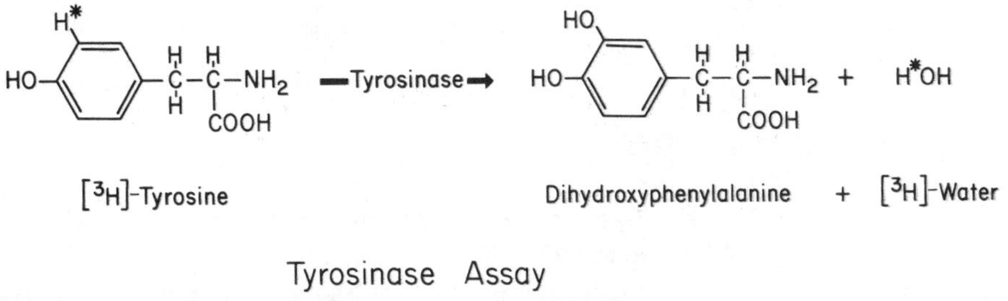

Figure 3.2 Radioisotope enzyme assay: tyrosinase assay.

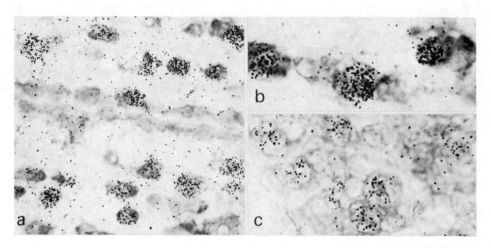

Figure 3.3 [^{3}H]estradiol labeling of neurons in the preoptic nucleus of the mouse brain. (From Warembourg, [23], with permission.)

Some hormones mediate their effects through stimulation of RNA synthesis. This is demonstrated by the use of tritium-labeled uracil which is incorporated specifically into RNA rather than DNA. Using giant chromosomes of the dipteran fly (midge), *Chironomus*, for example, it is possible to localize tritium uptake to specific Balbiani rings (Chapter 21) of the chromosomes [3], sites known to be responsible for very active RNA synthesis (Fig. 3.4).

Electrophysiological Methods

Most cells are excitable, that is, they will respond to stimuli by becoming depolarized or hyperpolarized [2]. These transmembrane potential changes can be monitored by intracellular or extracellular microelectrodes. The response of the cells to hormonal or other stimuli can therefore be detected. Most stimuli depolarize cells, but some chemical messengers—for example, gamma aminobutyric acid (GABA), a central nervous system neurotransmitter—hyperpolarize cells. Chemical messengers can be applied to the surface of a cell by *microionotophoresis* and resulting transmembrane potential changes recorded downstream by microelectrode recordings. Electrophysiological methods have been important in studying electrical properties of the neurosecretory neurons of the neurohypophysis (Fig. 7.3) and the response of pituitary cells to hormones (Fig. 6.16).

Pharmacological Methods

Many exogenous compounds interact with molecular components of cells, and they therefore can be utilized to study the endogenous physiological activity of cells or the mechanism by which chemical messengers stimulate or inhibit such activity [7]. For example, at the level of the plasmalemma, cardiac glycosides, such as ouabain, are used to inhibit the Na$^+$-K$^+$ pump. Certain hormone secretions are enhanced or inhibited by

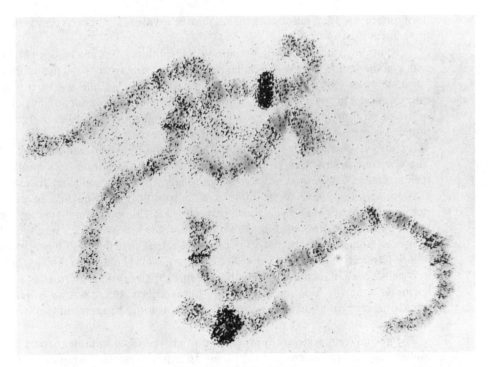

Figure 3.4 Pattern of [³H]uridine incorporation into RNA produced by larval salivary chromosomes of a dipteran fly. Note intense labeling of Balbiani rings 1 and 6. (From Beerman, [3], with permission.)

ouabain, and this suggests that active transport (Na⁺-K⁺ ATPase) systems may be involved in the mechanism of secretion of these hormones [4].

Many agents are inhibitors of intracellular enzyme activity. Of particular interest are the methylxanthines, such as theophylline and caffeine, which are phosphodiesterase inhibitors. These drugs mimic the actions of many hormones because they elevate intracellular cAMP and cGMP levels (Fig. 4.7).

There are a number of so-called metabolic inhibitors that affect utilization of substrates for ATP formation. Iodoacetic acid blocks glycolysis, dinitrophenol (DNP) uncouples oxidative phosphorylation, and oligomycin prevents mitochondrial phosphorylation of ADP to ATP. The false substrate, 2-deoxyglucose, can be utilized to slow down glucose utilization within cells. These inhibitors provide information on the degree to which the glycolytic (Embden-Myerhof) pathway or the citric acid cycle (Krebs cycle) contributes to cellular function [9].

Colchicine, a plant alkaloid, inhibits microtubule assembly by binding with tubulin, the protein subunit of microtubules. Inhibition of hormone action by colchicine or related microtubule inhibitors (vincristine and vinblastine) might suggest, therefore, that the hormone works through a cellular mechanism in which microtubules are involved. Insulin secretion is inhibited by colchicine suggesting that microtubules may function in the secretion of this hormone. Cytochalasin B is a fungal metabolite that specifically interferes with microfilament function and is without effect on microtubule integrity. Cytochalasin B is inhibitory to the secretion of a number of

Methods of Study

hormones; these filamentous organelles may be involved in the secretory processes of these hormones.

At the level of the nucleus, actinomycin D inhibits RNA production. Puromycin and cycloheximide, on the other hand, inhibit protein synthesis. Thus inhibition of hormone action by actinomycin D implies that the hormone works through the transcriptional process of RNA synthesis. Inhibition of hormone action by puromycin or cycloheximide, in contrast, is interpreted to implicate a translational process of protein synthesis in the mechanism of action of the chemical messenger.

Rather specific cation *ionophores* have been discovered and synthesized [15]. These organic cation transport molecules specifically incorporate certain cations into their structure. They apparently cross biological membranes and carry these ions into cells. Ionophore A23187, for example, is rather specific for calcium and, because many hormones activate cells by a calcium ion mechanism, this ionophore is in some systems hormone-mimetic. Valinomycin is an ionophore with relatively high specificity for K^+ transport. Some agents, on the other hand, are rather specific in inhibiting movement of ions into cells. Verapamil, a so-called calcium channel antagonist, blocks Ca^{2+} entry into cells. Used concomitantly with a hormone it may suggest that a particular hormone action is calcium dependent. Local anesthetics, such as procaine and tetracaine, may also block the action of some hormones by their antagonism of Ca^{2+} flux into cells.

Phospholipid vesicles (liposomes) have proved to be suitable carriers for many biologically active molecules [22]. These transport vehicles fuse with and become incorporated into the plasma membrane, thereby transferring their contents into the cytoplasm. Liposomes loaded with calcium, for example, are incorporated into mast cells which results in localized cell surface secretion of histamine [22]. Liposomes therefore provide a novel method of studying mechanisms of stimulus-secretion coupling, particularly as it relates to the release of a chemical messenger as histamine.

Some agents are hormone receptor agonists although in some cases they may not appear to bear any structural similarity to the true receptor agonist, the hormone. Certain ergot alkaloids, for example, stimulate dopamine receptors. MSH and prolactin secretion is inhibited by the hypothalamus, and ergot alkaloids are inhibitors of MSH and prolactin secretion, thus providing some evidence that dopamine may be the natural hypothalamic inhibitor of these hormones. Certain structures related to acetylcholine (e.g., carbachol) exhibit intrinsic cholinergic activity, and they are of particular usefulness because they have a longer duration of activity as they are somewhat more resistant to enzymatic degradation.

Hormone action can be blocked by compounds that specifically act with hormone receptors but lack intrinsic agonistic activity [1]. For example, chlorpromazine and related antidepressant drugs block dopamine receptors. Acetylcholine action can be blocked by atropine (on smooth muscle) and curare (on skeletal muscle) and other cholinergic receptor antagonists. Cimetidine is a specific inhibitor of histamine (H_2) receptors and markedly inhibits histamine-stimulated gastric acid secretion. Cyproterone acetate and spironolactone are specific antagonists (antihormones) of testosterone and aldosterone receptors, respectively. Cyproterone acetate is a valuable tool in the treatment of cancer of the prostate, abnormal behavior in the male and female, and precocious puberty in both sexes as these maladies are due to excess androgen secretion and action.

TABLE 3.2 Some Pharmaceutical and Other Agents Used In Cell Physiology Studies

Agent	Application
Actinomycin D	Inhibits RNA synthesis
Alloxan	Destroys beta (insulin-secreting) cells of pancreatic islets
Chlorpromazine	Dopamine receptor antagonist
Cobalt chloride	Destroys alpha (glucagon-secreting) cells of pancreatic islets
Colchicine	Disrupts microtubules
Cycloheximide	Inhibits protein synthesis
Cyproterone acetate	Testosterone receptor antagonist
Cytochalasin B	Disrupts microfilaments
2-Deoxy-D-glucose	Metabolic inhibitor: inhibits glucose uptake and utilization
Dexamethasone	Synthetic glucocorticoid agonist
Dinitrophenol	Metabolic inhibitor: uncouples oxidative phosphorylation
Ergot alkaloids (e.g., ergocryptine)	Dopamine receptor antagonist
Iodoacetic acid (or iodoacetamide)	Metabolic inhibitor: inhibits glycolysis
Ionophore A23187	Calcium transport carrier (ionophore)
Liposomes	Drug carrier
Local anesthetics (procaine, tetracaine)	Inhibits cellular uptake of calcium
Methylxanthines (theophylline, caffeine)	Phosphodiesterase inhibitors (elevates cAMP)
Spironolactone	Aldosterone receptor antagonist
Saralasin	Angiotensin II receptor antagonist
Thiouracil	Inhibits thyroid iodide uptake and $T_4 - T_3$ synthesis
Valinomycin	Potassium transport carrier (ionophore)
Verapamil	Inhibits cellular uptake of calcium
Puromycin	Inhibits protein synthesis
[^{3}H] Thymidine	Studies on DNA synthesis
[^{3}H] Uracil	Studies on RNA synthesis
Oligomycin	Metabolic inhibitor: inhibits phosphorylation of ADP to ATP

As mentioned earlier, cobalt chloride and alloxan can be used specifically to destroy the alpha (glucagon-secreting) or beta (insulin-secreting) cells, respectively, of the pancreas. Monosodium glutamate (MSG) administered neonatally causes degeneration of neurons of the arcuate nucleus of the hypothalamus[10]. The neurotoxicity of MSG appears to be useful for investigative purposes because it is difficult to produce such lesions by electrolytic and radiofrequency methods without damage to other neurons or fiber tracts. The use of MSG, therefore, offers the opportunity to study the endocrine and morphological manifestations of an apparently specific lesion of the hypothalamus. Some pharmaceutical agents used in endocrine studies are described in Table 3.2.

FUTURE PERSPECTIVES

Possibly the greatest contributions to recent advances in the field of endocrinology have derived from immunochemical methods. For example, it is now possible to produce antibodies against peptide hormones. Injected into an animal these proteins effectively produce an immunoneutralization. Thus an effective chemical ablation of a specific molecular component of the endocrine system can be provided. Most importantly the development of the radioimmunoassay (RIA) has allowed the detection of hormones in minute concentrations and with a high degree of specificity [27]. RIA has provided greatly increased accuracy of diagnosis of pathologic states which are characterized by hormonal excess or deficiency. Most of the information known about the regulation of hormone secretion is because of RIA. RIA has had an important role in the discovery of new forms of hormones in blood and tissues. The assay has provided new insights concerning the biosynthesis of peptide hormones, their precursors and metabolites. It is likely that many other insights into the synthesis, secretion, and function of hormones will be elucidated by RIA and immunocyto-chemistry.

Monoclonal Antibodies

Although the RIA is used extensively in diagnostic laboratories for a variety of purposes including measurement of hormone levels in blood and other tissues, these assays have always been plagued by the heterogeneity of the antibodies generated to the "pure" antigen utilized. Recent studies have led to a technology for the production of large quantities of homogeneous antibodies against a wide variety of antigens, including hormones [6]. These monoclonal antibodies are derived from a single parental cell type and recognize only one antigenic determinant, thus improving the quality and discriminating power of diagnostic methods for the detection and localization of hormones.

Recombinant DNA Techniques

Hormones play important roles in regulating the activity of most cells of the body; indeed, some hormones are necessary for life. Parathormone and aldosterone, two hormones that regulate the electrolyte composition of the body fluids, are examples. Somatotropin is necessary for growth, and its absence in the young animal results in dwarfism. Failure of the pancreas to produce insulin results in diabetes mellitus. Insulin replacement therapy requires obtaining these hormones from other animal sources, but some individuals develop antibodies to these nonhuman sources of the hormone. In the case of STH only pituitaries obtained from human cadavers or primates can be used as STH from other animals is ineffective. Recombinant DNA techniques offer the hope that a number of human hormones can be synthesized by bacteria in large amounts and at reasonable prices. Recombinant DNA techniques are essentially in vitro extensions of natural phenomena [24]. These methods involve purification or synthesis of genetic material and its insertion into a bacterial host. Several bacterial strains have been constructed that can produce human hormones, and it is probable that genetically engineered bacteria will provide important sources of peptide hormones [17]. Two methods have been used to provide the genetic material to be cloned. For shorter peptides (e.g., insulin, somatostatin), chemical DNA synthesis is used to make a gene of the desired hormone [11]. In the case of the two chains of insulin the 21 amino acid A chain and the 30 amino acid B chain are made in

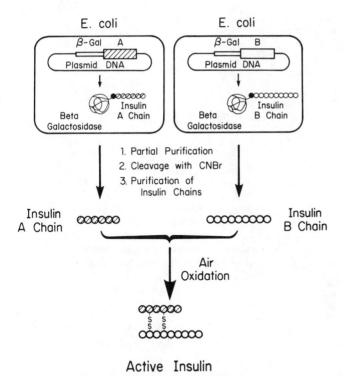

Figure 3.5 Recombinant DNA technique for the microbial production of insulin. (From Riggs and Itakura, [17], with permission.)

separate bacterial strains as tails on a larger precursor protein, the enzyme β-galactosidase. The individual insulin chains are then clipped from the precursor proteins and, after purification of the separate insulin chains, they are joined by air oxidation (Fig. 3.5). The other method used for larger proteins utilizes mRNA and reverse transcriptase to make a DNA copy which is then inserted into the bacterial genome and cloned [12].

For the diabetic there is the hope that pancreatic islet transplants may provide their needed insulin [21]. The implantation of insulin pumps may soon provide a method of delivering insulin at a constant rate. Unfortunately, unlike transplantable cells, pumps are not presently sensitive to circulating glucose levels. Nevertheless, new sources of previously scarce hormones with novel methods of delivery may provide cures for a considerable number of the world's population who suffer deficits in synthesis and secretion of hormones.

Genetic Engineering

The possibility of introducing foreign genes into mammalian embryos provides a powerful tool for use in endocrine research. It is now feasible to introduce foreign DNA into the mammalian genome by microinjection of DNA molecules of interest into pronuclei of fertilized cells, followed by the implantation of the eggs into the reproductive tracts of recipient mothers. The so-called transgenic animals that develop integrate the foreign DNA into one of the host chromosomes at an early stage of embryo development.

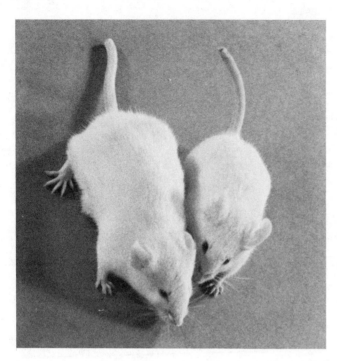

Figure 3.6 Photograph of gigantism produced in the mouse by injection of metallothionin-growth hormone fusion genes into the pronucleus of the fertilized egg followed by implantation within the uterus of a recipient mother. Giant mice (left) became almost twice as heavy as littermates (not bearing the STH gene). (Reprinted by permission from *Nature*, 300 (5893): 611–15. Copyright (c) 1982. Macmillan Journals, Limited.

Microinjection of the structural gene for rat growth hormone into the pronuclei of fertilized mouse eggs resulted in the development of some offspring that grew significantly larger than their littermates (Fig. 3.6). This methodology has important implications for studying the biological effects of growth hormone, as a way to accelerate animal growth, as a model for gigantism and possibly as a means of correcting genetic disease [13].

REFERENCES

[1] AGARWAL, M. K., ed. 1979. *Antihormones*. Amsterdam: Elsevier North-Holland, Inc.

[2] AIDLEY, D. J. 1978. *The physiology of excitable cells*. New York: Cambridge Univ. Press.

[3] BEERMANN, W. 1973. Direct changes in the pattern of Balbiani ring puffing in *Chironomus*: effects of sugar treatment. *Chromosoma* 4:297–326.

[4] BOWER, Sr. A., and M. E. HADLEY. 1972. Ionic requirements for melanophore stimulating hormone (MSH) release. *Gen. Comp. Endocrinol.* 19:147–58.

[5] BRANDENBURG, D., and A. WOLLMER, ed. 1980. *Insulin: chemistry, structure and function of insulin and related hormones*. Berlin: Walter de Gruyter.

[6] DIAMOND, B. A., D. E. YELTON, and M. D. SCHARFF. 1981. Monoclonal antibodies. *New Engl. J. Med.*, 304:1344–49.

[7] GILMAN, A. G., L. S. GOODMAN, and A. GILMAN. 1980. *Goodman and Gilman's The pharmacological basis of therapeutics*. 6th ed. New York: Macmillan, Inc.

[8] GURPIDE, E. 1975. *Tracer methods in hormone research*. New York: Springer-Verlag New York, Inc.

[9] HADLEY, M. E., and Sr. A. BOWER. 1976. Metabolic requirements for melanophore stimulating hormone (MSH) secretion. *Gen. Comp. Endocrinol.* 28:118–30.

[10] HOLZWARTH, M. A., J. R. SLADEK, Jr., and K. M. KNIGGE. 1976. Monosodium glutamate induced lesions of the arcuate nucleus. *Anat. Rec.* 186:197–205.

[11] ITAKURA, K., T. HIROSE, R. CREA, A. D. RIGGS, H. L. HEYNEKER, F. BOLWAR, and H. W. BOYER. 1977. Expression in *Escherichia coli* of a chemically synthesized gene for the hormone somatostatin. *Science* 198:1056–63.

[12] JOHNSON, I. S. 1983. Human insulin from recombinant DNA technology. *Science* 219:632-37.

[13] PALMITER, R. D., R. L. BRINSTER, R. E. HAMMER, M. E. TRUMBAUER, M. G. ROSENFELD, N. C. BIRNBERG, and R. M. EVANS. 1982. Dramatic growth of mice that develop from eggs microinjected with metallothionen-growth hormone fusion genes. *Nature* 300:611–15.

[14] POMERANTZ, S. 1964. Tyrosine hydroxylation catalyzed by mammalian tyrosinase; an improved method of assay. *Biochem. Biophys. Res. Commun.* 16:188–94.

[15] PRESSMAN, B. C. 1976. Biological applications of ionophores. *Ann. Rev. Biochem.* 45:501–30.

[16] RIGGS, A. D., and K. ITAKURA. 1979. Synthetic DNA and medicine. *Am. J. Hum. Genet.* 31:531–38.

[17] RIGGS, A. D., K. ITAKURA, R. CREA, T. HIROSE, A. KRASZEWSKI, D. GOLDDEL, D. KLEID, D. G. YANSURA, F. BOLIVAR, and H. L. HEYNEKER. 1980. Synthesis, cloning, and expression of hormone genes in *Escherichia coli*. *Rec. Prog. Horm. Res.* 36:261–76.

[18] SHIZUME, K., A. B. LERNER, and T. B. FITZPATRICK. 1954. In vitro bioassay for melanocyte stimulating hormone. *Endocrinology* 54:553–60.

[19] SÖNKSEN, P. H. 1974. Radioimmunoassay and saturation analysis. *Brit Med. Bull.* 30:1–103.

[20] STUMPF, W. E. 1970. Localization of hormones by autoradiography and other histochemical techniques. *J. Histochem. Cytochem.* 18:21–29.

[21] SUN, M. 1980. Insulin wars: new advances may throw market into turbulence. *Science* 210:1225–28.

[22] THEOHARIDES, T. C., and W. W. DOUGLAS. 1978. Secretion in mast cells induced by calcium entrapped within phospholipid vesicles. *Science* 201:1143–45.

[23] WAREMBOURG, M. 1976. Detection of diffusible substances. *J. de Microscopie et de Biologie Cellulaire* 27:277–80.

[24] WETZEL, R. 1980. Applications of recombinant DNA technology. *Am. Sci.* 68:664–75.

[25] WILLIAMS, L. T., and R. J. LEFKOWITZ. 1978. *Receptor binding studies in adrenergic pharmacology*. New York: Raven Press.

[26] WITORSCH, R. J. 1979. The application of immunoperoxidase methodology for the visualization of prolactin binding sites in human prostate tissue. *Human Pathol.* 10:521–32.

[27] YALOW, R. S. 1978. Radioimmunoassay: a probe for the fine structure of biologic systems. *Science* 200:1236–45.

[28] ZARROW, M. X., J. M. YOCHIM, J. L. MCCARTHY, and R. C. SANBORN. 1964. *Experimental endocrinology: a sourcebook of basic techniques*. New York: Academic Press, Inc.

4

General Mechanisms of Hormone Action

INTRODUCTION

Hormones stimulate or inhibit the activity of cells directly or indirectly through modulation of the actions of other chemical messengers. Some hormones, often referred to as first messengers, interact with the cell membrane to increase the production of intracellular second messengers, which are more directly responsible for activation of the cell. The second messenger is usually a cyclic nucleotide, either *cyclic adenosine monophosphate (cyclic AMP, cAMP)* or *cyclic guanosine monophosphate (cyclic GMP, cGMP)*. This first messenger-second messenger model of hormone action must now be expanded to include other messengers in the temporal sequence of hormone action. For example, some hormones require calcium for activation of cyclic nucleotide formation. In some cells the first messenger acting through induction of an inward calcium flux may activate prostaglandin biosynthesis. The newly synthesized prostaglandin activates the intracellular production of cAMP or cGMP. These cyclic nucleotides actually mediate their actions through stimulation of cellular enzymes—kinases—which phosphorylate cell-specific proteins; these phosphorylated proteins then function as the ultimate physiological effectors in the cell. Other first messengers interact with intracellular constituents of a cell to mediate their actions.

CELLULAR RECEPTORS AND HORMONE ACTION

Hormones regulate specific target tissues, not all cells in the body. One might ask what mechanism or characteristic of a cell determines whether it will be responsive to a particular hormone? Molecular components of cells, so-called *receptors*, provide the specificity for hormone-cell interaction. The receptor concept originated early in this century with the work of Langley [26]. Receptors may be components of the plasma membrane [20] or they may be cytosolic or nuclear elements [2, 23]. Receptors provide the means by which hormones initially interact with cells. If each type of cell did not possess specific hormone receptors, all cells might be expected to respond to all chemical messengers. Each time a single hormone was released, all cells in the body would respond, and this would result in uncoordinated muscle contraction and relaxation and the uncontrolled secretion of numerous cellular products such as hormones and enzymes. Therefore, cells do not possess receptors for all hormones, but rather, only a limited number of different receptors. Certain cellular elements may exhibit specific affinities for nonhormone agents, such as narcotics or other drugs; these affinities provide the basis for medicinal drug therapy. Some drugs interact with hormone receptors, which may result in activation of the cell, or, if the ligand (receptor-binding substance) lacks intrinsic biological activity, it may act as an antagonist to block the binding of a hormone.

Oxytocin and vasopressin (AVP) are related in structure, and both hormones stimulate uterine smooth muscle contraction and activate renal tubular cyclic AMP production. Uterine receptors are, however, more sensitive to oxytocin than to AVP, whereas renal receptors are more sensitive to AVP than oxytocin. Thus at normal circulating concentrations, each neurohypophysial hormone will only activate its appropriate target cell receptor. Vascular smooth muscle neurohypophysial hormone receptors are generally less sensitive to oxytocin or vasopressin than are uterine or renal tubular cells. During severe hemorrhage, however, large quantities of vasopressin are released from the neurohypophysis; the hormone may then be able to induce vasoconstriction and serve an important role in hemostasis.

Some hormones stimulate a number of tissues, which suggests that each of these diverse tissues possesses receptors for the hormone. Insulin is probably the best example of a hormone with multiple actions. Insulin stimulates glucose uptake by hepatocytes, fat cells, and certain muscle cells, and interacts with many other cell types. Insulin is thus able to lower rapidly extracellular glucose levels, which is one of its major functions. If more than one tissue responds to a particular hormone at one time, it might be expected that all these different physiological responses would complement the one physiological process being regulated. For example, parathormone elevates serum calcium levels by releasing Ca^{2+} from bone, stimulating Ca^{2+} uptake from the gut and preventing Ca^{2+} loss from the kidney. Each of these individual responses is important in elevating serum Ca^{2+} levels.

At normal physiological levels each hormone interacts with its own specific cellular receptor. Estradiol, for example, interacts with estrogen receptors, not with other steroid receptors such as those for cortisol or progesterone. Therefore hormone receptors possess a recognition function which must then be converted into an action function. Receptors recognize differences in hormone structure and thus provide receptor specificity. Norepinephrine and epinephrine are structurally similar (Fig. 14.3), but norepinephrine preferentially interacts with certain types of adrenergic receptors, whereas epinephrine interacts more specifically with other adrenergic receptors (Chapter 14). The pharmaceutical industry capitalizes on receptor specificity to provide hormone analogs that can be used medicinally to activate or inhibit certain tissue-specific receptors.

PLASMA MEMBRANE HORMONE RECEPTORS

With the exception of steroid and thyroid hormones, apparently all other hormones stimulate cells by an initial interaction with specific plasma membrane receptors. This initial receptor interaction results in *transduction* of signal to the cytoplasmic side of the membrane where *adenylate* or *guanylate cyclase* enzymes are activated, resulting in production of cAMP or cGMP, respectively. These membrane receptors are conceptually visualized as macromolecules, probably glycoprotein in nature, which display a high affinity for a specific hormonal ligand; only a few receptors have been well characterized. Most receptors studied thus far, such as those for insulin, LH, and TSH, contain carbohydrate moieties. Peptide hormone receptors are localized, at least partially, to the outer surface of the cells as shown by a number of experimental techniques. For example, ACTH covalently linked to a large polymer is still able to stimulate cyclic AMP-mediated adrenal steroidogenesis. Other hormones have also been linked to sepharose beads, which are too large to enter cells, and in all cases the hormones still activate cyclic AMP production in a variety of cells. In addition specific antisera to peptide hormones rapidly terminate their actions, again indicating that the site of action of the hormones is extracellular.

Regulation of Receptor Number

Receptors are not static components of the plasmalemma; indeed, receptor number is in a constant state of flux and may change with the state of cellular development or differentiation. A cell may therefore become more or less responsive to a hormone depending on its specific developmental or differentiated state. Cells may even lose their capacity to respond to a certain hormone, but gain the ability to respond to another, presumably because of the loss and gain of membrane receptors. Hormones may even regulate the number of their own (*homospecific*) or other (*heterospecific*) receptors. Homospecific receptor regulation may be negative or positive, resulting in so-called down or up regulation, respectively. Prolactin, for example, induces the appearance of prolactin receptors (up regulation) in the liver and certain other tissues [33]. Continuous exposure of lymphocytes to insulin results in decreased binding (down regulation) of the hormone to the cells [10]. Some obese individuals have high concentrations of insulin in their blood even though their blood sugar level is normal. Theoretically glucose levels should be diminished in the presence of insulin. The cells of these obese individuals apparently possess fewer insulin receptors. Increases in plasma insulin concentrations also decrease insulin receptor number in normal individuals.

When obese individuals diet, which lowers their blood insulin levels, their cells are able to bind increased amounts of insulin.

Most hormones, like insulin, produce the same effect (e.g., down or up regulation) on receptors in the various tissues that they regulate. Angiotensin II, however, appears to increase or decrease receptors depending on the particular cell type involved. For example, angiotensin II increases the number of its receptors on adrenal glomerulosa cells but decreases its receptor population on certain smooth muscles. TRH acts on pituitary thyrotrophs to release TSH which then stimulates thyroid hormone (T_4 and T_3) production by the thyroid gland. Thyroid hormones then decrease the sensitivity of thyrotrophs by stimulating a loss of TRH receptors, a good example of negative feedback. Glucocorticoids, on the other hand, increase the number of pituitary TRH receptors. The latter two examples of heterospecific receptor regulation demonstrate both down and up regulation. Changes in receptor number may provide an important mechanism for preventing hyperstimulation of cells to hormones under pathological states. Receptor modulation may also provide a mechanism by which hormones act in sequence to amplify or diminish responses to other hormones. The gonadotropins, FSH and LH, are secreted and act on the ovaries in a sequential manner; it appears that LH action is dependent on induction of LH receptors by FSH [9].

Choriogonadotropin, which has properties similar to luteinizing hormone, causes a marked loss of receptors from testicular Leydig cells with a resultant loss of cyclic AMP production. This process has also been described for the luteal cells of the ovary. In addition to Leydig cell receptor depletion further changes occur at a point distal to the receptor. There appears to be a biosynthetic defect in the steroidogenic pathway within Leydig cells which contributes to the marked loss of androgen production in response to gonadotropin stimulation and to cyclic AMP of endogenous or exogenous origin. This defect may prove to be characteristic of target cells for tropic peptide hormones that regulate both the state of differentiation as well as the acute responses of target cells [19].

Hormone Internalization and Hormone Action

Although the receptors for steroid and thyroid hormones are intracellular, there is evidence that certain peptide hormones may also enter cells [15, 24, 33]. The significance of this ligand internalization is controversial. It is strongly argued that internalization is one way for the cell to terminate hormone action. Peptide hormone receptors have been localized within cells, but these intracellular hormone receptors may have been synthesized for subsequent transport to the plasmalemma. On the other hand, there appear to be nuclear binding sites for insulin. Moreover, nerve growth factor, which is structurally related to insulin, is retrogradely transported within neuronal axons to the perikarya (cell body) of these cells. It is argued, therefore, that ligand internalization may provide a mechanism whereby hormones can stimulate relatively long-term (hours to days) effects, such as is characteristic of cell division and cell differentiation [13]. For example, insulin causes both a rapid membrane effect, resulting in glucose transport, and a subsequent delayed growth effect on fibroblasts. Epidermal growth factor (EGF) is also internalized in human fibroblasts grown in tissue culture. Prolactin (PRL) is internalized and concentrated in an intact state in the Golgi elements of rat liver cells, and these Golgi elements have been shown to contain PRL receptors [33].

Receptor Cooperativity and Hormone Action

Hormone receptor studies suggest that mechanisms of hormone-receptor interaction are compatible with negative or positive models of *cooperativity*. There are two major events which govern the response elicited by a hormone: hormone binding, and the coupling between the binding event and the first biochemical signal elicited. The binding event can be described as being *noncooperative*, *positively cooperative*, or *negatively cooperative* [3, 8]. These terms describe how binding of a hormone to its receptors affects subsequent binding of the hormone to other receptors possessed by the cells. Although it was originally believed that binding to one site did not affect binding to others, it is now realized that subsequent binding events can also be affected in a positive or negative manner. Positive cooperativity is the phenomenon observed where the initial binding of the hormone to its receptor enhances the affinity of other receptors to the hormone. This may be an important mechanism for sensitizing a cellular system when the hormone concentration occupies only a few of the available receptors. Negative cooperativity, where binding of the hormone reduces the affinity of receptors for subsequent binding events, may provide a mechanism for desensitizing cells to abnormal concentrations of a hormone. The kinetics of negative and positive cooperativity in hormone binding departs from the typical law of mass action behavior. The affinity of insulin receptors, for example, is not fixed, but decreases as occupancy increases [8].

Spare Receptors

In most cells a maximum biological response is achieved when only a small percentage of receptors is occupied. For example, maximal stimulation of steroidogenesis by Leydig cells occurs when only about 1% of LH receptors are occupied. The additional receptors are referred to as spare receptors and are considered to be fully functional. The role of this receptor reserve may be to increase the sensitivity of target cells to activation by low levels of hormone. It is recognized, however, that the term spare is used in a relative sense as the degree of receptor excess differs according to the particular biological response measured. Generally the magnitude of the adenylate cyclase activation is closely correlated with the degree of receptor occupancy, but the more distal physiological response, such as muscle contraction or hormone secretion, is evoked when only a small percentage of the receptor population is occupied [8].

Receptor Signal Transduction

Hormone binding to receptors located on the outer side of the plasmalemma results in an immediate activation of adenylate cyclase on the inner membrane of the cells. How does receptor occupation by hormonal ligands result in enzyme activation on the opposite side of the cell membrane? Receptor and enzyme were once thought to be structurally coupled, and binding of the hormone to the receptor then induced a conformational change in the enzyme, thus activating it. This hypothesis is no longer

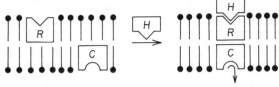

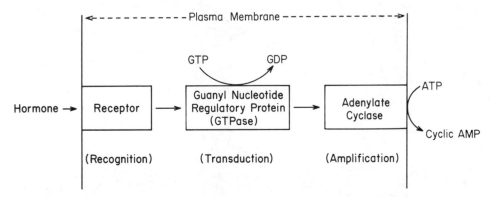

Cyclic Nucleotide Production

Figure 4.1 Mobile receptor model of peptide hormone action.

supported by most investigations; instead, the receptor unit may be "freely floating" in the membrane and in the unoccupied state may possess negligible affinity for the enzymatic unit [21]. Upon hormone binding, however, a conformational change occurs in the receptor thus establishing recognition sites for the enzyme; this may allow binding of the activated receptor to the enzyme to form an active complex (Fig. 4.1). This two-step mobile receptor model of hormone-receptor interaction with adenylate cyclase is sufficiently versatile to account for many if not all of the known events concerning hormone action at the membrane level [18, 20].

Convincing evidence accumulated from a variety of experimental methods also reveals that, indeed, hormone receptors are discrete units, not components of the inner membrane nucleotide cyclyzing enzymes. Fusion of cells, which lack receptors but possess adenylate cyclase activity, to a different species of cell, which possesses receptors but no adenylate cyclase activity, results in a hybrid cell which synthesizes cyclic AMP in response to hormone stimulation [35, 37]. Other evidence suggests that hormone receptors and adenylate cyclase are products of separate genes. The products of two separate genes would not be expected to result in the formation of a single protein.

Transduction of signal from receptor to adenylate and guanylate cyclases in some cells appears to involve the participation of monovalent and divalent cations as well as prostaglandin biosynthesis. In addition one or more regulatory proteins may be

Figure 4.2 Role of guanyl nucleotide regulatory protein (GTPase) in hormone-receptor signal transduction. In this model hormone occupancy of the receptor promotes association of the receptor moiety with the regulatory protein, which permits GTP to bind to the regulatory unit. The activated regulatory protein then dissociates from the receptor and interacts with the catalytic unit (adenylate cyclase) which is now able to convert ATP to cyclic AMP. Hydrolysis of GTP to ADP allows the regulatory unit to dissociate from the catalytic unit which becomes inactive [39].

components of the transduction signal [17]. One such regulatory protein may be an enzyme which exhibits GTPase activity (converts guanosine triphosphate to guanosine diphosphate) in the activated state (Fig. 4.2). Receptor signal transduction may, therefore, involve the mobilization and interaction of this protein with the mobile hormone receptor, an event which would then be requisite to adenylate cyclase activation [34, 39].

Cyclic Nucleotides and Hormone Action

Receptors provide the recognition site for hormone-cell interaction. This binding event must be translated into a cellular response. Most of the specific details are not known, but some data and hypotheses are available. Binding of hormone to its membrane receptor often results in the activation of one or more nucleotide-cyclyzing enzymes located on the inner surface of the membrane. Best studied is the enzyme adenylate cyclase which, upon stimulation by a chemical messenger, converts ATP (adenosine triphosphate) to 3',5'-cyclic adenosine monophosphate, cyclic AMP (cAMP). Some hormones, on the other hand, activate guanylate cyclase which converts guanosine triphosphate (GTP) to cyclic GMP (cGMP). Enzyme cleavage of the cyclic ring of the nucleotides by *phosphodiesterase* results in the production of inactive 5'AMP or 5'GMP which appears to be without subsequent significance to hormone action (Fig. 4.3).

Each of the cyclic nucleotides produced intracellularly combines with a specific *cyclic nucleotide-dependent protein kinase*. Cyclic AMP-dependent protein kinase, for example, is composed of two components, a *regulatory subunit* and a *catalytic*

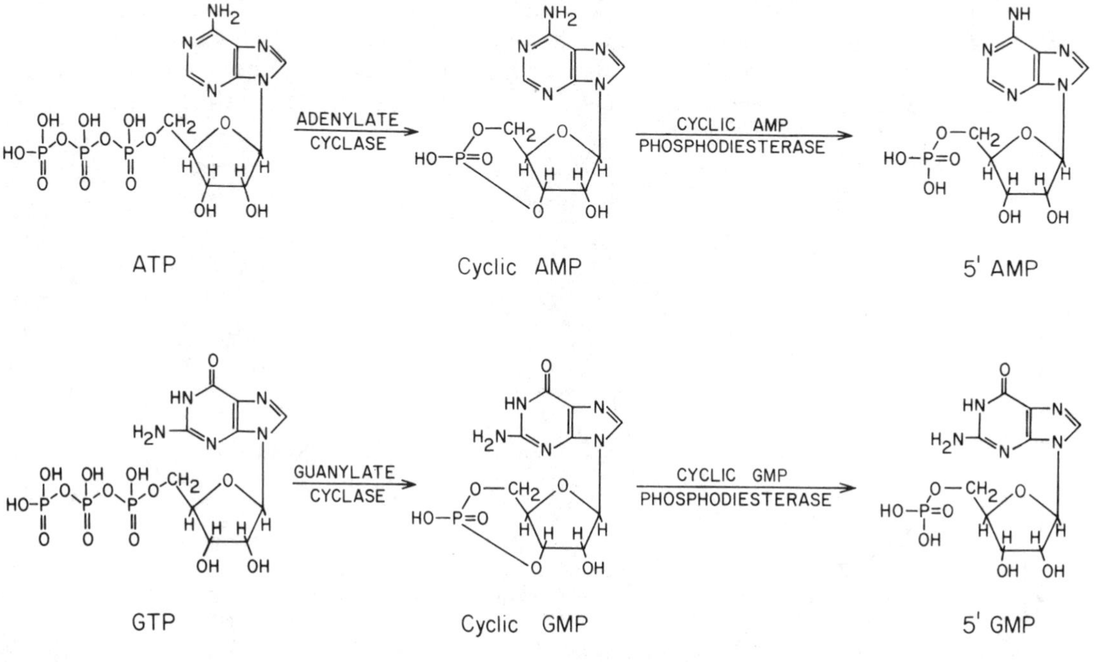

Figure 4.3 Cyclic nucleotide synthesis and inactivation.

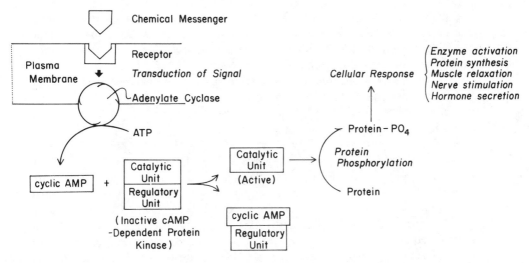

Figure 4.4 Cyclic AMP production and action.

subunit. Interaction of cAMP with the regulatory subunit results in the release of the catalytic unit (Fig. 4.4). The catalytic unit is now free to function as a *kinase*, that is, a phosphorylating enzyme. Cyclic nucleotides therefore function by causing phosphorylation of some cellular component (substrate protein) of the cell (Fig. 4.5), structural or enzymatic [29]. Enzyme phosphorylation leads to a cascade phenomenon whereby activation by phosphorylation of the first enzyme allows this enzyme to act as a kinase to phosphorylate a second enzyme, which may then phosphorylate another enzyme. At each step amplification occurs; thus a relatively few first messenger molecules acting on a limited number of receptors may produce a response several orders of magnitude greater. This cascade phenomenon has been studied in detail in the liver cell (Fig. 11.10), but may be common to a number of cellular systems.

Cyclic nucleotides produced by hormone action are rapidly metabolized. Cyclic AMP- and cGMP-specific phosphodiesterases cleave the cyclic bonds within cAMP

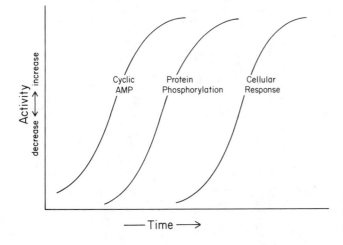

Figure 4.5 Temporal cellular events in hormone-mediated cyclic AMP production and action.

and cGMP to produce inactive 5'AMP and 5'GMP, respectively. *Phosphoprotein phosphatases* within the cell then dephosphorylate the proteins that were phosphorylated by the cyclic nucleotide-dependent protein kinases. Thus cellular activity is rapidly returned to basal level.

Sutherland was the first to demonstrate that extracellular chemical messengers, first messengers, activate production of intracellular cAMP, the so-called second messenger of hormone action [40]. This first messenger-second messenger hypothesis of hormone action must consider the role of another intracellular chemical messenger, cGMP [12], and possibly other cyclic nucleotides (e.g., cyclic uridine monophosphate, cUMP, and cyclic cytidine monophosphate, cCMP). In many tissues cyclic nucleotides function in contrasting roles, as in muscle contraction and relaxation (Fig. 4.6). As the concentration of one nucleotide goes up or down, the concentration of the other nucleotide is often, but not invariably, affected inversely. However, the exact events are as yet ill defined. The contrasting roles of the cAMP and cGMP have been formulated into the *yin yang* concept of hormone action [11]. This hypothesis is particularly applicable to tissues where cells can display a bimodal response, for example, to contract or to relax. Cyclic GMP is clearly correlated with smooth muscle contraction, whereas smooth muscle relaxation is correlated with cAMP elevation (Fig. 14.10). In excitable tissue, such as muscle or nerve, depolarization is correlated with cGMP formation, whereas increased cAMP is correlated with hyperpolarization. How or whether the two events are coupled is not clear.

Methylxanthines inhibit cAMP- and cGMP-dependent phosphodiesterase activity. Caffeine, theophylline, and theobromine are methylxanthines derived from coffee, tea, and cocoa, respectively (Fig. 4.7). Theophylline is the most potent of the three (but is less concentrated in tea than caffeine is in coffee). In the presence of relatively low concentrations of methylxanthines, effects of hormones that stimulate

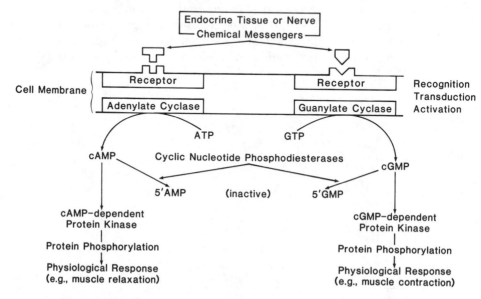

Figure 4.6 Cyclic AMP and cyclic GMP production and mechanisms of action.

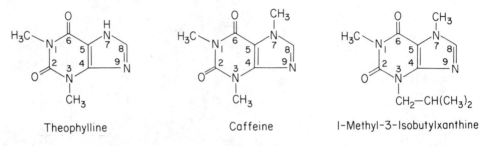

Figure 4.7 Methylxanthine structures: theophylline, caffeine, and 1-methyl-3-isobutylxanthine (a synthetic xanthine analog).

adenylate cyclase are potentiated as the cAMP generated by the hormones is not degraded by phosphodiesterase. At high concentrations (e.g., 10^{-3} M) theophylline or caffeine alone may evoke a maximal response in a particular tissue. This suggests that adenylate cyclase is always active, but that the cAMP generated is continually being destroyed.

Because many hormones interact with receptors to activate adenylate cyclase which then causes a physiological response, Sutherland [40] and his colleagues suggested criteria which should be satisfied before concluding that a particular effect of a hormone is mediated through cAMP. (1) The hormone should stimulate adenylate cyclase in broken cell preparations. (2) Physiological levels of the hormone should elevate cAMP before or concurrently with the physiological response. (3) There should be a correlation between the activity of hormone analogs that elevate cAMP and their ability to activate the particular cellular response. (4) Methylxanthines or other drugs which inhibit phosphodiesterase activity should potentiate and, at high concentrations, mimic the hormone response. (5) Exogenous cAMP or its analogs should mimic the effect of the hormone.

The criteria have been satisfied for many cells studied. There is no convincing reason, however, that the first criterion should be met as, in the intact cell, information is generated from the receptor on the outer side of the plasmalemma to adenylate cyclase on the inner surface. The ionic environments of these two compartments are not similar and cannot be duplicated in vitro for both compartments at any one time. Calcium, for example, is inhibitory to adenylate cyclase but may be necessary for transduction of signal from receptor to cyclase. It is difficult in vitro to provide Ca^{2+} for receptor binding or receptor signal transduction and at the same time not inhibit adenylate cyclase. The second criterion has been claimed not to have been satisfied in some systems. It is possible, however, that small changes in cAMP are undetectable or that in some tissues the increase in cAMP is compartmentalized to a few cells. Thus changes in cyclic nucleotide levels are not perceived among the larger cyclic nucleotide pool. The third and fourth criteria have generally been demonstrated in all cellular systems where cAMP plays a role as second messenger.

Cyclic AMP added to an in vitro preparation may induce the physiological response characteristic of the tissue but only at very high concentrations. This is apparently because the nucleotide does not easily enter cells through the plasmalemma. To satisfy the fifth criterion, certain lipophilic analogs of cAMP (e.g., dibutyryl

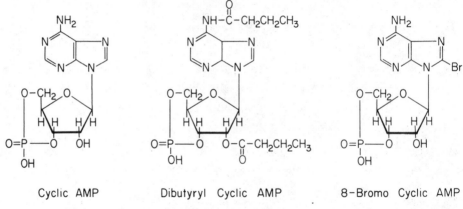

Figure 4.8 Cyclic AMP and related analogs.

cAMP) have been synthesized; they may produce a maximal response at relatively low concentrations in some tissues but only at higher levels in others (Fig. 4.8).

Separate Receptors for Hormone Action

The hormones epinephrine and glucagon stimulate glycogenolysis and the release of glucose by liver cells. Because glucagon and epinephrine are not similar in structure, they could not be expected to mediate their effects through the same receptor, although they both activate hepatic adenylate cyclase activity. This can be demonstrated by the use of antagonists which are specific for a receptor. Propranolol, a β-adrenergic receptor blocking agent, antagonizes epinephrine-induced liver glycogenolysis but not the glycogenolytic action of glucagon (Chapter 14). The action of glucagon, but not epinephrine, on the other hand, is blocked by specific antagonists of glucagon. Present evidence indicates that hormones which have similar actions do not stimulate separate cyclases. Maximal production of cAMP produced by one hormone generally is not augmented by the addition of another hormone. If individual cyclases were linked to each receptor, it would be expected that the maximal effects of each hormone would be additive (Fig. 4.9). Cholecystokinin, acetylcholine, and oxymetazoline (an α-adrenergic receptor agonist) stimulate guanylate cyclase activity in rabbit gall-bladder smooth muscle which leads to cGMP production. The action of acetylcholine or oxymetazoline is blocked by antagonists of their receptors, atropine or phentola-mine, respectively. These receptor blocking agents do not affect the stimulation of guanylate cyclase by CCK. The effects of the three agonists on cGMP production are also not additive [1]. These observations suggest that gallbladder smooth muscle cells possess more than one receptor type and each is sensitive to a specific agonist ligand. Nevertheless the action of the individual agonists is funneled through a single guanylate cyclase.

One might wonder why one cell, such as the hepatocyte (liver cell), possesses two separate receptors that activate the same ultimate physiological response. The reason may be that different hormones, such as glucagon and epinephrine, are released under different physiological states of an animal. Glucagon released from the pancreatic

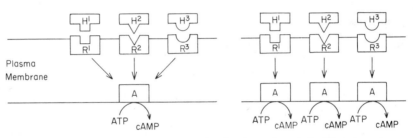

A. NON-ADDITIVE   B. ADDITIVE

Figure 4.9 Although many hormones (H^1, H^2, H^3) mediate their effects through separate membrane receptors, transduction of their signals is funneled through only one adenylate cyclase (A), *not* through different cyclases linked separately to each receptor (B).

islets regulates the moment-by-moment breakdown of liver glycogen whenever blood glucose levels become slightly depressed. Under conditions of stress, however, epinephrine is released from the adrenal chromaffin tissue. This hormone not only stimulates hepatic glycogen breakdown into glucose, but also increases vascular blood flow, respiratory rate, and many physiological processes that are associated with the stress response. Continuous stress would, over time, be detrimental to the welfare of the individual (Chapters 14 and 15).

KALLIKREIN-KININ SYSTEMS

Kallikreins are proteolytic enzymes present in the plasma or localized within specific tissues. These serine proteases act on substrate proteins, *kininogens*, to convert them to smaller biologically active peptide hormones. Kallikreins are derived from pro-enzymes referred to as *prekallikreins*. Prekallikreins become activated by hormones and possibly other stimuli (e.g., oxygen tension, pH). Thus a hormone may interact with a tissue to activate a prekallikrein, which will result in a tissue-specific activation of an enzyme. The kallikrein may then act on a circulating plasma protein substrate, a *kininogen*, to generate production of a local hormone, referred to as a *kinin*. The actions of the kinin might be expected to be limited to the tissues of their origin. An important local role of glandular kinins may be to regulate the local flow of blood by causing a vascular hyperemia. The effects of the kinins are subsequently abolished by proteolytic enzymes known as *kininases* which split the kinins into smaller, inactive fragments (Fig. 4.10). Bradykinin is an example of a kinin produced within the kidney in response to prekallikrein activation by the adrenal steroid hormone, aldosterone (Fig. 15.16). Bradykinin plays an important role in the control of vascular blood flow within the kidney (Chapter 15).

PROSTAGLANDINS AND HORMONE ACTION

In the early 1930s, it was noted that human semen and extracts of seminal vesicles from animals caused uterine tissue to contract or relax. The purified substance was given the

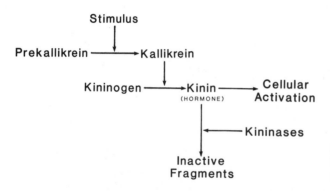

Figure 4.10 General outline for kallikrein activation and kinin production.

name *prostaglandin*, although it is now realized that the prostate glands are not a major source of prostaglandins. The prostaglandins are a family of chemically related substances that are produced by cells in response to a variety of extrinsic stimuli. They may be produced by cells in response to some hormones and can, therefore, be considered as intracellular second messengers in the actions of these hormones. The Nobel Prize in Physiology or Medicine for 1982 was awarded to Bergstrom, Samuelsson, and Vane for their "discoveries concerning prostaglandins and biologically related substances" [30, 31].

Prostaglandins are produced exclusively within the plasma membrane of cells and are derived mainly from arachidonic acid which is released from phospholipids by the action of phospholipases [31]. Arachidonic acid is formed from the essential fatty acid, linolenic acid, by elongation and desaturation. Hormones and other stimuli (e.g., local hypoxia) may activate phospholipase activity and liberate arachidonic acid to serve as substrate for prostaglandin biosynthesis. The arachidonic acid may be utilized in one or more different pathways depending on the tissue concerned and particular nature of the extrinsic stimulus. In one pathway arachidonic acid is converted to unstable endoperoxide intermediates by a group of enzymes termed the cyclooxygenase system (Fig. 4.11). Then, depending on the action of other tissue-specific enzymes, these intermediates may be converted to one of a number of related products: prostaglandin E_2 (PGE$_2$), prostaglandin $F_{2\alpha}$ (PGF$_{2\alpha}$), prostacyclin I_2 (PGI$_2$), or thromboxane (TXA$_2$). In some cells arachidonic acid metabolism follows a second pathway to produce a group of biologically active leukotrienes (Fig. 4.11).

Leukotrienes are formed by the enzyme 5-lipoxygenase which converts arachidonic acid to 5-hydroperoxy-6,8,11,14-eicosatetraenoic acid (5-HPETE). 5-HPETE is then converted to the epoxy acid, LTA$_4$, which is subsequently changed to LTB$_4$ by the addition of water, or to LTC$_4$ by the addition of glutathione. LTD$_4$ is then formed by the loss of glutamic acid and LTD$_4$ is converted to LTE$_4$ by the loss of the glycine residue (Fig. 4.11).

Each of these definitive products of arachidonic acid metabolism may then act on nucleotide cyclases within the plasma membrane to stimulate cyclic nucleotide formation. PGE$_2$ and PGI$_2$ invariably stimulate adenylate cyclase, whereas TXA$_2$ and PGF$_{2\alpha}$ activate guanylate cyclase. The actions of the leukotrienes appear to be also mediated through activation of guanylate cyclase. The cyclic nucleotides formed, cAMP and cGMP, respectively, then act within the cells to continue the cascade of events that follow the initial action of the first messenger. The actions of prosta-

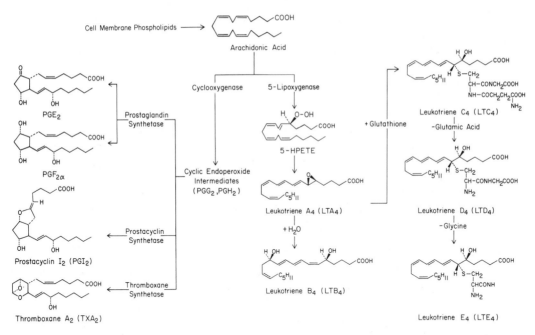

Figure 4.11 General scheme for prostaglandin, prostacyclin, thromboxane, and leukotriene biosynthesis.

glandins and thromboxanes may be confined within the cell membrane where they are synthesized. Leukotrienes and prostacyclins, on the other hand, are released from their cells of origin to act as humoral hormonal messengers. Nevertheless all the known actions of these biologically active derivatives of arachidonic acid are mediated via activation of membrane nucleotide cyclases (Fig. 4.12).

Aspirin and indomethacin inhibit cyclooxygenase activity, but not that of the

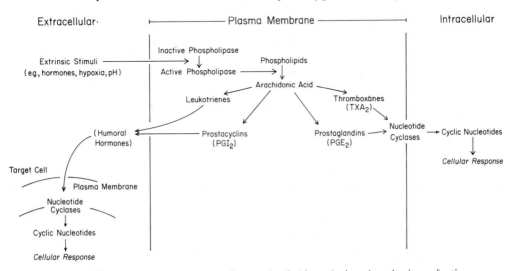

Figure 4.12 General scheme of prostaglandin biosynthesis and mechanisms of action.

Prostaglandins and Hormone Action

lipoxygenase system. Therefore these drugs may be used selectively to inhibit prostaglandin, prostacyclin, and thromboxane formation without a concomitant effect on leukotriene formation.

Prostaglandins

Prostaglandins were the first of the arachidonic acid products to be discovered. All the prostaglandins are variants of a basic 20-carbon carboxylic fatty acid (prostanoic acid) which is bent back on itself in the shape of a hairpin and is conformationally restricted by a five-membered cyclopentane ring. The number of double bonds present within the side chains determines whether the prostaglandin belongs to the 1, 2, or 3 series. Two particularly important prostaglandins of the E and F series are $PGF_{2\alpha}$ and PGE_2, which differ by the presence of a hydroxyl or a keto-group, respectively, at carbon 9 within the cyclopentane ring (Figs. 2.4 and 4.11).

A major physiological role of PGE_2 and $PGF_{2\alpha}$ is the control of vascular smooth muscle activity. Hormones that regulate smooth muscle relaxation or contraction stimulate the production of PGE_2 and PGI_2 or $PGF_{2\alpha}$, respectively (Fig. 14.10). In response to tissue hypoxia PGE_2 production may lead to a localized hyperemia in skeletal muscle. Thus prostaglandins, by their localized actions on the microcirculation, adjust local blood flow in response to changing metabolic requirements of the tissue [27].

Prostacyclins

Prostacyclins (PGI_2) are produced by the blood vessel wall, and PGI_2 is the most potent natural inhibitor known of blood platelet aggregation. PGI_2 binds to a specific platelet receptor and activates adenylate cyclase. Increased intracellular levels of cyclic AMP are then inhibitory to platelet aggregation. The vascular endothelium can therefore be considered as an endocrine tissue which produces a humoral hormone, PGI_2, whose role may be to prevent blood platelet aggregation and to maintain vascular flow through its action as a local vasodilator. Whether PGI_2 is released into the general circulation to function as a hormone on more distant blood platelets and vascular endothelia is presently unresolved.

It is hoped that selective inhibitors of thromboxane synthesis will be developed so that the tendency toward platelet aggregation is reduced while permitting normal rates of formation of the other prostaglandins.

Thromboxanes

Thromboxane A_2 is a specific product of the blood platelet. In response to stimuli known to induce clotting (collagen substrate, thrombin, epinephrine), platelet TXA_2 levels are elevated as are cGMP concentrations. It is believed that TXA_2 may act in some way as a Ca^{2+} ionophore to translocate this divalent Ca^{2+} from the extracellular environment or from sequestered intracellular organelles. The free cytosolic Ca^{2+} may then be responsible for inducing the cellular shape changes associated with the platelet aggregation phenomenon. As noted, PGI_2 is inhibitory to platelet aggregation through its action on increasing platelet cAMP levels. Inhibition of platelet aggregation may result from protein substrate phosphorylation and the subsequent uptake of Ca^{2+} into vesicular components of the cell.

Leukotrienes

Leukotrienes are so named because they are made by leukocytes and contain three conjugated double bonds. The subscript indicates the total number of double bonds in the molecule (Fig. 4.11). Leukotrienes are extremely potent in causing vascular contraction and inducing vascular permeability. Migratory leukocytes function in local inflammatory responses by releasing leukotrienes at the site of injury in response to noxious stimuli. The antiinflammatory actions of glucocorticoids (Chapter 15) may be because these steroids inhibit phospholipase activity and therefore restrict the availability of arachidonic acid for leukotriene formation. Certain leukocytes may be considered as wandering endocrine cells that release chemical messengers, leukotrienes, at sites of injury or invasion by foreign proteins to induce inflammatory or allergic responses, respectively.

CYTOSOLIC HORMONE RECEPTORS

In contrast to many polypeptide hormones, steroid and thyroid hormones initiate their actions by combining with intracellular receptors. The mechanisms by which these hormones cross the plasmalemma are unknown. It is likely that these hormones enter all cells but only manifest their action in those which possess receptors. Steroid hormones, for example, bind to specific cytoplasmic receptors of a proteinaceous nature, and the steroid-receptor complex then migrates to the nucleus where it interacts with specific chromosomal proteins [32, 36]. The binding of the receptor-steroid complex to chromatin results in derepression of a specific DNA sequence and increased messenger RNA synthesis (Fig. 4.13). The mRNA then codes for proteins specific to that cell type; in uterine muscle (myometrium), for example, estradiol induces the synthesis of actin and myosin, proteins necessary for the contractile machinery of the uterine myometrial cells.

Each steroid hormone has its own specific cytoplasmic receptor. Estrogens, but not androgens, bind to uterine cytoplasmic receptors. Thus, as for membrane receptors, receptor specificity determines whether a particular cell type will respond to the steroid. The synthesis of mRNA and the subsequent production of proteins require a matter of hours or days to be fully manifested (Chapter 18). The actions of most hormones are on membrane receptors and, in contrast, result in an immediate production of cyclic nucleotides followed by rapid protein phosphorylation and a subsequent cellular response.

Thyroid hormones also enter cells to initiate their actions by interacting with proteinaceous receptors which exist both free within the cytoplasm and as components of nuclear chromatin [2]. Like steroid hormones, thyroid hormones act on the genome to induce mRNA synthesis and subsequent protein synthesis (Fig. 13.10). Again the specific genes derepressed and the specific mRNA's and proteins synthesized depend

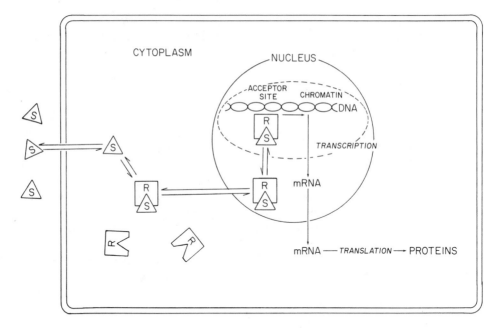

Figure 4.13 Mechanisms of steroid hormone action.

on the particular cell type that is stimulated. Thyroid hormones may affect other cellular mechanisms in addition to their action at the level of the nucleus (Chapter 13).

PERMISSIVE ACTION OF HORMONES

A number of hormones are said to exert a permissive action, that is, they must be present for other hormones to exert their effects. Because the majority of peptide hormones stimulate cells through activation of cAMP, one would not expect that the action of one peptide hormone could enhance the action of another peptide hormone other than in an additive manner. Rather it might be expected that for one hormone to potentiate the activity of another, the mechanisms of action of the two hormones would be different. The permissive effects of hormones are restricted mainly to the actions of steroid or thyroid hormones where the ligands enhance the action of each other or they enhance the action of other hormones working through membrane receptors. The following mechanisms, among others, could account for the permissive actions of steroid or thyroid hormones: (1) These hormones through their actions on specific mRNA synthesis could cause an increase in the number of membrane receptors, which might increase the production of cyclic nucleotides thus leading to an increased cellular response to hormones acting on the plasmalemma; (2) thyroid or steroid hormones could increase or decrease the amount of cyclic nucleotide-dependent protein kinases or the amount of substrate available for phosphorylation by cAMP- or cGMP-dependent protein kinases; (3) thyroid and steroid hormones could enhance the synthesis of a protein which could act as an inhibitor of another protein (e.g., phosphoprotein phosphatase) whose action is antagonistic to cyclic nucleotide action (Fig. 4.14).

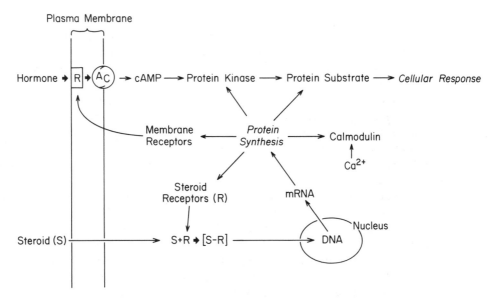

Figure 4.14   General scheme for the permissive actions of steroid hormones.

Synergism is a term often used to describe the physiological response of a tissue to a combination of two hormones that greatly exceeds the individual actions of either hormone. For example, FSH has no detectable effect on enzyme activity of testicular interstitial tissue and LH only minimally stimulates such activity. However, in the presence of FSH, the actions of LH are greatly enhanced (Fig. 17.5). This might be caused by an FSH-induced increase in LH receptors which is known to occur in other steroid-synthesizing tissue in response to these two gonadotropins. Methylxanthines, when used at low concentrations, may only slightly increase the basal activity of cells. Used at a low concentration, a hormone might also have a minimal effect. When used in combination, however, a hormone and a methylxanthine may produce a dramatic response. The action of the hormone is to increase cyclic nucleotide levels, whereas the action of the methylxanthine is to inhibit degradation of cAMP by phosphodiesterase.

In summary the action of one hormone may require the action of one or more other hormones that individually are relatively inactive, a phenomenon referred to as the permissive action of hormones. Synergism, on the other hand, is the enhanced response of a tissue to two or more hormones in combination which is greater in magnitude than the sum of the individual actions of the hormones. The permissive and synergistic actions of a hormone may not easily be separated into distinct physiological entities.

STIMULUS RESPONSE COUPLING

Most membrane-mediated hormone actions involve changes in the transmembrane potential. Because of the unequal distribution of ions between the extracellular and intracellular environments of a cell, a cell is generally 60 to 90 mv (millivolts) negative on the inside. The unequal charge distribution causes the cell to be electrically excitable. Muscle and nerve cells are particularly excitable as are some secretory cells. The excitability of certain cells is of pivotal importance in hormonal control of cellular function. In response to hormonal stimuli, cells may become *depolarized* or *hyperpolarized*. Acetylcholine, for example, depolarizes skeletal muscle cells which leads to contraction. Interaction of acetylcholine with membrane receptors causes Na^+ ion flow into the cell, thus depolarizing the muscle. Sodium ion flux into the cell is linked to an increase in cytosolic calcium; the Ca^{2+} ion interacts with the contractile proteins of the muscle and contraction ensues. This event is referred to as *stimulus-contraction coupling*. A similar *stimulus-secretion coupling* is responsible for hormone-induced cellular secretion. These phenomena are collectively termed *stimulus-response coupling*.

Substitution of Na^+ by other monovalent cations, such as Li^+ (lithium), provides information on the specificity of the cation requirement for hormone action. Magnesium (Mg^{2+}) or barium (Ba^{2+}) ions are often substituted for Ca^{2+} to determine the divalent cation specificity for hormone action. Although Ca^{2+} is of prime importance to stimulus-response coupling, this ion undoubtedly plays other more subtle roles in cellular responses to hormones. Calcium is inhibitory to adenylate cyclase activity and also appears to be stimulatory to cyclic nucleotide phosphodiesterase activity. The role of Ca^{2+} in relationship to these enzyme activities in hormone action will be clarified in time. Calcium is also required in some cellular systems for coupling between hormone receptors and nucleotide cyclase activity. Melanocyte stimulating hormone (MSH) action, for example, requires Ca^{2+} for activation of adenylate cyclase; this is a receptor-specific requirement as prostaglandin and epinephrine stimulation of melanocyte adenylate cyclase is without such a requirement [42]. In a number of cellular systems Ca^{2+} may also be specifically required for hormone activation of guanylate cyclase [14].

CALMODULIN—AN INTRACELLULAR CALCIUM RECEPTOR

Calcium, a divalent cation, is required for the actions of many hormones. Calcium may be essential for hormone activation of phospholipase A_2 and thus prostaglandin biosynthesis. Calcium may be directly required for transduction of signal between hormone receptor and adenylate or guanylate cyclase. Hormones may translocate Ca^{2+} into the cytosol to function in such processes as enzyme activation or cellular contraction. However, the precise mechanism of action of Ca^{2+} was for a long time an enigma. Ca^{2+} is now known to interact with its own cellular receptor, a protein referred to as *calmodulin*, or calcium-dependent regulatory protein (CDR). This ubiquitous protein is found in all eukaryotic cells and therefore in plants [5].

Calmodulin exists as a monomer of 148 amino acid residues. The primary sequence of CDR has been stringently conserved throughout phylogeny; for example, there are only seven conservative amino acid substitutions between vertebrate CDR's and that of a marine coelenterate. A distinctive feature of the protein is that the amino group of lysine 115 is posttranscriptionally trimethylated. Calmodulin possesses four Ca^{2+}-binding sites and the amino acid sequences within each domain contain a high degree of homology (Fig. 4.15). It is suggested that CDR may have evolved from a

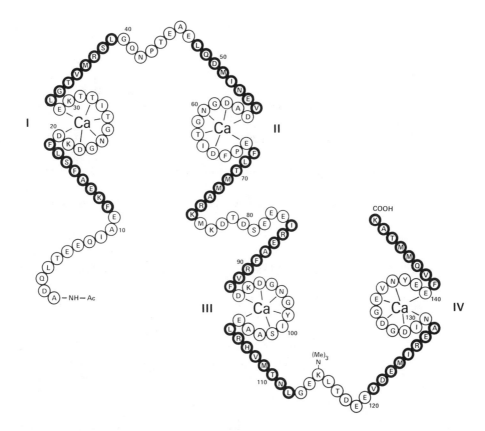

Figure 4.15 Primary structure of calmodulin, an intracellular calcium receptor. The following are one-letter codes for amino acid residues: A, Ala; D, Asp; E, Glu; F, Phe; G, Gly; H, His; I, Ile; K, Lys; L, Leu; M, Met; N, Asn; P, Pro; Q, Gln; R. Arg; S, Ser; T, Thr; V, Val; Y, Tyr. (Reproduced with permission, from *The Annual Review of Biochemistry*, Klee, et al., "Calmodulin". Vol. 49, pp. 480–515. © 1980 by Annual Reviews Inc.)

smaller precursor (which bound a single Ca^{2+}) by gene duplication [28]. The homology is greatest between domains 1 and 3 and 2 and 4, and it is possible that CDR may have arisen by two successive doublings of a primordial gene coding for a Ca^{2+}-binding domain [25]. Calmodulin is structurally related to troponin C found in skeletal and cardiac muscle.

The binding of Ca^{2+} to CDR results in a conformational change of the protein which may be required for the interaction of CDR with its substrate. Indeed each sequential interaction of Ca^{2+} with the four CDR Ca^{2+}-binding sites may confer a different conformational change in the protein. These variable conformations may provide a mechanism for multiple substrate specificities within a single cell.

Three major roles of CDR are regulation of intracellular Ca^{2+} levels, enzyme activation, and control of the activity of cellular filamentous organelles. The actions of CDR are direct and indirect; for example, CDR may activate an enzyme directly or indirectly through prior activation of another enzyme. A number of peptide and steroid hormones have been shown to be without effect on cellular levels of CDR;

levels of the Ca^{2+} regulatory protein hormone apparently remain constant regardless of the hormonal environment [28].

As an intracellular Ca^{2+} receptor CDR may play a pivotal role in cellular Ca^{2+} homeostasis [7]. The levels of Ca^{2+} within cells fluctuate due to fluxes of Ca^{2+} across the plasma membrane from or into storage depots within mitochondria and smooth endoplasmic reticulum, each of these pathways being of more or less importance depending on the cell type. In each case CDR stimulates a Ca^{2+}-Mg-dependent ATPase (Ca^{2+} pump) in the membranes of these organelles. In the presence of excessive cytosolic Ca^{2+}, CDR would become activated and would subsequently stimulate one or more of these membrane Ca^{2+} pumps which would bring Ca^{2+} levels back to normal.

Calmodulin may play an important role in the control of cyclic nucleotide levels. Calmodulin is stimulatory to adenylate cyclase and phosphodiesterase. Although these two actions of CDR may first appear to be opposed, the sensitivities of the two enzymes to CDR may differ considerably. In fact cAMP increases the affinity of phosphodiesterase for CDR, which may provide a cellular homeostatic mechanism, involving an initial activation of cAMP production, followed by a mechanism for the degradation of the cyclic nucleotide. In addition to a role for a cytosolic CDR in the control of adenylate cyclase activity, CDR may function by a Ca^{2+}-dependent mechanism in the transduction of signal between receptor and adenylate cyclase. Thus CDR can be envisioned to function at a number of sites in the control of cAMP levels. The possible relationship of CDR to the control of cellular cGMP levels is presently unclear. Activation of phosphodiesterase would, however, result in the degradation of cGMP (although the rates of such degradation may not be identical), which might provide a mechanism for the control of the relative levels of the two cyclic nucleotides. This may be of crucial importance to the function of a particular cyclic nucleotide.

Calmodulin regulates a variety of cellular contractile or motile processes. Actin and myosin are the major proteins responsible for cell motility, and they are present in both muscle and nonmuscle cells. Calcium is required for muscle contraction, and in smooth muscle it is now known that Ca^{2+} activates CDR which then binds to a regulatory subunit of an enzyme, myosin light chain kinase, whose catalytic domain phosphorylates the light chain protein of myosin. Activation of myosin ATPase provides the stimulus for formation of the actomyosin complex leading to the contractile process. In skeletal muscle an elevation of cytosolic Ca^{2+} is the stimulus to the contractile process resulting from actin and myosin interaction. Binding of Ca^{2+} to troponin C (which is structurally related to CDR) results in a conformational change in the troponin-tropomyosin-actin complex, which causes actomyosin formation.

Microtubules are filamentous components of cells and are involved in cellular activities involving motile processes, such as chromosome movement, axoplasmic flow, and neurite extension. Most interesting is the apparent role of calmodulin in chromosomal movement during mitosis. There is a major shift of calmodulin from a diffuse distribution within the cell during interphase to high local concentrations within the mitotic apparatus during mitosis. In this process CDR may perform such roles as regulating the concentration of Ca^{2+} in the microenvironment and thus affect microtubular assembly/disassembly. In addition CDR may activate other proteins or enzymes that may be involved in the mitotic machinery [28].

In skeletal muscle calmodulin regulates the activity of the enzyme phosphorylase kinase, which causes glycogen degradation to provide the glucose substrate necessary for mitochondrial ATP production. Calmodulin is an integral regulatory subunit of phosphorylase as the enzyme is completely dependent on Ca^{2+} for activity [25]. Phosphorylase kinase is composed of four different subunits, α, β, γ, and δ, and the δ subunit is calmodulin. In liver, skeletal, and cardiac muscle phosphorylase kinase plays a dual role in the control of glycogen metabolism. It activates the enzyme phosphorylase, which splits glycogen into its glucose subunits, and it may function as glycogen synthetase kinase, an enzyme that inactivates glycogen synthetase through phosphorylation of the enzyme.

PHOSPHORYLATED PROTEINS AS PHYSIOLOGICAL EFFECTORS

The membrane actions of most hormones involve generation of an intracellular cyclic nucleotide as second messenger. The immediate acceptor site for the action of cyclic AMP is the regulatory subunit of cyclic AMP-dependent protein kinase. Two forms of the enzyme with slightly different regulatory properties have been isolated and are referred to as type I and type II. Both consist of two regulatory (R) and two catalytic (C) subunits. The regulatory units may differ in structure, but the catalytic units are believed to be identical. Cyclic AMP acts as the positive effector and causes the dissociation of the oligomeric protein and an activation of the enzyme according to the following scheme:

$$R_2C_2 \text{ (inactive)} + 4 \text{ cyclic AMP} \rightleftharpoons (R\text{-cyclic AMP}_2)_2 + 2 \text{ C (active)}$$

The complete amino acid sequences of the catalytic and regulatory subunits of bovine cardiac muscle cyclic AMP-dependent protein kinase have been elucidated [38, 41].

Within each cell type one or more specific proteins act as substrate for phosphorylation by cyclic AMP-dependent protein kinase. For example the amino acid serine is a substrate for protein kinase action (Fig. 4.16). Little is known of the particular protein substrates of hormone target tissues. Specific nuclear histone proteins may be the targets of the enzyme within hepatocytes. Within smooth muscle and nerve, specific membrane proteins become phosphorylated through the actions of cyclic AMP or cyclic GMP. In neurons these substrate proteins may control the permeability of the postsynaptic membrane to ion flux [16]. In smooth muscle,

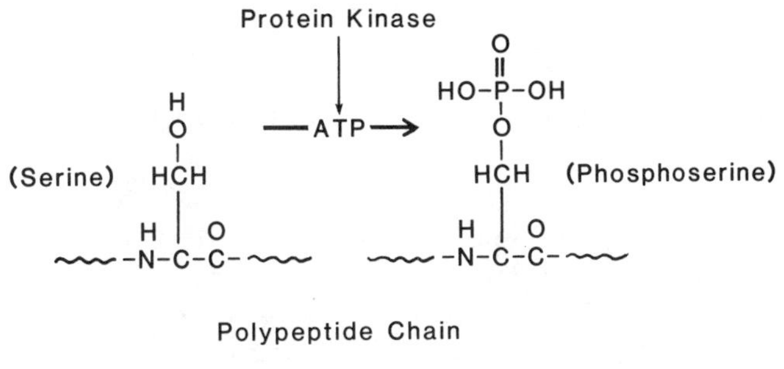

Figure 4.16   Protein kinase phosphorylation of a protein substrate.

phosphorylation of specific membrane substrate proteins in response to cyclic AMP or cyclic GMP generated by receptor-specific agonists may be related to the phenomena of membrane hyperpolarization and depolarization that accompany smooth muscle relaxation and contraction, respectively.

Cyclic nucleotide-independent substrate phosphorylation may be important in the actions of certain hormones (insulin and other growth factors). The intracellular effector molecules that activate the kinases involved in these substrate phosphorylations remain undetermined. The calcium ion may be shown to be a major stimulus to cyclic nucleotide-independent substrate phosphorylation. Through its interaction with calmodulin, skeletal muscle phosphorylase and myosin light chain kinase are activated by the divalent cation. Within neurons a Ca^{2+}-calmodulin-dependent kinase may regulate neurotransmitter release by phosphorylation of synaptic membrane proteins[6]. Even in plants there is evidence that a Ca^{2+}-calmodulin system may activate an NAD (niacin adenine dinucleotide) kinase.

TERMINATION OF HORMONE ACTION

Hormones that act at the plasmalemma are degraded within the blood by serum enzymes. The declining circulating level of a hormone would result in a decrease in further stimulation of membrane adenylate or guanylate cyclase activities. In the absence of cyclic nucleotide production the residual intracellular cyclic nucleotides would be destroyed rapidly by cytosolic phosphodiesterase action and cellular activity would return to basal levels. Effects of steroid and thyroid hormones and some peptide hormones may be of longer duration. The actions of these hormones involve DNA, RNA, and protein synthesis. In the absence of further hormone stimulation the newly synthesized RNA species and proteins are degraded by cytoplasmic enzyme actions.

After the initial stage in hormone-plasma membrane interaction, the hormone-receptor complexes cluster at specific sites on the cell membrane [15]. Clustering of hormone-receptor complexes apparently triggers vesiculation of the plasma membrane hormone-receptor complex followed by cellular internationalization by endocytosis (Fig. 4.17). What is unclear is whether the contents of the vesicle are degraded by lysosomal or other enzymes or whether plasmalemmal vesiculization and endocytosis provide a mechanism for hormone transport to intracellular target sites [13]. Both events may be operative, depending on the particular hormone and cellular species.

PATHOPHYSIOLOGICAL CORRELATES OF HORMONE ACTION

As noted, syndromes of hormone deficiency are often associated with increased sensitivity to the missing hormone, and this is correlated with increased concentrations of receptors for the hormone. Conversely, exposure of cells to elevated levels of a hormone may result in a decrease in target tissue receptors for the hormone. Clinical evidence suggests that receptor modulation by circulating hormone concentrations is an important physiological adaptation. There are examples of heterospecific receptor

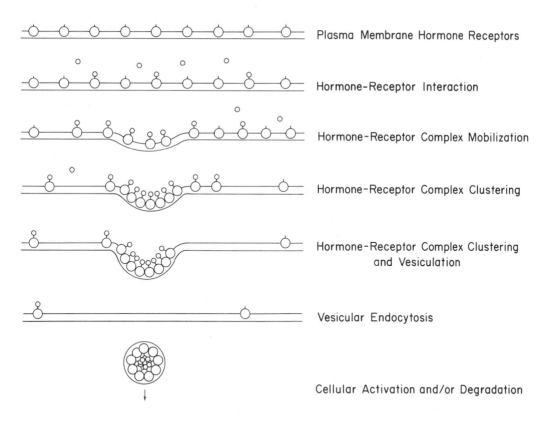

Figure 4.17 Scheme for hormone-receptor clustering and vesicular endocytosis.

modulation that can lead to adverse physiological responses. Thyroxine, for example, increases the number of β-adrenergic receptors in cardiac muscle and vascular tissues as well as having a direct effect on the heart. This accounts for the enhanced sympathetic nervous activity that is usually a symptom of hyperthyroidism.

Myasthenia gravis is an example of an *autoimmune disease* where antibodies to cholinergic receptors have been developed within the body. The antibodies block acetylcholine receptors at the neuromuscular junction. This, of course, leads to muscle dysfunction. In patients with *Graves' disease* there are circulating immunoglobulins which bind to thyrotropin receptors in the thyroid gland. This immunoglobulin, the so-called thyroid stimulating antibody (TSAb), enhances $T_4 - T_3$ production which results in hyperthyroidism (Chapter 13). A large number of human endocrinopathies are related to defects in hormone-receptor interaction [4, 22]. The hormone may be defective in structure, receptor number may be decreased, increased, or blocked as described, or there may be a defect in receptor-signal transduction. *Cholera* is a disease characterized by an enormous secretion of water and electrolytes by intestinal mucosal cells and often leads to death from dehydration. The affliction is caused by the cholera vibrio (*Vibrio cholerae*). The pathogen secretes a toxin (an antigen) which irreversibly binds to the guanyl nucleotide regulatory protein [43]. This leads to the continuous production of cyclic AMP and abnormal secretion of water and electrolytes.

SUMMARY AND PERSPECTIVES

The discovery of cAMP was crucial in understanding the mechanism of action of a large number of hormones. Many steps subsequent to cAMP formation, such as protein kinase activation and substrate phosphorylation, have been delineated. The role of cGMP in the mechanism of action of some hormones has provided a useful model of the relative roles of cyclic nucleotides in the biphasic responses of certain cells to hormone action. It is unclear whether the actions of all hormones on the plasma membrane are similarly linked to cyclic nucleotide production. Possibly other second messengers are yet to be discovered.

Clarification of the precise mechanisms involved in hormone action has contributed greatly to understanding the etiology of many disease states and aided in the clinical treatment of some of these endocrinopathies. In the future, antihormones may be generated and used clinically so that excess hormone stimulation can be blocked at the level of the cellular receptor. Glucagon is clearly implicated in the etiology of diabetes mellitus; it would be a boon if specific antagonists to glucagon could be produced for clinical use. Additional synthetic hormone analogs are being produced which are more effective in their actions than the native hormone. These analogs may possess greater intrinsic (inherent) activity or they may be more resistant to enzymatic degradation within the blood or at other sites. This latter phenomenon would prolong the activity of the hormone analog; lower doses or fewer injections of the hormone would be required, which would be of economic advantage to the patient.

Radiolabeled hormones are being utilized to determine the number of cellular hormone receptors in patients with certain endocrine disabilities, such as maturity onset diabetes, where the etiology of the disease is related to a decrease in cellular insulin receptor number. Radiolabeled somatotropin, for example, binds to its target tissue, the liver, but the liver fails to respond by producing growth factors (Chapter 12). Thus the etiology of Laron dwarfism is not due to any defect in the intrinsic nature of STH but rather at some more distal step in the mechanism of action of the hormone (Fig. 12.13). Again radiolabeled estradiol is utilized to determine the presence and number of estradiol receptors in breast cancer (mammary gland tumors). This information may provide the rationale for subsequent therapy. Ovariectomy and the subsequent decline in circulation of estradiol may be beneficial to those patients with hormone-dependent breast cancers (Chapter 19).

REFERENCES

[1] AMER, M. S. 1974. Cyclic guanosine 3', 5'-monophosphate and gallbladder contraction. *Gastroenterology* 67:333–37.

[2] BAXTER, J. D., and J. W. FUNDER. 1979. Hormone receptors. *New Engl. J. Med.* 301:1149–61.

[3] CATT, K. J., J. P. HARWOOD, G. AGUILERA, and M. L. DUFAU. 1979. Hormonal regulation of peptide receptors and target tissue responses. *Nature* 280:109–16.

[4] CHAN, L., and B. W. O'MALLEY. 1976. Mechanism of action of sex steroid hormones. *New Engl. J. Med.* 294:1322–28; 1372–81; 1430–37.

[5] CHEUNG, W. Y. 1982. Calmodulin. *Sci. Amer.* 246 (June): 62–70.

[6] COHEN, P. 1982. The role of protein phosphorylation in neural and hormonal control of cellular activity. *Nature* 296:613–20.

[7] DEDMAN, J. R., B. R. BRINKLEY, and A. R. MEANS. 1979. Regulation of microfilaments and microtubules by calcium and cyclic AMP. *Advan. Cyclic Nucl. Res.* 11:131–74.

[8] DE MEYTS, P., A. R. BIANCO, and J. ROTH. 1976. Site-site interactions among insulin receptors. Characterization of the negative cooperativity. *J. Biol. Chem.* 251:1877–88.

[9] ERICKSON, G. F., C. WANG, and A. J. W. HSUEH. 1979. FSH induction of functional LH receptors in granulosa cells cultured in a chemically defined medium. *Nature* 279:336–38.

[10] FLIER, J. S., C. R. KAHN, and J. ROTH. 1979. Receptors, antireceptor antibodies and mechanisms of insulin resistance. *New Engl. J. Med.* 300:413–19.

[11] GOLDBERG, N. D. 1974. Cyclic nucleotides and cell function. *Hospital Practice* May: 127–41.

[12] GOLDBERG, N. D., and M. K. HADDOX. 1977. Cyclic GMP metabolism and involvement in biological regulation. *Ann. Rev. Biochem.* 46:823–96.

[13] GOLDFINE, I. D., G. J. SMITH, K. Y. WONG, and A. L. JONES. 1977. Cellular uptake and nuclear binding of insulin in human cultured lymphocytes: evidence for potential intracellular sites of insulin action. *Proc. Natl. Acad. Sci.* 74:1368–72.

[14] GOMPERTS, B. D. 1976. Calcium cell activation. In *Receptors and recognition*, Series A, no. 2, eds. P. Cuatrecasas and M. F. Greaves, pp. 43–102. New York: Halstead Press.

[15] GORDEN, Ph., J. L. CARPENTIER, P. FREYCHET, and L. ORCI. 1980. Internalization of polypeptide hormones. *Diabetologia* 18:263–74.

[16] GREENGARD, P. 1979. Cyclic nucleotides, phosphorylated proteins, and the nervous system. *Fed. Proc.* 38:2208–17.

[17] HIRATA, F., and J. AXELROD. 1980. Phospholipid methylation and biological signal transmission. *Science* 209:1082–90.

[18] HOLLENBERG, M. D., and P. CUATRECASAS. 1978. Membrane receptors and hormone action: recent developments. *Neuro-Psychopharmac.* 2:287–302.

[19] HSUEH, A. J. W., M. L. DUFAU, and K. J. CATT. 1977. Gonadotropin-induced regulation of luteinizing hormone receptors and desensitization of testicular 3′:5′-cyclic AMP and testosterone responses. *Proc. Natl. Acad. Sci. USA.* 74:592–95.

[20] JACOBS, S., and P. CUATRECASAS. 1977. The mobile receptor hypothesis for cell membrane receptor action. *Trends in Biochem. Sci.* 2:280–82.

[21] KAHN, C. R. 1976. Membrane receptors for hormones and neurotransmitters. *J. Cell Biol.* 70:261–86.

[22] KAHN, C. R., K. MEGYESI, R. S. BAR, R. C. EASTMAN, and J. S. FLIER. 1977. Receptors for peptide hormones: new insights into the pathophysiology of disease states in man. *Ann. Intern. Med.* 86:205–19.

[23] KATZENELLENBOGEN, B. S. 1980. Dynamics of steroid hormone receptor action. *Ann. Rev. Physiol.* 42:17–35.

[24] KING, A. C., and P. CUATRECASAS. 1981. Peptide hormone-induced receptor mobility, aggregation, and internalization. *New Engl. J. Med.* 305:77–88.

[25] KLEE, C. B., T. H. CROUCH, and P. G. RICHMAN. 1980. Calmodulin. *Ann. Rev. Biochem.* 49:489–515.

[26] LANGLEY, J. N. 1906. On nerve endings and on special excitable substances. *Proc. Roy. Soc. B* 78:170–94.

[27] McGiff, J. C. 1981. Prostaglandins, prostacyclin, and thromboxanes. *Ann. Rev. Pharmacol. Toxicol.* 21:479–509.

[28] Means, A. R. 1981. Calmodulin: properties, intracellular localization, and multiple roles in cell regulation. *Rec. Prog. Horm. Res.* 37:333–67.

[29] Nathanson, J. A., and P. Greengard. 1977. Chemical messages between nerve cells are translated into messages within cells. *Sci. Amer.* 237 (Feb.) 108–19.

[30] Nelson, N. A., R. C. Kelly, and R. A. Johnson. 1982. Prostaglandins and the arachidonic acid cascade. *Chem. & Engin. News* Aug. 16:30–44.

[31] Oates, J. A. 1982. The 1982 Nobel prize in physiology or medicine. *Science* 218:765–768.

[32] O'Malley, B., and L. Birnbaumer, eds. 1978. *Receptors and hormone action.* New York: Academic Press, Inc.

[33] Posner, B. I., J. J. M. Bergeron, Z. Josefsberg, M. N. Khan, R. J. Khan, B. A. Patel, R. A. Sikstrom, and A. K. Verma. 1981. Polypeptide hormones: intracellular receptors and internalization. *Rec. Prog. Horm. Res.* 37:539–82.

[34] Ross, E. M., and A. G. Gilman. 1980. Biochemical properties of hormone-sensitive adenylate cyclase. *Ann. Rev.* 49:533–64.

[35] Schramm, M., J. Orly, S. Eimerl, and M. Korner. 1977. Coupling of hormone receptors to adenylate cyclase of different cells by cell fusion. *Nature* 268:310–13.

[36] Schulster, D., S. Burstein, and B. A. Cooke. 1976. *Molecular endocrinology of steroid hormones.* New York: John Wiley & Sons, Inc.

[37] Schulster, D., J. Orly, G. Seidel, and M. Schramm. 1978. Intracellular cyclic AMP production enhanced by a hormone receptor transferred from a different cell. *J. Biol. Chem.* 253:1201–1206.

[38] Shoji, S., D. C. Parmelee, R. D. Wade, S. Kumar, L. H. Ericsson, K. A. Walsh, H. Neurath, G. L. Long, J. C. Demaille, E. H. Fischer, and K. Titani. 1981. Complete amino acid sequence of the catalytic subunit of bovine cardiac muscle cyclic AMP-dependent protein kinase. *Proc. Natl. Acad. Sci.* 78:848–51.

[39] Spiegel, A. M., and R. W. Downs, Jr. 1981. Guanine nucleotides: key regulators of hormone receptor cyclase interaction. *Endocrine Rev.* 2:275–305.

[40] Sutherland, E. W. 1972. Studies on the mechanism of hormone action. *Science* 177:401–408.

[41] Takio, K., S. B. Smith, E. G. Krebs, K. A. Walsh, and K. Titani. 1982. Primary structure of the regulatory subunit of type II cAMP-dependent protein kinase from bovine cardiac muscle. *Proc. Natl. Acad. Sci. USA* 79:2544–48.

[42] Vesely, D. L., and M. E. Hadley. 1976. Receptor specific calcium requirement for melanophore stimulating hormone (MSH) control of melanophores. *Pigment Cell* 3:265–74.

[43] Vaughan, M. 1982. Cholera and cell regulation. *Hospital Practice* June: 145–52.

5

PITUITARY HORMONES

INTRODUCTION

The pituitary has often been referred to as the master endocrine gland of vertebrates. This perceived importance may have derived because the pituitary appeared to function autonomously and yet apparently controlled such important endocrine glands as the adrenals, thyroid, and the gonads. The pituitary gland is now known to be subservient to hormonal stimuli derived from the brain and from other endocrine glands.

The pituitary gland of the human male is somewhat smaller than the tip of the little finger and weighs between 0.5 to 1.0 g; its size in the human female becomes larger during pregnancy. The pituitary is recessed within the sella turcica of the sphenoid bone beneath the hypothalamus near the optic chiasm. In this position the pituitary is the most inaccessible of the mammalian endocrine glands. Early anatomists considered the pituitary to be a part of the brain and, in fact, the gland does consist of a neural component.

In 1886 Marie made an important observation that acromegaly often occurred along with a tumorous condition of the pituitary [14]. Other physicians noted that the pituitary gland of the male and the female often became enlarged following gonadectomy. Cushing was the first to note the association between basophil tumors of the pituitary and the resultant disease that bears his name. Much later it was established that pituitarigenic Cushing's disease was associated with elevated secretion of cortico-

85

tropin. Cushing showed in 1909 that partial removal of the anterior pituitary of an acromagalic resulted in rapid recovery.

Smith [14] noted that hypophysectomy of the rat resulted in complete stasis of growth and a rapid regression of the size of the adrenals (mainly the steroidogenic cortex), the thyroid, and the gonads. Ablation of the posterior lobe of the pituitary alone failed to produce these effects. Smith also observed that daily intramuscular injections of fresh rat or bovine anterior pituitary homogenates into hypophysectomized rats brought about a nearly normal growth rate. In addition this replacement therapy caused a partial restoration of the size of the adrenals, thyroid, and gonads. Evans and Long [14] noted that extracts of bovine pituitaries enhanced the growth rate of intact rats over that of their litter mates. Treatment of rats with such extracts for 9 months or more resulted in the production of experimental gigantism. This exaggerated increase in growth was due to generalized overgrowth of the skeleton and to an enlargement of most tissues and organs. These results provided experimental evidence for the existence of a growth hormone (somatotropin) of hypophysial origin.

Smith and Allen, working independently, demonstrated that growth and metamorphosis of larval amphibians (frog tadpoles) were prevented by extirpation of the anlage (tissue primordium) of the epithelial (nonneural component) pituitary [14]. The larval animals were also light in color compared to normal intact tadpoles. These early experiments provided evidence for the existence of a pituitary thyroid stimulating hormone and a melanophore stimulating hormone. Other researchers subsequently provided evidence for the existence of other pituitary hormones regulating adrenal and gonadal function and numerous physiological processes. This chapter will discuss the nature and endocrine role of the pituitary hormones.

ANATOMY OF THE PITUITARY GLAND

The pituitary gland (also known as the hypophysis) is composed of tissues that derive from two diverse origins. An understanding of the origin and development of the pituitary is critical to an understanding of the structure-function relationships of this endocrine gland. Early anatomists believed that the structural components of the pituitary (Latin: *pituita*, phlegm) gland were concerned with the removal of phlegm or mucus from the cavities of the brain. The comparative anatomy of the pituitary of many vertebrates has been reviewed in an important monograph by Holmes and Ball [18]. The ultrastructural characteristics of the cells of the anterior pituitary have been described in detail elsewhere [41].

Developmental Anatomy

The human pituitary is composed of an *adenohypophysis* (glandular or epithelial hypophysis) and a *neurohypophysis* (Fig. 5.1). The former derives from an inward

Pituitary Gland (Hypophysis)

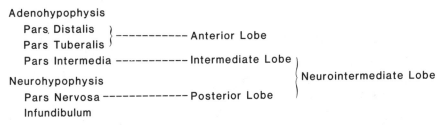

Adenohypophysis
   Pars Distalis ⎫
   Pars Tuberalis ⎭ ----------- Anterior Lobe
   Pars Intermedia ----------- Intermediate Lobe ⎫
Neurohypophysis   ⎬ Neurointermediate Lobe
   Pars Nervosa ------------ Posterior Lobe ⎭
   Infundibulum

Figure 5.1 Anatomical components of the pituitary gland.

evagination of the oral ectoderm of the stomodeum (primitive mouth cavity) known as Rathke's pouch (Fig. 5.2). The neuronal component arises from the neural ectoderm of the floor of the forebrain. Rathke's pouch elongates and becomes constricted at its attachment to the oral epithelium. A remnant of the connection between Rathke's pouch and the stomodeal ectoderm may persist as a "pharyngeal" pituitary. An infundibular process develops as a diverticulum of the floor of the diencephalon. The

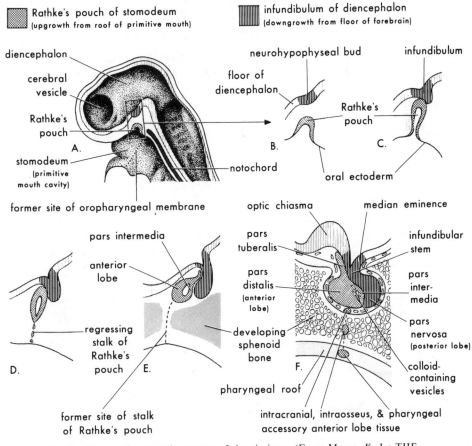

Figure 5.2 Developmental anatomy of the pituitary. (From Moore, K. L.: THE DEVELOPING HUMAN. Clinically Oriented Embryology, 2nd ed., 1977, Courtesy of W. B. Saunders Co.)

Anatomy of the Pituitary Gland

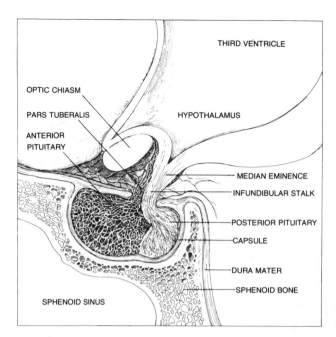

infundibulum increases in size because of neuroepithelial cell proliferation. Nerve fibers grow into the infundibulum from hypothalamic nuclei. The neuroepithelial cells then differentiate into *pituicytes* (neuroglial-like elements) which are dispersed between the neuronal endings within the infundibulum.

Cells of the anterior wall of Rathke's pouch proliferate to give rise to the pars distalis or anterior pituitary. Continued proliferation of these cells leads to reduction of the lumen of Rathke's pouch to a *residual cleft* and a separation of the cells of posterior wall from the anterior pituitary. Those cells adjacent to the infundibulum may proliferate to give rise to a pars intermedia of considerable size in some species. Failure of the adenohypophysis to contact the developing neurohypophysis results in the inability of the pituitary cells to form a pars intermedia. In birds the adenohypophysis is separated from the neurohypophysis by a layer of connective tissue and a pars intermedia does not develop. In humans the fetal pars intermedia regresses and is believed to be absent in the adult (Chapter 8). Dorsal extensions of the anterior pituitary surround the infundibular stalk to give rise to the *pars tuberalis*. The pars tuberalis may provide an important anatomical link between the pars distalis and the hypothalamus. The definitive pituitary in many species consists of the pars distalis, the pars intermedia, the pars tuberalis, and the pars nervosa (Fig. 5.3). The intimate anatomical relationship between the pituitary gland and the overlying brain provides an important clue to understanding the essential functional relationship of the brain-pituitary axis [17].

Lobation, Vascularization, Innervation

The size of each component of the pituitary gland varies within different species; the size of each hypophysial component may be related to the particular environmental niche occupied by the species. Animals that rapidly change color may possess a relatively large pars intermedia; the pars nervosa of aquatic species may be small, but relatively large in land-dwelling species, particularly those inhabiting arid climates. These size differences in components of the pituitary gland reflect the hormonal output of the glands required for successful adaptation to a particular habitat.

The pituitary gland receives its blood supply from the superior and inferior hypophysial arteries. The anterior and posterior branches of the superior hypophysial artery penetrate the hypophysial stalk as well as the hypothalamus (Fig. 5.4). The pars distalis is vascularized by hypophysial portal vessels which arise from the capillary beds within the median eminence of the hypothalamus. This hypophysial portal system provides an important link for carrying hormonal information from the CNS to the pituitary (Chapter 6). Whether the anterior lobe receives blood exclusively from the portal circulation or whether some additional direct arterial blood supply is available is unresolved. The pars nervosa receives a separate blood supply from the inferior hypophysial artery. The pars intermedia, if present, is relatively avascular. Physiologists have generally assumed that all hormones produced by the adenohypophysis are released directly into the efferent portal veins to be carried through the systemic circulation to distant target tissues. There is evidence that some adenohypophysial venous blood may be shunted to the neurohypophysis [2]. This circular path of blood flow may permit adenohypophysial venous blood to be carried up the infundibular process to the brain. This observation carries the important implication that pituitary hormones might be able to modify CNS function.

Except for neurovascular elements there is no evidence that neurons innervate or otherwise directly influence the activity of the cells of the pars distalis of humans or other mammals. Neuronal elements may affect cellular hormone secretion within the pars distalis of some teleost fishes. The cells of the pars intermedia of amphibians and some mammals are surrounded by a plexus of catecholaminergic neurons which

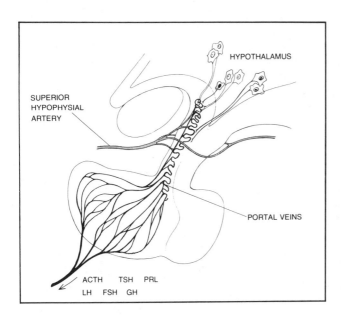

Figure 5.4 Vascular connections between the pituitary gland and the hypothalamus. (From R. Guillemin and R. Burgus, "The Hormones Of The Hypothalamus," with permission. Copyright 1979 by *Scientific American*, Inc., all rights reserved.)

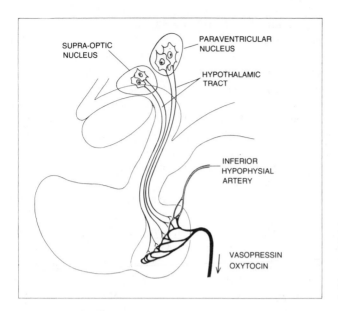

SUPRA-OPTIC
NUCLEUS

PARAVENTRICULAR
NUCLEUS

HYPOTHALAMIC
TRACT

INFERIOR
HYPOPHYSIAL
ARTERY

VASOPRESSIN
OXYTOCIN

Figure 5.5 Neural components of the pituitary gland of humans. (From R. Guillemin and R. Burgus, "The Hormones Of The Hypothalamus," with permission. Copyright 1979 by *Scientific American*, Inc., all rights reserved.)

regulate MSH secretion from the melanotrophs (MSH secreting cells). Such a direct neuronal innervation may be absent from the pars intermedia of some reptiles [44]. The pars nervosa is composed of axonal endings of neurons whose cell bodies are located in hypothalamic nuclei, in mammals, the paraventricular and supraoptic nuclei (Fig. 5.5).

The gross morphology of the pituitary differs considerably between the vertebrate classes and often between species of the same class. At the cytological level the individual cell types may be intermingled to varying degrees (as in tetrapods) or separated into zones (as in most teleost fishes) [39]. There is no distinct neural lobe in fishes. The neural lobe is, however, characteristic of tetrapods, and this may be related to the terrestrial manner of life of these vertebrates where one or both neurohypophysial hormones may be of adaptive importance (Fig. 8.2). The size of the pars intermedia varies considerably between species, and all birds lack a pars intermedia. This is not a unique feature as the pars intermedia is not present in some mammals (elephants, whales, adult humans).

Cytology

The cells of the pituitary are referred to as *acidophils*, *basophils*, or *chromophobes* depending on their affinity for certain dyes used in histological stains (Table 5.1). Histochemical and immunocytochemical methods have provided definitive information on the specific cellular sources of each pituitary peptide hormone. The cells of the pars distalis have been differentiated into somatotrophs, lactotrophs (mammotrophs), corticotrophs, thyrotrophs, and gonadotrophs. These terms relate to the particular hormonal product synthesized by each of these cells. Somatotrophs and lactotrophs are acidophils, whereas the thyrotrophs and the gonadotrophs are basophils. The corticotrophs are basophils but are often referred to as chromophobes. The cells of the

TABLE 5.1 Histochemical Classification of Pituitary Pars Distalis Cells

Cell type	Hormone	Staining Characteristic
Corticotroph[a]	Corticotropin (ACTH)	Basophil
Thyrotroph	Thyrotropin (TSH)	Basophil
Gonadotroph		
FSH-gonadotroph	Follitropin (FSH)	Basophil
LH-gonadotroph	Lutropin (LH)	Basophil
Lactotroph (mammotroph)	Prolactin (PRL)	Acidophil
Somatotroph	Somatotropin (STH)	Acidophil

[a]Cytological classification utilizes either the suffix -troph or -trope (e.g., corticotrope).

mammalian pars intermedia are also considered to be chromophobes. The extent to which a cell exhibits acidophilia, basophilia, or chromophobia may depend on the granular content (hormone-containing vesicles) of the cell, which often varies with the temporal secretory activity of the cell. These secretory vesicles may become depleted after continued secretory activity of the cells; in contrast, these granules may accumulate, at least transiently, if the cells stop releasing hormone. Granule synthesis may eventually decline if the cell is no longer stimulated to secrete its hormonal product. Except for the sparse pituicytes (glial-like cells), the pars nervosa only contains neuronal axonal endings.

Histochemical studies using the periodic acid-Schiff (PAS) reaction reveal the glycoprotein nature of the basophil cell secretory product. Other methods used in combination with the PAS reaction give evidence that the glycoprotein secreting cells as well as the acidophils consist of subclasses of cell types. One cannot, however, consistently distinguish between these cellular subtypes using present staining methods. One problem is that the chromophobe cells represent more than half the cells of the anterior pituitary. Many of these cells are corticotrophs, but it is extremely difficult to differentiate between them and other undifferentiated cells or cells that have released their secretory (vesicular) products. The electron microscope has revealed, however, that chromophobes do contain secretory granules. It is possible by use of electron microscopy to differentiate between each of the cells of the pars distalis by noting ultrastructural differences between the secretory granules present as well as unique organellar profiles within the different cells [17].

Nongranulated, presumably nonsecretory cells are also present in the pars distalis, pars intermedia, and neurohypophysis. These elements have been referred to as glial cells, glial-like cells, stellate cells, and follicular cells. The processes of these cells often separate one pituitary cell from contact with another. In some species they may form the lining of minute ductules or follicles within the adenohypophysis. A variety of putative functions have been suggested for these cells, and it is possible that they modulate pituitary hormone secretion in response to regulatory cues [40].

The utilization of peroxidase-labeled antibodies for the ultrastructural localization of hormones provides a method for identification of the specific hormone-producing cells of the pituitary and the intracellular sites of hormone synthesis. Antibodies to each of the pituitary peptides (antigens) are linked to the enzyme horseradish peroxidase. Thin sections of tissue are then exposed to the antibody-peroxidase conjugate and rinsed. The antibody interacts with its specific antigen (hormone) which is localized within the appropriate pituitary cells. The peroxidase is then localized histochemically by providing a substrate (peroxide) and a dye. The peroxidase reacts with the peroxide to yield molecular oxygen which then produces a particular color depending on the dye present. Different dyes provide differently colored end products. By this method one can note that the reaction product is specifically localized to the secretory granules of the cells. One cell can be differentiated from another by the sequential addition of different antibody-peroxidase conjugates and by the use of different dyes. Differentiation of one gonadotroph from another utilizes antisera raised specifically against the β-subunit of follitropin or lutropin.

Although each of the pituitary hormones is localized to a particular cell type, as determined by ultrastructural and immunocytochemical analysis, most gonadotrophs (at least in rats) contain lutropin and follitropin. Nevertheless, subpopulations of gonadotrophs contain only one of the gonadotropins [4]. This may account for the nonparallel release of gonadotropins in response to certain stimuli (Fig. 18.9). Individual gonadotrophs vary in their staining intensity for labeled antibodies to each of the gonadotropins suggesting that gonadotrophs may represent a fluid, heterogeneous population of cells capable of synthesizing and storing both or one of the hormones [4]. Immunocytochemical observations have revealed that all cell types of the pars distalis are present within the pars tuberalis of the human and monkey. The hormonal function of the pars distalis may therefore be augmented by secretory contributions from the pars tuberalis [1].

HORMONES OF THE PITUITARY

A number of peptide hormones are produced by the pituitary. These hormones regulate such target organs as the gonads, the adrenals, and the thyroid gland. The mammary glands, uterus, kidneys, and other tissues are also controlled by hypophysial hormones. Two gonadotropins are present: *follicle stimulating hormone* (FSH), or follitropin, and *luteinizing hormone* (LH), or lutropin. A *thyroid stimulating hormone* (TSH), or *thyrotropin*, and an *adrenal cortical stimulating hormone* (ACTH), or *adrenocorticotropin* (*corticotropin*), regulate thyroid and adrenal activity, respectively. A *somatotropin* (STH), or *growth hormone* (GH), which has generalized growth-promoting effects, and a *prolactin* (PRL, mammotropin), which has more specific growth-promoting action on the mammary glands, are also present in some species. A melanocyte stimulating hormone (α-MSH, α-melanotropin) is produced by cells of the pars intermedia, or possibly by cells within the pars distalis (of birds). The neurohypophysial hormones, *oxytocin* and the *vasopressins*, are elaborated within neurons of the neurohypophysis whose cell bodies originate within the hypothalamus. The pituitary hormones are released into the bloodstream where they circulate to interact with their target organs.

Families Of Pituitary Hormones

The hormones of the pituitary can be classified into four groups based on their structural similarity and presumed evolutionary origin. Somatotropin and prolactin possess numerous similar sequences of amino acids within their individual structures, and they are also structurally related to placental lactogen (also known as somato-mammotropin). Thyrotropin, follitropin, and lutropin are glycoproteins and are related in structure to each other and to chorionic gonadotropin (choriogonado-tropin), a hormone of placental origin. α-Melanotropin and corticotropin contain a sequence of amino acids in common which accounts for their overlapping actions and suggests a related evolutionary origin.

Somatotropin And Prolactin

These hormones of the pituitary exert profound effects on body growth. In the young animal STH plays an essential role in general body growth, whereas PRL stimulates the growth of specialized tissues as the mammary gland during pregnancy and lactation.

Somatotropin. The existence of a hormone that is responsible for general somatic growth was suggested by the early experiments of Evans and Long (1922) and Smith (1926) (see [14] for references). Hypophysectomized young rats failed to grow to adult size, but extracts of the pituitary stimulated growth in these rats and in rats of normal growth. It is well established that human STH is also effective in promoting linear growth in children with congenital STH deficiency. In young animals the epiphyses of the long bones are separated from the bones by an epiphyseal cartilaginous plate. Chondrogenesis is accelerated by STH, which results in a widening of the epiphyseal plates as more extracellular matrix (chondroitin sulfate) is synthesized and released by chondrocytes. This widening has been utilized as a bioassay for STH (tibia test).

Somatotropin accounts for 4% to 10% (5 to 10 mg per gland) of the wet weight of the anterior pituitary in the human adult [8]. STH circulates in the plasma in an unbound form, and basal (resting or nonstressed) levels of immunoassayable STH in the plasma range from 1 to 5 ng per milliliter. The circulating levels of the hormone decline during the first 2 or 3 weeks after birth to reach the basal levels characteristic of the adult human. Age-related changes in total 24-hour secretion of STH have been described. Although STH levels remain rather constant during the period of accelerated growth in early childhood, there is an appreciable increase during the period of maximal growth in adolescence. Interestingly, a substantial part of the 24-hour secretion of STH occurs during the first 90 minutes of nocturnal sleep.

Both a hypothalamic STH releasing factor, somatocrinin, as well as an STH release-inhibiting factor have been implicated in the control of STH secretion (Chapter 6). The chemical nature of a putative STH releasing factor has been determined (Fig. 6.8). The structure of the inhibiting factor, more commonly referred to as *somatostatin* (or somatotropin release-inhibiting factor, SRIF), has been determined (Fig. 6.6). This tetradecapeptide is found in other anatomical sites where it may subserve a number of diverse biological functions.

Somatotropin is a polypeptide synthesized by certain acidophils (somatotrophs) of the pars distalis. STH is derived from a prohormone in the pituitary cells but is rapidly converted to STH by proteolysis. The human hormone consists of 191 amino acids with two intramolecular disulfide bonds. The hormone is strikingly similar in structure to prolactin and placental lactogen. The latter molecule also contains 191 amino acids and possesses S—S bonds in exactly the same locations as in STH; in 161 positions the amino acids are identical. The structural homologies suggest a single progenitor molecule that arose early in vertebrate evolution (Fig. 12.4).

Somatotropins of human and primate origin have intrinsic prolactinlike activity, and for years STH and PRL were considered to be the same hormone because separation of the two hormones proved very difficult. STH of mammalian origin is active in many species, but human subjects are only responsive to human or primate STH. The large size of STH makes it impractical to synthesize the hormone on a large scale, and at present the only readily available source of STH is from pituitaries taken from humans at autopsy. However, STH may be commercially produced by gene-splicing techniques within bacteria (Chapter 3).

The two disulfide bridges of STH are easily reduced and then reoxidized to the native state. Human STH maintained in the reduced state by chemical modification retains biological activity as the secondary and tertiary structures remain indistinguishable. Human plasmin (fibrinolysin, a plasma peptidase) does not change the biological properties of STH although the hormone is cleaved at positions 134–135 and 140–141 of the molecule. Apparently removal of the hexapeptide sequence (residues 135–140) from the structure of STH does not alter the conformation of the molecule. The reduced 1–134 and 141–191 fragments of STH individually exhibit some biological activity. Full biological activity of STH is restored by noncovalent interaction of these two reduced fragments of the hormone. Combination of the NH$_2$-terminal sequence of human STH with a synthetic COOH-terminal fragment regenerates full biological activity. This may provide a method for the synthesis of the hormone by the noncovalent combination of synthetic NH$_2$- and COOH-terminal fragments. These methods also provide a means for determining the minimum structure of STH required for full biological activity [23, 24].

STH is important in growth through its effects on metabolism and cellular proliferation. The reported biological actions of STH are, however, confusing. The effects of the hormone are mediated directly on certain tissues and indirectly through the production of somatomedins. These effects are biphasic, that is, immediately insulinlike followed soon after by an antiinsulin action. The initial in vivo responses to STH include: a fall in blood glucose levels, amino acids, and free fatty acids; the enhanced uptake of amino acids by muscle; and the enhanced uptake and utilization of glucose by adipose tissue, cardiac and skeletal muscle. These responses are followed by mobilization of nonesterified fatty acids from adipose tissue. Somatotropin activation of lipolysis is accomplished through the regulation of protein synthesis. These proteins may maintain the lipolytic machinery of adipose tissue cells at optional levels so that fast-acting lipolytic agents, such as epinephrine, may elicit rapid, maximal mobilization of FFA's in times of need (Chapter 14).

Somatotropin stimulates hepatic glycogenolysis and inhibits the effect of insulin on glucose uptake by peripheral tissues (muscle and adipose tissue). The actions of STH are obviously diabetogenic in nature, and the hyperglycemic effect of STH is stimulatory to insulin secretion. In addition STH sensitizes, or in some way enhances, the secretion of insulin to most secretogogues (e.g., arginine). Nevertheless, in the face of increased insulin secretion the response of insulin target tissues to the hormone is blunted by STH. The mechanism by which STH mediates its antiinsulin effects on hepatic glycogenolysis in liver and muscle cells is not well understood. There may be a down regulation (Chapter 4) of target tissue insulin receptors due to the increased circulating levels of insulin (hyperglycemia from the actions of STH).

STH is a protein anabolic hormone in that it enhances amino acid incorporation into muscle protein and stimulates extracellular collagen deposition. Thus it produces a positive nitrogen and phosphorus balance and a concomitant fall in blood urea nitrogen and amino acid levels. Urinary excretion of sodium and potassium is also decreased, probably due to the increased uptake of these ions by growing tissue. These effects of STH on protein metabolism and electrolyte balance are mediated indirectly through the actions of the somatomedins which are released from the liver in response to STH stimulation of hepatocytes. These somatomedins stimulate cellular growth in a variety of tissues and organs (Fig. 12.12).

The absence of STH secretion leads to dwarfism in the young child, whereas overproduction of STH during early postnatal development leads to gigantism. In the adult excess STH secretion leads to acromegaly. Dwarfism may result from a pituitary failure of STH production (hypopituitary dwarfism) or from a failure of the liver to respond to STH and synthesize somatomedins (Laron dwarfism). The pathogenesis of acromegaly has been explained by an adenohypophysial and a hypothalamic hypothesis. In the former view overproduction of STH may result from STH secreting tumors of the adenohypophysis (intrasellar tumors). The hypothalamic hypothesis implicates the defect as residing within the central nervous system, possibly from an overproduction of an STH releasing hormone or an underproduction of somatostatin. The secretion of either of these factors is controlled by other neural inputs (e.g., dopaminergic neurons) which may contribute indirectly to the etiology of acromegaly. Nevertheless, the vast majority of patients with acromegaly have identifiable pituitary tumors, but whether these tumors arise from long-term overstimulation by the hypothalamus or are independent of hypothalamic influence, possibly due to cellular mutagenesis of somatotrophs or a related stem cell, is still in doubt [43].

The acromegalic characteristics of STH overproduction probably result from the direct effects of STH on target tissues as well as growth effects mediated through the somatomedins. The growth changes in bones and soft tissues are most noticeable in the hands, feet, and face. Proliferation of connective tissue and interstitial fluid results in thickening of the skin and an increase in subcutaneous tissues. The viscera and related organs as the lungs, liver, heart, and kidneys are usually enlarged. Acromegalics may display increased metabolic rates, and the lipolytic actions of STH on adipose tissue combined with antiinsulin actions on other tissues result in hyperglycemia as a symptom of a developing diabetes mellitus.

The etiology of STH deficiency may also relate to a pituitary or hypothalamic dysfunction [7]. Intrasellar tumors or other destructive processes as well as familial (genetic) or congenital (birth) defects may result in a lack of STH production and which could lead to dwarfism if initiated at a young age. Lack of STH secretion may be accompanied by a total lack of pituitary hormone production (panhypopituitarism) or may be an example of an isolated STH deficiency of unknown etiology. Dwarfism may also result from pituitary deficiency secondary to hypothalamic dysfunction, possibly related to an absence of the putative STH releasing factor. Suprasellar (CNS) lesions may also result in STH deficiency, and there are even examples of psychosocial dwarfism.

Evidence for a pituitary somatotropin in fish pituitaries is well established. Hypophysectomy, for example, causes a cessation of growth which can be reestablished by replacement therapy with fish pituitary extracts or mammalian STH. Results based on RIA of purified somatotropins and pituitary extracts from diverse vertebrate species indicated a close immunochemical relatedness between the preparations of the species studied. These somatotropins and extracts also possess significant biological activity (rat tibia test). None of the extracts from the bony fishes tested, however, showed any immunological or biological relationship to the somatotropins of other vertebrate species. Extracts from primitive fishes, holosteans (lung fishes), and cartilaginous fishes, however, showed immunological and biological relatedness. Thus the structures of somatotropins have been conserved throughout evolution, except apparently in modern bony fishes which diverged early from the main line of vertebrate evolution [16]. More recent studies on teleost somatotropins indicate low but significant biological activity in the rat tibia test and some immunological relatedness to mammalian STH [9, 10].

Prolactin. Mammary growth and development and lactogenesis in the human female are regulated, in part, by a hormone from the pituitary [12]. This prolactin plays diverse roles in other vertebrates [19]. No other known polypeptide hormone has such a repertoire of biological actions. Because the varied effects of this hormone usually bear some relationship to physiological responses essential for reproductive success, PRL has been referred to as the "hormone of maternity." Only recently has a role for PRL in the male and nonpregnant female been recognized (Chapters 17 and 18).

In 1928 Stricker and Grueter discovered that an extract of the anterior pituitary gland could stimulate milk secretion in rabbits. The control of mammary gland development and the stimulation of milk synthesis are complex processes that involve the participation of many hormones. The mammotropic action of PRL requires the participation of several hormones which in some species include estrogens, insulin, glucocorticoids, progesterone, and STH. The direct action of PRL on the mammary gland was shown in ovariectomized rabbits first given estrogen and progesterone to produce lobuloalveolar growth (Chapter 19). When PRL was injected into the individual ducts of the mammary gland, only the alveoli connected to the injected duct produced milk Riddle, Bates, and Dykshorn [35] discovered that a specific fraction of bovine pituitary extracts, which they named prolactin, stimulated crop sac growth in pigeons. The hormone is also referred to as mammotropin or lactogenic hormone.

Prolactin is synthesized within acidophilic (lactotroph) cells that are not easily distinguished from somatotrophs by conventional staining methods. Newer methods which employ immunofluorescent and immunoenzymatic methods can differentiate the individual cell types. Prolactin cells are also distinguished from somatotrophs by their ultrastructural features. During pregnancy or in the postpartum lactational period prolactin cells comprise as much as 50% of the acidophil population of the pituitary. Observations reveal, using an electron microscope, that the secretory granules of the lactotrophs are released by vesicular exocytosis.

The primary structures of ovine, bovine, porcine, and human prolactins have been determined [26]. Although 141 of 199 amino acids are in identical positions in these prolactins, the nonhuman hormones are not active in humans. Digestion of ovine PRL with fibrinolysin (a plasma enzyme) revealed that a major cleavage site was located between position 53–54 of the hormone which yielded an N-terminal 1–53 fragment and C-terminal 54–199 fragment. These two PRL fragments could be noncovalently recombined to yield a product that was immunologically and biologically indistinguishable from the native hormone. These results suggest that the three-dimensional conformation of PRL is determined by intrachain charge interactions that, under experimental conditions, do not require the intact molecule for expression.

Serum PRL levels increase at puberty, but only modestly compared to the rises in FSH and LH concentrations that also occur. Estrogen infusions are stimulatory to PRL secretion which may explain the increase in PRL secretion at puberty, a time when ovarian steroid biosynthesis is enhanced. During pregnancy there is a progressive increase in serum PRL concentrations reaching maximal values at term. In mothers who do not nurse their young the postpartum concentrations of PRL fall rapidly back to normal by 3 weeks unless breast feeding is commenced. Concentrations of PRL in the amniotic fluid exceed those in the maternal or fetal circulation early in pregnancy and at term. By biological, chemical, and immunological criteria, human amniotic fluid PRL is similar or identical to that in the pituitary hormone. The chorion-decidua may be the source of amniotic lactogen but the possible physiological function of the placental prolactin is unknown.

Progesterone production by the ovarian corpus luteum is required for growth and development of the uterus and for suppression of further ovum maturation and ovulation (Chapter 19). Prolactin is luteotropic in some mammalian species, and it may act in concert with LH or FSH on the corpus luteum. Prolactin has a profound effect on the growth, differentiation, and function of a number of integumental structures: hair and sebaceous glands in mammals; brood patch and feather development in certain birds; epidermal sloughing in lizards; and integumental mucous gland secretion in certain teleosts. Because the mammary gland is an integumental derivative and is considered to be phylogenetically related to sweat glands, one may conclude that the highly specialized mammotropic action of PRL in humans and most mammals may have evolved from the more generalized action of PRL on a variety of integumentary functions.

In certain birds (pigeons and doves) PRL controls the production of a so-called crop sac milk. In response to PRL the epithelium of the two lateral lobes of the crop wall thicken in both the male and the female at the time the eggs are hatched. The epithelium proliferates and the cells accumulate lipid and begin to degenerate. The layers of cells are sloughed off to form a mass of material which is regurgitated to feed the young birds. Besides its effect on the integument, PRL controls many other physiological processes. Considering its versatility of actions, the name given to the hormone, prolactin, is obviously restrictive and only refers to one of its many roles [5].

Although the major role of PRL in humans is the control of lactation, recent evidence suggests that PRL may control testicular function, at least in some rodents [45]. Hypophysectomy of adult rats causes a loss of testicular LH receptors and this, as expected, is associated with a loss in testicular responsiveness to LH. Inhibition of LH or FSH secretion from the pituitary is not, however, associated with a loss of LH receptors. Pituitary hormones other than gonadotropins are essential for maintenance of testicular LH receptors. Inhibition of pituitary PRL release, on the other hand, is associated with a loss of testicular LH receptors. Thus PRL may be essential for the maintenance of LH receptors. This view is substantiated by the observation that PRL treatment increases LH receptor number in the gonads of dwarf male mice and in atrophic testes of light-deprived hamsters (Chapter 20). Prolactin also stimulates growth of the testosterone-stimulated prostate gland of the castrated rat.

Plasma levels of PRL in humans are slightly higher in females than males, although there is considerable overlap of the ranges of PRL concentration in the two sexes. PRL is secreted episodically and has a half-life in the blood of about 15 to 20 minutes. There is a nighttime surge of PRL secretion which, like STH, is associated with sleep (Fig. 5.6). The times of onset and duration of the PRL peak are not identical to those of STH [12]. The most potent stimulus to PRL secretion is nursing. Release of the hormone is mediated by cutaneous sensations arising from the breast and nipple, not by psychic factors associated with the presence of the infant. Breast stimulation of the human male has no effect on PRL release. Secretion of PRL from the pituitary is controlled by a PRL inhibiting factor, PIF [29]. This inhibitory control is somehow diminished during late pregnancy and lactation. The existence of a PRL releasing factor has been suggested in mammals, and PRL secretion in birds is mainly under a stimulatory control (Chapter 6).

Studies using ^{125}I-labeled prolactin reveal that mammary cells possess PRL receptors on their surface membranes. Antibodies prepared against mammary gland cell receptors block the binding of PRL to these receptors and also selectively block PRL-stimulated casein synthesis and amino acid transport into mammary tissue in culture. These results support a functional role for PRL receptors in mediating some actions of the hormone on lactogenesis. Other evidence suggests that PRL may enter

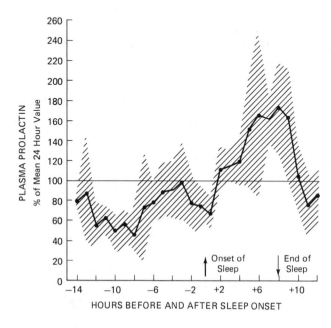

Figure 5.6 Human plasma levels of PRL during a 24-hour period. (Reprinted, by permission of *The New England Journal of Medicine*, Frantz, A. G, "Prolactin", vol. 298, pp. 201–207, 1978.)

intact mammary cells, possibly to be degraded by lysosomal enzymes. Although PRL manifests part of its action at the level of the plasma membrane, there is strong evidence that cAMP is *not* a second messenger in the action of PRL on mammary gland cells. Experimental evidence indicates, however, that cGMP may mediate some of the actions of PRL, at least on casein production (Chapter 19).

Although PRL and STH share structural similarity, their physiological actions in humans are discrete. Acromegalic patients with elevated STH levels only occasionally develop galactorrhea; individuals with galactorrhea or women who are breast-feeding have normal serum STH concentrations. Some patients with a hereditary form of isolated growth hormone deficiency (ateliotic dwarfism) lactate normally although STH is absent.

A pituitary hormone apparently similar to prolactin is present in all vertebrate groups with the possible exception of the cyclostomes. Mammalian, teleost, amphibian, and reptilian PRL's are related structurally to somatotropins from a biological and an immunological standpoint. Teleost PRL shares common structural features with mammalian PRL's and STH's as well as to teleost STH's. Teleost (*Sarotherodon mossambicus*) PRL possesses significant lactogenic activity (stimulates rabbit mammary gland casein synthesis). These observations support the hypothesis that PRL and STH originated from a common ancestral molecule [19]. Although the structure of STH has apparently been strongly conserved throughout evolution, the PRL molecule appears to have been more labile, which may account for the large diversity of actions reported for PRL in the vertebrates.

The Glycoprotein Hormones

Three hormones of the anterior pituitary are glycoproteins [32, 33]. Thyrotropin (TSH), follicle stimulating hormone (FSH), and luteinizing hormone (LH) contain covalently bound carbohydrate moieties at one or more positions within their structures. Each of these pituitary glycoproteins is composed of two chains, so-called α- and β-subunits. The α-subunits of the three pituitary glycoproteins within a species are virtually identical to each other, whereas the β-subunit of each hormone is structurally distinct. The α- and β-subunits of the glycoprotein hormones are independently synthesized; some pituitary tumors, for example, exhibit isolated or unbalanced α-subunit secretion. Also, isolated or unbalanced ectopic secretion of α- or β-subunits of choriogonadotropin by malignant uterine neoplasms has been noted. Two separate mRNA species from mouse thyrotropic tumors have been identified, each coding for a different subunit of the hormone [42]. There is evidence for a single gene per haploid DNA complement that codes for the α-subunits of the glycoprotein family of hormones in any one species [3]. The peptide component of the glycoproteins is first synthesized under direct genetic control. Glycosylation, the attachment of carbohydrate moieties, is believed to be a postribosomal event which is controlled by glycosyltransferase enzymes localized in the Golgi cisternae of the cells.

The constituent sugars of glycoprotein hormones are D-mannose, D-galactose, L-fucose, N-acetyl neuraminic acid, D-glucosamine, and N-acelylated D-galactosamine [33]. All α-subunits contain two oligosaccharides which are N-linked to asparagines. All pituitary glycoprotein hormones may contain O-sulfated (attached through serine to the peptide chain) hexosamines. The biological role of the carbohydrate moieties of pituitary glycoprotein hormones remains unknown; they might conceivably function in receptor recognition and affect the rate of inactivation or clearance of the hormones by the blood. In addition the carbohydrate moieties may be important for antirecognition, such as protection of certain groups in the glycoprotein from proteolysis, self-aggregation, and antigenicity [32].

One may question the individual roles of each of the subunits of the glycoprotein hormones in cellular interaction. It has been suggested that the α-subunit endows the hormone-specific β-subunit with a conformation necessary for binding to the receptor and that the α-subunit itself is necessary for stimulation of adenylate cyclase. It has also been proposed that domains on the α-subunit, in combination with domains on the β-subunit or alone, are responsible for interaction with receptors. In the latter case conformational changes contributing to the specificity of binding could also be induced in the α-subunit by the β-subunit [32]. Molecular hybridization studies involving recombinations of α-subunits with β-subunits demonstrate that hormonal specificity is conferred upon the hybrid by the β-subunit (Fig. 5.7). Amino acid sequences that are identical in the glycoprotein β-subunits have been suggested to represent intersubunit contact sites, whereas the nonidentical residues contribute to interaction with target tissue receptors and therefore provide hormonal specificity.

Thyrotropin. The early work of Allen and of Smith (see [14], for references) demonstrated that thyroidectomy resulted in failure of tadpoles to metamorphose into frogs. This effect could also be duplicated by hyphophysectomy of tadpoles. Metamorphosis of thyroidectomized tadpoles could be accomplished, however, by addition of thyroid gland extracts to the water in which the larvae swam. Pituitary extracts stimulated metamorphosis of hypophysectomized but not thyroidectomized tadpoles. These observations suggested that the pituitary gland might be the source of a substance which was stimulatory to thyroid production of a metamorphic hormone. Thyroxine and triiodothyronine are the hormones produced by the thyroid (Chapter 13). A thyroid-stimulating hormone (TSH, thyrotropin) has been isolated from the

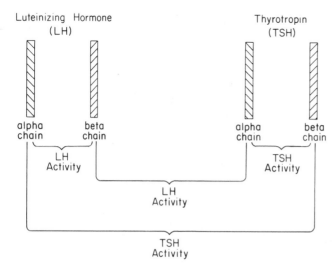

Figure 5.7 Glycoprotein subunit hybridization studies.

pituitary and its structure determined in a number of mammalian species. Thyroid-stimulating activity has also been found in pituitaries of all vertebrates examined. Thyrotropin is synthesized within basophilic thyrotrophs of the pars distalis. The number of secretory granules present within the thyrotrophs is increased if animals are treated with thyroxine, suggesting that thyroid hormones exert a negative feedback to TSH secretion.

The complete primary structure of human TSH has been determined [37]. The α-subunit of TSH consists of 89 amino acid residues and the β-subunit is 112 amino acids in length. The hTSH-α-subunit is similar in length to that of hLH-α; the α-hFSH- and α-hCG-subunits are 92 amino acids in length. Human TSH-α is shorter than bovine or ovine TSH-α by seven residues. There is, however, nearly 70% homology between the linear sequences of the human and the ovine and bovine α-subunits. The human α-subunit differs considerably, however, from the bovine hormone in its carbohydrate content, quantitatively and qualitatively. Two oligosaccharide chains are linked to asparagine residues at positions 49 and 75 of the human TSH-α molecule.

The 112 amino acids comprising hTSH-β reveal very great homology to the structure of bovine TSH-β. The attachment of the carbohydrate moiety to asparagine at position 23 is the same and the location of the 12 half-cystine residues is identical. Altogether there are only 11 residue positions that differ (90% homology) and these can be considered as conservative (for example, phenylalanine for tyrosine). There is also homology between the β-subunits of human TSH, FSH, and LH, with 27 identical residues. There are, however, differences in the number of carbohydrate moieties attached to the polypeptide chains. FSH-β has two compared to the single carbohydrate moiety in TSH-β- and LH-β-subunits. The β-subunit of human chorionic gonadotropin is also similar to the β-subunit of the pituitary glycoproteins, but hCG contains five attached oligosaccharide chains.

As the name implies, the most important role of TSH is the control of thyroid gland function. Thyrotropin may have several extrathyroidal functions. Highly purified bovine thyrotropin causes exophthalmos (abnormal protrusion of the eyes). It has been suggested that the human exophthalmos, often characteristic of Graves' disease, is due to TSH or a degradative derivative of the hormone. The lipolytic activity of thyrotropin is not shared by any other glycoprotein hormones. The physiological significance of this finding is unclear. By its action on the thyroid to liberate thyroid hormones, TSH is responsible for the control and coordination of many biological processes. In the amphibian, for example, the action of TSH on the thyroid is responsible for inducing metamorphosis; in the mammal TSH plays an important role in thermogenesis.

A number of in vivo bioassays measure TSH activity. The effect on amphibian metamorphosis is absolutely specific but is difficult to quantitate. Another method monitors the release of ^{131}I in response to TSH from the thyroid glands of mice or chicks pretreated with T_4 to inhibit the secretion of endogenous TSH from the pituitary gland. The depletion by TSH of stored radiolabeled iodide from thyroid slices is the basis for an in vitro assay of the hormone. Thyrotropin binds to thyroid cell plasma membranes. This binding correlates with adenylate cyclase activation and cyclic AMP formation thus implicating this second messenger in the biological action of this hormone. The role of TSH in the control of thyroid function and the details of its mechanism of action are discussed in Chapter 13.

Thyrotropins of mammalian origin stimulate thyroid activity in all vertebrates except cyclostomes, and pituitary extracts of nonmammalian vertebrates stimulate mammalian thyroid glands. The amino acid composition of turtle TSH is strikingly similar to that of bovine TSH [28]. Purified lutropin of mammals possesses intrinsic TSH activity when tested on teleost thyroid glands. This observation supports the suggestion that the primitive glycoprotein may have been an LH-like molecule that became modified during evolution into a TSH-like molecule [11].

Lutropin. The gonads—the ovaries and the testes—secrete steroid hormones that regulate the growth and development of a variety of target tissues. In many animals hypophysectomy leads to atrophy of the gonads and extracts of the pituitary cause recrudescence of the gonads of hypophysectomizd animals. These experiments implicate the pituitary gland in the control of gonadal function. Originally two pituitary fractions possessing gonadotropic activity were obtained. One of these stimulated follicular growth in the ovaries and increased spermatogenic activity in the testes. This hormone is now referred to as follicle stimulating hormone (FSH) or follitropin. The other factor, referred to as luteinizing hormone (LH) or lutropin, stimulated corpora lutea formation and ovulation in the female and stimulated testosterone secretion and development of secondary sexual characteristics in the male.

Like TSH, LH is composed of two chemically dissimilar glycoprotein subunits which individually are inactive. These subunits may, however, be recombined with resultant regeneration of full biological activity of the hormone. The α-subunit of ovine LH consists of 96 amino acids and is identical in structure to that of bovine TSH-α. Two carbohydrate moieties are linked to asparagine residues within the two proteins. Although ovine LH-α and LH-β differ considerably in their primary amino acid sequence, there are, nevertheless, many sequence similarities between the two subunits. Both contain a large number of disulfide bonds which suggest that their structures are tightly coiled. Ovine LH-β is 120 amino acids in length and is similar to bovine TSH-β which consists of 113 residues. The two structures are likely derived from a common ancestral molecule. The biological activities of the LH-α- and LH-β-subunits are negligible in comparison to the intact LH molecule.

LH stimulates testosterone synthesis by the interstitial cells of Leydig of the testes. The action of LH is dependent on FSH induction of Leydig cell LH receptors. Indirectly LH stimulates spermatogenesis by way of its effect of testosterone biosynthesis which is required for maturation of the germ cells. In the human female LH induces ovulation and is necessary for the initial development of the corpus luteum (Chapters 18 and 19).

Follitropin. After many initial difficulties, a gonadotropic hormone separate from LH was obtained. FSH is responsible for the early development of the ovarian follicle in the female and for the initial steps of spermatid maturation in the male. The role of FSH in the male is twofold: (1) To increase the LH receptor population of testicular Leydig cells so that they are sensitive to the actions of LH; (2) To act in concert with LH to stimulate spermatogenesis. Specifically FSH stimulates synthesis of a testicular (Sertoli cell) androgen-binding protein. FSH interacts with granulosa cells of the developing follicle, and its actions are mediated through cAMP. The biological roles and mechanisms of action of FSH are discussed later (Chapters 17 and 18).

The α-subunit of human FSH consists of 92 amino acids and contains two carbohydrate moieties [36]. The primary amino acid sequence of hFSH-β is 118 residues long, and there are two carbohydrate moieties attached to asparagine at positions 7 and 24. The total carbohydrate content of hFSH is 27.2%. The structure of the carbohydrate moiety attached to position 78 of the α-subunit of hFSH has been determined. Removal of sialic acid and other carbohydrate moieties from hFSH-α results in loss of biological activity of the recombinant hormone. The primary structures of the ovine follitropin α- and β-subunits have been determined. The α-subunit structure of ovine FSH is identical to that of ovine LH [36]. The amino acid sequence of the follitropin β-subunit is very similar to that of the β-subunit of human, porcine, and equine origin [38]. Many amino acid residues of the ovine follitropin β-subunit are identical to those in ovine lutropin and thyrotropin β-subunits.

Nonmammalian Gonadotropins.   Two chemically distinct gonadotropin molecules have been isolated from the pituitaries of representatives of each class of tetrapods [27]. Members of certain orders or vertebrates may possess only one functional gonadotropin. The two gonadotropic hormones of nonmammalian tetrapods appear to be homologous to the FSH and LH of mammals. Although biochemical data suggest structural conservatism of FSH and LH among different species, important differences in their biological activities are apparent. Nonmammalian gonadotropins, for example, are without significant activity on mammalian tissues and mammalian hormones are not always fully active on nonmammalian species. Phylogenetic specificity is related, in part, to differing affinities of the various gonadotropins for binding sites on target tissues. Present evidence suggests that each gonadotropin may not play the same physiological role in all tetrapods.

Pro-opiomelanocortin: Corticotropin and Melanotropin

Corticotropin and α-melanotropin are hormones of the pituitary that share some structural similarity. Although ACTH has been associated with the corticotroph cells of the pars distalis, this hormone can also be demonstrated within cells of the pars intermedia by immunocytochemical methods. The pars intermedia is the major source of a melanotropin that controls integumental melanocyte melanin production in many vertebrates. Nevertheless melanotropins have been found within the corticotroph cells of the pars distalis. A β-lipotropin (β-LPH) of pars distalis origin was first described by Li in 1964, but the physiological significance of this polypeptide (Fig. 21.3) was not discerned until many years later [25]. β-LPH is now realized to be a component of an even larger precursor molecule referred to as pro-opiomelanocortin (Fig. 8.4). Within the structure of this precursor protein is the amino acid sequence of ACTH and possibly other hormonally important peptides [22]. In addition within the molecule of β-LPH is found the amino acid sequence of a so-called β-melanotropin (β-melanocyte stimulating hormone, β-MSH). There is no evidence, however, that this melanotropic peptide is cleaved from the parent molecule and plays any normal hormonal role (Chapter 8). The C-terminal 61–93 sequence of bovine β-LPH is referred to as β-endorphin and the smaller 61–65 sequence is referred to as methionine enkephalin (Fig. 21.3). Both β-endorphin and met-enkephalin function within the nervous system as neurohormones, perhaps as the analgesic hormones of humans (Chapter 21). Within the pars distalis enzymes within corticotrophs split the ACTH sequence from the precursor protein. In the pars intermedia, on the other hand, enzymes release the tridecapeptide sequence of α-MSH (Fig. 8.3) from the pro-opiomelanocortin molecule. The remaining components of the precursor protein are released with ACTH or α-MSH during vesicular exocytosis. The presence of pro-opiomelanocortin within corticotrophs of the pars distalis and melanotrophs of the pars distalis accounts for the confusion of MSH and ACTH together within each of these cell types.

Both α-MSH and ACTH possess similar sequences within their structures (Fig. 8.1), which is why each hormone stimulates the target tissues of the other hormone, melanocytes, and adrenal glands, respectively. As in the mammalian pituitary, there is evidence in other species for the biosynthesis of a pro-opiomelanocortin. The salmon pituitary, it has been found, produces two precursor molecules that are coded on two separate genes. A calcitoninlike substance is present in porcine pituitary glands, as demonstrated by RIA and immunohistochemistry. It is interesting that a number of amino acids in the pro-opiomelanocortin precursor are homologous with the structure of calcitonin. The observed homology between the precursor and calcitonin may suggest the evolution of some neuropeptides from a precursor molecule common also to the evolution of the calcitonins. β-Lipotropin has been isolated from the fin whale pituitary and chemically characterized [20]. The proposed primary structure of whale β-LPH differs from the ovine LPH only at four amino acid residues. The β-endorphin segment (residues 61–91) is identical to that of ovine β-LPH. The total number of residues in β-LPH differs among species: human (89), ovine (91), bovine (93), porcine (91), ostrich (90), fin whale (91).

Corticotropin. The steroidogenic tissues of the adrenal glands secrete a number of steroid hormones that profoundly affect carbohydrate and mineral metabolism. In most mammals steroidal tissue surrounds the adrenal medulla to form the so-called adrenal cortex. Hypophysectomy results in atrophy of the adrenal cortex. The steroidogenic tissue of the hypophysectomized animal is restored in animals receiving replacement therapy with pituitary extracts. Purification of pituitary preparations led to the isolation and structural characterization of an adrenal cortical stimulating hormone (ACTH), adrenocorticotropin or corticotropin, as it is also designated.

Corticotropin is synthesized within basophils of the pars distalis. Unlike the glycoprotein-containing basophils that synthesize TSH, FSH, and LH, the corticotroph cells are often chromophobic, and are sometimes considered to be chromophobes. Certain chromophobic basophils may represent very active corticotrophs that are essentially degranulated. Certain adenoma cells associated with Cushing's disease are, on the other hand, intensely PAS-positive. The glycoprotein present within these cells is not directly related to ACTH but is apparently a component of the precursor molecule of ACTH.

Corticotropin is the smallest peptide hormone of the anterior pituitary and is composed of a single linear chain consisting of 39 amino acids [34]. Thus far this chain length is a consistent feature of all species of ACTH. Structural differences between species are only found between residues 24–33, and these differences in mammals only amount to one or two residue differences (at position 31 and 33) between any two species (Fig. 5.8). A shark (*Squalus acanthias*) corticotropin is also 39 amino acids long but differs at 11 positions from the human hormone. Ostrich (*Struthio camelus*) ACTH is similar in length to other corticotropins and differs from human ACTH at only five residues.

The synthesis of a biologically active nonadecapeptide, corresponding to the first 19 amino-terminal residues of ACTH, and the subsequent total synthesis of the porcine ACTH were landmarks in the field of peptide hormone synthesis. $ACTH_{1-24}$ is commercially available and is the form generally used for studies on ACTH action, as the biological activity resides within this invariant 1–24 sequence of the hormone.

As its name implies the major role of ACTH is to stimulate steroid biosynthesis within adrenal steroidogenic tissue. Cortisol and corticosterone are the major glucocorticoids produced by the adrenal gland in response to ACTH stimulation. These steroid hormones are important in carbohydrate metabolism. Excessive secretion of ACTH in humans leads to Cushing's disease, which is characterized by excessive plasma levels of cortisol and, therefore, pathological alterations in glucose metabolism (Fig. 15.15). The absence or diminished secretion of ACTH results in Addison's disease, a disorder characterized by deficits in cortisol production with severe consequences relative to altered cellular metabolism. Because the first 13 amino acids are similar to those comprising α-MSH, it is not surprising that ACTH possesses considerable melanotropic activity. Nevertheless there is no evidence that ACTH plays any normal role in the control of integumental melanocyte function. On the other hand, in primary Addison's disease and in Cushing's syndrome of secondary origin, where ACTH is secreted in excessive amounts, hyperpigmentation is also a visually obvious symptom. In these diseases the hyperpigmentation is probably due to the excessive levels of circulating ACTH. The heptapeptide sequence, -Met-Glu-His-Phe-Arg-Trp-Gly-, the active site of α-MSH, is responsible for the melanotropic activity of ACTH. In some species ACTH also possesses lipolytic activity, an action shared by other melanotropins. It is doubtful, however, whether this so-called adipokinetic action represents a physiological role of the hormone.

The action of ACTH on adrenal cortical cells, melanocytes, and adipose tissue

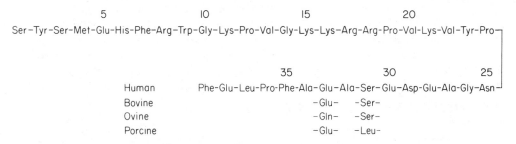

Figure 5.8 Comparative primary structures of the adrenocorticotropins.

cells is mediated through stimulation of adenylate cyclase and the subsequent formation of cyclic AMP. Older methods of bioassay for ACTH measured the effect of the hormone on the weight of the adrenals or on depletion of ascorbic acid in adrenals of hypophysectomized rats. More modern methods involve measuring the effect of the peptide on steroid synthesis by adrenal slices or by isolated adrenocortical cells. Corticotropin is also localized to certain neurons within the brain where it may function as a neuropeptide in processes related to memory and learning.

Melanotropin.   The pars intermedia is the source of a melanocyte stimulating hormone (α-MSH, α-melanotropin). The pituitary gland of the adult human lacks a pars intermedia, and this is correlated with the absence in humans of α-MSH in the pituitary and plasma. α-Melanotropin is present in the pituitary of other vertebrates and plays an important role in the skin coloration of many animals. α-MSH is composed of 13 amino acids (Fig. 8.1). The physiological roles of α-melanotropin are discussed in Chapter 8.

Neurohypophysial Hormones

Two nonapeptides, oxytocin and arginine vasopressin (AVP), are present in the neurohypophysis of humans. Each of these hormones is separately synthesized in different neurohypophysial neurons. Each neurohypophysial hormone is derived from a prohormone, oxyphysin or pressophysin, which is synthesized within cell bodies located within the paired paraventricular and paired supraoptic nuclei of the hypothalamus (Fig. 5.5). Oxytocin- and AVP-containing vesicles travel from the sites of synthesis within the hypothalamic nuclei by axoplasmic flow to axon terminals within the pars nervosa where they are stored until released.

The neurohypophysial hormones are released into the circulation to travel to their distant target tissues. Oxytocin plays an instrumental role in stimulating milk release from the mammary gland through an action on contractile elements (myoepithelial cells) of the breasts. Oxytocin may also stimulate uterine contraction at term and therefore provide a major endocrine stimulus to the process of parturition. Vasopressin plays an essential role in water retention (and therefore blood pressure) by its action on the collecting tubules of the kidney. Two or more neurohypophysial hormones are present in the neurohypophysis of each vertebrate species except cyclostomes (lampreys and hagfishes) which possess but a single such principle, arginine vasotocin (AVT). The structures of the individual neurohypophysial hormones (oxytocin, lysine and arginine vasopressin, vasotocin, mesotocin, isotocin, and others) from a number of species have been determined and the possible pathways of their structural evolution described. The roles and actions of the neurohypophysial hormones are discussed in Chapter 7.

PITUITARY PATHOPHYSIOLOGY

Pituitary dysfunction may involve undersecretion of oversecretion of one or more hypophysial hormones. Hyposecretion of pituitary hormones may result from destruction of normal glandular cells within the pituitary by an expanding tumor, disruption of hypothalamo-pituitary vascular connections, or damage or disease of the hypothalamus. Hypersecretion, on the other hand, may result from neoplasia (pituitary tumors) or from hypertrophy and hyperplasia, resulting from enhanced hypothalamic stimulation of the pituitary. Hypersecretion of α-MSH or PRL could result plausibly from loss of a tonic hypothalamic inhibitory input to the pituitary (Chapter 6).

Panhypopituitarism, which involves total loss of hypophysial hormone secretion, could be due to a congenital dysfunction—failure of the pituitary to develop—or to destruction of the already present pituitary at a later stage in life. It is also possible that the pars distalis might fail to secrete only one of its many hormones. Hypopituitary dwarfism may result, for example, from the specific failure of the pituitary to secrete STH, although the etiological basis for such a discrete endocrinopathy is not well understood. Microadenomas, on the other hand, may be responsible for the excess secretion of a particular pituitary hormone. Microadenomas composed of PRL-secreting cells are the most common pituitary neoplasms of rats and humans. Although some patients may have astronomical levels of serum PRL, not all develop galactorrhea. Other hormones, such as estrogens and corticosteroids, along with PRL may be responsible for its development. Amenorrhea, anovulation, and galactorrhea are all common sequelae of excess PRL secretion, and hypogonadism occurs in many hyperprolactinemic adult females. Hypersecretion of PRL is inhibitory to pituitary gonadotropin secretion, which accounts for the loss of gonadal function associated with the galactorrhea-amenorrhea syndrome. If PRL-secreting adenomas are selectively removed by surgical techniques, normal menses return.

The pivotal role of PRL in mammary gland growth and differentiation is well established [21]. In addition there is substantial evidence that PRL is a causative factor in mammary gland neoplasia of rodents and possibly of humans [6]. Nevertheless at present the possible role of PRL in the development and progression of breast cancer is little understood. There is evidence that PRL in conjunction with sex steroids contributes to accelerated malignant mammary growth as indicated by the more fulminant course of breast cancer during pregnancy [31].

There are no reported examples of overproduction or underproduction of oxytocin. Vasopressin secretion may, however, be excessively secreted or not secreted at all. In the Brattleboro strain of rats, for example, the animals do not secrete any vasopressin, and this defect is correlated with an absence of AVP within neurons of the neurohypophysis. In the syndrome of inappropriate ADH (AVP) secretion, excess amounts of AVP are secreted without relationship to plasma osmolality (Chapter 7).

Although excess secretion of pituitary hormones may result from a defect at the pituitary or hypothalamic level, pituitary hormones may be secreted by tumors of nonpituitary origin. Thus *ectopic* production of excessive amounts of ACTH by certain lung tumors may be responsible for the etiology of Cushing's disease where the adrenal cortex releases excessive amounts of cortisol in response to the ACTH of ectopic tumor origin. Elevated plasma levels of β-LPH and ACTH are frequently observed in blood and tumor tissue of patients with various types of carcinoma. Because β-LPH and ACTH are components of a larger pro-opiomelanocortin precursor, it is not surprising that these peptides are elaborated together by neoplastic tissues. A common cause of excessive AVP secretion is malignancy, where AVP is secreted from a carcinoma of the lung.

Pituitary Pathophysiology

TABLE 5.2.   Some Examples of Pituitary Pathophysiology

Hormone	State of Hormone Secretion	Symptom
All hormones	No pituitary hormones (empty sella syndrome)	Panhypopituitarism
Somatotropin (STH)	Deficiency (childhood)	Dwarfism
	Excess	
	child	Gigantism
	adult	Acromegaly
Prolactin (PRL)	Deficiency	No disease states reported
	Excess	Hyperprolactinemia-galactorrhea-amenorrhea syndrome
Thyrotropin (TSH)	Deficiency	
	child	Hypothyroidism (cretinism)
	adult	Hypothyroidism (myxedema)
	Excess	Hyperthyroidism (thyrotoxicosis, Graves' disease)
Follitropin (FSH)	Deficiency	Hypogonadism, failure of germ cell maturation
	Excess	No information available
Lutropin (LH)	Deficiency	Hypogonadism, failure of sexual maturation
	Excess	No information available
Corticotropin (ACTH)	Deficiency	Addison's disease
	Excess	Cushing's disease (hypercortisolism)
α-Melanotropin (MSH)	Not present in the adult human	
Oxytocin	Deficiency	No information available (necessary for milk secretion)
	Excess	No disease states reported
Vasopressin (AVP, ADH)	Deficiency	Diabetes insipidus (excessive water loss, dehydration)
	Excess	Syndrome of inappropriate ADH secretion (hypertension)

Tumors of patients with acromegaly may secrete STH and PRL, which suggests that these tumors may represent discrete mixed adenomas. There is no evidence that a common pituitary stem cell persists beyond the prenatal period. When more than one hormone is found within a certain tumor, they are usually those most related structurally, that is, PRL and GH or TSH, FSH, and LH. During the induction and progression of pituitary neoplasms, secretion of more than one hypophysial hormone is common. Ectopic secretion of PRL occurs from cancers of nonhypophysial origin (e.g., brochogenic or nephrogenic sources). Table 5.2 summarizes the major physiological defects related to the pathophysiology of the pituitary gland.

REFERENCES

[1] BAKER, B. L. 1977. Cellular composition of the human pars tuberalis as revealed by immunocytochemistry. *Cell Tiss. Res.* 182:151–63.

[2] BERGLAND, R. M., and R. B. PAGE. 1979. Pituitary-brain vascular relations: a new paradigm. *Science* 204:18–24.

[3] BOOTHBY, M., R. W. RUDDON, C. ANDERSON, D. McWILLIAMS, and I. BOIME. 1981. A single gonadotropin α-subunit gene in normal tissue and tumor-derived cell lines. *J. Biol. Chem.* 256:5121–27.

[4] CHILDS (MORIARITY), G. W., D. G. ELLISON, and L. L. GARNER. 1980. An immunocytochemist's view of gonadotropin storage in the adult male rat: cytochemical and morphological heterogeneity in serially sectioned gonadotropes. *Am. J. Anat.* 158:397–409.

[5] CLARKE, W. C., and H. A. BERN. 1980. Comparative endocrinology of prolactin. In *Hormonal proteins and peptides*, vol. VIII, ed. C. H. Li, pp. 105–97. New York: Academic Press, Inc.

[6] CLIFTON, K. H., and J. FURTH. 1980. Mammotropin effects in tumor induction and growth. In *Hormonal proteins and peptides*, vol. VIII, ed. C. H. Li, pp. 75–103. New York: Academic Press, Inc.

[7] DAUGHADY, W. H., and P. E. CRYER. 1978. Growth hormone hypersecretion and acromegaly. *Hosp. Prac.* August: 75–80.

[8] ELLIS, S., M. A. VODEAN, and R. E. GRINDELAND. 1978. Studies on the bioassayable growth hormone-like activity of plasma. *Rec. Prog. Horm. Res.* 34:213–38.

[9] FARMER, S. W., H. PAPKOFF, T. HAYASHIDA, T. A. BEWLEY, H. A. BERN, and C. H. LI. 1976. Purification and properties of teleost growth hormone. *Gen. Comp. Endocrinol.* 30:91–100.

[10] FARMER, S. W., H. PAPKOFF, T. A. BEWLEY, T. HAYASHIDA, R. S. NISHIOKA, H. A. BERN, C. H. LI. 1977. Isolation and properties of teleost prolactin. *Gen. Comp. Endocrinol.* 31:60–71.

[11] FONTAINE, Y. A., and E. BURZAWA-GERARD. 1977. Esquisse de l'évolution des hormones gonadotropes et thyrotropes des vertébrés. *Gen. Comp. Endocrinol.* 32:341–47.

[12] FRANTZ, A. G. 1978. Prolactin. *New Engl. J. Med.* 298:201–7.

[13] GREEN, J. D. 1951. The comparative anatomy of the hypophysis with special reference to its blood supply and innervation. *Amer. J. Anat.* 88:225–311.

[14] GREEP, R. O. 1974. History of research on anterior hypophysial hormones. In *Handbook of physiology*, section 7, vol. 4, part 2, eds. R. O. Greep and E. B. Astwood, pp. 1–27. Washington, D.C.: Am. Physiological Soc.

[15] GUILLEMIN, R., and R. BURGUS. 1972. The hormones of the hypothalamus. *Sci. Amer.* 227:24–33.

[16] HAYASHIDA, T. 1975. Immunochemical and biological studies with antisera to pituitary growth hormones. In *Hormonal properties and peptides*, Vol. III, ed. C. H. Li, pp. 40–146.

[17] HERLANT, M. 1964. The cells of the adenohypophysis and their functional significance. *Intern. Rev. Cytol.* 17:299–382.

[18] HOLMES, R. L., and J. N. BALL. 1974. *The pituitary gland*. Cambridge, England: Cambridge Univ. Press.

[19] JAFFE, R. B., ed. 1981. *Prolactin*. New York: Elsevier North-Holland, Inc.

[20] KAWAUCHI, H., D. CHUNG, and C. H. LI. 1980. Isolation and characterization of β-lipotropin from fin whale pituitary glands. *Int. J. Peptide Protein. Res.* 15:171–76.

[21] KIM, U., and J. FURTH. 1976. The role of prolactin in carcinogenesis. *Vitamin Horm.* 34:107–36.

[22] KRIEGER, D. T., A. S. LIOTTA, M. J. BROWNSTEIN, and E. A. ZIMMERMAN. 1980. ACTH, β-lipotropin, and related peptides, in brain, pituitary, and blood. *Rec. Prog. Horm. Res.* 36:277–344.

[23] LEWIS, V. J., R. N. P. SINGH, G. F. TRITWILER, M. B. SIGEL, E. F. VANDERLAAN, and W. P. VANDERLAAN. 1980. Human growth hormone: a complex of proteins. *Rec. Prog. Horm. Res.* 36:477–508.

[24] LI, C. H. 1975. The chemistry of pituitary growth hormone: 1967–1973. In *Pituitary proteins and peptides*, vol. III, ed. C. H. Li, pp. 1–40. New York: Academic Press, Inc.

[25] ———. 1978. The chemistry of melanotropins. In *Hormonal proteins and peptides*, vol. V, ed. C. H. Li, pp. 1–13. New York: Academic Press, Inc.

[26] ———. 1980. The chemistry of prolactin. In *Hormonal proteins and peptides*, vol. VIII, ed. C. H. Li, pp. 1–36. New York: Academic Press, Inc.

[27] LICHT, P. H., H. PAPKOFF, S. W. FARMER, C. H. MULLER, H. W. TSUI, and D. CREWS. 1977. Evolution of gonadotropin structure and function. *Rec. Prog. Horm. Res.* 33:169–248.

[28] MacKENZIE, D. S., P. LICHT, and H. PAPKOFF. 1981. Purification of thyrotropin from the pituitaries of two turtles: the green sea turtle and the snapping turtle. *Gen. Comp. Endocrinol.* 45:39–48.

[29] MARTIN, J. B. 1973. Neural regulation of growth hormone secretion. *New Engl. J. Med.* 288:1384–93.

[30] MOORE, K. L. 1973. *The developing human*. Philadelphia: W. B. Saunders Company.

[31] NAGASAWA, H. 1979. Prolactin and human breast cancer: a review. *Europ. J. Cancer* 15:267–79.

[32] PARSONS, T. F., and J. G. PIERCE. 1979. Biologically active covalently cross-linked glycoprotein hormones and the effects of modification of the COOH-terminal region of their α subunits. *J. Biol. Chem.* 254:6010–15.

[33] PIERCE, J. G., and T. F. PARSONS. 1981. Glycoprotein hormones: structure and function. *Ann. Rev. Biochem.* 50:465–95.

[34] RAMACHANDRAN, J. 1973. The structure and function of adrenocorticotropin. In *Hormonal proteins and peptides*, vol. II, ed. C. H. Li, pp. 1–28. New York: Academic Press, Inc.

[35] RIDDLE, O., R. W. BATES, and S. W. DYKSHORN. 1933. The preparation, identification and assay of prolactin—a hormone of anterior pituitary. *Am. J. Physiol.* 105:191–216.

[36] SAIRAM, M. R. 1981. Primary structure of the ovine pituitary follitropin α-subunit. *Biochem. J.* 197:535–39.

[37] SAIRAM, M. R. and C. H. LI. 1978. Chemistry of human pituitary thyrotropin. In *Hormonal proteins and peptides*, vol. VI, ed. C. H. Li, pp. 1–56. New York: Academic Press, Inc.

[38] SAIRAM, M. R., N. G. SEIDAH, and M. CHRÉTIEN. 1981. Primary structure of the ovine pituitary follitropin β-subunit. *Biochem. J.* 197:541–52.

[39] SCHREIBMAN, M. P., J. F. LEATHERLAND, and B. A. McKEOWN. 1973. Functional morphology of the teleost pituitary gland. *Amer. Zool.* 13:719–42.

[40] SEMOFF, S., and M. E. HADLEY. 1978. Localization of ATPase activity to the glial-like cells of the pars intermedia. *Gen. Comp. Endocrinol.* 35:329–41.

[41] TIXIER-VIDAL, A., and M. G. FARQUHAR, eds. 1975. *The anterior pituitary*. New York: Academic Press, Inc.

[42] VAMVAKOPOULOS, N. C., and I. A. KOURIDES. 1979. Identification of separate mRNA's coding for the α and β subunits of thyrotropin. *Proc. Natl. Acad. Sci.* 76:3809–13.

[43] VAN WYK, J. J., and L. E. UNDERWOOD. 1980. Growth hormone, somatomedins, and

growth failure. In *Neuroendocrinology*, eds. D. T. Kreiger and J. C. Hughes, pp. 299–309. Sunderland, Ma.: Sinauer Associates Inc.

[44] WEATHERHEAD, B. 1978. Comparative cytology of the neuro-intermediate lobe of the reptilian pituitary. *Zbl. Vet. Med. C., Anat. Histol. Embryol.* 7:84–96.

[45] ZIPF, W. B., A. H. PAYNE, and R. P. KELCH. 1978. Prolactin, growth hormone, and luteinizing hormone in the maintenance of testicular luteinizing hormone receptors. *Endocrinology* 103:595–606.

6

The Endocrine Hypothalamus

INTRODUCTION

In the embryonic development of the pituitary gland, ectoderm from the oral cavity and neuroectoderm from the brain evaginate and move toward each other to form the pituitary gland. There must be some physiological significance in that these two different tissues have become integrated into one functional component. As we have noted (Chapter 5) the pituitary gland is a rich source of hormones that controls a variety of physiological functions. Adrenocorticotropin secretion exhibits a diurnal (daily) rhythm and is also released in response to a variety of stresses. FSH and LH secretion fluctuates in a predictable pattern throughout the female menstrual cycle and, midway through the cycle, there is a pulsatile burst of LH release which is responsible for initiating ovulation. Oxytocin is released from the pituitary in response to suckling or sometimes during coitus. Somatotropin is secreted due to the ingestion of certain metabolic substrates.

Pituitary hormone secretions are clearly adaptive in nature as hormones play essential roles under conditions of special need. For example, the reproductive cycles of many animals are linked to seasonal changes in day length. The pelage color of the weasel is white in winter and brown the rest of the year. The weasel's coat color is regulated by pituitary melanocyte stimulating hormone. What are the cues which dictate whether or not a particular pituitary hormone will be secreted? Metabolic substrates, such as glucose, fatty acids, and amino acids, might serve as intrinsic cues to inform the pituitary of circulating levels of these substrates. But in vitro studies reveal that the pituitary is not directly sensitive to these substrates. Cold temperature is a stimulus to TSH secretion, and day length affects pituitary gonadotropin secretion. Obviously these extrinsic stimuli must be initially intercepted by the nervous system. A vast body of experimental data supports the view that the control of secretion of each of the pituitary hormones is regulated by the brain. This would explain the embryological processes related to the early development of the pituitary. In this chapter the evidence for a central nervous system control of pituitary function is reviewed and the specific roles of the *hypophysiotropic hormones* that control pituitary hormone secretion are examined.

THE NEUROVASCULAR HYPOTHESIS

Removal of the pituitary gland leads to atrophy of the adrenal cortex, thyroid, and gonads. Transplantation of the pituitary to an *ectopic* site in an animal, such as in the eye or under the kidney capsule, leads to a similar end-organ atrophy. Retransplantation of the pituitary back under the hypothalamus, however, is followed by revascularization and functional reactivation of the pituitary. Transection of the pituitary stalk or placement of a barrier between the hypothalamus and the pituitary leads to atrophy of the pituitary and its target organs. Subsequent revascularization of the pituitary leads to functional reactivation of the gland and its target organs. From these observations Harris concluded that it is "difficult to escape from the conclusion that the hypophysial portal supply has some specific effect in activating anterior pituitary tissue" [19]. Transplantation of pituitary tissue from young immature rats under the pituitary stalk of adult female rats resulted in the recurrence of normal, regular estrus cycles at a time when the donor young were still immature. The onset of pituitary-gonadotropic activity, it was concluded, probably depends on a hypothalamic influence rather than a maturation of pituitary or ovarian tissues. Even a pituitary from a young male animal could reactivate the pituitary-gonadal axis when transplanted into a female. According to Harris, the anterior pituitary tissue is plastic in nature and "its pattern of secretory activity is not due to any intrinsic property of the tissue itself, but to some outside 'drive' or stimulus, derived probably from the central nervous system."

These observations led Harris to elaborate the *neurovascular hypothesis*. He suggested that humoral factors released by the hypothalamus were carried by the portal blood vessels to the pituitary to regulate hormone secretion. Extacts of the brain, specifically the hypothalamus, will stimulate or inhibit secretion from the pituitary whether studied in vivo or in vitro. Lesions of specific areas of the hypothalamus, as induced by electrocautery, lead to specific defects in pituitary hormone secretion. Electrode stimulation of these same anatomical sites within the hypothalamus, on the other hand, leads to the release of a particular pituitary hormone.

Crude extracts of the hypothalamus provided early evidence that the hypothalamus contained factors which were inhibitory or stimulatory to pituitary hormone secretions. These extracts were further purified to yield subfractions that by bioassay inhibited somatotropin release or stimulated thyrotropin or gonadotropin secretion. Still further purification and physical methods of analysis provided information on the definitive structures of the so-called *hypophysiotropic factors* present in these extracts. The data from these studies have revolutionized the field of endocrinology [15, 43, 44].

STRUCTURE-FUNCTION OF THE ENDOCRINE HYPOTHALAMUS

The hypothalamus is the basal part of the diencephalon lying below the thalamus, as its name implies. The hypothalamus forms the walls and lower part of the third ventricle of the brain (Fig. 6.1). It includes the optic chiasm, the tuber cinereum, the infundibulum, and the mammillary bodies. The tuber cinereum is the part of the floor of the third ventricle which extends downward toward the infundibulum. The lower part of the tuber cinereum, which is richly supplied with blood vessels that drain into the pituitary stalk and then in turn empty into a secondary plexus in the anterior pituitary, is referred to as the *median eminence*. The vascular link between the median eminence and the pituitary is known as the *hypophysial portal system* (Fig. 6.2). Within the hypothalamus are clusters of neurons, *hypothalamic nuclei*, which are symmetrically located around the third ventricle. The supraoptic (SON) and paraventricular nuclei (PVN), for example, are composed of cell bodies whose axons extend into the median eminence and then into the neurohypophysis (Fig. 5.5). This particular nerve tract consisting of neuronal axons from the SON and PVN is the *supraopticoparaventriculohypophysial tract*. Other major nuclear groups within the hypothalamus include the ventromedial nuclei, the arcuate nucleus, lateral tuberal nuclei, and dorsomedial nuclei (Fig. 6.1).

The endocrine hypothalamus consists of *neurosecretory neurons* whose secretory activity provides the neurohormones (hypophysiotropic factors) that regulate adeno-hypophysial function [24]. These neurons are the elements of the *parvicellular* (Latin:

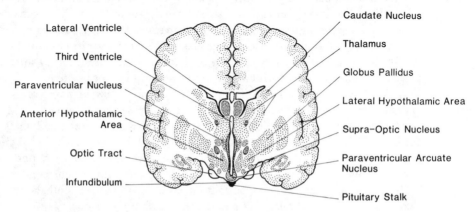

Figure 6.1 Frontal section through the cerebral hemispheres of the human brain: The principal hypothalamic nuclei present within the plane of transect are indicated.

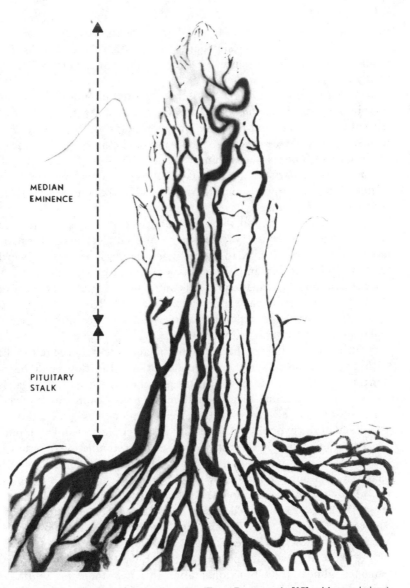

MEDIAN
EMINENCE

PITUITARY
STALK

Figure 6.2. Hypophysial portal system. (From Porter et al., [37], with permission.)

parvus, small) *neurosecretory system* and are distinguished from the *magnocellular system* of neurosecretory neurons that compose the supraoptic and paraventricular neurons which synthesize oxytocin and vasopressin. In contrast to the large cellular elements of the magnocellular system, the smaller parvicellular neuronal elements synthesize and secrete a number of hypophysiotropic hormones. These small hormone-secreting cells are distributed diffusely throughout the hypothalamus, and their specific anatomical distribution has not been easy to delineate. The neurons of the parvicellular neurosecretory system converge toward the pituitary stalk to form the

Structure-Function of the Endocrine Hypothalamus

tuberoinfundibular tract. These neurons abut on the endothelium of the primary plexus of the portal system of the median eminence. Immunocytochemical methods have demonstrated hypophysiotropic factors within these neurons. Electron microscopic studies provide evidence that these cells release their chemical messengers into the hypophysial portal system.

When pieces of pituitary tissue were grafted into various regions of the basal forebrain of rats, the *medial basal hypothalamus* (MBH) was capable of maintaining the normal structure and function of the pituitary grafts. The MBH was therefore named the *hypophysiotropic area* [18]. Apparently the integrity and secretory activity of pituitary cells implanted within this area is due to the local release of hypophysiotropins from the parvicellular neurons. The hypophysiotropic area extends from the median eminence upward and forward through the anterior hypothalamus to the suprachiasmatic region.

The endocrine hypothalamus is connected to the rest of the central nervous system by synaptic contacts from other neuronal elements. Information flow from other brain centers is relayed to hypothalamic parvicellular neurons which then secrete their hypophysiotropins into the pituitary portal vasculature of the median eminence. The median eminence can therefore be considered the final point of convergence of the CNS upon the peripheral endocrine system [24]. The hypophysial portal system provides a restricted vascular link between the neurosecretory cells of the hypothalamus and the anterior pituitary gland [51].

The most rigid proof that the hypothalamus does indeed release hormones into the hypophysial portal system to regulate pituitary function would be the demonstration that such hormones are found in the portal vessels in higher concentrations than in the systemic circulation. Elegant methods involving cannulation of the hypophysial portal system and selective collection of portal blood has verified this thesis (Fig. 6.3) [37]. Each of the hypophysiotropins has been demonstrated within portal blood; the concentration of these hormones is increased after stimulation of certain hypothalamic sites. In addition infusion of hypophysiotropins by portal cannulation induces secretion of pituitary hormones.

To determine the functional relationship of the medial basal hypothalamus to the rest of the brain, a knife was designed by Halász and colleagues that cut all the neural connections between the MBH and the remainder of the forebrain. This knife left the MBH in continuity with the pituitary gland and supposedly left most of the blood supply to the MBH and the pituitary intact. Nevertheless, the hypophysiotropic area remained almost fully functional after this *hypothalamic deafferentation.* This suggests that the cells of origin of the hypophysiotropins reside mostly if not entirely within the MBH [18].

The importance of hypothalamic humoral factors in the control of pituitary function was uniquely demonstrated by ectopic transplantation of the adenohypophysis under the kidney capsule [9]. Although the adenohypophysis becomes well vascularized in this site, most of the gland atropies due to generalized hypoactivity of most cellular elements of the gland. The prolactin cells, however, become hyperplastic. The systemic effects of adenohypophysial inactivity include end-organ atrophy of the gonads, adrenals, and thyroid gland. On the other hand, there is "functional reactivation and cytological restoration of pituitary grafts by continuous local

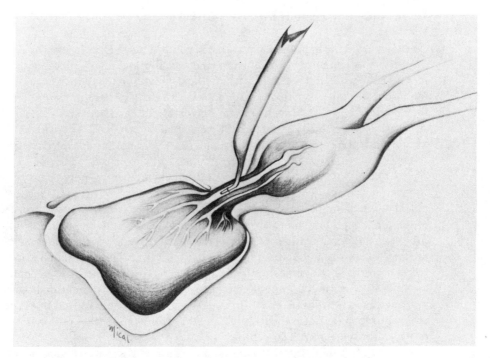

Figure 6.3 Technique for cannulation of the hypophysial portal system. (From Porter et al., [37], with permission.)

intravascular infusion of median eminence extracts." It was concluded that hypothalamic humoral factors of median eminence origin control the structure and function of the pituitary gland. This information has been reviewed extensively [29, 30, 32, 47].

THE HYPOPHYSIOTROPIC HORMONES

Stimulatory and inhibitory factors of hypothalamic origin are implicated in the control of pituitary hormone secretion. There is overwhelming evidence for a gonadotropin releasing hormone, thyrotropin releasing hormone, somatotropin release inhibiting hormone, and prolactin and MSH release inhibiting hormones. There is less information available relative to the existence of putative STH, PRL, and MSH releasing factors. In many cases the distribution of these hypophysiotropins within the CNS has been determined by radioimmunoassay of brain tissue. Brain tissue can be cut in a rostral-caudal direction and also laterally from side to side to provide a series of tissue slices. A small round (Palkovits) punch is used to obtain small samples of tissue from the brain slices. By radioimmunoassay one may determine the concentration of hypophysiotropins within these punch biopsies and then map the distribution of the neuropeptides within the brain. Using immunohistochemical methods involving antibodies against neuropeptides, one can localize hypophysiotropins to specific neurons within the brain.

Thyrotropin Releasing Hormone (TRH)

The structure of the hypothalamic hormone controlling TSH secretion was determined in 1969 independently by Guillemin and Schally and their colleagues. For this monumental work and the elucidation of the structures of the growth hormone release inhibiting hormone (somatostatin) and the gonadotropin releasing hormone (GnRH), they received a Nobel Prize in Physiology or Medicine. The task of elucidating the structure of TRH was not easy, but its eventual determination provides important insights into present-day methods of endocrine research. The episodes relating to the so-called race to Stockholm have been dramatically described [53].

From about 250,000 ovine and an equal number of porcine hypothalamic fragments, 1 mg each of TRH was obtained. These purified preparations, extremely potent in stimulating TSH release from the pituitary, both in vivo and in vitro, consisted of a simple peptide composed of three amino acids: glutamic acid, histidine, and proline in equimolar ratios. What was the exact sequence of the amino acids in the peptide? There was not enough material left to answer this essential question. It was therefore decided to synthesize the six possible putative isomers of the peptide (Fig. 6.4). Most surprisingly, none of the tripeptides possessed the chromatographic or biologic characteristics of TRH. It was discovered that there was no free N-terminal amino group in the natural tripeptide; in other words, the amino terminal group was protected in some way. The peptides were then treated with acetic anhydride in an effort to protect the NH_2-terminus, as in the natural TRH which lacked a free NH_2 group (Fig. 6.5). Only one of the peptides, Glu-His-Pro-OH, possessed biological activity that was, however, lower than that of the natural TRH. This product proved to be pyro-Glu-His-Pro-OH. The α-amino group of glutamic acid had condensed with the carboxyl group of the glutamic acid to give the pyroglutamic acid form of the peptide. This structure, however, was not identical to natural TRH which was more basic in nature. A more basic, less acidic compound could be obtained by protecting the free carboxyl group of the proline. Amidation of the C-terminal proline then yielded pyro-Glu-His-Pro-NH_2, whose activity was indistinguishable from that of natural TRH (Fig. 6.5). The structures of porcine, ovine, bovine, and human TRH proved to be identical in structure. The arduous task just outlined for the determination of the structure of TRH illustrates the important contributions of chemistry to the emerging field of neuroendocrinology.

Rat hypothalamic fragments synthesize TRH in vitro; synthesizing activity is present in the stalk median eminence and ventral hypothalamus. The TRH-synthesizing system appears to be enzymatic and involves a glutamic acid cyclase. Direct documentation of de novo TRH synthesis was obtained by incubating rat

NH_2–His–Pro–Glu—OH

NH_2–Pro–Glu–His—OH

NH_2–Pro–His–Glu—OH

NH_2–His–Glu–Pro–OH

NH_2–Glu–Pro–His —OH

NH_2–Glu–His–Pro–OH

(pyro)–Glu–His–Pro–NH_2

Figure 6.4 Six synthetic peptides related to thyrotropin releasing hormone (TRH).

The Endocrine Hypothalamus   Chap. 6

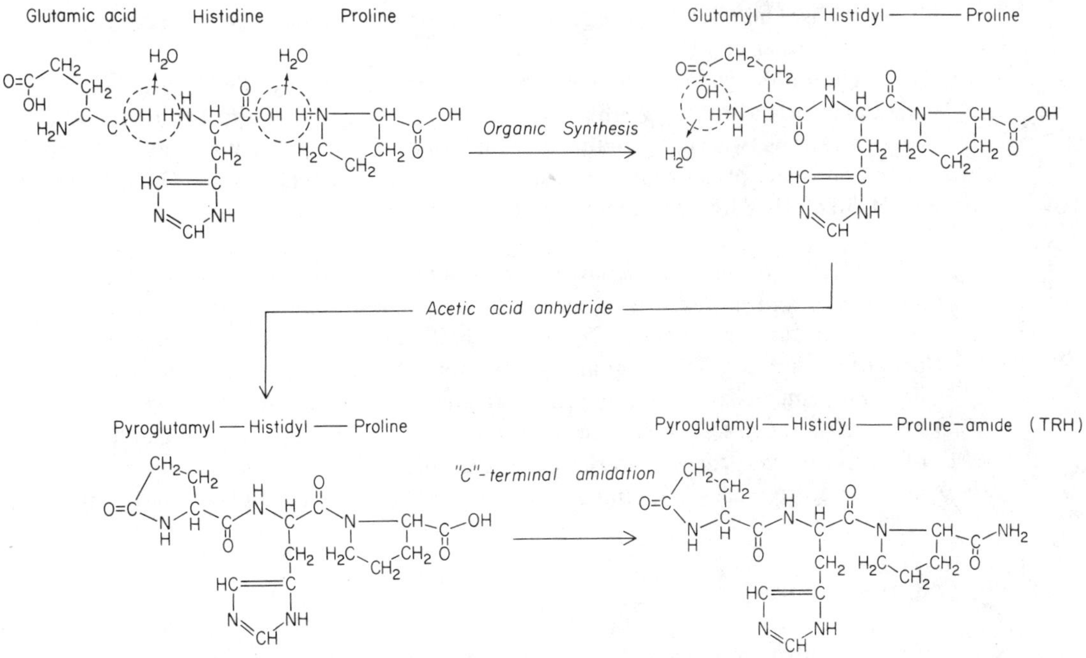

Figure 6.5 Synthesis of thyrotropin releasing hormone. (Modified from Studer, [48].)

hypothalamic fragments with radiolabeled precursor amino acids of TRH. The mechanism by which TRH is synthesized is special in that synthesis occurs enzymatically rather than by peptide translation from a messenger RNA. TRH immunoactive cell bodies have been localized within the brain. The highest concentration of TRH cells is found in the medial part of the external layer of the median eminence and extends laterally with high concentrations also found in the pituitary stalk. Electrical stimulation of the medial basal hypothalamus of the rat elevates plasma TRH levels, suggesting that there are neural structures within the hypothalamus which release preformed TRH.

TRH also stimulates the release of PRL in humans, cattle, sheep, and rats. TRH stimulates STH secretion in cattle and rats under certain specific conditions and in humans with acromegaly or chronic renal insufficiency. It is not known whether the TRH effect on PRL and STH secretion is physiological. TRH is rapidly degraded by plasma of adult rats but not by plasma from young (4- to 16-day-old) rats. The development of an active peptidase in rat plasma suggests that this may represent the physiological mechanism for the inactivation of TRH.

Although TRH is present in the CNS of teleosts, this tripeptide has not been clearly demonstrated to have hypophysiotropic activity in fishes. TRH can be detected in neural tissues of representatives of most classes of vertebrates, but its ability to promote TSH release is less universal than its occurrence [7]. TRH has been shown to cause prolactin release by the adenohypophysis of representatives of all tetrapod groups as well as teleosts and birds. The ability of TRH to stimulate TSH release, on the other hand, appears to be restricted to homeotherms. The ability of thyrotrophs to respond to TRH may be a recent evolutionary acquisition relative to that of the

The Hypophysiotropic Hormones   **119** lactotrophs. The TSH-releasing activity of the tripeptide may have emerged coincident with homeothermy [7].

The amphibian hypothalamus contains large amounts of TRH. In addition TRH circulates in the blood of the frog (*Rana pipiens*) and is present in the skin in concentrations twice those in the hypothalamus. The frog skin might be considered a huge endocrine organ that synthesizes and secretes this hormone. Thus the role of TRH, like other hypothalamic peptides, may not be limited to the central nervous system [22].

TRH is present in the larval lamprey (a cyclostome) and in the head end of amphioxus and has even been localized to the circumesophageal ganglia of a snail. Because the lamprey lacks TSH and the snail and amphioxus a pituitary, it has been proposed that the TSH-regulating function of TRH may be a late evolutionary development, an example where an organism acquires a new function for a preexisting hormone or chemical substance [21]. In addition TRH appears to regulate a variety of physiological processes in the CNS; the presence of the peptide in the brain does not, therefore, necessarily implicate its role in TSH secretion and thyroid function (Chapter 21).

Somatostatin

There is ample physiological and clinical evidence that the hypothalamus controls the secretion of somatotropin. A hypothalamic peptide that inhibits the release of STH from the anterior pituitary has been isolated and its primary structure determined [5]. This tetradecapeptide, referred to as somatostatin (SS) (or somatotropin release-inhibiting hormone), has been synthesized and determined to be chemically and biologically identical to the hypophysiotropic peptide (Fig. 6.6). The oxidized (ring) and the reduced (linear) forms of the peptide have full biological activity in vitro and in vivo.

Somatostatin has been localized by electron microscopic immunohistochemistry to secretory granules of neurons located within the hypothalamus. Although originally isolated from the hypothalamus, this peptide has been shown to have widespread effects on brain, endocrine and exocrine pancreas, and gut function. Furthermore, SS has a widespread distribution in the CNS and is also found localized to the D cells of the gut and exocrine pancreas. Somatostatin has an inhibitory effect on STH released in response to every known stimulus. The action of SS is directly on the pituitary somatotrophs.

A 28-residue prosomatostatin, a putative somatostatin precursor from the porcine hypothalamus, has been isolated, chemically characterized, and its primary structure determined (Fig. 6.7). After synthesis it was found to be chemically and biologically identical to the prosomatostatin isolated from the brain and gut [45]. This peptide possesses high somatotropin and prolactin release-inhibiting activity and may, in time, be shown to be a hormone in its own right.

Somatostatin also inhibits TRH-induced TSH secretion and at the same time

Ala–Gly–Cys–Lys–Asn–Phe–Phe–Trp–Lys–Thr–Phe–Thr–Ser–Cys

Figure 6.6 Primary structure of mammalian somatostatin.

Ser–Ala–Asn–Ser–Asn–Pro–Ala–Met–Ala–Pro–Arg–Glu–Arg–Lys–

                                                                     28
–Ala–Gly–Cys–Lys–Asn–Phe–Phe–Trp–Lys–Thr–Phe–Thr–Ser–Cys

Figure 6.7 Primary structure of
porcine prosomatostatin.

does not affect the concomitant secretion of prolactin triggered by TRH. This suggests
that the inhibitory action of SS is specifically on the thyrotrophs, not the lactotrophs.
A physiologic inhibitory role for SS in the regulation of TSH secretion in some species
is supported by the demonstration that anti-SS serum administered to rats enhances
the release of TSH due to cold or to exogenous TRH [51]. Somatostatin lowers blood
glucose levels and this is associated with an inhibition of glucagon and insulin
secretion. Other studies have shown that SS also inhibits secretion of the following:
renin, parathormone, calcitonin, gastric HCl, acetylcholine, adrenergic neurotransmitters, and TRH secretion from organ cultures of the rat hypothalamus. Somatostatin also inhibits blood platelet aggregation, brain cell electrical activity, and
parathormone receptor binding and other less clearly defined physiological processes.

Plasma STH levels fall and remain low for several hours after stress. Administra-
tion of SS antiserum to rats prior to stress partially restores the STH secretory pulses.
These results indicate that somatostatin plays a role in stress-induced inhibition of
STH secretion in the rat.

Somatostatin has been found in the brain and pancreas of the frog, catfish,
torpedo (an elasmobranch), and hagfish (a cyclostome). It is also present in the skin
and bladder of the frog. Incubation of pituitary glands of the teleost, tilapia
(*Sarotherodon mossambicus*), in the presence of synthetic SS resulted in a dose-
dependent decrease in STH secretion. These results suggest that STH secretion in
teleosts may be controlled by SS or an SS-like peptide [12]. An SS-like, but
structurally different peptide, has indeed been isolated from nervous tissue (urophysis)
of a teleost fish (Chapter 21).

Somatotropin Releasing Hormone (Somatocrinin)

A 44 amino acid peptide has been isolated from a human pancreatic tumor which
specifically stimulates STH secretion both in vitro and in vivo from the rat pituitary
gland (Fig. 6.8) The synthetic replicate has full biological activity and appears to be
similar in physicochemical properties to a still uncharacterized STH releasing peptide

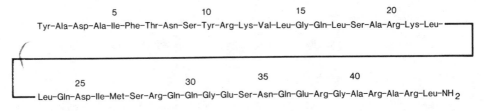

                    5   10   15   20
Tyr–Ala–Asp–Ala–Ile–Phe–Thr–Asn–Ser–Tyr–Arg–Lys–Val–Leu–Gly–Gln–Leu–Ser–Ala–Arg–Lys–Leu–

                  25   30   35   40
Leu–Gln–Asp–Ile–Met–Ser–Arg–Gln–Gln–Gly–Glu–Ser–Asn–Gln–Glu–Arg–Gly–Ala–Arg–Ala–Arg–Leu–NH$_2$

Figure 6.8 Primary structure of a putative somatotropin releasing hormone.

The Hypophysiotropic Hormones   **121** present in hypothalamic tissues [16, 40]. This peptide, hpGRF, or somatocrinin, possesses sequence homologues to several gut peptides of the secretin-glucagon family.

Gonadotropin Releasing Hormone (GnRH)

A vast amount of experimental evidence has established that the hypothalamus is stimulatory to pituitary gonadotropin secretion. GnRH has been detected in the nerve fibers and terminals in proximity to the portal vessels in the median eminence of the hypothalamus. The anatomical site of the cell bodies of these neurons has not been determined; they may reside outside the MBH, possibly in the medial preoptic area. The structure of GnRH was determined from extracts of 250,000 porcine hypothalami. The peptide was subsequently synthesized and found to act in an identical physiological manner to the putative hypothalamic peptide in all animals studied. Mammalian GnRH is a decapeptide whose primary structure appears to be similar between mammalian species (Fig. 6.9).

Deafferentation of the rat hypothalamus causes a marked reduction in the GnRH content of the MBH, which suggests that GnRH arises from or is controlled by cells elsewhere in the brain [6]. GnRH has been found in hypophysial portal blood in higher concentrations than in the systemic circulation. Portal GnRH levels are elevated after castration and following electrochemical stimulation of the hypothalamus. The role of GnRH in the control of pituitary gonadotropin secretion has been further confirmed by the use of immunization techniques. Injections of antibodies to GnRH are followed by testicular atrophy. Similarly, when GnRH antiserum is injected into female rats on the morning of proestrus, the preovulatory surge of LH release that normally follows in the afternoon does not occur, and ovulation is prevented (Chapter 18). Furthermore, administration of anti-GnRH serum administered to normal or castrated rats lowers LH and FSH levels, thus revealing the key role of the hypophysiotropin in maintaining the secretion of both gonadotropins [51].

Many questions surround the mechanism by which GnRH differentially stimulates FSH and LH secretion from folliculotrophs and luteotrophs at different times during the ovulatory cycle. There is strong experimental support for the view that only one GnRH (sometimes referred to as FSH/LH-RH) regulates the secretin of both LH and FSH. Nevertheless, the secretory ratio of FSH/LH differs considerably during the reproductive cycle. For example, GnRH mainly stimulates the secretion of

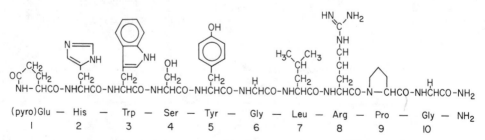

Figure 6.9 Primary structure of mammalian gonadotropin releasing hormone (GnRH).

LH at the time of ovulation, whereas at menstruation FSH release in response to GnRH occurs without a concomitant rise in LH. These results suggest that other modulators (e.g., steroid hormones, hypothalamic neurotransmitters) may act on pituitary FSH and LH cells in a differential way, thus altering the secretory FSH/LH ratio.

In the intact rhesus monkey GnRH appears to be released in a pulsatile manner. Although intermittent administration of GnRH may be optimal for reestablishing gonadotropin secretion in monkeys with hypothalamic lesions, constant infusions of GnRH fail to do so. Constant GnRH may lead to a desensitization or down regulation of the processes responsible for gonadotropin release (Chapter 18).

Crude hypothalamic extracts from birds, reptiles, teleosts, and amphibians contain significant GnRH activity. Hypothalamic extracts from lower vertebrates are biologically active in higher vertebrates, which suggests a lack of species specificity. Nevertheless, although amphibian GnRH may be identical to the mammalian peptide, GnRH's from birds, reptiles, teleosts, and elasmobranchs are structurally different. These latter peptides appear, however, to be identical to each other [23].

Synthetic GnRH has significant gonadotropic activity in mammals, birds, and amphibians. In the amphibian hypothalamic concentrations of GnRH vary with the seasonal reproductive cycle. A physiological role for GnRH has been demonstrated in teleosts [8]. Because GnRH may function in physiological processes in mammals, the demonstration of the presence of the peptide in the brain of nonmammalian species need not restrict its function to a reproductive role.

Corticotropin Releasing Hormone (CRH)

The first of the hypophysiotropic hormones to be investigated with great vigor was the putative corticotropin releasing hormone (CRH). The hypothalamus does contain a peptide factor which enhances ACTH release from the pituitary whether administrated in vivo or added to pituitaries incubated in vitro. Nevertheless, the chemical identification of this factor has remained elusive. The CRH-producing neurons have not been identified; they may reside outside the hypothalamus and CRH may be stored within their axon terminals within the medial basal hypothalamus [35]. Stimulation of the neural lobe, which provokes the release of neurohypophysial hormones, results in a significant increase in plasma ACTH levels [1]. In contrast, such stimulation elicits no significant change in circulating levels of ACTH in Brattleboro rats that have a hereditary diabetes insipidus due to a lack of vasopressin. Other experimental data suggested that vasopressin and CRH were similar but not identical in structure.

A peptide with high potency and intrinsic activity for stimulating the secretion of ACTH-like activity from cultured rat pituitaries has been isolated from ovine hypothalami and synthesized [52]. The structure of this 41-residue peptide, a putative CRH, is shown (Fig. 6.10) and is partially similar in structure to urotensin I, a peptide found within the spinal cord (urophysis) of a teleost fish (Fig. 21.11). Hypophysial portal blood obtained from rats contains a substance which is bound to an antiserum against synthetic ovine CRH. Antisera to the putative ovine CRH significantly lowers ACTH levels in adrenalectomized rats, suggesting that an endogenous CRH plays a physiological role in regulating pituitary ACTH secretion [39]. A peptide with CRH activity has also been isolated from porcine hypothalami [46].

```
1                                                                    20
Ser-Gln-Glu-Pro-Pro-Ile-Ser-Leu-Asp-Leu-Thr-Phe-His-Leu-Leu-Arg-Glu-Val-Leu-Glu-Met ─┐
                                                                                        │
                                                                                        │
                            30                                    41                    │
  ┌─ Thr-Lys-Ala-Asp-Gln-Leu-Ala-Gln-Gln-Ala-His-Ser-Asn-Arg-Lys-Leu-Leu-Asp-Ile-Ala-NH₂ ┘
```

Figure 6.10   Primary structure of a putative corticotropin releasing hormone (CRH).

Prolactin Release Inhibiting Factor (PIF)

There is abundant evidence that PRL secretion from the pars distalis is under an inhibitory control by the hypothalamus. When female rat anterior pituitaries are autotransplanted to extracranial sites, they selectively maintain functional corpora lutea while the remainder of the ovary atrophies, as do the adrenals and thyroid gland [33, 34]. In the rat, PRL is required for functional activation of the corpora lutea and progesterone biosynthesis. These results demonstrate that PRL secretion continues uninterrupted, whereas FSH, LH, and other anterior pituitary hormones are discontinued following ectopic transplantation. If after being autotransplanted under the kidney capsule for a month pituitaries are retransplanted back into close anatomical relationship with the median eminence, female rats return to normal cycling, which includes ovulation. If these recycling rats are mated, they will successfully carry litters to term.

Patients with pituitary stalk section or hypothalamic lesions also have elevated plasma levels of PRL. In the rat electrolytic lesions in the median eminence result in a large increase in PRL secretion. If anterior pituitary glands are incubated in vitro, PRL secretion commences immediately and continues uninterrupted almost indefinitely. Cytologically the lactotrophs hypertrophy under such conditions. None of the other hormones of the pars distalis is secreted and, with the exception of the lactotrophs, the other secretory elements of the glands atrophy and disappear from the incubated glands. Taken together, all these observations, both in vivo and in vitro, support the hypothesis that the hypothalamus is the source of a prolactin inhibiting factor, a so-called PIF.

The evidence is overwheming that this PIF is dopamine (DA) [11]. The presence of DA in hypophysial portal blood as well as in the anterior pituitary gland has been demonstrated. DA inhibits PRL secretion from pituitary glands incubated in vitro. In addition apomorphine or ergot alkaloids (e.g., ergocryptine), known DA receptor agonists, are inhibitory to PRL secretion in vitro or in vivo. This inhibition by DA and related agonists can be antagonized by chlorpromazine, haloperidol, and other DA receptor antagonists. In vivo injections of DA receptor antagonists result in increased PRL secretion. On the other hand, injections of L-dopa, a substrate for DA biosynthesis, are inhibitory to PRL secretion.

Prolactin Releasing Factor (PRF).   There is some experimental evidence for the existence of a PRL releasing factor. TRH, for example, is a potent stimulus to PRL secretion in virtually every vertebrate species studied [4]. It is unclear, however, whether TRH is the physiological PRF; there is evidence for a PRF of hypothalamic origin that is not TRH.

MSH Release Inhibiting Factor (MIF) (Melanostatin)

The role of the pars intermedia as the source of a melanotropin (α-MSH) that regulates color change in many animals is well established (Chapter 8). Like PRL, MSH is under an inhibitory control by the hypothalamus. Stalk transection or damage to the hypothalamus results in enhanced MSH secretion. Transplantation of the pars intermedia to an ectopic site in the animal also leads to enhanced MSH secretion. In addition incubation of neurointermediate lobes in vivo results in a sustained secretion of MSH. These results suggest that the hypothalamus exerts a tonic inhibitory control of MSH secretion.

What is the mechanism by which the hypothalamus tonically represses MSH secretion? In many vertebrates (e.g., frog and mouse) the pars intermedia is penetrated by aminergic neurons whose cell bodies are located within the hypothalamus. The axons of these neurons form a plexus around and between the pars intermedia cells. The release of a neurotransmitter, most likely dopamine, from these neurons is apparently responsible for inhibition of MSH secretion. In vitro, DA is inhibitory of MSH secretion from isolated pituitary glands (Chapter 8). Present evidence suggests that DA is the physiological MSH release-inhibiting factor (MIF, melanostatin). Contrary to some early reports, there is no evidence that Pro-Leu-Gly-NH$_2$, the tripeptide side chain of oxytocin, or any other peptide functions as an MIF[17]. There is minimal evidence for the existence of any putative hypothalamic MSH releasing factor (MRF) of peptidergic nature. In some species serotonin may be a factor regulating pars intermedia MSH secretion (Chapter 8).

CONTROL OF HYPOTHALAMIC-HYPOPHYSIAL HORMONE SECRETION

In response to cold many mammals release TSH, and in response to stress, ACTH is secreted from the pituitary gland. Suckling of the mammary gland stimulates PRL secretion, and somatotropin is released in response to intake of certain dietary metabolic substrates. These pituitary responses, as discussed, are regulated by hypophysiotropic factors. What factors and mechanisms regulate the secretion of the hypophysiotropins? Because the brain is composed mainly of neurons and supporting elements, other neurons within the brain would be expected to regulate the hypophysiotropin-secreting neurons [25]. These other neurons in turn may be linked to yet other neuronal inputs or to sensory neurons that are receptive to endogenous and exogenous cues.

Role of CNS Neurohormones

Extrinsic and intrinsic stimuli received through sensory neurons are conducted through neuronal routes to the brain where this information may be inhibitory or stimulatory to hypophysiotropic hormone secretion. Conduction of sensory information involves neuronal elements, and each one must release a neurotransmitter to affect synaptic transmission. These neurohormones include the well-studied monoamine neurotransmitters (Fig. 6.11) and the less characterized amino acid neurotransmitters

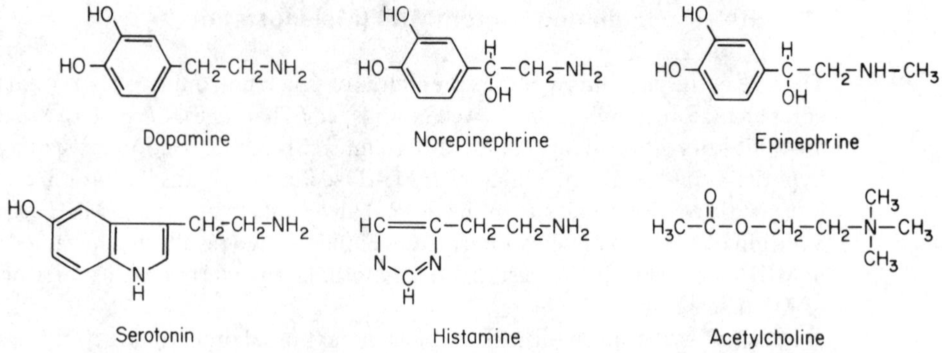

Figure 6.11   The monoamine neurotransmitters.

(Fig. 6.12) [54]. There are well-defined aminergic (monoamine) pathways within the brain which are composed of serotonergic, dopaminergic, noradrenergic, and even epinephrine-containing neurons. Axons from these neurons project from extra-hypothalamic sites into the hypothalamus where they innervate hypophysiotropic hormone-producing cells. Depending on the nature of the receptors possessed by these neurons, the neurotransmitters may inhibit or stimulate hypophysiotropin secretion from these peptidergic neurons. This will then be reflected in enhanced or inhibited pituitary hormone secretion. For example, inhibitory inputs to hypophysiotropic neurons containing inhibitory factors (MIF, PIF, SS) would be expected to enhance pituitary secretion of MSH, PRL, and STH.

Histamine is synthesized within the brain where it interacts with receptors (H_1 or H_2-type histamine receptors). Whether histamine is derived from histaminergic neurons to act as a neurotransmitter or released from mast cells is unclear. Nevertheless, histamine injected into the brain does affect the secretion of certain pituitary hormones, presumably through its action at the level of the hypothalamus. One method of partially determining the role of various neurotransmitters in the regulation of hypophysiotropin secretion is by *microiontophoresis*. This involves pipetting microliter quantities of a substance onto a group of neurons. *Single-unit iontophoresis* involves application of the agent onto single neurons.

Neurohormonal Control of Hypophysiotropin Secretion

Control of CRH Secretion.   It is unclear which transmitters and pathways play important regulatory roles in ACTH secretion, but there is evidence that a number of different neurotransmitters are involved [13]. Stress is a potent stimulus to ACTH

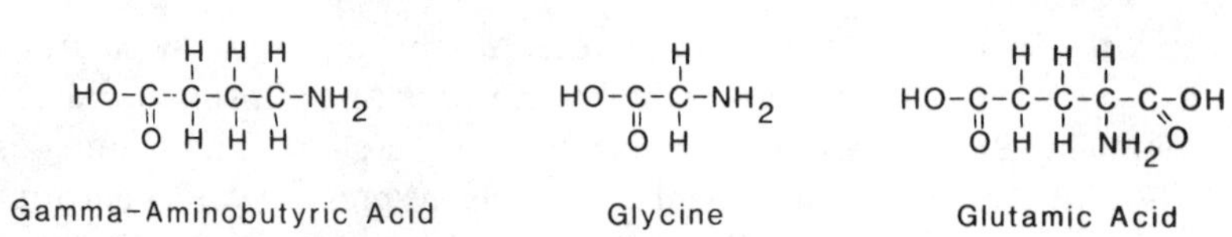

Figure 6.12   The amino acid neurotransmitters.

The Endocrine Hypothalamus   Chap. 6

secretion. This response is diminished by atropine implantations at sites within the hypothalamus thus implicating one or more cholinergic pathways (involving acetylcholine as neurotransmitter) in the control of ACTH secretion. Stimulation of CNS cholinergic structures provokes pituitary ACTH release. The particular cholinergic pathways have not been definitively determined [35]. Norepinephrine and epinephrine inhibit stress-induced ACTH secretion, which is blocked by the α-adrenergic antagonist clonidine. The actions of drugs or neurotransmitters that might affect CRH secretion can be studied by the addition of drugs to hypothalamic tissue incubated in vitro. The amount of CRH released into the medium from the tissue can then be determined by subsequent addition to pituitary glands incubated in vitro. The ACTH released from the pituitary corticotrophs can be monitored by radioimmunoassay or by its action on glucocorticoid production and release by cultured adrenal tissue (Fig. 6.13).

Control of PIF Secretion. During suckling direct tactile breast stimulation is the normal stimulus to PRL secretion. This neuroendocrine reflex involves the inhibition of dopaminergic neurons whose release of PIF maintains a tonic inhibition of PRL secretion. A number of neurotransmitters participate in the control of PRL secretion. PRL secretion increases during sleep and is entrained to sleep as a shift in the sleep cycle will shift the rhythm of PRL secretion (Fig. 5.6). The nocturnal rise in PRL secretion apparently involves activation of hypothalamic serotonergic (5-HT) neurons because administration of the 5-HT blocking agent, methysergide, blunts the increase in PRL secretion. In addition inhibitors of serotonin synthesis (e.g., p-chlorophenylalanine) abolish suckling-induced PRL release. There is an increased metabolism of brain 5-HT in suckled female rats and PRL secretion is enhanced following administration of 5-HT receptor agonists.

Gamma aminobutyric acid (GABA) may also function in the control of PRL secretion. Injections of GABA stimulate or inhibit PRL secretion depending on the concentrations employed. The stimulating effect of large doses of GABA is blocked by

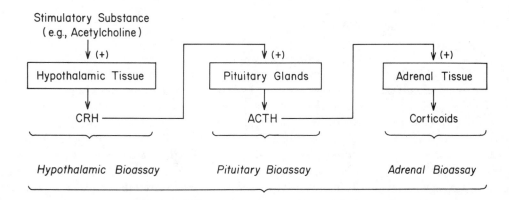

(*Corticotropin Releasing Hormone Bioassay*)

Figure 6.13 In vitro test system for the detection of corticotropin releasing hormone (CRH).

Control of Hypothalamic-Hypophysial Hormone Secretion

the GABA receptor antagonist, bicuculline. Vasoactive intestinal peptide (VIP) has been localized to nerve endings in the hypothalamus and is present in the hypo-thalamohypophysial portal blood. VIP receptors have been identified in a PRL-secreting tumor; the peptide stimulates cAMP production in the pituitary gland while stimulating PRL secretion. VIP may play a physiological role in the control of PRL secretion. There is some evidence for the role of the histaminergic system in the regulation of PRL secretion because intraventricular injections of histamine stimulate PRL secretion in rats, whereas blockage of histamine H_1 receptors prevents stimulation of PRL secretion in response to stress or suckling.

Control of Somatotropin Secretion. A variety of stimuli are stimulatory to STH secretion, presumably through inhibition of somatostatin secretion or by an enhancement of somatocrinin secretion. The participation of dopaminergic, nor-adrenergic and serotonergic systems in the control of STH has been reviewed [25], but the precise relationship of these neurotransmitter systems to somatostatin or to a putative STH-releasing hormone is presently unclear. Gastrin of GI tract or hypothalamic origin has been implicated in STH secretion (Chapter 10). α-Melano-tropin and related peptides are found in the hypothalamus, and α-MSH has also been implicated in the control of STH secretion (Chapter 8).

Control of GnRH Secretion. Catecholamines, most likely norepinephrine and dopamine, participate in the control of GnRH secretion. It is uncertain whether DA functions as an inhibitory or stimulatory neurotransmitter. The particular temporal action of DA on LH secretion may be dependent on the presence or absence of gonadal steroids. It is believed that noradrenergic neurons play a stimulatory role in the induction of the preovulatory surge of LH secretion. The role of 5-HT and histamine in the control of LH secretion is uncertain [38].

Control of TRH Secretion. Noradrenergic neurons stimulate TSH secretion apparently by a stimulatory action on TRH-secreting neurons. Little is known about the role of other neurohormones in the control of TRH secretion (see Chapter 21).

Feedback Mechanisms

In response to a hypophysiotropin, adenohypophysial hormones, such as TSH, ACTH, and the gonadotropins, are released into the general circulation where they circulate to their target tissues. Target tissue stimulation results in increased secretion of target tissue hormones, such as thyroid hormones (T_4 and T_3), adrenal glucocorti-coids (e.g., cortisol), and gonadal steroids (e.g., estradiol, testosterone, progesterone). These hormones then circulate to their respective target tissues to mediate their actions. The pituitary gland and the hypothalamus are themselves target organs of these steroid or thyroid hormones (Fig. 6.14). Three mechanisms of feedback control of hypophysiotropin and hypophysial hormone secretion are recognized. Peripheral target tissue hormones may feed back through a so-called *long-loop* system to act at the level of the pituitary or at the level of the hypothalamus or even higher brain centers (Fig. 6.15). Hypophysial hormones may also circulate by retrograde portal system blood flow to affect hypothalamic hypophysiotropic hormone secretion by a so-called *short-loop* mechanism. There is even evidence that secreted hypophysial hormones

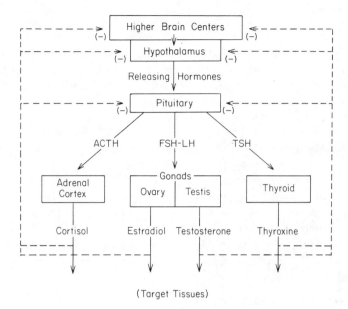

Figure 6.14 Feedback control of pituitary hormone secretion.

may feed back on their cells of origin to inhibit their own secretion, referred to as *autoinhibition* or *autofeedback inhibition* (Fig. 6.15).

Although some of the pituitary hormones, such as PRL, the neurohypophysial hormones, and α-melanotropin, stimulate peripheral target tissues, these target tissues do not themselves secrete hormones. The secretion of these hypophysial hormones therefore is not controlled by long-loop hormonal feedback mechanisms. The

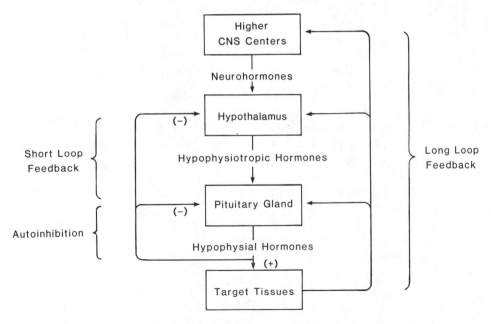

Figure 6.15 Model of long-loop and short-loop mechanisms and autoregulation of pituitary hormone secretion.

Control of Hypothalamic-Hypophysial Hormone Secretion

129

secretion of these hormones may, however, be controlled by reflex mechanisms and other sensory stimuli reaching the hypothalamus from sensory receptors. For example, suckling of the breast by the infant leads to secretion of oxytocin from the neurohypophysis. A decreased blood volume or increase in plasma electrolyte concentration is stimulatory to vasopressin secretion. It is becoming more evident that certain metabolic substrates (e.g., glucose, amino acids, FFAs) may also act at the level of the hypothalamus to affect hypophysiotropin secretion.

Steroid hormones implanted in the hypothalamus also modulate pituitary hormone secretion [28]. It can be demonstrated, using autoradiographic methods, that steroid hormones localize to specific sites within the CNS [10]. These feedback sites for steroid hormones may also represent production sites of the hypophysiotropins. Indeed, immunocytochemical methods have localized hypophysiotropins, such as GnRH and somatostatin, to these same hypothalamic steroid-binding sites. Neural steroid hormone receptors appear to be similar and probably identical to receptor systems from nonneural target tissues [28]. Steroid interaction with these receptors, as in peripheral tissues, is presumed to involve a subsequent action at the level of the gene, involving activation of RNA and protein synthesis (Chapters 4, 9, and 18).

Corticotropin Secretion. ACTH stimulates adrenal glucocorticoid production and secretion. Glucocorticoids, such as cortisol and corticosterone, and dexamethasone (a synthetic glucocorticoid) exert a negative feedback on ACTH secretion. Their locus of action is apparently at the level of both the pituitary and the hypothalamus as determined by the following experiments. Dexamethasone injected into the adenohypophysis inhibits ACTH secretion. Given prior to microinjection of exogenous CRH or hypothalamic extract directly into the pituitary, dexamethasone abolishes ACTH release in response to the hypophysiotropin. Finally CRH stimulation of ACTH secretion from pituitary glands incubated in vitro is inhibited by addition of corticosterone to the medium. CRH levels in the brain are increased after bilateral adrenalectomy; this change can be prevented by administration of exogenous glucocorticoids. Thus glucocorticoids act on the hypothalamus to modulate the turnover of hypothalamic CRH as well as acting directly on the pituitary.

Gonadotropin Secretion. Gonadectomy of an animal, such as the rat, results in an increased secretion of gonadotropins. Injections of gonadal steroids—estrogens or androgens—result in decreased circulating levels of gonadotropins in gonadectomized animals. These results suggest that gonadal steroids exert a negative feedback inhibition of gonadotropin secretion. Where are the sites of action of gonadal steroids in this feedback mechanism? This question has been partially answered by the use of radiolabeled gonadal steroids. Injections of [^{3}H]-estradiol, for example, result in an accumulation of the ligand within the hypothalamus; autoradiographic studies demonstrate that the hormone localizes over the nuclei of neurons in specific hypothalamic sites (Fig. 3.3). The radiolabeled hormone localizes to the same hypothalamic neurons that have been implicated in the control of pituitary gonadotropin secretion [49]. These results indicate that gonadal steroids regulate pituitary gonadotropin secretion through long-loop feedback to the hypothalamus. Gonadal steroids may also exert positive and negative feedback effects directly at the level of pituitary gonadotrophs (Chapter 18).

Implantation of luteinizing hormone (LH) or follicle stimulating hormone (FSH) into specific sites within the hypothalamus is reported to depress hypophysial LH and FSH secretion. These effects are suggested to be an example of a short-loop feedback mechanism. There is even evidence that secreted gonadotropins may feed back at the level of the pituitary to establish an autoinhibition: Both in vivo and in vitro, acute increases in blood or medium concentrations of LH inhibit basal and GnRH-stimulated LH secretion. This effect is gonadotropin specific as there is no inhibition of GnRH-stimulated LH secretion by FSH [36].

Prolactin Secretion. Injection of PRL or implantation of PRL into the median eminence of rats reduces the secretion of PRL from the pituitary. In some of these studies the hypothalamic content of PIF was found to be increased; these results suggested that a short-loop feedback system might regulate pituitary PRL secretion. There is other evidence that PRL can inhibit its own secretion by a direct action on the lactotrophs of the anterior pituitary gland.

Somatotropin Secretion. The central nervous system control of pituitary somatotropin (STH) secretion is believed to be mediated by a balance between somatostatin and somatocrinin. There is evidence that STH acts at the level of the hypothalamus to stimulate the synthesis and release of SS. Somatotropin mediates most of its effects indirectly through the stimulation of somatomedin production and release by the liver. The somatomedins then act on many tissues and organs to enhance growth. There is evidence that somatomedin *C* acutely stimulates SS release by the hypothalamus. Somatomedin *C* also exerts a much slower direct inhibitory effect on pituitary STH secretion. These observations suggest that somatomedin *C* participates in a long-loop negative feedback action on SS secretion by the hypothalamus as well as a slower long-loop action at the level of the pituitary [2].

Rhythms of Hypophysiotropin Secretion

During the process of evolution certain physiological processes of animals have become regulated by endogenous rhythms that are closely attuned to the daily periodicities of the light-dark cycle. The term *circadian* (Latin: *circa*, about; *dies*, day) was coined to describe these diurnal rhythms of activity. These endogenous rhythms undoubtedly evolved in response to the daily environmental light cycle; daily exogenous light cues, however, no longer act as the immediate cause of the *biologic rhythm*, but only as a synchronizing mechanism or *Zeitgeber* (time-givers). In the absence of environmental information the biological rhythm free-runs with its own frequency and can be entrained to a range of frequencies, however limited, that differ from the 24-hour cycle.

The control of biological rhythms is regulated by a so-called *biological clock* whose anatomical site may be the *suprachiasmatic nuclei* of the hypothalamus [31]. Because seasonal changes in animals may be triggered by changes in the length of the day, some mechanism must exist whereby the duration of the daylight period can be measured and translated into changes in pituitary hormone secretion. The mechanisms involved in measurement and translation are unknown, but they must involve neural inputs to hypophysiotropin-secreting cells (Chapter 20).

In humans the plasma concentration of cortisol rises in the morning and declines in the afternoon and evening. A similar adrenocortical rhythm, present in many mammalian species, may be associated with a 24-hour variation in secretion rates of CRH and ACTH as the plasma concentration of ACTH and the hypothalamic content of CRH exhibit a similar circadian rhythm.

Neuropharmacology

Pharmacological methods have been used with success to determine the particular neural components involved in hypophysiotropin regulation of pituitary hormone secretion [54]. For example, it was demonstrated that reflex ovulation in the rabbit could be blocked by rapid postcoital intravenous injections of Dibenamine, an α-adrenergic (Chapter 13) blocking agent [42]. Infusions of norepinephrine into the third ventricle of the brain resulted in an ovulatory surge of pituitary gonadotropins which was blocked by an α-receptor blocker and also by pentobarbital (a CNS-acting anesthetic), indicating that norepinephrine was acting within the brain.

Many drugs are available that can specifically modify neuronal activity and, in turn, hormonal secretion. The neuronal events are classified as presynaptic, synaptic, and postsynaptic. There are drugs that can modify the presynaptic events by affecting availability of neurotransmitter precursors, synthesis of neurotransmitters, transport of neurotransmitters along the axon, storage of neurotransmitters within secretory vesicles, exocytotic release of neurotransmitters from these vesicles, and inhibition of reuptake of neurotransmitters by presynaptic neurons. There are drugs that specifically interfere with the synaptic event by inhibiting the action of enzymes normally responsible for neurotransmitter inactivation, thereby prolonging the action of neurotransmitters. Drugs can also affect postsynaptic events by blocking neurotransmitter receptors, by mimicking the receptor-mediated actions of the neurotransmitter, and by interfering with cAMP production and degradation with presynaptic or postsynaptic neurons. Increased or decreased release of a pituitary hormone by one of these drugs is interpreted to imply that a particular neurotransmitter is involved somewhere in the hypothalamic pathway of control of the hormone.

MECHANISMS OF HYPOPHYSIOTROPIN ACTION

Attempts to determine the mechanisms of action of hypophysiotropic hormones on pituitary target cells are complicated due to the heterogeneity of the pituitary cell population. Nevertheless, the action of hypophysiotropins directly on hypophysial cells has been demonstrated [50]. Electrophysiological recordings of individual pituitary cells have been monitored. Application of TRH by micropipette to individual dissociated anterior pituitary cells elicited action potentials in previously silent cells and increased the frequency of such potentials in spontaneously active cells (Fig. 6.16). The respondent cells probably represent thyrotrophs (or possibly lactotrophs). TRH-induced depolarization of thyrotrophs is Ca^{2+} dependent, which suggests that the hypophysiotropic factor stimulates thyrotropin secretion through a stimulus-secretion coupling mechanism.

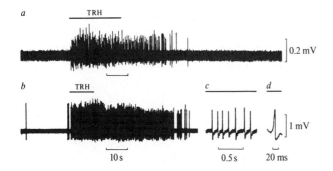

Figure 6.16 TRH-induced action potentials from pituitary thyrotrophs. (From Taraskevich and Douglas, [50], with permission.)

Further evidence that hypophysiotropins mediate their action on the pituitary by a modulation of membrane action potentials was demonstrated on prolactin-secreting cells of a fish. In some teleost fishes the PRL-secreting cells are segregated to a specific region of the pituitary, making it possible to study a pure population of cells. These cells, as in the mammal, are under an inhibitory hypothalamic dopaminergic control. Isolated cells removed from this inhibitory influence spontaneously depolarize which results in PRL secretion. Addition of dopamine to these cells inhibits the spontaneous discharge of the action potentials. Dopamine, the putative MIF, has a similar action on cells of the pars intermedia and is inhibitory of MSH secretion (Chapter 8). Taken together these results provide evidence that the stimulatory and inhibitory effects of hypophysiotropins are mediated through their immediate actions at the level of the plasma membrane.

Methylxanthines and cyclic AMP derivatives stimulate secretion of each of the six anterior pituitary hormones [26, 27]. Thus cyclic AMP is considered to be the intracellular messenger regulating adenohypophysial cell hormone secretion in response to hypophysiotropic factors. Somatostatin, whose action is inhibitory to STH secretion, inhibits pituitary cAMP production, which is accompanied by an inhibition of both STH and TSH secretion. Somatostatin also inhibits theophylline-induced hormone secretion, which suggests that the hypothalamic hormone mediates its action at the level of adenylate cyclase production. In addition somatostatin elevates adenohypophysial cGMP levels by an activation of guanylate cyclase. Cellular secretions are generally correlated with an elevation in cAMP levels, whereas inhibition of secretion is most often correlated with decreased levels of the cyclic nucleotide. Therefore it would be expected that dopamine, the hypophysiotropic PIF and MIF, mediates its inhibitory action on pituitary PRL and MSH secretion through a depression of cAMP production.

Modulation of Pituitary Hormone Secretion by Thyroid and Steroid Hormones

Thyroid hormones and adrenal and gonadal steroids secreted in response to hypophysial hormones feed back at the level of the pituitary to modulate the action of hypophysiotropins. Thyroid hormones, thyroxine and triiodothyronine, are inhibitory to TSH secretion through their actions mainly at the level of the pituitary gland. For example, TRH is stimulatory to TSH release from pituitary glands incubated in vitro, but the release of TSH from pituitaries is prevented by prior incubation of the glands in the presence of T_4 or T_3. The inhibitory effects of these thyroid hormones are in turn abolished by concomitant incubation of the glands in the presence of actinomycin or cycloheximide (inhibitors of RNA and protein synthesis, respectively), suggesting that the thyroid hormones stimulate the synthesis of an inhibitor of TRH action [3].

CRH stimulation of pituitary ACTH secretion is abolished by the synthetic glucocorticoid dexamethasone, both in vivo and in vitro. The negative feedback of adrenal glucocorticoids therefore is mediated, in part, directly at the level of the pituitary. Androgens have an inhibitory action on LH release at the hypothalamic and pituitary levels; their inhibitory effect on FSH release is restricted to the hypothalamus [26]. Progesterone can exert stimulatory and inhibitory effects on gonadotropin secretion at the pituitary and hypothalamic levels. Modulation of hypophysiotropin action can occur by an alteration of hypophysial cell receptor number (and possibly receptor sensitivity). Estradiol increases the sensitivity of FSH- and LH-secreting cells to GnRH by a direct action at the level of the pituitary. The effect of estradiol can be stimulatory or inhibitory, depending on the dose and time of administration of the estrogen. The number of pituitary GnRH receptors is positively correlated with concentrations of estradiol in the serum. Modulation of gonadotroph GnRH receptors may be a necessary component of increased pituitary sensitivity to the hypophysio-tropin during the estrous cycle [41]. Estradiol may also increase PRL secretion in the human and the rat, and the steroid is also stimulatory to TSH secretion in the rat. Daily injections of estradiol increase the number of pituitary TRH binding sites (Fig. 19.8). Thyroxine injections in the rat, on the other hand, lead to a progressive decrease in pituitary TRH binding sites. Binding of the TRH to thyrotroph plasma membranes is enhanced by prior treatment with propythiouracil, a drug which reduces thyroid hormone production by the thyroid (Chapter 13).

PATHOPHYSIOLOGY OF HYPOTHALAMIC DYSFUNCTION

Because each of the hormones of the pituitary is under stimulatory or inhibitory control by hormones of the hypothalamus, adrenal, thyroidal, and gonadal hypo-activity or hyperactivity may often relate to defects at the level of the hypothalamus rather than at the pituitary gland. Abnormal pituitary hormone secretion may be related to defects in hypophysiotropic hormone synthesis and secretion or to altered activity of the neuronal inputs to hypophysiotropin neurons. Overproduction or underproduction of dopamine within CNS neurons, for example, is believed responsible for the etiology of schizophrenia and Parkinson's disease, respectively. Because synthetic hypophysiotropic hormones are commercially available, one can differentiate hypothalamic dysfunction from defects related to pituitary patho-physiology. For example, TRH is a potent stimulator of TSH release in humans and is a useful diagnostic peptide in testing for pituitary TSH reserve. Thus one can diagnose hypothyroidism in patients with secondary hypothyroidism (due to pituitary rather than thyroid dysfunction). Hypothalamic and pituitary causes of hypothyroidism may be distinguished as release of TSH by TRH stimulation would indicate that the pituitary was fully functional.

An anomalous release of ACTH in response to TRH has been noted in some untreated patients with elevated glucocorticoid levels. TRH also stimulates ACTH release from certain neoplastic pituitary cells but not normal pituitary cells in tissue culture. A primary abnormality in some cases of these clinical syndromes may be intrinsic to the ACTH cells themselves. Neoplastic human ACTH-secreting cells may synthesize receptors for TRH, which are coupled to ACTH release, and allow direct stimulation by TRH [14].

[Phe^4]-somatostatin is twice as active as somatostatin (SS) in suppressing rat STH release in vitro but is only a weak antagonist of glucagon release in vivo. These results suggest a fundamental difference in SS receptors of pituitary and pancreas. The [Phe^4]-analog of SS may, therefore, possess properties that are useful in the development of agents for the treatment of acromegaly or other disorders associated with increased STH levels.

GnRH has been used therapeutically to induce ovulation in amenorrheic females. The hormone has also been used to treat oligospermia and hypogonadotropic hypogonadism in males. Highly potent analogs of GnRH have been developed for use in the treatment of hypogonadal function in the male and the female. Although administration of GnRh causes an initial large release of gonadotropins in females, prolonged treatment results in disturbances in gonadotropin secretion, irregular follicular maturation, and a low incidence of ovulation (Chapter 18). A single dose of certain long-acting GnRH analogs is effective in decreasing gonadotropin secretion. These peptides may prove useful as antifertility (contraceptive) agents.

Some ectopic tumors may secrete hypothalamic hormones. For example, ectopic secretion of a CRH-like peptide may be responsible for certain cases of Cushing's disease. A number of mechanisms may be invoked to explain the hyperprolactinemia associated with pituitary prolactinomas. First a hypothalamic disorder, involving decreased secretion of PIF or increased secretion of a PRL-releasing factor, could lead to eventual tumor formation. A second possibility is that PRL is produced autonomously by a tumor whose cells, by loss of dopamine receptors or other mechanisms, have become partially or wholly independent of hypothalamic control [11].

CONCLUSIONS AND SPECULATIONS

The hypothalamus, the coordinating center of the brain, controls endocrine, behavioral, and autonomic nervous system functions. Specifically, it plays an important role in thermoregulation, feeding and drinking behaviors, cardiovascular activity, pituitary gland regulation, and certain types of motivation and learning [20]. The experimental affirmation of the neurovascular hypothesis of Harris [19] was particularly important in establishing the functional role of hypothalamic hypophysiotropic factors in the control of endocrine function. Indeed, the hypothalamus provides the final common neuroendocrine pathway in the control of the peripheral endocrine system. The endocrine hypothalamus is itself regulated by the peripheral endocrine system as well as by autonomic nervous system afferent inputs. Thus the concept of neuroendocrinology has emerged which emphasizes the reciprocal integrated roles of

TABLE 6.1 Experimental Evidence Supporting a Hypothalamic Control of Pituitary Hormone Secretion.

1. Pituitary stalk section or placement of a mechanical barrier between the hypothalamus and the pituitary leads to diminished or enhanced secretion of certain pituitary hormones.
2. Ectopic transplantation of the pituitary gland leads to decreased or increased secretion of pituitary hormones.
3. Retransplantation of ectopically transplanted pituitaries under the hypothalamus leads to reactivation of pituitary hormone secretion (and, e.g., reestablishment of ovulatory cycles).
4. Specifically placed discrete lesions in the hypothalamus lead to diminished or enhanced secretion of specific hypophysial hormones.
5. Electrode stimulation of discrete hypothalamic sites leads to inhibition or release of certain pituitary hormones.
6. Pituitary hormone secretion is inhibited by implantation of target organ tissues or hormones into discrete sites within the hypothalamus.
7. Hypothalamic extracts injected into intact animals or added to pituitary glands incubated in vitro enhance or inhibit pituitary secretions.
8. Ectopic pituitary grafts are reactivated (after partial atrophy) by local infusions of extracts of the median eminence.
9. Fragments of the pituitary glands transplanted within a specific site (hypophysiotropic area) of the hypothalamus remain functionally active.
10. Administration of pharmaceutical agents, which enhance or inhibit neurotransmitter production by hypothalamic neurons, leads to enhanced or inhibited pituitary hormone secretion.
11. Synthetic peptides identical in structure to the putative hypophysiotropic hormones mimic the activity of the hypothalamic peptides on pituitary hormone secretion when administered in vivo or in vitro.
12. Putative hypophysiotropic hormones are found in the hypophysial portal blood in greater concentration than in the systemic circulation.
13. Radiolabeled gonadal steroids localize to hypothalamic sites known to control pituitary gonadotropin secretion.
14. Electrode stimulation of hypothalamic tissue in vitro leads to a Ca^{2+}-dependent release of putative hypophysiotropins.
15. Electrical stimulation of the hypothalamus elevates plasma levels of hypophysiotropins.
16. Adrenalectomy, gonadectomy, and thyroidectomy, procedures that alter levels of pituitary hormone secretion, also alter hypothalamic levels of hypophysiotropins.
17. Immunocytochemical techniques localize hypophysiotropins to specific hypothalamic neurons.
18. Antisera to hypophysiotropic hormones lead to enhanced or inhibited pituitary hormone secretion.
19. Radiolabeled amino acids are incorporated into hypophysiotropins within hypothalamic tissue fragments.

the nervous and endocrine systems in the control of physiological processes. Table 6.1 summarizes the evidence for a role of hypothalamic hypophysiotropins in the control of pituitary function.

The progressive elucidation of the presence and precise distribution of neurohormones within the hypothalamus and other brain centers may provide the exact neuroanatomical-neurohormonal correlates related to normal and abnormal neuroendocrine physiology [43, 44]. The knowledge of the structure of the hypophysiotropins and their subsequent synthesis has provided the clinician with new tools for enhancing pituitary hormone secretion under conditions of hypothalamic dysfunction.

Of great interest is the discovery that the hypophysiotropins are not restricted to the hypothalamus, but rather are found throughout the nervous system, the gut, and other peripheral organs. Each of these hypophysiotropins may function in the control of a diverse number of physiological processes. A study of the comparative endocrinology of these peptides reveals that their role in the hypothalamus may indeed be a rather late evolutionary acquisition.

REFERENCES

[1] BAERTSCHI, A. J., P. VALLET, J. B. BAUMANN, and J. GIRARD. 1980. Neural lobe of pituitary modulates corticotropin release in the rat. *Endocrinology* 106:878–82.

[2] BERELOWITZ, M., M. SZABO, L. A. FROHMAN, S. FIRESTONE, and L. CHU. 1981. Somatomedin-C mediates growth hormone negative feedback by effects on both the hypothalamus and the pituitary. *Science* 212:1279–81.

[3] BOWERS, C. Y., K.-L. LEE, and A. V. SCHALLY. 1968. Effect of actinomycin on hormones that control the release of thyrotropin from the anterior pituitary glands of mice. *Endocrinology* 82:303–10.

[4] BOYD, A. E. III, and S. REICHLIN. 1978. Neural control of prolactin secretion in man. *Psychoneuroendocrinology* 3:113–30.

[5] BRAZEAU, P., W. VALE, R. BURGUS, N. LING, M. BUTCHER, J. RIVIER, and R. GUILLEMIN. 1973. Hypothalamic polypeptide that inhibits the secretion of immunoreactive pituitary growth hormone. *Science* 179:77–79.

[6] BROWNSTEIN, M. J., A. ARIMURA, A. V. SCHALLY, M. PALKOVITS, and J. S. KEZER. 1976. The effects of surgical isolation of the hypothalamus on its luteinizing hormone-releasing hormone content. *Endocrinology* 98:662–65.

[7] CLEMONS, G. K., S. M. RUSSELL, and C. S. NICOLL. 1979. Effect of mammalian thyrotropin releasing hormone on prolactin secretion by bullfrog adenohypophysis *in vitro. Gen. Comp. Endocrinol.* 38:62–67.

[8] CRIM, J. W., W. W. DICKHOFF, and A. GORBMAN. 1978. Comparative endocrinology of piscine hypothalamic hypophysiotropic peptides: distribution and activity. *Amer. Zool.* 18:411–24.

[9] EVANS, J. W., and M. B. NIKITOVITCH-WINER. 1969. Functional reactivation and cytological restoration of pituitary grafts by continuous local intravascular infusion of median eminence extracts. *Neuroendocrinology* 4:83–100.

[10] FINK, G. 1979. Feedback actions of target hormones on hypothalamus and pituitary, with special reference to gonadal steroids. *Ann. Rev. Physiol.* 41:571–86.

[11] FRANTZ, A. G. 1978. Prolactin. *New Engl. J. Med.* 298:201–207.

[12] FRYER, J. N., R. S. NISHIOKA, and H. A. BERN. 1979. Somatostatin inhibition of teleost growth hormone secretion. *Gen. Comp. Endocrinol.* 39:244–46.

[13] GANONG, W. F. 1980. Neurotransmitters and pituitary function: regulation of ACTH secretion. *Fed. Proc.* 39:2923–30.

[14] GERSHENGORN, M. C., C. O. AREVALO, E. GERAS, and M. J. REBECCHI. 1980. Thyrotropin-releasing hormone stimulation of adrenocorticotropin production by mouse pituitary tumor cells in culture. *J. Clin. Invest.* 65:1294–1300.

[15] GUILLEMIN, R., and R. BURGUS. 1972. The hormones of the hypothalamus. *Sci. Amer.* 227:24–33.

[16] GUILLEMIN, R., P. BRAZEAU, P. BÖHLEN, E. ESCH, N. LONG, and W. B. WEHRENBERT. 1982. Growth hormone-releasing factor from a human pancreatic tumor that caused acromegaly. *Science* 218:585–87.

[17] HADLEY, M. E., and V. J. HRUBY. 1977. Neurohypophysial peptides and the regulation of melanophore stimulating hormone (MSH) secretion. *Amer. Zool.* 17:809–21.

[18] HALÁSZ, B., L. PUPP, and S. UHLARIK. 1962. Hypophysiotropic area in the hypothalamus. *J. Endocrinol.* 25:147–54.

[19] HARRIS, G. W. 1955. *Neural control of the pituitary gland.* London: Edward Arnold Ltd.

[20] HAYWARD, J. N. 1977. Functional and morphological aspects of hypothalamic neurons. *Physiol. Rev.* 57:574–658.

[21] JACKSON, I. M. D. 1978. Phylogenetic distribution and function of the hypophysiotropic hormones of the hypothalamus. *Amer. Zool.* 18:385–99.

[22] JACKSON, I. M. D., and S. REICHLIN. 1979. Thyrotropin-releasing hormone in the blood of the frog, *Rana pipiens*: its nature and possible derivation from regional locations in the skin. *Endocrinology* 104:1814–21.

[23] KING, J. A., and R. P. MILLAR. 1980. Comparative aspects of luteinizing hormone-releasing hormone structure and function in vertebrate phylogeny. *Endocrinology* 106:707–17.

[24] KNIGGE, K. M., and A. J. SILVERMAN. 1974. Anatomy of the endocrine hypothalamus. In *Handbook of physiology*, vol. 4, part 1, eds. R. O. Greep and E. B. Astwood, pp. 1–32. Washington, D.C.: Amer. Physiol. Soc.

[25] KRULICH, L. 1979. Central neurotransmitters and the secretion of prolactin, GH, LH, and TSH. *Ann. Rev. Physiol.* 41:603–16.

[26] LABRIE, F., J. DROUIN, L. FERLAND, L. LAGACÉ, M. BEAULIEU, A. DE LEAN, P. A. KELLY, M. G. CARON, and V. RAYMOND. 1978. Mechanism of action of hypothalamic hormones in the anterior pituitary gland and specific modulation of their activity by sex steroids and thyroid hormones. *Rec. Prog. Horm. Res.* 34:25–93.

[27] LABRIE, F., L. LAGACÉ, M. BEAULIEU, L. FERLAND, A. DE LEAN, J. DROUIN, P. BORGEAT, P. A. KELLY, L. CUSAN, A. DUPONT, A. LEMAY, T. ANTAKLY, G. H. PELLETIER, and N. BARDEN. 1979. Mechanisms of action of hypothalamic and peripheral hormones in the anterior pituitary gland. In *Hormonal proteins and peptides*, vol. 7, ed. C. H. Li, pp. 205–77. New York: Academic Press, Inc.

[28] MCEWEN, B. S. 1980. Binding and metabolism of sex steroids by the hypothalamic-pituitary unit: physiological implications. *Ann. Rev. Physiol.* 42:97–110.

[29] MEITES, J., ed. 1969. *Hypophysiotropic hormones of the hypothalamus: assay and chemistry.* Baltimore, Md.: The Williams & Wilkins Company.

[30] MEITES, J., B. T. DONOVAN, and S. M. MCCANN, eds. 1975. *Pioneers in neuroendocrinology.* New York: Plenum Publishing Corporation.

[31] MOORE, R. Y. 1978. Central neural control of circadian rhythms. *Front. Neuroendocrinol.* 5:185–206.

[32] MOTTA, M., ed. 1980. *The endocrine functions of the brain.* New York: Raven Press.

[33] NIKITOVITCH-WINER, M., and J. W. EVERETT. 1958. Comparative study of luteotropin secretion by hypophysial autotransplants in the rat. Effects of site and stages of the estrous cycle. *Endocrinology* 62:522–32.

[34] ——. 1959. Histologic changes in grafts of rat pituitary on the kidney and upon re-transplantation under the diencephalon. *Endocrinology* 65:357–68.

[35] PALKOVITS, M. 1977. Neural pathways involved in ACTH regulation. *Ann. New York Acad. Sci.* 297:455–76.

[36] PATRITTI-LABORDE, N., A. R. WOLFSEN, D. HEBER, and W. D. ODELL. 1979. Site of short-loop feedback for luteinizing hormone in the rabbit. *J. Clin. Invest.* 64:1066–69.

[37] PORTER, J. C., R. S. MICAL, I. A. KAMBERI, and Y. R. GRAZIA. 1970. A procedure for the cannulation of a pituitary stalk portal vessel and perfusion of the pars distalis in the rat. *Endocrinology* 87:197–201.

[38] PORTER, J. C., D. D. NANSEL, G. A. GUDELSKY, M. M. FOREMAN, N. S. PILOTTE, C. R. PARKER, JR., G. H. BURROWS, G. W. BATES, and J. D. MADDEN. 1980. Neural control of gonadotropin secretion. *Fed. Proc.* 39:2896–2901.

[39] RIVIER, C., J. RIVIER, and W. VALE. 1982. Inhibition of adrenocorticotropic hormone secretion in the rat by immunoneutralization of corticotropin-releasing factor. *Science* 218:377–79.

[40] RIVIER, J., J. SPIESS, M. THORNER, and W. VALE. 1982. Characterization of a growth hormone-releasing factor from a human pancreatic islet tumor. *Nature* 300:276–78.

[41] SAVOY-MOORE, R. T., N. B. SCHWARTZ, J. A. DUNCAN, and J. C. MARSHALL. 1980. Pituitary gonadotropin releasing hormone receptors during the rat estrous cycle. *Science* 209:942–44.

[42] SAWYER, C. H., and D. K. CLIFTON. 1980. Aminergic innervation of the hypothalamus. *Fed. Proc.* 39:2889–95.

[43] SCHALLY, A. V. 1978. Aspects of hypothalamic regulation of the pituitary gland. *Science* 202:18–28.

[44] SCHALLY, A. V., D. H. COY, C. A. MEYERS, and A. J. KASTIN. 1979. Hypothalamic peptide hormones: basic and clinical studies. In *Hormonal proteins and peptides*, vol. 71, ed. C. H. Li, pp. 1–54. New York: Academic Press, Inc.

[45] SCHALLY, A. V., W. Y. HUANG, R. C. C. CHANG, A. ARIMURA, T. W. REDDING, R. P. MILLAR, M. W. HUNKAPILLER, and L. E. HOOD. 1980. Isolation and structure of pro-somatostatin: a putative somatostatin precursor from pig hypothalamus. *Proc. Natl. Acad. Sci. USA* 77:4489–93.

[46] SCHALLY, A. V., R. C. C. CHANG, A. ARIMURA, T. W. REDDING, J. B. FISHBACK, and S. VIGH. 1981. High molecular weight peptide with corticotropin-releasing-factor activity from porcine hypothalami. *Proc. Natl. Acad. Sci. USA* 78:5197–5201.

[47] SÉTÁLÓ, G., B. FLERKÓ, A. ARIMURA, and A. V. SCHALLY. 1978. Brain cells as producers of releasing and inhibiting hormones. *Intern. Rev. Cytol.* Suppl. 7:1–51.

[48] STUDER, R. O. 1972. Chemistry of TRH. *Front. Horm. Res.* 1:4–10.

[49] STUMPF, W. E., and M. SAR. 1977. Steroid hormone target cells in the periventricular brain: relationship to peptide hormone producing cells. *Fed. Proc.* 36:1973–77.

[50] TARASKEVICH, P. S., and D. W. DOUGLAS. 1977. Action potentials occur in cells of the normal pituitary gland and are stimulated by the hypophysiotropic peptide thyrotropin-releasing hormone. *Proc. Natl. Acad. Sci. USA* 74:4064–67.

[51] VALE, W., C. RIVIER, J. RIVIER, and M. BROWN. 1978. Adenohypophysial and other extracentral nervous system roles of hypothalamic regulatory peptides. In *Psychopharmacology: a generation of progress*, eds. M. A. Lipton, A. DiMascio, and K. F. Killam, pp. 403–21. New York: Raven Press.

[52] VALE, W., J. SPIESS, C. RIVIER, and J. RIVIER. 1981. Characterization of a 41-residue ovine hypothalamic peptide that stimulates secretion of corticotropin and β-endorphin. *Science* 213:1394–97.

[53] WADE, N. 1978. Guillemin and Schally. *Science* 200:279–82; 411–15; 510–13.

[54] WEINER, R. I., and W. F. GANONG. 1978. Role of brain monoamines and histamine in regulation of anterior pituitary secretion. *Physiol. Rev.* 58:905–76.

7

Neurohypophysial
Hormones

INTRODUCTION

As early as 1895 extracts of pituitaries were discovered to cause a rapid rise in blood pressure when injected into animals [26]. An important advance was made with the subsequent discovery by Howell (1898) that the pressor principle of pituitary extracts resided in the posterior lobe [19]. Dale, an eminent English pharmacologist, was the first to note that an extract of dried bovine pituitary glands caused a contraction of the uterus in addition to an elevation in blood pressure [8]. In 1909 posterior pituitary extracts were first used in clinical obstetrics to induce labor at term. In the years following, it was discovered that posterior lobe extracts caused a rapid flow (release) of milk. *Antidiuresis* in response to injections of posterior pituitary extracts was demonstrated in 1913. The injections reduced urine flow, increased the osmolality of the urine, and alleviated thirst. Extracts of the neurohypophysis then became established as the clinical method of controlling the polyurea of diabetes insipidus, although the etiology of the syndrome was not yet understood.

In the early 1950s the two physiologically active principles of the posterior pituitary, oxytocin and vasopressin, were completely separated so that their individual activities could be studied. Du Vigneaud and his colleagues determined the structures of the oxytocic and antidiuretic principles of the neurohypophysis [20]. Among the first peptide hormones to be completely chemically characterized, oxytocin and vasopressin were then synthesized, and for this work du Vigneaud was awarded a Nobel Prize. This merging of pure chemistry with physiology provided the foundation for modern endocrinology.

THE NEUROHYPOPHYSIS

Unlike the adenohypophysis, which derives from an upward evagination of the oral (buccal) epithelium, the posterior pituitary develops from a downward growth of the neural ectoderm. The neurohypophysis mainly consists therefore of neural endings and associated blood vessels (Chapter 5). There are only a few cellular elements present within the pars nervosa. The cells that are within the neurohypophysis are referred to as *pituicytes*, and their function is unknown. They are probably glial cells and may function like the neuroglia of the central nervous system. This paucity of cell bodies was a puzzling observation to the early investigators who ascribed an endocrine role to the pars nervosa. Where or what were the secretory elements of the posterior pituitary?

Lesions within specific areas of the hypothalamus led to degeneration of the pars nervosa and to a disturbance in water balance. These and other observations revealed that the neurons of the pars nervosa originate in two pairs of hypothalamic nuclei. These neurons contain a stainable material that allows easy identification of the pathways from the hypothalamic nuclei through the median eminence and down the infundibular stalk of the neurohypophysis (Fig. 7.1). The stainable material is composed of granules which are now known to contain the hormones of the neurohypophysis. These large granules are referred to as *neurosecretory granules*; the process of granule formation and release is termed *neurosecretion*.

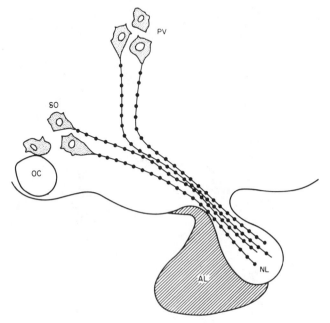

Figure 7.1 Diagram of a sagittal section through the pituitary gland. The relationship of the neurons which compose the supraoptic nuclei (SO) and the paraventricular nuclei (PV) to the hypothalamo-hypophysial tract and the neurohypophysis (NL) is revealed. (From Pickering, [28], with permission.)

The discovery that the neurohypophysis is the terminal organ of a CNS neurosecretory system and is mainly composed of hormone-containing nerve terminals, and that these axonal endings secrete their products into the bloodstream to act as hormones on distant target tissues, was an important landmark in understanding the role of neurons in endocrine function [3]. Thus the discipline of vertebrate neuroendocrinology was established. The concept of neurosecretion in the vertebrate provided information that furthered understanding the role of the brain in the control of pituitary and other endocrine functions. Neuroendocrinology in the vertebrate began with the study of the neurohypophysis and its hormones.

The vertebrate neurohypophysis is considered anatomically to be a storage organ for the products of individual neuronal syntheses. As with other endocrine organs, the stored hormones are released into the adjacent vascular network. Such a functional unit is referred to as a *neurohemal organ* and is structurally analogous to the *corpus cardiacum* of some invertebrates. The study of these depot-release structures, the neurohypophysis and corpus cardiacum, and their release of neurohormones has been crucial in understanding brain-endocrine relationships in vertebrates and invertebrates.

SYNTHESIS AND CHEMISTRY

Two nonapeptides, oxytocin and vasopressin (the latter also referred to as antidiuretic hormone, ADH), are found within the pars nervosa of most mammalian species. These neurohypophysial hormones are closely related structurally, but serve quite

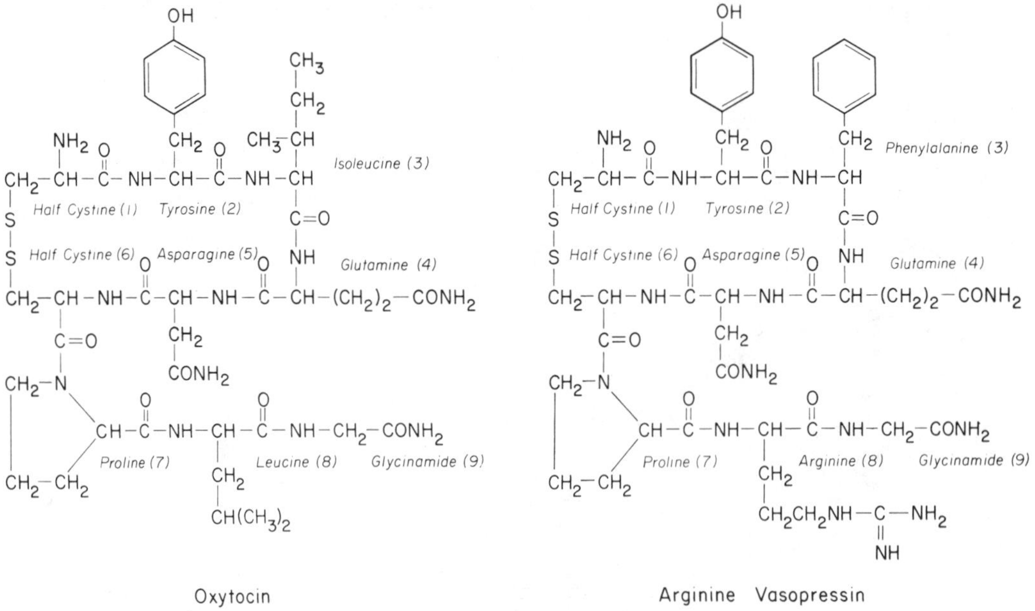

Oxytocin

Arginine Vasopressin

Figure 7.2 Primary structures of oxytocin and vasopressin. The individual amino acids are numbered by the conventional method.

different physiological roles. Oxytocin, for example, controls milk release from the mammary gland and contraction of the uterus, whereas vasopressin is concerned with water balance. The neurohypophysial hormones consist of nine amino acids folded into a ring through a disulfide bridge at positions 1 and 6 of the molecule, leaving a terminal tripeptide side chain (Fig. 7.2). Vasopressin differs from oxytocin in possessing a phenylalanine and an arginine at the 3 and 8 positions, respectively, of the molecule and is usually referred to as arginine vasopressin (AVP). Other structurally different neurohypophysial principles are found within the neurohypophysis of nonmammalian vertebrates (Table 7.1).

The neurohypophysial hormones are localized within the axonal endings that make up the pars nervosa. These hormones are, however, synthesized within the cell bodies of these neurons which are located a relatively long distance away in the hypothalamus. In mammals, birds and reptiles these cell bodies are found principally within the paired supraoptic nuclei (SON) and paraventricular nuclei (PVN) of the magnocellular neurosecretory system (Fig. 7.1). In other vertebrates this system consists of a single group of neurons in the anterior hypothalamus, the *preoptic*

TABLE 7.1 Primary structures of the Vertebrate Neurohypophysial Hormones[a]

Hormone	Positions of amino acid residues	Animal Group
Ancestral molecule	1 2 3 4 5 6 7 8 9 Cys-Tyr-X-X-Asn-Cys-Pro-X-Gly-(NH₂)	
Oxytocin	1 2 3 4 5 6 7 8 9 Cys-Tyr-Ile-Gln-Asn-Cys-Pro-Leu-Gly-(NH₂)	Mammals
Arginine vasopressin	1 2 3 4 5 6 7 8 9 Cys-Tyr-Phe-Gln-Asn-Cys-Pro-Arg-Gly-(NH₂)	Mammals (except domestic pigs)
Lysine vasopressin	1 2 3 4 5 6 7 8 9 Cys-Tyr-Phe-Gln-Asn-Cys-Pro-Lys-Gly-(NH₂)	Suiformes: peccaries, wart hogs, hippopotami
Arginine vasotocin	1 2 3 4 5 6 7 8 9 Cys-Tyr-Ile-Gln-Asn-Cys-Pro-Arg-Gly-(NH₂)	Birds, reptiles, amphibians, bony fishes, and possibly cartilaginous fishes
Isotocin (Ichthyotocin)	1 2 3 4 5 6 7 8 9 Cys-Tyr-Ile-Ser-Asn-Cys-Pro-Ile-Gly-(NH₂)	Some bony fishes
Mesotocin	1 2 3 4 5 6 7 8 9 Cys-Tyr-Ile-Gln-Asn-Cys-Pro-Ile-Gly-(NH₂)	Birds, reptiles, amphibians, lungfishes
Glumitocin	1 2 3 4 5 6 7 8 9 Cys-Tyr-Ile-Ser-Asn-Cys-Pro-Gln-Gly-(NH₂)	Cartilaginous fishes (rays)
Valitocin	1 2 3 4 5 6 7 8 9 Cys-Tyr-Ile-Gln-Asn-Cys-Pro-Val-Gly-(NH₂)	Cartilaginous fishes (sharks)
Aspargtocin	1 2 3 4 5 6 7 8 9 Cys-Tyr-Ile-Asn-Asn-Cys-Pro-Leu-Gly-(NH₂)	Cartilaginous fishes (sharks)

[a]Modified from [1].

nucleus. In the amphibian, immunocytochemical studies have demonstrated separate hormone-producing neurons within the magnocellular preoptic nucleus, suggesting that the two types of hormone-producing neurosecretory neurons are intermingled. Although there is evidence that individual neurons synthesize only one species of hormone, both types of neurons are found intermingled within each of the hypothalamic nuclei [49]. Oxytocin-synthesizing cells predominate in the PVN and vasopressin-synthesizing cells in the SON [44]. In the rat the number of neurosecretory neurons is, however, more than three times greater in the SON than the PVN, and the contribution of oxytocin from the former structure may be several times greater than that from the latter during reflex stimulation of oxytocin release [14]. The relative contribution of oxytocinergic and vasopressinergic neurons within the PVN and SON varies considerably between species; the individual contributions of these two nuclear centers to neurohypophysial hormone secretion therefore remain unresolved.

Radioisotope studies using [^{35}S]-cysteine injected into the third ventricle reveal that incorporation of the radiolabel into protein occurs first within the cell bodies of the neurosecretory neurons. The label is then transported rapidly (2.5 mm/hr) down the axons to terminals within the pars nervosa. Studies revealed that radioactive amino acids injected into the supraoptic nucleus appear in the posterior pituitary incorporated into vasopressin and its precursors within 2 hours of injection. In vitro studies showed that hypothalamo-median eminence tissue, but not neurohypophysial tissue, incorporated [^{35}S]-cysteine into vasopressin. These experimental observations documented the origin of the neurosecretory material of the pars nervosa [35].

Each of the hormones is found in close association with a larger protein, referred to as a *neurophysin*, the Van Dyke protein of the older literature [34]. There is a specific neurophysin for each hormone, oxytocin-neurophysin (*oxyphysin*) and vasopressin-neurophysin (*pressophysin*). Additional neurophysins have been identified: They may be derived enzymatically from one of the other neurophysins and may therefore be artifacts of extraction, or they may be neurophysins for as yet unidentified peptides. Neurophysins and their associated hormones are derived from the posttranslational cleavage of precursor proteins, propressophysin and pro-oxyphysin [6]. Inhibitors of neurophysin formation also repress formation of the associated hormones. In the homozygous state the Brattleboro strain of rat, which has hereditary diabetes insipidus, demonstrates an absolute lack of vasopressin but no comparable defect in oxytocin synthesis and secretion. Pressophysin is also absent from the hypothalamus of these rats, providing further evidence for the common origin of the neurophysin and its associated neurohypophysial hormone. The concept that peptide hormones may arise from the proteolytic cleavage of a precursor *prohormone* (in this case a *proneurophysin*) is now recognized to be of more general significance for the production of most other peptide hormones.

The amino acid sequences of the two neurophysins are similar within and between species. This suggests that they have arisen from a common ancestral neurophysin by gene duplication. These two neurophysins have been found in the pituitary of each of the mammals studied. A neurophysin from the cod (*Gadus morrhua*) has also been isolated and the N-terminal sequence determined [27]. The precursor molecule, with associated proteolytic enzymes, is present within the granules of the neurosecretory cells. These enzymes may be necessary to split the neurophysin from the precursor molecule because cleavage of the precursor occurs inside the granule after it begins migration from the Golgi regions in the hypothalamic perikarya to the axon terminals in the neural lobe. Vasopressin and oxytocin bind noncovalently in a specific manner to neurophysins. Thus the neurophysins are believed to function as transport proteins for the neurohypophysial hormones. Neurophysin is secreted with its hormone into the bloodstream in response to physiologic stimulation. The secreted neurophysins are considered to function only as intraneuronal carrier proteins for the hormones and to lack any hormonal function.

The early work of Bargmann and Scharrer[3], which utilized staining techniques for neurosecretory material, established the site of origin of the hormones of the pars nervosa. It was noted that some axons of the supraoptico-hypophysial tract project to the external zone of the median eminence and also to the third ventricle. Both AVP and neurophysin are present in granules of axons that are in contact with the hypophysial portal system, and these peptides are secreted into the portal blood in high concentrations [18]. These observations support the established view for a possible role of AVP or similarly derived peptide in the control of anterior pituitary function. Neurohypophysial hormone secretion into the cerebrospinal fluid may also be important physiologically, for example, in the regulation of cerebrospinal electrolyte balance.

MECHANISMS OF RELEASE

Stimuli received by sensory receptors in the breast or vascular system result in release of oxytocin or AVP, respectively, from the neurohypophysis. Neural afferents to the spinal cord connect with other neural pathways to the neurosecretory cell bodies localized within the paraventricular and supraoptic nuclei. The neurosecretory neurons are in synaptic contact with neurons from these afferent pathways. There may be excitatory (cholinergic) and inhibitory (noradrenergic) connections from the rostral midbrain to the neurosecretory neurons. Destruction of noradrenergic neurons in the rabbit brainstem, for example, elevates plasma AVP, resulting in hypertension [5]. There may also be interneurons that synchronize the activity of the neurosecretory neurons within the hypothalamic nuclei. Release of the excitatory neurotransmitter from afferent neurons onto the neurosecretory neurons results in depolarization of the cells. Action potentials can be recorded from mammalian neurosecretory cells of the SON and PVN. The pattern of firing of oxytocin cells can be distinguished from that of AVP-secreting cells during appropriate stimulation, such as suckling or hemorrhage, respectively [10, 29]. The putative AVP-secreting cells show a rhythmic bursting-type discharge that is increased by high osmotic pressure, whereas oxytocin-producing cells appear to discharge continuously and in a random fashion. This pattern of firing, characteristic of the rat, may not be typical in all species [48].

Depolarization of neurosecretory cell bodies is propagated along the axons of the hypothalamo-hypophysial tract to the neuron terminals in the pars nervosa. Calcium ions apparently enter the neurosecretory neurons during depolarization; they are responsible for initiating some undefined event related to the secretory process, as neurohypophysial hormone secretion is inhibited in the absence of Ca^{2+} [9].

Neurosecretory granules fuse with the plasmalemma of the cells and are extruded via exocytosis. Following secretory granule discharge by exocytosis, the vesicular membrane fragments incorporated into the axonal plasmalemma, or membrane fragments of equivalent area, are internalized by *inverse exocytosis*. Filaments (possibly microfilaments or microtubules) may in some way be involved in vesicle transport to the plasma membrane, and calcium may affect this neurofilament transport process. The secreted hormone and associated neurophysin enter the bloodstream in the vessels passing out of the neurohypophysis. The specific mechanisms related to neurohypophysial hormone secretion have been described by Douglas [9].

PHYSIOLOGICAL ROLES

Oxytocin is involved in the control of milk release and uterine contraction during labor. Vasopressin, or antidiuretic hormone as its name implies, is important in the homeostatic control of the extracellular fluid volume. The antidiuretic response is of lifetime survival value to individuals of both sexes. Oxytocin, on the other hand, functions only during specific times in the reproductive cycle of the adult female. No function for oxytocin in the male has been clearly established.

Oxytocin

Milk release (let-down).   Oxytocin functions in the control of milk release (milk let-down) after parturition. Sensory nerve endings, which are localized mainly to the areolae and nipples of the breasts, are stimulated by suckling (Fig. 7.3), and afferent neural pathways conduct these stimuli to the neurohypophysis [22, 23]. From studies on different animals, the various components of these neural pathways have been traced. The pathways are ipsilateral (same side) to the teat being suckled. Neural impulses conducted along the sensory neurons enter the spinal column and ascend via dorsal, lateral, and ventral spinothalamic tracts to the mesencephalon of the brain.

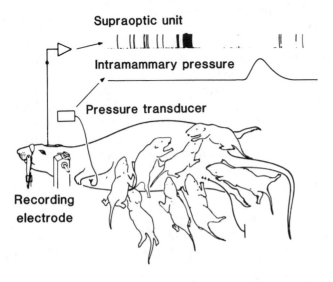

Figure 7.3 Scheme for measuring the electrical activity of hypothalamic neurosecretory neurons associated with reflex release of oxytocin during suckling in the rat. The upper trace (supraoptic unit: SO) shows the action potentials recorded from a cell in the supraoptic nucleus while the lower trace is a recording of intramammary pressure. Note the burst of potentials which occurs 12 seconds before the increase in pressure. (From J. B. Wakerley, [22], with permission.)

These stimuli are then transmitted via a diencephalic route to the hypothalamus. The neural pathways controlling oxytocin secretion have been determined by electrode stimulation and lesioning experiments [30, 43]. Stimulation of the supraoptico-hypophysial tract in anesthetized animals results in ejection of milk. On the other hand, lesions in the supraoptic nuclei in lactating animals result in marked diminution in the quantity of milk released from the mammary gland. Electrophysiological recordings from putative oxytocinergic neurons in unanesthetized, freely moving rats established that the electrical activity displayed by these magnocellular neurons, some 10 to 12 seconds before milk ejection, is responsible for oxytocin release under normal physiological conditions [23, 42].

At parturition dilation of the cervix (vaginal stretching) may also be a stimulus to oxytocin secretion. Cross-circulation experiments have been carried out with pairs of unanesthetized ewes in which the jugular veins were crossed so that each member of a pair received blood only from its partner. Mechanical distension of the vagina in one of the ewes resulted in a milk-ejection response in only the other ewe. Similar results were obtained when the roles were reversed. There is increased uterine activity during mating, and milk ejection during coitus in the human female and other animals has been reported. Auditory and optic sensory stimuli also affect milk let-down in some animals.

Ovarian hormones affect the levels of neurohypophysial hormones in the pituitary of the rat. The firing rates of paraventricular neurons are increased during proestrus and estrus and after estrogen treatment in ovariectomized rats. Estrogen treatment also facilitates the activation of paraventricular secretory cell units and the reflex release of oxytocin by genital tract stimulation. Therefore, ovarian hormones may not only promote the expression of sexual receptivity (Chapter 18), but may also increase levels of neurohypophysial hormones and facilitate release of these hormones during mating. Because these hormones have potent stimulating effects on uterine and oviduct smooth muscle, they might also enhance the likelihood of fertilization by promoting sperm transport.

Oxytocin released from the pars nervosa elicits contraction of cellular musclelike elements [24, 31], myoepithelial cells (Fig. 7.4), which results in increased intra-mammary pressure and the expression of milk from the alveoli and ducts out through the teats (Fig. 7.5). The effect of oxytocin on milk release from isolated mammary gland tissue in vitro is easily demonstrated [4]. High affinity sites that bind [^{3}H]-labeled oxytocin are present in membrane fractions of mammary gland from the lactating rat [39]. Oxytocin binding activity is specifically localized by autoradiography to the myoepithelial cells of mammary tissue; the binding sites are localized to the plasma membrane of the myoepithelial cells (Fig. 7.6).

Uterine contraction. Oxytocin has been used for years to induce labor in human females at term. Oxytocin contracts the myometrium (uterotropic action), which can be demonstrated in vitro. Whether oxytocin is responsible for initiating labor has been debated. Although oxytocin is found in the maternal circulation throughout pregnancy, oxytocin concentrations in the blood increase only during the final stages of labor, not before. It is suggested that parturition may not only be triggered by an increase in oxytocin secretion per se, but also by an increase in the

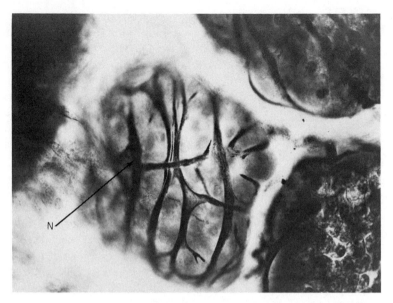

Figure 7.4 Silver-stained section of lactating mammary gland of the goat. A surface view of a contracted alveolus shows a myoepithelial cell with nucleus (N) and branching processes. (From Richardson, [31], with permission.)

sensitivity of the myometrium of the uterus to the hormone [41]. The response of the myometrium to oxytocin is maximal at or near parturition.

It has been demonstrated that specific binding of tritium-labeled [^{3}H]-oxytocin to uterine receptors of pregnant rats increases dramatically at term and is maximal during labor [41]. In contrast, there is only a gradual increase in binding of [^{3}H]-oxytocin to mammary tissue, but this binding does become maximal during lactation. Changes in the ratio of plasma estradiol to progesterone concentration closely parallel the changes in oxytocin binding: Estradiol is elevated and progesterone diminished. Estrogens increase myometrial sensitivity to oxytocin and increase the number of oxytocin receptors in the uterus. Progesterone, an estrogen antagonist, may, on the

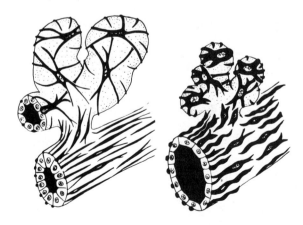

Figure 7.5 Disposition of myoepithelial cells (black) around alveoli and ducts. *Left*: myoepithelial cells relaxed, alveoli full. *Right*: myoepithelial cells contracted, alveoli emptied, ducts widened. (From Linzell, [24], by permission of John Wright & Sons.)

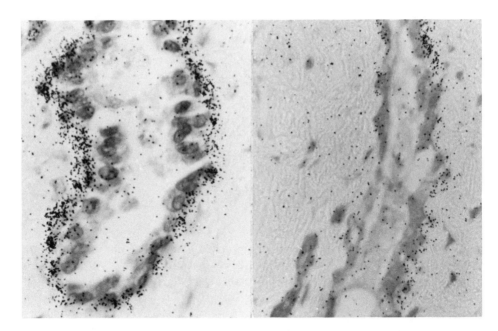

Figure 7.6 Autoradiographic localization of tritium-labeled oxytocin to myoepithelial cells of the mammary gland. (From Soloff et al., [39], with permission.)

other hand, suppress the appearance of oxytocin receptors. Decreased synthesis of progesterone may, therefore, indirectly increase production of oxytocin receptors. Thus it appears that parturition is preceded by a dramatic increase in myometrial oxytocin receptors, which may render the myometrium more sensitive to oxytocin. The meager number of oxytocin receptors before term might make the myometrium insensitive to the circulating hormone. Parturition may therefore be triggered by an increase in myometrial receptor number as well as an increase in oxytocin levels in the blood during labor. This hypothesis unites many observations and arguments on the role of oxytocin in parturition.

Vascular smooth muscle actions. Neurohypophysial hormones contract or relax vascular smooth muscle. The exact type of response depends on species, vascular bed, and region within a vascular bed [2]. Thus within a single species of animal the neurohypophysial peptides can exert vasoconstrictor actions in one peripheral vascular bed and vasodilator actions in another. There may be two distinct kinds of neurohypophysial hormone receptors: one which subserves contraction and the other which subserves relaxation. There may even be different relative proportions of both receptors which vary in number depending on blood vessel segment and species. In addition oxytocin may act on a distinctly different vascular receptor from that for AVP. For example, oxytocin is highly effective in contracting human umbilical arteries and veins, whereas vasopressin is relatively inactive. Rat aortic strips, in contrast, are extremely sensitive to the contractile effects of AVP but are insensitive to oxytocin. Synthesis of neurohypophysial analogs can provide peptides with unique and selective microcirculatory effects that may be clinically useful in the treatment of low vascular flow rates.

Physiological Roles

Other functions or effects.   Oxytocin is released during coitus, and it has been suggested that the induced uterine contractions might facilitate the transport of sperm toward the ova. It is believed that the ascent of sperm in the female tract is too rapid to occur by flagellar activity alone. Thus the rapid transport of sperm may be due to the propulsive forces generated from uterine contractions induced by oxytocin released from the neurohypophysis as a result of the mechanical stimulation of the vagina during coitus. The nonpregnant human uterus is, however, very insensitive to oxytocin; in addition hypophysectomy does not influence the incidence of pregnancy after mating in rats and guinea pigs. Also, catecholamines may be liberated during coitus, and they may augment uterine activity. The role of oxytocin in sperm transport thus remains speculative [25].

Vasopressin (AVP)

Vasopressin has two major physiological actions: It induces the contraction or relaxation of certain types of smooth muscle, and it promotes the movement of water (and sodium) across responsive epithelial tissues, notably the distal tubule of the mammalian kidney and the skin and urinary bladder of amphibians. Radioimmunoassay of circulating AVP under varying experimental conditions and pathophysiological states has now provided detailed information on the role of vasopressin in the control of water balance [33].

Osmoregulation.   Blood osmolality is important in the control of AVP secretion [45], and injections of small volumes of hypertonic solution into the carotid artery of the dog result in an immediate antidiuresis [16]. Osmoreceptors are localized in the anterior hypothalamus. These osmoreceptors were thought to be near or identical to the cell bodies of the neurohypophysis. It is now believed that the osmoreceptor function is not performed by the neurosecretory cells. An antidiuretic response is evoked only when hypertonic saline is infused in small volumes at sites some distance from the supraoptic nucleus. Small lesions in the medial preoptic area of the hypothalamus, which do not involve the neurohypophysis, prevent AVP secretion in response to fluid deprivation. In addition in the rare clinical syndrome of adipsic hypernatremia, patients have a complete lack of osmotically mediated vasopressin secretion, but they secrete AVP in response to hemodynamic stimuli. The osmoreceptors in humans would therefore appear to be totally separate from the neurosecretory cells and are apparently not an integral component of the neuronal pathways by which AVP secretion is affected by hemodynamic variables [33].

In summary, the physiologically important osmoreceptor control mechanism is near but neither identical to nor intermixed with the cell bodies of the neurohypophysial neurons (Fig. 7.7, A_1). Because osmotically mediated vasopressin release can be totally ablated without altering in any way the hormonal response to hypotension, this excludes the possibility that hemodynamic stimuli are transmitted to the neurohypophysis by way of osmoreceptor neurons (Fig. 7.7, A_1 and A_2). Possibly the AVP-secreting cells of the neurohypophysis are functionally heterogeneous; that is, they are divided into different units that receive afferents from the osmoregulatory or baroregulatory systems (Fig. 7.7, B). One might expect that the function of one unit

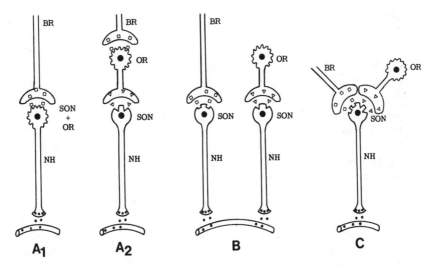

Figure 7.7 Schematic representation of possible modes of organization of the neurohypophysis (NH) and its regulatory afferents from osmoreceptors (OR) and baroreceptors (BR). Supraoptic and paraventricular nuclei are designated as SON. (From Robertson, Athar, and Shelton, [33], with permission.)

should have no effect on the other. This is not the case. In addition electrophysiological recordings from neurosecretory cells in the anterior and lateral hypothalamus revealed firing rates that could be altered by *both* volume and osmotic stimuli. Thus the control system may be organized as depicted (Fig. 7.7, C).

In normal individuals the *osmostat* appears to be set so that AVP secretion is suppressed to low or undetectable levels whenever plasma osmolality falls to 280 mOsm/kg or below [32]. Above this concentration AVP secretion rises (Fig. 7.8 A) in direct proportion to the osmolality, affecting maximal antidiuresis at a plasma

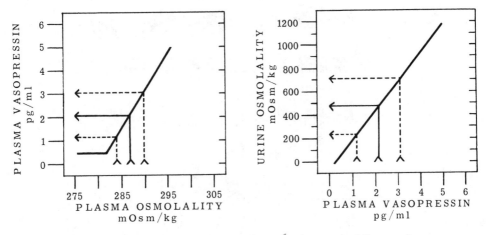

Figure 7.8 Effect of small alterations in basal plasma osmolality on plasma vasopressin and urine osmolality in normal humans. (From Robertson, Shelton, and Athar, [32], with permission.)

osmolality around 295 mOsm/kg. Changes in plasma osmolality as small as 1% will increase or decrease plasma AVP levels and affect urinary osmolality (Fig. 7.8 B), suggesting that the osmoreceptors are extraordinarily sensitive to changes in blood electrolyte concentration. Osmoreceptors exhibit a specificity for certain solutes. For example, hypertonic saline or sucrose, but not urea or glucose, induces an antidiuresis. Because well over 90% of the osmotic activity of plasma is normally contributed by sodium and its anions, the osmoreceptors would be expected to function mainly in the detection of changes of sodium osmolality [33]. Oral saline intake reduces the AVP content of the SON and PVN but is without effect on the vasopressin content of the median eminence. This supports the concept for an independent control and role of AVP in the median eminence [34].

Blood volume-pressure regulation. Changes in blood volume and pressure affect AVP secretion [21]. Hemodynamic influences are exerted via neural afferents originating in pressure-sensitive receptors (baroreceptors) in the left atrium of the heart, aortic arch, and the carotid sinus ([47], Fig. 7.9). Afferent stimuli in response to changing blood volume or pressure reach the brainstem through the vagal and glossopharyngeal nerves. The central pathways integrating these signals are unidentified, but they may involve a primary synapse in the nucleus tractus solitarius with a secondary relay in the posteriormedial nucleus of the hypothalamus.

Significant increases in plasma AVP are not detected (in rats) until blood volume is reduced by more than 8%. Other experimental data suggest that the relationship between vasopressin and blood volume in humans follows an exponential pattern similar to that of the rat. Under more unphysiological conditions, as in excessive hemorrhage, AVP causes maximal antidiuresis and may exert significant pressor effects on certain vascular beds. In humans and other animals there is an exponential relationship between plasma AVP levels and the degree of hypotension produced. Enhanced AVP secretion ensues after a reduction in mean arterial pressure as small as

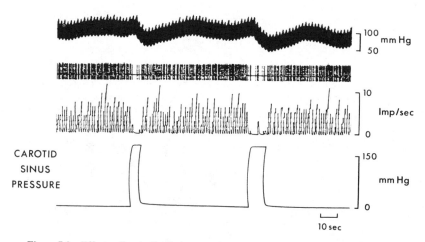

Figure 7.9 Effects of periodically increased pressure in the isolated carotid sinus on the activity of a SON neuron. Upper, middle, and bottom traces show the blood pressure, unit activity, integrated record of the number of spikes/sec, and carotid sinus pressure. (From Yamashita, [47], with permission.)

5%. Volume and sodium concentration may also affect AVP secretion through the renin-angiotensin system (Chapter 15). Angiotensin II, an octapeptide, may act on the brain to stimulate AVP secretion (Chapter 21). Thus a complex set of factors control AVP secretion and subsequently water and electrolyte balance. Much remains to be clarified to define completely the complex events in water-mineral homeostasis.

Vasopressin as CRH. Vasopressin has been suggested to serve as a corticotropin releasing hormone (CRH). In the monkey AVP is present in high concentrations in the portal blood of the anterior pituitary. There is an increase in neurosecretory material in the median eminence of the rat after adrenalectomy. Specifically there is an increase in both neurophysin and AVP, but not oxytocin, in the external zone of the median eminence, and the increase appears to be due to a lack of glucocorticoids. These data support the view that AVP may serve as a CRH in certain situations, particularly the acute response to stress [36]. AVP may be a natural CRH, but its action on the pituitary corticotrophs is modulated by other synergistic factors [15].

Vasopressin and behavior. Vasopressin is said to play a role in behavior (Chapter 21). Unless the hormone is transported retrogradely from the pars nervosa directly to the brain, one may wonder how this neurohypophysial hormone could play such a role if secreted directly into the peripheral circulation. If, on the other hand, this hormone is secreted from neurons within the brain, then it or other neurohypophysial peptides might indeed act as a neurotransmitter or, more likely, as a neuromodulator.

METABOLISM

Removal of AVP and oxytocin from the plasma may be reversible, by diffusion out of the plasma into interstitial fluid or other compartments, or irreversible, by degradation at or near target organ receptors and at clearing sites not related to target organ functions and also by urinary excretion. A number of enzymes exist in a variety of tissues which can degrade the neurohypophysial hormones in a specific manner. For example, an enzyme capable of inactivating oxytocin appears in human blood during pregnancy. It is produced in the placenta and is referred to as plasma *oxytocinase*. This amino peptidase produces a rupture of the ring of oxytocin by hydrolysis of the hemicystinyl-tyrosyl bond. The colostrum also contains enzymes, apparently produced in the mammary gland, which inactivate neurohypophysial hormones. The kidney, which is also a target organ for neurohypophysial hormones, contains a variety of enzymes which degrade and inactivate these hormones. A major question is whether these enzymatic inactivating processes are of any physiological significance. In addition many studies on neurohypophysial hormone degradation have been conducted with tissue homogenates containing intracellular enzymes which never come in contact with the hormones under normal physiological conditions.

MECHANISMS OF HORMONE ACTION

As for other peptide hormones, oxytocin and AVP interact with target tissue cellular membrane receptors. It would be expected that this initial receptor interaction would be followed by intracellular cyclic nucleotide production. Some of the earliest evidence for a role of cyclic nucleotides in hormone action did derive from studies on the mechanism of AVP action. The understanding of how oxytocin mediates its effects has come to light only recently.

Oxytocin

Uterine contraction.   Oxytocin not only interacts with myometrial receptors but also with endometrial tissue, an important event in the control of myometrial activity. Oxytocin stimulates the synthesis of $PGF_{2\alpha}$ in the ovine uterus, possibly by interacting with the endometrium, which is the principal source of uterine prostaglandins [40]. Estrogens may also enhance uterine synthesis of prostaglandins by increasing the activity of prostaglandin synthetase. Estrogens also increase the number of endometrial and myometrial oxytocin receptors. Progesterone antagonizes these effects of estrogens [38]. Thus estrogen-induced development of endometrial oxytocin receptors would enhance endometrial $PGF_{2\alpha}$ production in the presence of oxytocin. Myometrial contractions, a mechanical event, also induce endometrial $PGF_{2\alpha}$ production; thus oxytocin may affect $PGF_{2\alpha}$ synthesis directly and indirectly.

Prostaglandins of uterine origin are believed to control luteolysis in some species of mammals. Oxytocin could induce luteal regression via regulation of uterine synthesis of prostaglandins. The normal course of labor might depend on an early increase in uterine synthesis of prostaglandins to inhibit luteal or placental production of progesterone. Decreased progesterone levels would remove the block to oxytocin-induced uterine contractions, which are maintained up to that time by the steroid (Chapter 19).

Vasopressin

The mechanism of action of AVP has been determined from studies on a variety of epithelia—frog skin, toad bladder, and mammalian nephron. The toad bladder, a storage organ for water, is a useful and simple model system and responds to AVP somewhat similarly to the distal tubule of the mammalian nephron. The organ is a relatively large sheet of thin epithelium which survives for long periods in vitro. Exposure of isolated toad bladder to AVP results in an increase in sodium and water transport from the outer (mucosal or luminal) to the inner (serosal) side. Increased water movement is not, however, dependent on the presence of sodium ion in the mucosal medium. The significance of sodium ion transport and water movements is unclear. Vasopressin may or may not translocate sodium (or urea), depending on the species studied. Vasopressin can only affect water permeability if applied to the serosal side of the bladder, and it can only act on the kidney collecting duct when applied to the peritubular (serosal) side. The barrier to the penetration of water across such membranes is in the mucosal (luminal) side. This barrier is decreased in the presence of AVP, and water is moved across the cells and leaves at the basal (serosal) margins. Water is believed to move through pores in the epithelial cells and AVP may increase the size of these pores. The response may reflect an increase in the number of the pores, not an increase in pore radius. Whether the increase in flow is due to an increase in the number of pores or in their diameter, or to both, remains unclear.

Interaction of AVP with toad bladder serosal plasmalemmal receptors activates adenylate cyclase and intracellular levels of cyclic AMP are elevated [40, 46]. An increased permeability to water of the mucosal membrane then results. Cyclic AMP or its analogs as well as phosphodiesterase inhibitors (e.g., theophylline) enhance water permeability, thus supporting a role for cyclic AMP as the intracellular messenger of AVP. Vasopressin and cyclic AMP stimulate epithelial cell protein kinases, and phosphorylation or dephosphorylation (by phosphorylation activation of phospho-protein phosphatases) of membrane proteins may be responsible for the ultimate effect of vasopressin, working through cyclic AMP, on membrane water permeability [46]. The site of action of these effects is the membrane of the mucosal surface. Structural changes (intramembranous particle aggregation) occur in this barrier to render the membrane more permeable to water. Microtubules have been implicated in mucosal cell structural changes in response to AVP. Vasopressin stimulates prostaglandin synthesis in the toad urinary bladder and rabbit renal tubular cells [17]. The prostaglandin produced is then inhibitory to toad bladder adenylate cyclase activity. The significance of this observation is unclear, but might represent a negative feedback mechanism. The actions of AVP on frog skin and the mammalian nephron also involve elevations in cyclic AMP levels.

PATHOPHYSIOLOGY

The control of vasopressin release and regulation of fluid balance occurs primarily in response to alterations in blood tonicity and blood volume so that a relative constancy of these two parameters is maintained. This finely adjusted homeostatic system can be disrupted by disease states which affect neurohypophysial or renal function and in which vasopressin is produced independent of normal regulatory influences. The resulting clinical disturbance of body water balance will be manifest by hypernatremia or hyponatremia and by excessive water loss or retention.

Diabetes insipidus.   Impairment of the neurohypophysial system to synthesize or release vasopressin results in a diminished ability of the kidney to conserve water, resulting in pituitary (neurogenic) diabetes insipidus. The pituitary form of diabetes insipidus may result from a defect present at birth or later in life. Failure to synthesize AVP can also occur as a result of disease processes which destroy hypothalamic or posterior pituitary tissue. Diabetes insipidus can also result from traumatic or surgical injury to the hypothalamus.

In the normal individual plasma osmolality is maintained in a range of 285 to 290 mOsmol/kg with associated plasma AVP levels of 1 to 3 μU/ml and urinary AVP levels of 11 to 30 mU/24 hours [32, 33]. In patients with severe diabetes insipidus plasma osmolality may rise to more than 330 mOsmol/kg; under this severe osmotic stress, plasma and urinary AVP remain well below the normal range.

In *nephrogenic* (vasopressin-resistant) diabetes insipidus, there is a defect in the urinary concentration mechanism at the level of the kidney. Pituitary diabetes insipidus can be treated by replacement therapy with vasopressin, but the hormone is without effect in the nephrogenic disease type. In fact, greater than normal levels of

AVP are present in this condition. The antidiuretic response of the kidney to AVP is used clinically to diagnose the specific type of defect responsible for the diuresis. Females may have a subclinical form of the disease or the more severe form which is characteristic in males. A dominant sex-linked inheritance with variable penetrance is suggested. The defect appears to involve a failure to generate intracellular levels of cyclic AMP within distal tubular cells of the kidney in response to AVP.

Syndrome of inappropriate vasopressin secretion. The state of continual release of AVP without relationship to plasma osmolality or volume is referred to as the syndrome of inappropriate vasopressin secretion. The syndrome is characterized by an inability to excrete a maximally dilute urine, which results in retention of water, an expansion of the extracellular fluid volume, and a resultant dilutional hyponatremia. The most common cause of excessive AVP secretion is malignancy: AVP is secreted from a carcinoma of the lung, and is secreted with its neurophysin. Although plasma and urinary levels of AVP may be markedly elevated, the amount of hormone in the blood or urine may be similar to that of normal individuals. However, these levels are excessive considering that the hypotonicity should have inhibited AVP secretion.

Genetic defect in vasopressin synthesis. Transplantation of vasopressin neurons from normal rat fetuses into the adult Brattleboro rat, which congenitally lacks AVP-producing neurons, alleviates the polydipsia and polyuria that are symptomatic of this genetic defect. Apparently the axons of the grafted fetal neurons make appropriate and functional connections within the brain of the host. The ability of transplanted neurons to correct a CNS deficiency has important theoretical and clinical implications [13].

COMPARATIVE ENDOCRINOLOGY

Determination of the structure of the neurohypophysial peptides, present within the pars nervosa of different vertebrate classes, has provided a remarkable understanding of the evolution of the neurohypophysial hormones [1, 37]. This information has also given insight into the structural requirements for neurohypophysial hormone action. From these studies a variety of hormone analogs for detailed analysis of hormone-receptor interaction have been designed.

Neurohypophysial hormones have been characterized in representatives of all vertebrate classes [1]. The neurohypophysis of each vertebrate species contains at least two principles, except in the cyclostomes where only a single peptide, arginine vasotocin (AVT), has so far been detected. In the species studied the same two hormones are usually present in the neurohypophysis of each of the members of a particular vertebrate group. Only one or two residues differ between the hormones of any two different vertebrate classes. Sequence differences occur only at positions 3, 4, and 8 of the nonapeptides. Structural differences at these positions apparently account for the differing receptor affinities and activities of the neurohypophysial peptides.

Nine of the neurohypophysial hormones have been characterized: six are regarded as oxytocinlike and the remaining three as vasopressinlike. An early gene duplication apparently led to two lines of neurohypophysial principles. Gene mutation following gene duplication may have resulted in one line originating with isotocin, found in bony fishes, which gave rise by further base mutations to the oxytocin-related structures. The other line originating directly from AVT gave rise much later in evolution to the vasopressins. Although the oxytocic and antidiuretic roles of neurohypophysial hormones are well documented in mammals, there is no convincing evidence that the neurohypophysial or related peptides subserve these functions in nonmammalian vertebrates. Vasotocin is intermediate in structure between oxytocin and arginine vasopressin and is considered to be phylogenetically the oldest neurohypophysial hormone. AVT was synthesized and found to have properties identical to the naturally occurring amphibian water balance principle [20]. Chemical analysis of the amphibian neurohypophysis revealed that the natural peptide was AVT. This provided a unique example where a synthetic hormone was synthetically prepared before its natural homologue had been identified.

Some members of the piglike mammals (pigs, peccaries, wart hogs, and hippopotami) contain a vasopressin with a lysine rather than arginine at the 8 position of the molecule [12]. It has been suggested that lysine vasopressin (LVP) arose as a single-step mutation from arginine vasopressin. This genetic transformation apparently took place in an ancestor of this family before the hippopotami diverged from the pig-peccary stock. AVP and LVP may both be present in individual members of the pig family according to a Hardy-Weinberg distribution [11]. Homozygotes contain one peptide and the heterozygotes contain both, suggesting the gene for vasopressin is present in two allelic forms. Only LVP is present in the domestic pig which may have resulted from the restrictive and selective force of domestication by humans. Both LVP and AVP are present in individual pituitaries of both Australian macropodian (kangaroos and wallabies) and American didelphian (opossums) marsupials [1]. The constant presence of two pressor principles within individual pituitaries suggests that these peptides arose by gene duplication. A new neurohypophysial peptide, phenypressin ([Phe^2, Arg^8]-vasopressin) has been found in the pituitary of two marsupials, the red kangaroo and the tammar [7].

REFERENCES

[1] Acher, R. 1980. Molecular evolution of biologically active polypeptides. *Proc. R. Soc. Lond.* B210:21–43.

[2] Altura, B. M., and B. T. Altura. 1977. Vascular smooth muscle and neurohypophysial hormones. *Fed. Proc.* 36:1853–60.

[3] Bargmann, W., and E. Scharrer. 1951. The site of origin of the hormones of the posterior pituitary. *Am. Sci.* 39:255–59.

[4] Bisset, G. W. 1974. Milk ejection. In *Handbook of physiology*, Section 7, Endocrinology, eds. R. O. Greep and E. B. Astwood, vol. 4, part 1, pp. 493–520. eds. E. Knobil and W. H. Sawyer. Washington, D.C.: Am. Physiol. Soc.

[5] Blessing, W. W., A. F. Sved, and D. J. Reis. 1982. Destruction of noradrenergic neurons in rabbit brainstem elevates plasma vasopressin, causing hypertension. *Science* 217:661–62.

[6] Brownstein, M. J., J. T. Russell, and H. Gainer. 1980. Synthesis, transport, and release of posterior pituitary howmones. *Science* 207:373–78.

[7] Chauvet, M. T., D. Hurpet, J. Chauvet, and R. Acher. 1980. Phenypressin (Phe^2-Arg^8-vasopressin), a new neurohypophysial peptide found in marsupials. *Nature* 287:640–42.

[8] Dale, H. H. 1906. On some physiological actions of ergot. *J. Physiol.* 34:163–206.

[9] DOUGLAS, W. W. 1974. Mechanism of release of neurohypophysial hormones; stimulus-secretion coupling. In *Handbook of physiology*, Section 7, Endocrinology, eds. R. O. Greep and E. B. Astwood, vol. 4, part 1, pp. 191–224, eds. E. Knobil and W. H. Sawyer. Washington, D.C.: Am. Physiol. Soc.

[10] DREIFUSS, J. J., E. TRIBOLLET, and M. MUHLETHALER. 1981. Temporal patterns of neural activity and their relation to the secretion of posterior pituitary hormones. *Biol. Reprod.* 24:51–72.

[11] FERGUSON, D. R. 1969. The genetic distribution of vasopressins in the peccary (*Tayasau angulatus*) and warthog (*Phacochoerus aethiopicus*). *Gen. Comp. Endocrinol.* 12:609–13.

[12] FERGUSON, D. R., and B. T. PICKERING. 1964. Arginine and lysine vasopressins in the hippopotamus neurohypophysis. *Gen. Comp. Endocrinol.* 13:425–28.

[13] GASH, D., J. R. SLADEK, JR., and C. D. SLADEK. 1980. Functional development of grafted vasopressin neurons. *Science* 210:1367–69.

[14] GEORGE, J. M., S. STAPLES, and B. M. MARKS. 1976. Oxytocin content of microdissected areas of rat hypothalamus. *Endocrinology* 98:1430–33.

[15] GILLIES, G., and P. LOWRY. 1979. Corticotropin releasing factor may be modulated by vasopressin. *Nature* 278:463–64.

[16] HALTER, J. B., A. P. GOLDBERG, G. L. ROBERTSON, and D. PORTE, JR. 1977. Selective osmoreceptor dysfunction in the syndrome of chronic hypernatremia. *J. Clin. Endocrinol. Metab.* 44:609–16.

[17] HANDLER, J. S., and J. ORLOFF. 1981. Antidiuretic hormone. *Ann. Rev. Physiol.* 43:611–24.

[18] HAYWARD, J. N. 1975. Neural control of the posterior pituitary. *Ann. Rev. Physiol.* 37:191–210.

[19] HOWELL, W. H. 1898. The physiological effects of extracts of the hypophysis cerebri and infundibular body. *J. Exp. Med.* 3:235–58.

[20] KATSOYANNIS, P. G., and V. DU VIGNEAUD. 1958. Arginine-vasotocin, a synthetic analogue of the posterior pituitary hormones containing the ring of oxytocin and the side chain of vasopressin. *J. Biol. Chem.* 233:1352–54.

[21] KIRCHHEIM, H. R. 1976. Systemic arterial baroreceptor reflexes. *Physiol. Rev.* 56:100–77.

[22] LINCOLN, D. W., and J. B. WAKERLEY. 1974. Electrophysiological evidence for the activation of supraoptic neurones during the release of oxytocin. *J. Physiol.* 242:533–54.

[23] LINCOLN, D. W., and A. C. PAISLEY. 1982. Neuroendocrine control of milk ejection. *J. Reprod. Fertil.* 65:571–86.

[24] LINZELL, J. L. 1961. Recent advances in the physiology of the udder. *Vet. Ann.* 2:44–53.

[25] MARSHALL, J. M. 1974. Effects of neurohypophysial hormones in the myometrium. In *Handbook of physiology*, Section 7, Endocrinology, eds. R. O. Greep and E. B. Astwood, vol. 4, part 1, pp. 469–92, eds. E. Knobil and W. H. Sawyer. Washington, D.C.: Am. Physiol. Soc.

[26] OLIVER, G., and E. A. SCHAFER. 1895. On the physiological actions of extracts of the pituitary body and certain other glandular organs. *J. Physiol.* 18: 277–79.

[27] PICKERING, B. T. 1968. A neurophysin from cod (*Gadus morrhua*) pituitary glands: isolation and properties. *J. Endocrinol.* 42:143–52.

[28] ———. 1978. The neurosecretory neurone: a model system for the study of secretion. *Essays in Biochem.* 14:45–81.

[29] POULAIN, D. A., J. B. WAKERLEY, and R. E. J. DYBALL. 1977. Electrophysiological differentiation of oxytocin- and vasopressin-secreting neurones. *Proc. Roy. Soc. Lond.*, B. 196:367–84.

[30] RICHARD, P. 1972. The reticulo-hypothalamic pathway controlling the release of oxytocin in the ewe. *J. Endocrinol.* 53:71–83.

[31] RICHARDSON, K. C. 1949. Contractile tissues in the mammary gland with special reference to myoepithelium in the goat. *Proc. Roy. Soc. Lond.* B 136:30–45.

[32] ROBERTSON, G. L., R. L. SHELTON, and S. ATHAR. 1976. The osmoregulation of vasopressin. *Kidney Int.* 10:25–37.

[33] ROBERTSON, G. L., S. ATHAR, and R. L. SHELTON. 1977. Osmotic control of vasopressin function. In *Disturbances in body fluid osmolality*, pp. 125–48. Washington, D.C.: Am. Physiol. Soc.

[34] ROBINSON, A. G. 1978. Neurophysins, an aid to understanding the structure and function of the neurohypophysis. *Front. Neuroendocrinol.* 5:35–59.

[35] SACHS, H., and Y. TAKABATAKE. 1974. Evidence for a precursor in vasopressin biosynthesis. *Endocrinology* 75:943–48.

[36] SAFFRAN, M., and A. V. SCHALLY. 1977. The status of the corticotropin releasing factor (CRF). *Neuroendocrinology* 24:359–75.

[37] SAWYER, W. H. 1977. Evolution of the neurohypophysial hormones. *Amer. Zool.* 17:727–37.

[38] SMALL, M. G. P., J. E. GAVAGAN, and J. S. ROBERTS. 1978. Oxytocin-stimulated production of prostaglandin $F_{2\alpha}$ by isolated endometrium of rabbit: modulated by ovarian steroids. *Prostaglandins* 15:103–12.

[39] SOLOFF, M. S., H. D. REES, M. SAR, and W. E. STUMPF. 1975. Autoradiographic localization of radioreactivity from [^{3}H]-oxytocin in the rat mammary gland and oviduct. *Endocrinology* 96:1475–77.

[40] SOLOFF, M. S., and A. F. PEARLMUTTER. 1979. Biochemical actions of neurohypophysial hormones and neurophysin. In *Biochemical actions of hormones*, vol. 6, ed. G. Litwack, pp. 265–333. New York: Academic Press, Inc.

[41] SOLOFF, M. S., M. ALEXANDROVA, and M. J. FERNSTROM. 1979. Oxytocin receptors: triggers for parturition and lactation. *Science* 204:1313–14.

[42] SUMMERLEE, A. J. S., and D. W. LINCOLN. 1981. Electrophysiological recordings from oxytocinergic neurones during suckling in the unanaesthetized lactating rat. *J. Endocrinol.* 90:255–65.

[43] TINDAL, J. S., and G. S. KNAGGS. 1971. Determination of the detailed hypothalamic route of the milk-ejection reflex in the guinea pig. *J. Endocrinol.* 50:135–52.

[44] VANDESANDE, F., K. DIERICKX, and J. DEMEY. 1975. Identification of the vasopressin-neurophysin II and the oxytocin-neurophysin I producing neurons in the bovine hypothalamus. *Cell Tiss. Res.* 156:189–200.

[45] VERNEY, E. B. 1947. The antidiuretic hormone and the factors which determine its release. *Proc. Roy. Soc. Lond.*, B. 135:25–106.

[46] WALTON, R. G., R. J. DELORENZO, P. F. CURRAN, and P. GREENGARD. 1975. Regulation of protein phosphorylation and sodium transport in toad bladder. *J. Gen. Physiol.* 65:153–77.

[47] YAMASHITA, H. 1977. Effect of baro- and chemoreceptor activation on supraoptic nuclei neurons in the hypothalamus. *Brain Res.* 126:551–56.

[48] YAMASHITA, H., K. KOIZUMI, and C. MCC. BROOKS. 1979. Rhythmic patterns of discharge in hypothalamic neurosecretory neurons of cats and dogs. *Proc. Natl. Acad. Sci.* 76:6684–88.

[49] ZIMMERMAN, E. A., and A. G. ROBINSON. 1976. Hypothalamic neurons secreting vasopressin and neurophysin. *Kidney Int.* 10:12–24.

8

The Melanotropins

INTRODUCTION

The early studies of Smith and Allen clearly implicated the pituitary gland as the source of a hormone that controlled color changes in amphibians. These color changes were found to be due to the response of certain *chromatophores* (pigment-bearing cells), particularly *melanophores* (melanin-containing cells), found within the skin. The melanotropic substance was specifically localized to the neurointermediate lobe (pars intermedia) of the pituitary [1, 11]. This substance is now referred to as *melanocyte-stimulating hormone* (MSH) or sometimes as *intermedin*. MSH and other structurally related peptides found within the pituitary and the brain are referred to generically as *melanotropins* (Fig. 8.1). Although research on MSH dates to the early part of this century, it is only recently that the origin, chemistry, and secretion of this hormone have become more fully clarified.

There have been some confusing interludes in the story of the melanotropins. It was generally believed that the vertebrate pituitary contains an α-MSH and a β-MSH. Human pituitaries, however, were said to lack an α-MSH but to contain a β-MSH, which consisted of more amino acids than the melanotropins of other mammalian β-MSH's. More confusing was that the pars intermedia of the pituitary gland of the adult human and some other primates is rudimentary in structure, although a fetal zona intermedia is present and may produce a melanotropin. This chapter will review the interesting story of the melanotropins and their newly suggested roles in vertebrate physiology.

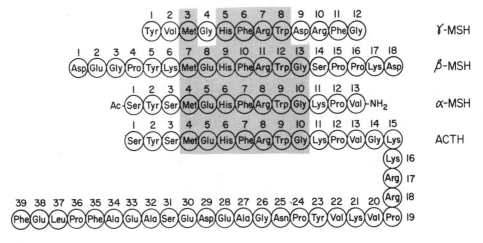

Figure 8.1 Amino acid sequences of bovine γ-, β-, and α-MSH compared to ACTH. (From Sawyer et al., [39], with permission.)

THE PARS INTERMEDIA

The pars intermedia apparently develops as a result of contact between the infundibulum and the adenohypophysial analage [9]. In cyclostomes, amphibians, reptiles, and most mammals, the MSH-secreting cells (melanotrophs) form a well-defined pars intermedia or intermediate lobe (Fig. 8.2). Although the pars intermedia of certain mammals is absent (cetaceans: whales, dolphins), a zona intermedia does exist in the human fetus, though it subsequently becomes modified or rudimentary (Fig. 5.1). Birds lack a pars intermedia, but it is claimed, on cytological and bioassay evidence, that MSH-secreting cells are present within the pars distalis [20]. In elasmobranchs and teleosts the MSH cells are localized caudally but are contiguous with other cells of the pars distalis (Fig. 8.2). The pars nervosa and the pars intermedia of tetrapods are inseparable from each other; this anatomical unit is often referred to as the neuro-intermediate lobe.

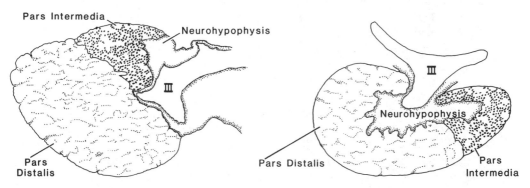

Figure 8.2 Sagittal sections of (left) an amphibian (salamander) pituitary and (right) a teleost pituitary gland. The three lobular components of the glands are indicated: neurohypophysis, pars intermedia, and pars distalis. The third ventricle (III) is also indicated.

The size of the pars intermedia is usually positively correlated with whether or not an animal is able to change color in conformity with the background of the immediate environment. The pars intermedia of the lizard, *Anolis carolinensis*, is very large, and this reptile has an outstanding ability for color change, being a bright green or dark brown on light or dark backgrounds, respectively. In some mammals, on the other hand, the size of the pars intermedia is said to be correlated with the nature of the environment, large in mammals living in dehydrating conditions [19]. In rats injection of hypertonic saline or dehydration results in hypertrophic changes in the cells of the pars intermedia, thus suggesting some possible role for the pars intermedia in ion regulation.

The pars intermedia is relatively avascular compared to the other components of the pituitary gland and other endocrine tissues. Nevertheless, an extravascular, multibranched transport system penetrates the parenchyma of the pars intermedia and may provide a pathway for the passage of secretory products and regulatory factors to and from the gland [34]. In some species the pars intermedia differs from the pars distalis in that it is penetrated by neurons from the hypothalamus. Neurosecretory and catecholamine-containing neuronal elements may be present; the latter may form a plexus around the secretory cells. These aminergic neurons play a dominant role in the control of MSH secretion as will be discussed. Neurons are absent from the neurointermediate lobe of the few lizards that have been studied [36, 49].

The pars intermedia of many teleost fishes contains two cell types. One stains selectively with lead hematoxylin (PIPbH cell) and the other with periodic acid-schiff (PIPAS cell) [4]. Immunocytochemical studies indicate that the PIPbH cell is the source of MSH. Depending on the species, the PIPbH cell or the PIPAS cell or both control the darkening response of the skin of fishes adapted to a black background. The chemical nature of the secretory product of the PIPAS cell is unknown [3].

SYNTHESIS AND CHEMISTRY OF MELANOTROPINS

The history of research related to the present understanding of the chemistry and proposed roles of the vertebrate melanotropins began with investigations which established that the pituitary gland contained a number of melanotropic peptides. A rather pure MSH (α-MSH) was indeed subsequently isolated from the pituitary of a number of mammalian species. Soon after the discovery of α-MSH, another chemically different MSH, β-melanotropin (β-MSH), was also isolated from the pituitary of these same species.

Human pituitaries were said to lack α-MSH but to contain a β-MSH that was longer (22 amino acids) than the β-MSH's (18 amino acids) isolated from other mammalian pituitaries. Radioimmunoassays revealed that in normal humans and those with certain pathological conditions the plasma concentrations of β-MSH and ACTH were always correlated. It was therefore thought that β-MSH was the principal melanotropic hormone of humans. Subsequently the α-MSH's from a number of mammalian pituitaries were chemically characterized and found to be identical in structure. The structure of α-MSH, however, differs slightly in the few poikilotherms that have been studied [21, 27]. Shark (*Squalus acanthias*) and salmon (*Oncorhynchus keta*) α-MSH's are also tridecapeptides, but the N-terminal serine is unacetylated in these species. In addition in the dogfish shark the C-terminal amino acid, which is valine in all mammalian α-MSH's, is replaced by methionine.

Eventually it was discovered that pituitaries of a number of species contained a melanotropic peptide that was larger than that of any known pigmentary peptide. The ovine molecule was shown to contain 91 amino acids and was referred to as β-lipotropic hormone, β-LPH (Fig. 21.3). The complete structure of β-MSH is contained within the 41–58 sequence of this peptide [7]. Further work revealed that the so-called β-MSH of humans is merely a fragment of β-LPH, artifactually formed during extraction of the tissue. Thus the earlier radioimmunoassay measurements of β-MSH in humans were measurements of the β-LPH present within the plasma. The adult human pituitary may therefore produce only two melanotropic peptides, ACTH and β-LPH, and these are probably not involved, under normal conditions, in the control of melanocyte activity. There is no evidence that β-MSH serves any peripheral physiological function other than as a necessary secretory by-product of other hormones derived from the melanotrophs.

Subsequent to these early studies a corticotropinlike peptide, CLIP, was discovered in the pars intermedia of rat and pig pituitaries. This peptide is composed of the 18–39 amino acid sequence of ACTH. It has been proposed that CLIP and α-MSH are products of the intracellular cleavage of ACTH, and that ACTH serves as the prohormone for α-MSH [26]. No clear function for CLIP has been shown; CLIP may simply be a necessary cleavage product of MSH secretion. Similarly a larger protein (31,000 MW) has been isolated from both the pars distalis and the pars intermedia (Chapter 21). This protein, pro-opiomelanocortin, contains the sequences of ACTH and β-LPH. In the pars distalis ACTH is released under certain physiological conditions to regulate adrenocortical function. In the pars intermedia, on the other hand, enzymes are present within the secretory granules and are responsible for the enzymatic cleavage of pro-opiomelanocortin to α-MSH (Fig. 8.3). Following cleavage from the precursor protein, posttranslational amidation and acetylation of the C-terminus and N-terminus, respectively, of the MSH molecule then occurs [7, 22].

α-MSH has also been localized to the hypothalamus where it is found within the perikarya of neurons of the arcuate nucleus. These α-MSH-containing cell bodies in the ventral hypothalamus send multiple projections to numerous extrahypothalamic regions of the brain. Destruction of the arcuate nucleus lowers the α-MSH content

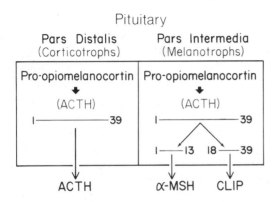

Figure 8.3 Prohormone theory of ACTH and α-MSH biosynthesis [26]. It is unclear whether in the pars distalis ACTH is first enzymatically released from pro-opiomelanocortin to yield α-MSH and CLIP or the latter two peptides are liberated directly from pro-opiomelanocortin. (Modified from Lowry and Scott, [26].)

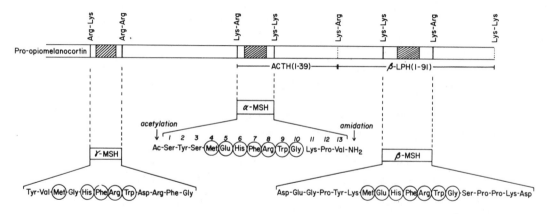

Figure 8.4 Schematic representation of the known biologically active peptides derived from pro-opiomelanocortin which is found in the vertebrate pituitary (corticotrophs and melanotrophs) and hypothalamus. (Reprinted with permission from Sawyer et al., [38]. Copyright 1982, American Chemical Society.)

of extrahypothalamic regions (Chapter 21). Neuronal perikarya of the arcuate region also contain ACTH and β-endorphin, and the reduction in levels of these peptides (including α-MSH) after various treatments suggests that these neuronal peptides are derived from a common precursor, pro-opiomelanocortin, similar to ACTH and α-MSH in the pituitary gland. A γ-MSH is also present within the pituitary gland and hypothalamus as a component of pro-opiomelanocortin in some mammalian species (Fig. 8.1). Thus the precursor protein pro-opiomelanocortin contains within its primary structure the sequences of five melanotropic peptides: α-MSH, β-MSH, γ-MSH, ACTH, and β-LPH (Fig. 8.4).

A heptapeptide sequence has been conserved within the structures of α-MSH, β-MSH, and ACTH. The first 13 amino acids of ACTH are identical to those of α-MSH. Unlike the other melanotropins, the N-terminus of α-MSH is acetylated and the C-terminus is amidated. There is a great species heterogeneity in structure of the β-MSH's, which may further support the suggestion that β-MSH serves no functional role other than as a structural component of pro-opiomelanocortin.

CONTROL OF MSH SECRETION

Disruption of the normal anatomical relationships between the pars intermedia and the hypothalamus results in the release of MSH. The endocrine implications of this observation were first appreciated in the early studies of Etkin [10]. Ectopic transplantation of the entire pituitary gland or the isolated neurointermediate lobe usually leads to hypertrophy of the pars intermedia cells and to an increased (uninhibited) release of MSH. These experiments and others involving hypothalamic lesions or pituitary stalk transection have yielded similar results in a variety of vertebrates. The observations suggest that the hypothalamus exerts an inhibitory control over MSH release [17].

Hypothalamic extracts have been claimed to inhibit MSH secretion in vitro but in most cases this inhibition was due to enzymes present within the extracts that degrade MSH. As yet no MSH release-inhibiting hormone (melanostatin) has been isolated from the hypothalamus. Nevertheless there is strong evidence that inhibition of MSH secretion by the hypothalamus is controlled by a catecholamine, most likely dopamine. Catecholamines, such as norepinephrine, epinephrine, and dopamine, are inhibitory to MSH secretion from the isolated neurointermediate lobe of the pituitary [6]. The inhibitory actions of these catecholamines are antagonized by chlorpromazine, a dopaminergic receptor antagonist. Dopaminergic receptor agonists, such as certain ergot alkaloids, on the other hand, are inhibitory to pars intermedia MSH secretion both in vivo and in vitro [30].

In animals that change color in response to a light- or to a dark-colored background, the following model has been proposed from early studies on the frog. The amount of light that is reflected from the background substratum (albedo) to the dorsal aspect of the retina relative to the amount that reaches the bottom of the retina from the light source overhead determines whether MSH will be secreted. On a black background very little light is reflected to the upper aspect of the retina compared to the amount reflected from a light-colored substratum. In either case the amount reaching the lower part of the retina remains the same. The differential stimulation of the two retinal components therefore determines the chromatic response. On a black background animals turn dark in color due to the release of MSH from the pars intermedia, whereas animals become light on a white background due to an inhibition of MSH secretion.

In the absence of any tonic hypothalamic inhibitory input melanotrophs and lactotrophs exhibit spontaneous electrical activity in vitro. They both provide informative model systems for determining the relationship between cellular secretion and membrane bioelectrical activity. For example, hormones that affect MSH or PRL secretion do so by mechanisms that modify the membrane electrical activity of the melanotrophs and lactotrophs [8].

From a large amount of data obtained from a variety of species the following events are possibly involved in the control of MSH release from the pars intermedia, at least in animals that change color [16]. Environmental photic cues received by the lateral eyes are relayed via neuronal circuits to the hypothalamus. These neurons of inhibitory or stimulatory nature may terminate and synapse with other neurons within the hypothalamus. Aminergic and peptidergic neurons originating in the postoptic nucleus and preoptic nucleus, respectively, have been shown (in the skate) to course through the basal hypothalamus, as a pair of lateral aminergic fiber tracts and a central neurosecretory tract, to penetrate the pars intermedia [29]. The catecholamine-containing neurons make synaptic contact with the individual melanotrophs. The neurosecretory neurons penetrate only to the pars nervosa-pars intermedia border. Other cholinergic neurons of unknown hypothalamic origin may also penetrate into the pars intermedia of some species.

Dopamine released from the aminergic neurons interacts with dopaminergic receptors possessed by the membranes of the pars intermedia cells. The tonic release of the catecholamine maintains the cells in the hyperpolarized state, and this release is inhibitory to MSH secretion. The cholinergic neurons may antagonize the aminergic neurons by release of acetylcholine at synapses on the aminergic neurons themselves or by direct synaptic contact with the pars intermedia cells. MSH release would then result from presynaptic inhibition (of dopamine release) or by a direct depolarizing input to the doubly innervated melanotrophs. Release would result if the cholinergic depolarizing input were able to override the aminergic hyperpolarizing inhibitory input. Fine adjustments between the two opposing synaptic events might then modulate the amount of MSH to be secreted.

In those vertebrates where a direct aminergic innervation is absent (e.g., lizards), neurotransmitters released from the median eminence or pars nervosa may be delivered to the pars intermedia by way of vascular or other routes [36, 49]. In the few nonmammalian species studied serotonin appears to exert a stimulating effect on MSH secretion [32]. Administration of 5-hydroxytryptophan, a precursor of serotonin, is indirectly stimulatory to melanophore dispersion in the skin of some fishes and amphibians. There is cytological evidence that pituitary melanotrophs are stimulated by serotonin. Serotonin stimulates MSH secretion from the isolated neurointermediate lobe of some species, and the frequency of pars intermedia action potentials (depolarizations) is enhanced coincident to MSH secretion. It is possible that in some species (e.g., the lizard, *Anolis carolinensis*), where an inhibitory hypothalamic control is lacking and there is minimal autonomous secretion of MSH, serotonin subserves a function as a hypophysiotropin, a so-called MSH releasing hormone (melanocrinin).

PHYSIOLOGICAL ROLES OF MSH

The role of the pars intermedia and MSH in the control of color changes in poikilothermic vertebrates is the one clearly documented physiological function of the hormone and one of the earliest described roles for a vertebrate hormone. Only recently have other putative functions been ascribed to MSH [11].

Melanin Pigmentation of the Skin

The one unquestionable role of MSH is to control melanin pigmentation of the skin of most vertebrate species [14]. In mammals and many other vertebrates melanin-containing pigment cells are found in the basal layers of the epidermis. These *melanocytes* (also referred to as melanophores) utilize the precursor amino acid, tyrosine, and through a number of biochemical events controlled by one or more enzymes, produce a colored polymer called *melanin*. This melanin is incorporated into a subcellular structure referred to as a *premelanosome*. When this organelle becomes fully melanized, it is known as a *melanin granule* or *melanosome*. Brown and black melanins are referred to as *eumelanins*, whereas red or lighter colored melanins are known as *phaeomelanins*. Mammals with differently colored pelage patterns produce specifically colored melanins in different anatomical areas of the skin.

The melanin produced within the melanocytes is released into surrounding cells of the skin by a secretory (cytocrine) mechanism that is not fully understood. The functional unit of epidermal pigmentation, comprised of a melanocyte and its associated epidermal cells, is referred to as an *epidermal melanin unit* [15]. Melanotropins enhance melanin production within melanocytes, and the melanosomes produced migrate into the dendritic processes of the cells where they are released into the surrounding cells of the epidermis (Fig. 8.5). The melanocytes in haired parts of the skin

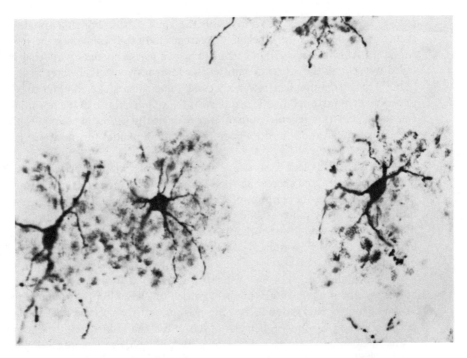

Figure 8.5 Epidermal melanin units of the frog *Rana pipiens*. Melanosomes synthesized by the melanocytes are released into adjacent keratinocytes where they function, at least in humans, as a sunscreen against ultraviolet radiation [15].

are localized to the hair follicles, and synthesis of melanin by these follicular melanocytes is responsible for pigmentation of the hair; a similar process is responsible for melanin pigmentation of feathers. MSH and steroid hormones may sequentially or in combination affect the production of eumelanins and phaeomelanins within individual follicular melanocytes, which can lead to hairs which contain black, brown, or white bands, or an *agouti pattern*. Although MSH affects hair pigmentation in some mammals, the hormonal basis of melanin pigmentation of feathers is not clearly understood, particularly because birds lack a pars intermedia.

Seasonal alterations in pigment cell activity are an important aspect of the ability of an animal to conform to yearly changes in environmental conditions. Control of integumental pigmentation is generally a dynamic rather than a static process. An animal, such as the varying hare (*Lepus americanus*), is thus able to change color from a brown summer pelage to a white winter coat. Suntanning in humans is another example. Ontogenic changes in integumental pigmentation occur as in the development of the nuptial coloration of the skin that is associated with the sexual activity of such vertebrates as birds. The graying of hair of humans and other mammals is a common phenotypic characteristic of older age, but its physiological significance and etiology is not well understood.

Morphological color changes, which involve alterations in the amount of pigment present within the skin, are generally manifest in response to seasonal changes in background conditions. Rabbits and ptarmigans, for example, develop a white pelage or plumage in conformity with the snow of the winter habitat. During the spring and summer a dark pelage or feather change accompanies the melting of the snows. MSH is implicated in the white to brown pelage changes that occur in the short-tailed weasel and the Siberian hamster in conformity with the winter to spring change [25, 37]. That mammalian melanocytes of some species can respond to MSH is dramatically demonstrated by the response of the yellow mouse to the hormone (Fig. 8.6). Phenotypically this genetic strain of mice is normally yellow in color [13]; the response to MSH is unnatural, but does demonstrate the potential for melanogenic activity in the mammal.

Because birds lack a pars intermedia, it is possible that certain cells of the pars distalis synthesize and secrete an MSH or some other melanotropin. However, MSH has been shown to be without effect on feather pigmentation in the few species of birds studied. Not much is known about the neuroendocrine control of avian pigmentation. One would like to know, for example, what endocrine or other chemical messengers control winter-to-spring and fall-to-winter plumage color changes, particularly in ptarmigans.

Morphological color changes result from changes in the number and synthetic activity of the integumentary pigment cells. For example, frogs maintained on light- or dark-colored backgrounds for long periods of time become light or dark in color (Fig. 8.7), and the number of melanocytes in the epidermis from these animals differs dramatically (Fig. 8.8). This morphological color change is controlled by MSH and clearly demonstrates hypertrophy and hyperplasia of melanocytes in response to the hormone [15]. In vitro studies demonstrate that melanotropins are clearly stimulatory to melanoblast cytodifferentiation and proliferation [47].

Because MSH is apparently absent from the pituitary of adult humans, the stimulus for enhanced melanogenic activity during suntanning is not known. Repeated injections of MSH into darkly pigmented individuals, however, increase epidermal pigmentation which is readily visible after a few days. This demonstrates the capability of the human melanocyte system, at least in dark-skinned individuals, to respond to hormonal activation by MSH [33]. Pigmentation of humans is genetically con-

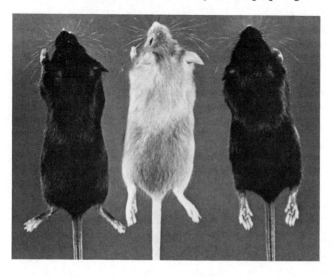

Figure 8.6 Effect of injected α-MSH on melanin pigmentation of the hair of the yellow (C57BL/6J-A^y strain) mouse (From Geschwind, Huseby, and Nishioka, [13], with permission.)

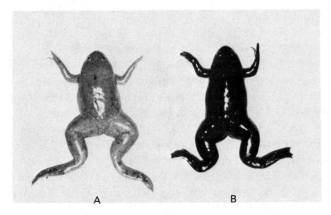

Figure 8.7 Morphological color change. Effect of long-term (9-week) adaptation of frogs, *Xenopus laevis*, to a white (A) or black (B) background [15].

trolled, and radiant energy from the sun may directly activate melanogenic activity within melanocytes. It is also possible that cholecalciferol (vitamin D₃) or other vitamin D metabolites produced within the skin in response to solar radiation stimulate melanogenesis directly or synergistically in concert with other endogenous hormonal factors.

During pregnancy the areolae of the nipples of the breast in the human female may become more darkly pigmented. The darkening of the skin is most pronounced in the last trimester and diminishes slowly after parturition. This increased pigmentation has been considered to be due to elevated levels of a melanotropin. It must be pointed out, however, that gonadal steroid levels are also elevated, and steroid hormones are clearly melanogenic in some species. The MSH-like activity of the blood and urine is increased during pregnancy, and indeed, the frog skin bioassay for MSH was originally designed to measure an elevation of the hormone as an index for predicting pregnancy in the human [42]. The source and nature of the MSH-like activity of the blood and urine during pregnancy is unknown. It is interesting to speculate that it might be of fetal origin as the fetal, but not the adult pituitary, is thought to produce a melanotropin. There is, however, one report that α-MSH may be synthesized by the pars intermedia of the pregnant female [44].

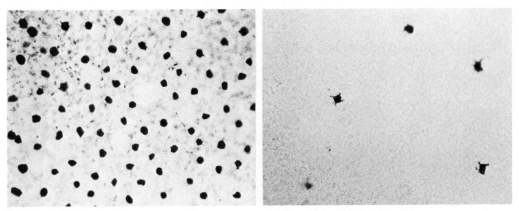

Figure 8.8 Photomicrograph of melanophores in the epidermis of frogs, *Xenopus laevis*, adapted to a white (left) or a black (right) background for a 10-week period.

Physiological Roles of MSH

169

Chromatophores and Color Changes

The only known function of MSH in nonmammalian vertebrates is the control of integumental pigmentation [1]. Present evidence implicates α-MSH as the only physiological melanotropin controlling this chromatic behavior. Many poikilothermic vertebrates, for example fishes, amphibians, and reptiles, rapidly adapt to the color of the background over which they reside. The American anole, *Anolis carolinensis*, can change, chameleon-like, from a bright green to a darker brown in a matter of minutes after moving from a light- to a dark-colored surface. Rapid *physiological color changes* do not involve changes in the amount of pigment in the skin, but rather, changes in the morphology of dermal chromatophores (Fig. 8.9). The chromatophores of poikilotherms are the xanthophores, iridophores, and melanophores. The xanthophores may contain carotenoids and pteridines; these pigments may be yellow, orange, or red, and xanthophores may therefore contain combinations of these pigments. The iridophores contain reflecting crystals of purines and related molecules. These three chromatophore types are often functionally grouped together in a *dermal chromatophore unit* (Fig. 8.10). The individual chromatophores of this functional unit respond to MSH by aggregating or dispersing their pigments; in this way the skin becomes light or dark or even yellow or green in color [2, 45].

A radioimmunoassay for α-MSH has been successfully utilized to determine pituitary and plasma levels of α-MSH in frogs adapted to various background (albedo) conditions. The results verified what might be expected (although never confirmed before) that plasma levels of MSH were elevated in toads on a black background compared to animals maintained on a gray or especially a white background. The inverse relationship was observed for α-MSH levels within the neurointermediate lobe of the pituitary [50].

Other Putative Roles Of Melanotropins

Many other physiological roles have been suggested for MSH. A few of these putative functions are discussed, but more information is needed to substantiate them fully.

Fetal pituitary-adrenal axis. The discovery that the pituitary gland produces a family of related hormonal peptides is most interesting [43]. We have seen how α-MSH is derived from a larger (31,000 MW) protein which also contains β-LPH

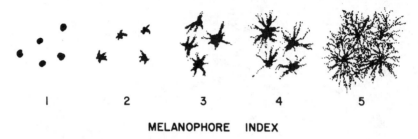

| 1 | 2 | 3 | 4 | 5 |

MELANOPHORE INDEX

Figure 8.9 A melanophore index is used to evaluate melanosome movements, centrifugal (dispersion) or centripetal (perinuclear aggregation), in response to MSH or other stimuli.

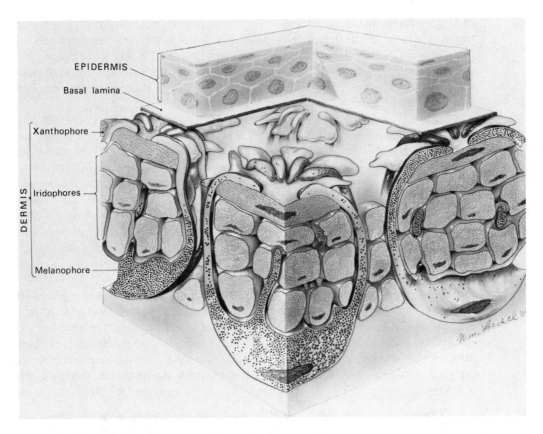

EPIDERMIS

Basal lamina

Xanthophore

Iridophores

DERMIS

Melanophore

Figure 8.10 Dermal chromatophore unit of the lizard *Anolis carolinensis.* (From Taylor and Hadley, [45], with permission.)

within its structure. Possibly the most exciting recent discovery in endocrinology is that the pituitary and brain contain opiatelike peptides. These peptides interact with so-called opiate receptors of neurons and are believed by some investigators to be the analgesic hormones (endorphins) of humans (Chapter 21). These endorphins (endogenous morphinelike substances) are derived from the β-LPH sequence within pro-opiomelanocortin. The sequence 61–91 of β-LPH is β-endorphin, and smaller sequences (enkephalins) within this peptide also possess potent analgesic activity. Thus the interesting situation exists where a whole family of hormonal peptides is derived from a common precursor molecule (Fig. 21.3).

Significant alterations in the synthesis of the family tree of hormonal peptides derived from pro-opiomelanocortin may occur during different stages of development. For example, pituitary α-MSH and CLIP predominate during the fetal life of humans and monkeys but disappear in the adult; the levels of β-endorphin may also be more prominent during fetal life. The presence of these pituitary peptides is suggested to reflect a physiological function in the fetus which is not present in postnatal life. In this regard, then, it is important to discuss current thoughts about the pituitary-adrenal axis in development. The human adrenal cortex possesses a so-called *fetal zone* which is of great size during gestation (Chapter 15). This steroidogenic zone

Physiological Roles of MSH

undergoes rapid involution at parturition, whereas the outer cortical zone hypertrophies to produce the definitive cortical zone. There is evidence that the fetal zone of some animals is responsive to α-MSH rather than ACTH and that the definitive cortical zone is responsive to ACTH but not α-MSH. Near the time of parturition there is a sharp increase in ACTH production relative to the smaller peptides such as α-MSH and CLIP.

A key event preceding parturition (at least in sheep) is a surge of cortisol from the fetal adrenal cortex. Infusion of ACTH or cortisol into the ewe will induce premature delivery any time during the second half of pregnancy [23]. The fetal adrenal cortex of some species (e.g., rabbit) is said to be responsive to α-MSH but not to ACTH. It is postulated, therefore, that the increase in ACTH relative to smaller peptides (α-MSH, endorphins) at parturition is responsible for the increasing production of cortisol by the definitive adrenal cortex. Thus the key mechanism in the chain of events controlling parturition may be the switch in pituitary peptide synthesis from α-MSH production in the pars intermedia to ACTH synthesis in the pars distalis [43].

The levels of β-endorphin are also more prominent in fetal than in adult pituitaries; there is, for example, a dramatic increase of β-endorphin in the pituitary of the newborn monkey. Silman and colleagues speculate that because the process of parturition may be a time of intense psychological trauma for the fetus and the fetus may need to be rendered insensitive to the assault of parturition, "the high levels of plasma β-endorphin present at delivery may serve to protect the infant against a necessary but otherwise intolerable event" [43]. A corticotropin releasing hormone (CRH) is reported to stimulate ACTH and α-MSH secretion. It was surmised, therefore, that α-MSH may play a role in the physiological response to stress [35].

Somatotropin secretion. MSH injected into rat fetuses in utero (with brains and pituitaries removed) stimulates their growth. Other adenohypophysial hormones as well as choriogonadotropin and oxytocin are without such an effect [44]. Specific antibodies against α-MSH, but not ACTH, induce a decrease in fetal body weight. There is no effect of α-MSH on body growth during the first 2 weeks after birth. There is also a positive correlation between fetal pituitary content of MSH and fetal body weight in humans. Thus α-MSH or other melanotropins may function directly or indirectly as growth-promoting hormones during fetal growth and development [44].

In one study the intravenous injection of α-MSH into constitutionally small prepuberal children caused an immediate but variable release of somatotropin (STH). Children with hypopituitarism uniformly show no STH secretory response to insulin or arginine stimulation. α-MSH, on the other hand, causes a significant increase in STH secretion in children with severe multiple hormone deficiency caused by craniopharyngioma. It was speculated that MSH acts directly on the pituitary gland and is effective because somatostatin, the STH release-inhibiting hormone of the hypothalamus, was absent [5]. This suggestion is supported by the observation that somatostatin blocks α-MSH-induced STH release in humans when administered with the melanotropin. In addition somatostatin inhibits MSH-induced STH release from human pituitary fragments in vitro [51]. The arcuate nucleus has been implicated as a source of an STH-releasing hormone, and α-MSH has been found within the hypothalamus where it is localized to perikarya of cells within the arcuate nucleus. Because α-MSH is capable of releasing STH, both in vivo and in vitro, a hypothalamic melanotropin may, indeed, function as an STH-releasing hormone. Melanotropins may therefore control STH secretion as well as have intrinsic growth-promoting activity in the fetus.

Melanotropins and aldosterone secretion. Angiotensin II is the hormone mainly concerned with the control of adrenocortical aldosterone biosynthesis (Chapter 15). Nevertheless, one form of primary hyperaldosteronism, bilateral adrenal hyperplasia, appears to be regulated by pituitary ACTH or some other pituitary factor. Although it is too early to describe clearly the mechanism involved, some component of pro-opiomelanocortin acting in combination with ACTH or individually may be involved [28]. β-Melanotropin directly stimulates aldosterone secretion, and this steroidogenic action can be blocked by an inactive β-MSH analog which is without an inhibitory effect on ACTH- or angiotensin II-stimulated aldosterone production. This observation demonstrates that β-MSH mediates its action through a separate adrenocortical receptor and suggests that β-MSH, its precursor, β-LPH, or an even longer pro-opiomelanocortin fragment may normally regulate adrenal aldosterone production. Most interesting is the observation that another fragment of pro-opiomelanotropin, which is devoid of direct steroidogenic activity, enhances aldosterone secretion in response to ACTH. This synergistic action could be mimicked by γ-MSH. α-MSH has also been implicated in the control of adrenal aldosterone secretion. Taken together, these observations suggest that some factor incorporating a common feature of the active site of α-MSH, γ-MSH, or β-MSH may play a role in the control of adrenal zona glomerulosa aldosterone biosynthesis and secretion.

Melanotropins and behavior. Melanotropins have been reported to affect central nervous system activity in laboratory animals and humans (Chapter 21). These effects include arousal, increased motivation, longer attention span, memory retention, and increased learning ability [31]. Immunocytochemical studies have localized melanotropic activity to specific neurons within the brain. The potency of melanotropin action on CNS-related activity is enhanced when administered directly into the ventricles of the brain. It is suggested, therefore, that α-MSH or related melanotropins may function as a neurotransmitter or neuromodulator within the brain (Chapter 21).

Thermoregulation. Certain lizards (e.g., *Sceloporus jarrovi*) orient themselves such that their dorsal surface is maximally exposed to the early morning sun. During this time they are generally dark in color compared to later in the day when temperatures are elevated. It can be speculated that this adaptive chromatic response is regulated by MSH and that the skin is able to absorb more radiant energy. Experimental verification is needed as it is possible, at least in some species, that skin darkening could be regulated through direct neural innervation of the melanophores.

A melanotropin may be involved in the central control of body temperature and fever. Both α-MSH and ACTH cause dose-related hypothermia when injected into the cerebral ventricles of the rabbit [24]. α-MSH and ACTH have been immunocytochemically isolated to neurons within areas of the brain (preoptic-anterior hypothalamus) known to be of paramount importance in temperature regulation. Table 8.1 summarizes the established and suggested physiological roles and effects of the melanotropins.

TABLE 8.1. Established and Suggested Physiological Roles and Effects of Melanotropins[a]

Source of melanotropin	Site of action	Physiological response
Pars intermedia α-MSH	Propigment (stem) cells	Melanoblast cytodifferentiation
	Epidermal melanocytes	Melanin biosynthesis (morphological color change): skin, hair, and pelage pigmentation
	Dermal chromatophores melanophores iridophores	Physiological color change melanosome dispersion reflecting platelet perinuclear aggregation
	xanthophores/erythrophores	carotenoid and pterinosome dispersion
	Sebaceous (dermal) glands	Sebum production
	Preputial glands	Lipogenesis and pheromone production
	Fetal adrenal cortex	Steroidogenesis (fetal growth and development?)
	Unknown	Stress adaptation
Pituitary melanotropin[b]	Adrenal zona glomerulosa	Aldosterone synthesis and secretion
Brain neurons (α-MSH or [desacetyl]-α-MSH)	Other brain neurons	Inhibition of opiate peptide-induced analgesia
		Neurotransmitter or neuromodulator functions: arousal, attention, learning, memory retention
		Central temperature control
	Anterior pituitary	Stimulation of ACTH secretion
		Stimulation of STH secretion
Pineal gland (epiphysis cerebri)	Unknown	Circadian processes of the pineal (rat)

[a]See [11, 46] for a fuller description of the known and putative roles of melanotropins.
[b]Cellular source and putative melanotropin are presently undetermined.

MECHANISM OF MSH ACTION

Studies on the mechanism of action of MSH have utilized both in vitro and in vivo methods to monitor responses of integumental melanocytes to the hormone. The frog skin and lizard skin assays monitor the mechanical movements of pigment granules within dermal melanophores and other chromatophores. A few in vivo studies have monitored melanin synthesis within epidermal melanocytes in response to MSH. When melanocytes become cancerous they are referred to as malignant melanoma. Mouse melanoma cells have been successfully grown in tissue culture and, because these relatively undifferentiated cells respond to MSH, the intracellular biochemical parameters of hormone action have been studied [33].

Melanosome Movements

Melanophores are found within the dermis of the skin of most poikilothermic vertebrates. Like melanocytes these specialized pigment cells synthesize melanosomes (melanin granules); instead of being secreted into surrounding cells these organelles can be rapidly translocated into the dendritic processes of the cell and back toward the cell center. These movements, centrifugal dispersion and centripetal aggregation, result in the skin becoming dark or light in color, respectively. The responses in the skin can be monitored microscopically by using a so-called melanophore index (Fig. 8.10). These changes in skin color can be objectively monitored in response to MSH or other chemical messengers using photoelectric reflectance methods [42]. The endocrine mechanisms controlling melanosome movements are well detailed but nevertheless incomplete [1, 16, 18].

MSH induces an outward dispersion of melanosomes into the dendritic processes of melanophores. Melanosome dispersion in response to MSH can be mimicked by methylxanthines (caffeine, theophylline) and by cyclic AMP or its dibutyryl derivative. MSH increases the concentration of cyclic AMP in frog skins concomitant with melanosome dispersion and darkening of the skins. These results implicate cyclic AMP as the intracellular second messenger of MSH action. Epinephrine and norepinephrine also affect melanosome movements within melanophores. Classical pharmacological studies using a variety of adrenergic agonists and antagonists have established that melanosome dispersion in response to these catecholamines is mediated through melanophore β-adrenergic receptors (Chapter 14). These receptors are distinct from MSH receptors as demonstrated by the preferential blockade of one receptor while the functional response of the other is maintained. Melanosome dispersion in response to MSH or a catecholamine (acting through β-adrenergic receptors) is inhibited or reversed by catecholamines acting through α-adrenergic receptors possessed by the melanophores. This antagonism of MSH by α-adrenergic receptor stimulation involves a decrease in cyclic AMP formation (Chapter 14).

The involvement of adrenergic receptors controlling melanophore responses has been demonstrated in teleosts, amphibians, and reptiles. The melanophores of some amphibians lack α-adrenergic receptors but possess β-adrenergic receptors. Catecholamines therefore fail to inhibit MSH action in these species. Stimulation of β-adrenergic receptors in all vertebrate tissues studied results in increased cyclic AMP production and a similar increase of the cyclic nucleotide probably occurs within melanophores. Melatonin, an indoleamine synthesized within the pineal, antagonizes the action of MSH on melanophores. The possible role of the pineal and melatonin in the control of vertebrate pigmentation shall be discussed (Chapter 20).

Prostaglandins also disperse melanosomes within fishes and amphibian melanophores. As expected, the action of prostaglandins is not inhibited by MSH receptor or β-adrenergic receptor blockade. MSH and epinephrine (or isoproterenol), but not prostaglandins, darken lizard (*Anolis*) skins. It has been suggested that some hormones may mediate their effects indirectly by stimulating cellular prostaglandin biosynthesis. The failure of melanophores of some species to respond to prostaglandins would argue against such a generalized role for prostaglandins in the control of vertebrate melanophores.

There is a calcium ion requirement for MSH action but not for melanosome movements per se because melanosome dispersion proceeds in a Ca^{2+}-free medium in response to theophylline or to dibutyryl cyclic AMP [48]. Calcium is the only cation required for MSH action as the sodium and potassium of the medium can be replaced by lithium, cesium, or rubidium, other monovalent cations. Epinephrine or isoproterenol acting through melanophore β-adrenergic receptors or prostaglandins does not require Ca^{2+} for its activation of melanophore cyclic AMP production [48]. These results demonstrate a receptor-specific Ca^{2+} requirement for MSH action.

It is interesting that ACTH and MSH elevate cyclic AMP levels of cells by receptor mechanisms separate from β-adrenergic receptors, which similarly increase the production of this cyclic nucleotide. Adrenocorticotropin and epinephrine, for example, stimulate lipolysis, but through different receptors. As for MSH, ACTH requires Ca^{2+} for its mechanism of action, whereas epinephrine, acting through β-adrenergic receptors of adipose cells, does not.

There is evidence that both ACTH and MSH acting as first messengers stimulate adrenal cortical cells and melanophores, respectively, by interacting with the plasma membrane receptors of these cells. ACTH stimulation of adenylate cyclase, but not the ACTH-receptor interaction, requires Ca^{2+} [40]. Thus there is a Ca^{2+}-dependent step between the binding of ACTH to its receptor and the subsequent activation of adrenal adenylate cyclase. Adrenal cortical cells are more responsive to ACTH as the concentration of Ca^{2+} is increased. It has been suggested that the strength of the signal generated by the interaction of ACTH with its receptor and transmitted to the adenylate cyclase compartment is proportionately increased as the Ca^{2+} concentration is increased [40]. This model for adrenocortical control by ACTH appears to be appropriate as a model for MSH control of melanophores. Because both hormones are related structurally, and presumably evolutionarily, it would seem plausible that they might share a common mechanism of action as each is capable of stimulating adrenocortical cells and melanophores.

The biochemical events underlying melanophore melanosome dispersion are analogous to those for smooth muscle relaxation: Both processes result from increases in cyclic AMP levels as mediated, for example, by catecholamine stimulation of β-adrenergic receptors. An increase in cyclic AMP production results in a sequestering of Ca^{2+} from the cytoplasm to the plasma membrane of the smooth muscle cell. Because melanosome dispersion proceeds in the absence of the Ca^{2+} ion and is enhanced under such conditions [48], a similar Ca^{2+} transport mechanism may also be requisite for melanosome dispersion. Such a model would require the presence of extracellular Ca^{2+} for MSH (but not catecholamine or prostaglandin) action, but the cyclic AMP generated would mediate melanosome dispersion by a subsequent sequestering of cytoplasmic calcium [39].

Microtubules, microfilaments, and microtrabeculae [41] are abundant in some but not all melanophores. There is no clear consensus for a definitive role of these cytoskeletal organelles within melanophores. The different functions of melanocytes, such as synthesizing and secreting melanin or, as in melanophores, rapidly translocating melanosomes, belie a single role for these organelles in pigment cell functions. Their presence in some melanophores is, however, striking and suggests some important role. A hypothetical model for the control of melanophore melanosome movements is shown (Fig. 8.11).

Melanogenesis

The understanding of the mechanisms of α-MSH action has traditionally derived from studies on the integumental chromatophores of frogs, lizards, and fishes. Because of the possible malignancy of melanocytes, it is hoped that the results gleaned from

The Melanotropins   Chap. 8

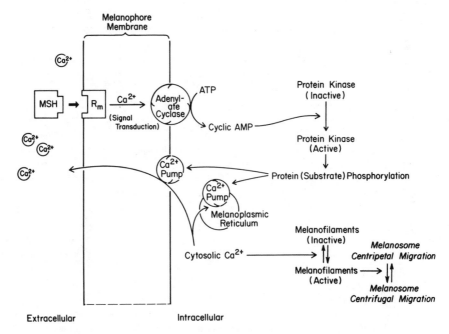

Figure 8.11 Hypothetical model for a role of MSH and Ca²⁺ ions in the control of melanosome movements within melanophores [39].

these studies may be extrapolated to mammalian melanocytes. Melanocytes and melanoma cells differ from melanophores in that they are undifferentiated cells. Mouse melanocytes, both normal and abnormal (melanoma), possess MSH receptors and also respond to prostaglandins. These agonists activate adenylate cyclase and elevate intracellular levels of cyclic AMP, which results in enhanced tyrosinase activity and increased melanogenesis. MSH action is blocked by actinomycin *D* and cycloheximide, thus implicating transcriptional and translational effects of the hormone [12]. Although MSH activates cyclic AMP production, and this cyclic nucleotide activates a cyclic AMP-dependent protein kinase, the mechanism by which this cyclic nucleotide activates nuclear transcriptional processes leading to increased enzyme activity is unknown. A model based on present knowledge of the control of melanogenesis by MSH is shown (Fig. 8.12).

Melanotropin Structure-Function Studies

Numerous analogs of α-MSH and related melanotropins have been synthesized for structure-function studies [38, 39]. The natural melanotropins share a common heptapeptide sequence, -Met-Glu-His-Phe-Arg-Trp-Gly- (Fig. 8.1); because these peptides (α-MSH, β-MSH, ACTH, β-LPH) possess melanotropic activity, it is believed that this sequence represents the active site of the molecule. Minimal contribution is nevertheless provided by the C-terminal tridecapeptide sequence, -Lys-Pro-Val-NH₂, as well as the N-terminal sequence, Ac-Ser-Tyr-Ser-, in some species. Insight into the three-dimensional requirements of α-MSH structure related to its biologically-active conformation at its receptor has been provided [39].

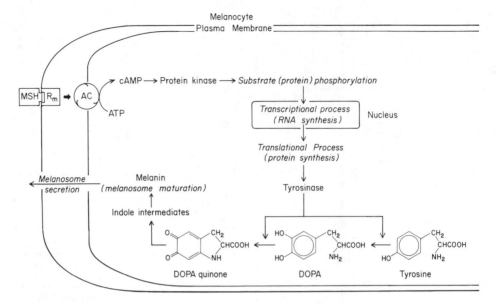

Figure 8.12 Model for MSH activation of melanocyte tyrosinase and melanin synthesis. *The substrate for cyclic-AMP-dependent protein kinase is unknown. Phosphorylation may take place outside or within the nucleus, or at both sites. (Modified from Hadley et al., [18], with permission.) **Protein synthesis is required for MSH action on melanocytes, but it is not clear whether this requirement involves de novo synthesis of tyrosinase or is related to a number of alternative mechanisms.

PATHOPHYSIOLOGY

Because the pituitary of the adult human lacks a pars intermedia, it is not surprising that, unlike most hormones, no pathophysiological states related to overproduction or underproduction of MSH have been described. The discovery that α-MSH is present in the fetal pituitary and may function in the control of fetal growth and development within the uterus should alert the clinician to possible postnatal defects resulting from pars intermedia dysfunction in the fetus. Because α-MSH may function as a neurohormone within the brain, α-MSH may eventually be implicated in the etiology of certain behavioral pathologies. The evidence for hypothalamic α-MSH as a possible regulator of somatotropin secretion may further implicate this melanotropin in certain cases of abnormal growth and development.

In Addison's disease destruction of the adrenal cortex results in a subsequent failure of adrenal steroid hormone production. Because of an absence of circulating levels of cortisol, there is a lack of negative feedback inhibition to the hypothalamus and pituitary, which results in enhanced pituitary secretion of ACTH (Chapter 15). The hyperpigmentation that follows, a cardinal symptom of Addison's disease, is because excessive circulating levels of ACTH or other melanotropic sequences are stimulatory to melanogenesis within epidermal melanocytes. In Cushing's syndrome of pituitary origin where excessive amounts of ACTH are secreted, hyperpigmentation is often noted and may be due again to elevated circulating levels of pro-opiomela-nocortin-derived melanotropic peptides. Hyperpigmentation may also occur in the *ectopic ACTH syndrome* where excessive amounts of ACTH or other melanotropins are secreted by tumors of nonpituitary origin.

Vitiligo is a malady of the skin where melanocytes in certain areas are absent or fail to become pigmentogenic. Areas of the integument are thus unpigmented. There was hope that melanogenesis within these affected areas might be restored by injections of MSH or related melanotropins. Unfortunately, MSH only increases the pigment in the adjacent normal areas, thus, in effect, accentuating the pigmentary problem.

REFERENCES

[1] BAGNARA, J. T., J. D. TAYLOR, and M. E. HADLEY. 1968. The dermal chromatophore unit. *J. Cell Biol.* 38:67–79.

[2] BAGNARA, J. T., and M. E. HADLEY. 1972. *Chromatophores and color change: comparative physiology of animal pigmentation.* Englewood Cliffs, N.J.: Prentice-Hall Publishing Co., Inc.

[3] BAKER, B. I. 1981. Biological role of the pars intermedia in lower vertebrates. In *Peptides of the pars intermedia*, Ciba Foundation Symposium 81, eds. D. Evered and G. Lawrenson, pp. 166–75. Bath, England: Pitman Medical.

[4] BALL, J. N., and T. F. C. BATTEN. 1981. Pituitary and melanophore responses to background in *Poecilia latipinna* (Teleostei): role of the pars intermedia PAS cell. *Gen. Comp. Endocrinol.* 44:233–48.

[5] BARNASCONI, S., T. TARRESANI, and R. ILLIG. 1975. The effect of α-MSH on plasma growth hormone, cortisol and TSH in children. *J. Clin. Endocrinol. Metab.* 40:759–63.

[6] BOWER, A., M. E. HADLEY, and V. J. HRUBY. 1974. Biogenic amines and control of melanophore stimulating hormone release. *Science* 184:70–72.

[7] CHRÉTIEN, M., and M. LIS. 1978. Lipotropins. In *Hormonal proteins and peptides*, ed. C. H. Li, pp. 75–102. New York: Academic Press, Inc.

[8] DAVIS, M. D., and M. E. HADLEY. 1978. Pars intermedia electrical potentials: changes in spike frequency induced by regulatory factors of melanocyte stimulating hormone (MSH) secretion. *Neuroendocrinology* 26:277–82.

[9] EAKIN, R. M., and F. E. BUSH. 1957. Development of the amphibian pituitary with special reference to the neural lobe. *Anat. Rec.* 129:279–95.

[10] ETKIN, W. 1962. Hypothalamic inhibition of the pars intermedia activity in the frog. *Gen. Comp. Endocrinol.* Suppl. 11:148–59.

[11] EVERED, D., and G. LAWRENSON, eds. 1981. *Peptides of the pars intermedia*, Ciba Foundation Symposium 81. Bath, England: Pitman Medical.

[12] FULLER, B. B., and D. VISKOCHIL. 1979. The role of RNA and protein synthesis in mediating the action of MSH on mouse melanoma cells. *Life Sci.* 24:2405–15.

[13] GESCHWIND, I. I., R. A. HUSEBY, and R. NISHIOKA. 1972. The effect of melanocyte-stimulating hormone on coat color in the mouse. *Rec. Prog. Horm. Res.* 28:91–130.

[14] HADLEY, M. E. 1972. The significance of vertebrate integumental pigmentation. *Amer. Zool.* 12:63–76.

[15] HADLEY, M. E., and W. C. QUEVEDO, JR. 1967. The role of epidermal melanocytes in adaptive color changes in amphibians. *Advan. Biol. Skin* 8:337–59.

[16] HADLEY, M. E., and J. T. BAGNARA. 1975. Regulation of release and mechanism of action of MSH. In *Trends in comparative endocrinology*, Amer. Zool. Suppl. 1975, ed. E. J. W. Barrington, pp. 81–104. New York: Thomas J. Griffiths Sons.

[17] HADLEY, M. E., and V. J. HRUBY. 1977. Neurohypophysial peptides and the regulation of melanophore stimulating hormone (MSH) secretion. *Amer. Zool.* 17:809–21.

[18] HADLEY, M. E., C. B. HEWARD, V. J. HRUBY, T. K. SAWYER, and Y. C. S. YANG. 1981. Biological actions of melanocyte-stimulating hormone. In *Peptides of the pars intermedia*, Ciba Foundation Symposium 81, eds. D. Evered and G. Lawrenson, pp. 244–62. Bath, England: Pitman Medical.

[19] HOLMES, R. L., and J. N. BALL. 1974. *The pituitary gland: a comparative account*. Cambridge, England: University Press.

[20] ITURRIZA, F. C., F. E. ESTIVARIZ, and H. P. LEVITIN. 1980. Coexistence of α-melanocyte-stimulating hormone and adrenocorticotropin in all cells containing either of the two hormones in the duck pituitary. *Gen. Comp. Endocrinol.* 42:110–15.

[21] KAWAUCHI, H., Y. ADACHI, and M. TSUBOKAWA. 1980. Occurrence of a new melanocyte stimulating hormone in the salmon pituitary gland. *Biochem. Biophys. Res. Commun.* 96:1508–17.

[22] LI, C. H. 1978. The chemistry of melanotropins. In *Hormonal proteins and peptides*, ed. C. H. Li, pp. 1–33. New York: Academic Press, Inc.

[23] LIGGINS, G. C., R. J. FAERCLOUGH, S. A. GRIEVES, J. Z. KENDAL, and B. S. KNOX. 1973. The mechanism of initiation of parturition in the ewe. *Rec. Prog. Horm. Res.* 29:111–59.

[24] LIPTON, J. M., J. R. GLYN, and J. A. ZIMMER. 1981. ACTH and α-melanotropin in central temperature control. *Fed. Proc.* 40:2760–64.

[25] LOGAN, A., and B. WEATHERHEAD. 1980. Pelage colour cycles and hair follicle tyrosinase activity in the Siberian hamster. *J. Invest. Dermat.* 75:192–95.

[26] LOWRY, P. J., and A. P. SCOTT. 1975. The evolution of vertebrate corticotropin and melanocyte stimulating hormone. *Gen. Comp. Endocrinol.* 26:16–23.

[27] LOWRY, P. J., J. HOPE, and R. E. SILMAN. 1976. The evolution of corticotropin, melanotropin and lipotropin. *Excerpta Med. Intern. Congress* ser. no. 402:71–76.

[28] MATSUOKA, H., P. J. MULROW, R. FRANCO-SAENZ, and C. H. LI. 1981. Effects of β-lipotropin and β-lipotropin derived peptides on aldosterone production in the rat adrenal gland. *J. Clin. Invest.* 68:752–59.

[29] MEURLING, P., and A. BJÖRKLUND. 1970. The arrangement of neurosecretory and catecholamine fibres in relation to the pituitary intermedia cells of the skate, *Raja radiata*. *Z. Zellforsch. Mikroskop. Anat.* 108:81–92.

[30] MORGAN, C. M., and M. E. HADLEY. 1976. Ergot alkaloid inhibition of melanophore stimulating hormone secretion. *Neuroendocrinology* 21:10–19.

[31] O'DONOHUE, T. L., and D. M. DORSA. 1982. The opiomelanotropinergic neuronal and endocrine systems. *Peptides* 3:353–95.

[32] OLIVEREAU, M., J.-M. OLIVEREAU, and C. AIMAR. 1980. Responses of MSH and prolactin cells to 5-hydroxytryptophan (5-HTP) in amphibians and teleosts. *Cell Tiss. Res.* 207:377–85.

[33] PAWELEK, J. M., and A. M. KÖRNER. 1982. The biosynthesis of mammalian melanin. *Amer. Sci.* 70:136–45.

[34] PERRYMAN, E. K., and J. T. BAGNARA. 1978. Extravascular transfer within the anuran pars intermedia. *Cell Tiss. Res.* 193:297–313.

[35] PROULX-FERLAND, L., F. LABRIE, D. DUMONT, J. COTE, D. H. COY, and J. SVEIRAF. 1982. Corticotropin-releasing factor stimulates secretion of melanocyte-stimulating hormone from the rat pituitary. *Science* 217:62–63.

[36] RODRÍGUEZ, E. M., and J. LAPOINTE. 1970. Light and electron microscopy of the pars intermedia of the lizard, *Klauberina riversiana*. *Z. Zellforsch. Mikroskop. Anat.* 104: 827–37.

[37] RUST, C. C., and R. K. MEYER. 1969. Hair color, molt, and testis size in male, short-tailed weasels treated with melatonin. *Science* 165:921–22.

[38] SAWYER, T. K., V. J. HRUBY, B. C. WILKES, M. T. DRAELOS, M. E. HADLEY, and M. BERGSNEIDER. 1982. Design and comparative biological activities of highly potent analogues of α-melanotropin$_{4-10}$. *J. Med. Chem.* 25:1022–27.

[39] SAWYER, T. K., V. J. HRUBY, M. E. HADLEY, and M.H. ENGEL. 1983. α-Melanocyte stimulating hormone: chemical nature and mechanism of action. *Amer. Zool.* 23: *In press.*

[40] SAYERS, G., R. J. BEAL, and S. SEELIG. 1972. Isolated adrenal cells: adrenocorticotropic hormone, calcium, steroidogenesis, and cyclic adenosine monophosphate. *Science* 175: 1131–32.

[41] SCHLIWA, M., M. OSBORN, and K. WEBER. 1978. Microtubule system of isolated fish melanophores as revealed by immunofluorescence microscopy. *J. Cell. Biol.* 76:229–36.

[42] SHIZUME, K., A. B. LERNER, and T. B. FITZPATRICK. 1954. *In vitro* bioassay for the melanocyte stimulating hormone. *Endocrinology* 54:553–60.

[43] SILMAN, R. E., D. HOLLAND, T. CHARD, P. J. LOWRY, J. HOPE, L. H. REES, A. THOMAS, and P. NATHANIELSZ. 1979. Adrenocorticotropin-related peptides in adult and fetal sheep pituitary glands. *J. Endocrinol.* 81:19–34.

[44] SWAAB, D. F., and J. T. MARTIN. 1981. Functions of α-melanotropin and other opiomelanocortin peptides in labour, intrauterine growth and brain development. In *Peptides of the pars intermedia*, Ciba Foundation Symposium 81, eds. D. Evered and G. Lawrenson, pp. 196–217. Bath, England: Pitman Medical.

[45] TAYLOR, J. D., and M. E. HADLEY. 1970. Chromatophores and color change in the lizard *Anolis carolinensis*. *Z. Zellforsch. Mikroskop. Anat.* 104:282–94.

[46] THODY, A. J. 1980. *The MSH peptides*. New York: Academic Press, Inc.

[47] TURNER, W. A., JR., S.-T. CHEN, H. WAHN, L. T. LIGHTBODY, J. T. BAGNARA, J. D. TAYLOR, and T. T. TCHEN. 1977. Tropic effects of MSH. *Front. Horm. Res.* 4:105–16.

[48] VESELY, D. L., and M. E. HADLEY. 1979. Ionic requirements for melanophore stimulating hormone (MSH) action on melanophores. *Comp. Biochem. Physiol.* 62A:501–508.

[49] WEATHERHEAD, B. 1978. Comparative cytology of the neuro-intermediate lobe of the reptilian pituitary. *Zbl. Vet. Med. C., Anat. Histol. Embryol.* 7:84–96.

[50] WILSON, J. F., and M. A. MORGAN. 1979. α-Melanotropin-like substances in the pituitary and plasma of *Xenopus laevis* in relation to colour change responses. *Gen. Comp. Endocrinol.* 38:172–82.

[51] ZAHND, G. R., and A. VECSEY. 1977. Stimulation of growth hormone release *in vivo* and *in vitro* by α-MSH. *Front. Horm. Res.* 4:188–92.

9

HORMONAL CONTROL
of CALCIUM HOMEOSTASIS

INTRODUCTION

The calcium ion Ca^{2+} is a key element in numerous physiological functions. Derived from the structural component of bone, this divalent cation is important in bone growth, and it is readily available to serve in a variety of intracellular and extracellular roles. Ca^{2+} is necessary for normal blood clotting, and, with sodium and potassium, it aids in maintaining the transmembrane potential of cells. Ca^{2+} may be necessary for the transduction of signal between hormone receptor and adenylate and guanylate cyclases. Stimulus-secretion and stimulus-contraction coupling also require Ca^{2+}.

Three hormones are of prime importance in the control of calcium homeostasis and a number of other hormones indirectly affect the availability of this cation. *Parathyroid hormone* (PTH), or parathormone, derived from the parathyroid glands, increases circulating levels of Ca^{2+}, whereas *calcitonin*, derived from the *parafollicular cells* of the mammalian thyroid, lowers the circulating levels of the ion. A metabolite of vitamin D, 1,25-dihydroxyvitamin D_3, also increases serum levels of Ca^{2+}. These three hormones interact to maintain normal plasma Ca^{2+} levels. Because of the importance of Ca^{2+} to normal bodily function and due to the complex number of interactions between the hormones regulating Ca^{2+} homeostasis, a large number of endocrinopathies related to Ca^{2+} homeostasis and bone mineral metabolism have been described.

CALCIUM AND BONE PHYSIOLOGY

Cytosolic and extracellular fluid concentrations of Ca^{2+} must be maintained within narrow limits despite the wide fluctuations in Ca^{2+} intake. In humans the Ca^{2+} level of plasma and extracellular fluid is maintained at about 10 mg/100 ml. Serum Ca^{2+} derived from the diet is delivered to the blood after being actively transported across the intestinal mucosa. Urinary Ca^{2+} loss is partially prevented by active transport of the cation back across the renal tubular epithelium. Bone serves as the immediate source of Ca^{2+} to maintain serum Ca^{2+} homeostasis. Half of the Ca^{2+} present in blood is in the free ionized form and half is bound to albumin. The free ionized form of Ca^{2+} is readily available and important in physiological processes. Three factors can alter the distribution of Ca^{2+} in plasma: albumin concentration, acid-base disturbances, and protein abnormalities.

To understand the actions of hormones on skeletal formation and resorption, it is necessary to review the cellular processes involved in the mineralization and demineralization of bone. Bone is covered by the periosteum which consists of connective tissue fibers. A layer of *osteoblasts* within the deeper layer of the fibrous periosteum synthesizes and releases molecules of collagen. The individual collagen molecules become oriented in a specific molecular architecture to form an extracellular matrix around the osteoblasts. Calcium and phosphate ions are stereochemically bound to specific sites on the collagen matrix where they are precipitated as $Ca_{10}(PO_4)_6(OH)_2$, hydroxyapatite. Precipitation of calcium phosphate depends on the product of the concentrations of Ca^{2+} and PO_4^{-3}. Whenever the concentration of $[Ca^{2+}] \times [PO_4^{-3}]$ exceeds the solubility product at the local site of ossification, calcium phosphate precipitates. Precipitation of bone mineral may be enhanced under conditions of local alkalinization resulting from osteoblastic activity. After calcification of the collagen matrix, the embedded cells are referred to as *osteocytes*. Demineralization of bone is effected by large multinucleate cells or *osteoclasts* which release acid phosphatase and hyaluronic acid. Local decreases in pH caused by the osteoclasts favor the solubilization of hydroxyapatite with the resulting release of Ca^{2+} and PO_4^{-3} from the collagen matrix.

PARATHORMONE

Historically, parathormone was the first of the trio of hormones controlling Ca^{2+} homeostasis to be discovered. Because of the essential role of Ca^{2+} in cellular function, PTH is acutely necessary for life. Although other hormones may be required for normal body function, with the exception of aldosterone (Chapter 15), they are not absolutely essential for survival.

The Parathyroid Glands

Parathormone is derived from the parathyroids which in most mammals are embedded on the surface of the thyroid gland. In humans four parathyroid glands are present and they are located on the back side of the thyroid gland, one near each pole of the two lobes of the thyroid gland (Fig. 9.1). The parathyroid glands are derived from the third and fourth pharyngeal pouches, the two superior glands

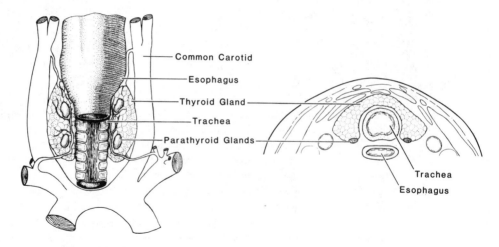

Figure 9.1 Posterior (left) and transverse (right) views of the human thyroid with attached parathyroids.

from the fourth and the two inferior glands from the third. Removal of the thyroid usually leads to death in animals; it was subsequently discovered, however, that the lethal effects of thyroidectomy could be duplicated by removal of the parathyroids rather than the thyroid itself. In mammals other than humans there may be one or two pairs of parathyroids which may or may not be associated with thyroid tissue. The parathyroids are composed of two cell types, the *chief* cells which are the source of PTH and the *oxyphil* cells of unknown function. The chief cells are most numerous and in some mammals may be the only cells present. Oxyphil cells in humans appear around puberty and increase in number with age; they contain an eosinophilic granular cytoplasm.

Removal of the parathyroids results in a drop in plasma Ca^{2+} levels, which usually results in tetanic convulsions and death. In 1925 Collip isolated a biologically active fraction from bovine parathyroid glands which could restore Ca^{2+} levels in parathyroidectomized dogs. This active substance of the parathyroid glands was appropriately named parathyroid hormone, or as it is more commonly known, parathormone (PTH).

Synthesis, Chemistry, and Metabolism

Parathormone, a polypeptide 84 amino acids in length, is derived from a precursor molecule of 115 amino acid residues. This so-called preproparathyroid hormone (PreProPTH) then undergoes two proteolytic cleavages to yield a proPTH of 90 amino acids from which six residues are then removed within the cell to yield the definitive hormonal product. In an in vitro translation system (for the production of protein from messenger RNA) PreProPth has been synthesized and shown to be converted to PTH in the Golgi zone of the chief cells by a trypsinlike protease. The hormone is then packaged into secretory vesicles which migrate to the periphery of the cell where the hormone is secreted by a mechanism of vesicular exocytosis [21, 23].

The primary structures of human PTH as well as those of the pig and the cow

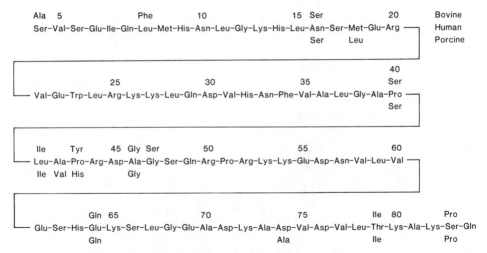

Figure 9.2 Comparative structures of parathormone.

have been determined (Fig. 9.2). There is extensive sequence homology among the three species of hormone. A variation in the structure of human PTH has been reported where glutamine, lysine, and leucine are at the 22, 28, and 30 positions of the peptide [7]. The 84-amino acid sequence appears to be the major form of the hormone secreted from the parathyroids. In the peripheral circulation the intact hormone is cleaved into two major fragments, one of which, PTH-(1-34), retains biological activity. Studies using radiolabeled bovine PTH in calves showed an initial rapid disappearance of most of the hormone with a half-life of 3 to 4 minutes. In humans PTH has approximately the same half-life as measured after parathyroidectomy. In the isolated perfused kidney intact PTH is taken up and cleaved into its N- and C-terminal fragments. The kidney may not be the only site of hormone degradation, and metabolism of the hormone may vary from person to person.

Control of Secretion

The release of PTH from the parathyroid glands is controlled by circulating levels of calcium. Parathyroid cells apparently possess recognition sites for Ca^{2+} as incubation of parathyroid slices in a low concentration of Ca^{2+} increases PTH release, whereas incubation in the presence of high concentrations of the cation decreases PTH release. These results demonstrate that the concentration of Ca^{2+} bathing the parathyroid cells controls the release of PTH. Theophylline stimulates PTH release as does dibutyryl cyclic AMP, thus suggesting that cyclic AMP is involved in the mechanism of PTH release. Much information is available on the cellular mechanisms involved in PTH secretion [8]. There is also evidence that parathyroid gland secretion of PTH may be controlled by a pituitary parathyroid stimulating hormone [30].

Physiological Roles

Parathormone acts on a number of tissues; in most cases elevating, directly or indirectly, plasma levels of Ca^{2+} and decreasing circulating concentrations of PO_4^{-3}.

Parathormone

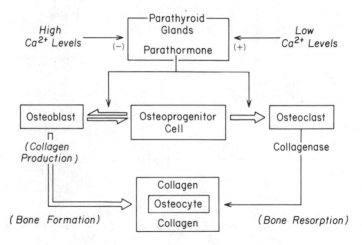

Figure 9.3 Parathormone effects on osteoblast-osteoclast-osteocyte activity.

Bone mineral metabolism. According to one hypothesis, PTH has a dual physiological role on bone mineral metabolism; the hormone is responsible for bone remodeling and the control of plasma Ca^{2+} levels by effecting bone demineralization. In this model (Fig. 9.3) low or basal levels of PTH would stimulate the proliferation and maturation of undifferentiated (osteoprogenitor cells) or partially differentiated cells toward formation of osteoclasts and osteoblasts. The activities of these two populations of cells would be responsible for simultaneous bone destruction and formation, processes necessary for bone remodeling. At higher concentrations of the hormone there would be an increase in osteoclast formation. In addition PTH may inhibit osteoblast formation or actually favor the dedifferentiation of osteoblasts back to undifferentiated cells which would then, through cellular fusion, become osteoclasts [41]. This would favor bone demineralization rather than bone formation, and increased osteoclastic activity would enhance Ca^{2+} transfer from bone to body fluids. There is strong evidence that osteoblasts transform into osteoclasts spontaneously during the egg-laying cycle of birds [41]. The initial rapid response of bone to PTH is independent of an increase in the number of osteoclasts and is unrelated to the bone-remodeling system. The early hypercalcemic response is mediated mainly at the level of the osteocyte and may only involve removal of mineral from the collagen matrix.

Renal reabsorption of calcium. A major physiological role of PTH is to increase renal tubular reabsorption of calcium. Parathyroidectomy, for example, leads to calciuria which can be corrected immediately by injections of PTH.

Renal excretion of phosphate. Parathyroidectomy leads to a decrease in urinary phosphate levels. Injections of PTH, on the other hand, cause an immediate increase in urinary phosphate concentration (phosphaturia). PTH mediates its effect at the level of the proximal convoluted tubule. Increased renal excretion of PO_4^{-3} in response to PTH would enhance the ionization of plasma Ca^{2+} through a lowering of the $[Ca^{2+}] \times [PO_4^{-3}]$ solubility product.

Intestinal absorption of calcium.   Parathormone enhances intestinal uptake of Ca^{2+}, but this action, as discussed later, may be mediated indirectly through its action on vitamin D metabolism.

Control of vitamin D synthesis.   A major role of PTH in Ca^{2+} homeostasis is to stimulate the biosynthesis of 1,25-dihydroxyvitamin D_3 from vitamin D precursors by the kidney. Thus, some of the actions of PTH are mediated indirectly through the action of this steroid hormone.

Other possible actions of PTH.   Parathormone increases the rate of mitosis of red cell progenitors (reticulocytes) and thymic lymphocytes. Mitotic activity is also increased by regenerating rat liver following partial hepatectomy in response to PTH. The physiological significance, if any, of these observations on the mitogenic actions of PTH is unknown.

More recently PTH and its fragments were shown to produce vasodilation in the coronary and other vascular beds in the dog. The blood-pressure lowering effect of the bPTH is not blocked by α- or β-adrenergic, cholinergic, or histaminergic blocking agents, thus suggesting direct effects of the peptide on vascular smooth muscle receptors. This vasodepressor response has been demonstrated in a variety of species [40]. Because PTH regulates blood Ca^{2+} levels and Ca^{2+} is important in the control of smooth muscle contractility, studies on other cellular systems may provide important insights into other physiological roles of PTH as yet unrecognized.

In reptiles, birds, and some mammals there are one or two pairs of glands which are found free from association with thyroid tissue. There is evidence that in tetrapods calcium homeostasis is under the control of PTH and calcitonin. Parathyroidectomy, for example, results in hypocalcemia and tetanic muscular contractions in several species of snakes and lizards [10], and PTH has a hypercalcemic effect in hypocalcemic lizards. In several species of birds there is convincing evidence that PTH plays an important role in regulation of calcium and phosphate [11]. In teleost fishes, on the other hand, PTH has no observable effect on serum Ca^{2+} levels or on changing bone or muscle mineral content. Parathyroid glands are absent in bony fishes and, when first encountered in amphibians, they are usually present as two pairs of glands which are closely associated with branches of the jugular vein.

CALCITONIN

The plasma concentration of Ca^{2+} is maintained at a very precise level. PTH functions to maintain plasma Ca^{2+} levels by its action on a number of target tissues. As seen, the levels of PTH are affected by the circulating levels of Ca^{2+}. Although Ca^{2+} is directly inhibitory to PTH release from the parathyroids, this is not the only means of protecting the animal against the elevated Ca^{2+} levels that occur, for example, after a meal. If plasma Ca^{2+} levels are elevated by injecting Ca^{2+} salts, plasma Ca^{2+} rapidly returns to normal. Infusion of a Ca^{2+} chelator, on the other hand, effectively lowers Ca^{2+} levels which soon return to normal after cessation of the infusion. It was discovered, however, that depressed or elevated Ca^{2+} levels fail to return to normal in thyroidectomized animals. This failure could partly be explained by the absence of PTH which was caused by the removal of the parathyroids and the thyroid glands. The solution, however, was not so simple. It was concluded that the thyroid might also produce a hormone whose role is to lower Ca^{2+} levels under conditions where the cation is elevated. Although this hypocalcemic factor, referred to as calcitonin (CT), was initially believed to be derived from the parathyroids, other experimental evidence pointed toward the thyroid [13, 35, 36].

The Parafollicular Cells

The thyroid gland is mainly composed of follicular cells (Fig. 13.2) whose function is to synthesize and store thyroid hormones (Chapter 13). Another cell nestled among the follicular cells of the thyroid had been identified and referred to as a C (clear) cell whose function was unknown. Immunohistochemical staining techniques have demonstrated that these C cells synthesize and secrete CT. In mammals including humans these cells are derived from the ultimobranchial bodies which develop from the most posterior branchial pouch. Of interest was the discovery that cells of the neural crest migrate to the posterior branchial pouch to form the *ultimobranchial glands* early in development [32]. In nonmammalian vertebrates (cartilaginous and bony fishes, amphibians, reptiles, birds) the ultimobranchial glands persist and are the source of CT in the adult animal. In the human fetus the appearance of functional activity of parafollicular cells at the onset of calcification may suggest an important role for CT in fetal bone growth. The parafollicular cells also form and store 5-hydroxytryptamine (serotonin) in the same granules which contain CT. The physiological significance of this observation is unclear.

Synthesis, Chemistry, and Metabolism

Calcitonin was purified in 1967 and its amino acid sequence determined in 1968 [42]. The primary sequence of CT from a number of species has been determined and the peptides are all similar (Fig. 9.4). All contain 32 residues, have a 1-7 intrachain disulfide ring, and the carboxyterminal group of all is prolinamide. There is evidence that, as for many peptide hormones, CT is derived from a larger precursor molecule. Human calcitonin (Fig. 9.5) has been isolated only from medullary carcinoma of the thyroid because the low levels of the hormone found in normal human thyroid tissue have so far prevented isolation of CT from nonmalignant tissue. Circulating human CT appears by immunological and chemical criteria to be structurally similar to CT isolated from thyroid medullary carcinoma. Analysis of calcitonin from four separate species of salmon reveals that each species produces two forms of the molecule, a salmon I plus a salmon II or salmon III variant of the molecule. These molecular varieties of CT represent *isohormonal* forms of the hormone; that is, the primary structure of these forms varies slightly from one to another.

Control of Secretion

Perfusion of hypercalcemic blood through the thyroid is a stimulus to CT secretion and incubation of thyroid tissue in a hypercalcemic medium also results in secretion

		1	2	3	4	5	6	7	8	9	10	11	12	13	14	15	16
Human	H$_2$N	Cys	Gly	Asn	Leu	Ser	Thr	Cys	Met	Leu	Gly	Thr	Tyr	Thr	Gln	Asp	Phe
Salmon	H$_2$N	Cys	Ser	Asn	Leu	Ser	Thr	Cys	Val	Leu	Gly	Lys	Leu	Ser	Gln	Glu	Leu
Ovine	H$_2$N	Cys	Ser	Asn	Leu	Ser	Thr	Cys	Val	Leu	Ser	Ala	Tyr	Trp	Lys	Asp	Leu
Bovine	H$_2$N	Cys	Ser	Asn	Leu	Ser	Thr	Cys	Val	Leu	Ser	Ala	Tyr	Trp	Lys	Asp	Leu
Porcine	H$_2$N	Cys	Ser	Asn	Leu	Ser	Thr	Cys	Val	Leu	Ser	Ala	Tyr	Trp	Arg	Asn	Leu

17	18	19	20	21	22	23	24	25	26	27	28	29	30	31	32	
Asn	Lys	Phe	His	Thr	Phe	Pro	Gln	Thr	Ala	Ile	Gly	Val	Gly	Ala	Pro	NH$_2$
His	Lys	Leu	Gln	Thr	Tyr	Pro	Arg	Thr	Asn	Thr	Gly	Ser	Gly	Thr	Pro	NH$_2$
Asn	Asn	Tyr	His	Arg	Tyr	Ser	Gly	Met	Gly	Phe	Gly	Pro	Glu	Thr	Pro	NH$_2$
Asn	Asn	Tyr	His	Arg	Phe	Ser	Gly	Met	Gly	Phe	Gly	Pro	Glu	Thr	Pro	NH$_2$
Asn	Asn	Phe	His	Arg	Phe	Ser	Gly	Met	Gly	Phe	Gly	Pro	Glu	Thr	Pro	NH$_2$

Figure 9.4 Comparative structures of some calcitonins. Three molecular species of salmon CT exist; the structure of salmon I calcitonin is shown, which differs from eel CT at only three residues (eel: 26, Asp; 27, Val.; 29, Ala).

of the hormone. Is there evidence that elevated levels of Ca^{2+} are also a stimulus to CT secretion in humans? Changes in plasma Ca^{2+} (caused by oral ingestion of Ca^{2+}) within the physiological range are indeed associated with parallel changes in CT levels in humans [4].

The increase in CT release in response to calcium infusion is greater in males than in females, and the basal levels of CT and the response to calcium wane with age in both sexes [14]. Animal studies indicate that estrogens and androgens enhance calcitonin secretion, and the progressive decreases in gonadal function may therefore contribute to the age and sex-related changes in CT secretion in humans. There is evidence that cyclic AMP is the second messenger controlling CT secretion.

Physiological Roles

If a very small amount of Ca^{2+} is delivered to the stomach (of the pig) so as not to produce a detectable hypercalcemia, plasma CT still increases severalfold. It was hypothesized that some gastrointestinal factor in addition to Ca^{2+} might be a CT secretogogue [12]. Gastrin is a potent stimulator of CT secretion, and analogs of

```
  ┌S─────────────S┐
Cys-Gly-Asn-Leu-Ser-Thr-Cys-Met-Leu-Gly-Thr-Tyr-Thr-Gln-Asp-Phe-Asn-
 1   2   3   4   5   6   7   8   9  10  11  12  13  14  15  16  17
```

```
Lys-Phe-His-Thr-Phe-Pro-Gln-Thr-Ala-Ile-Gly-Val-Gly-Ala-Pro-NH2
 18  19  20  21  22  23  24  25  26  27  28  29  30  31  32
```

Figure 9.5 Primary structure of human calcitonin.

gastrin (Chapter 10) exhibit a potency profile similar to their effectiveness in stimulating gastric acid secretion. Cholecystokinin is also effective, due most likely to its partial structural similarity to gastrin. Physiological stimuli that increase gastrin levels in the blood cause a parallel increase in CT secretion. Gastrin does not, however, evoke CT release in the rat. In some patients with Zollinger-Ellison syndrome (hypergastrinemia) there is an elevation in circulating calcitonin.

Because CT is released from the parafollicular cells in direct relation to the circulating level of Ca^{2+}, it has been suggested that CT functions in the prevention of hypercalcemia. In particular CT may prevent the postprandial hypercalcemia that results from the absorption of Ca^{2+} from foods during a meal. Calcitonin might also promote mineralization of skeletal bone via Ca^{2+} absorbed from milk in pre-weanling animals. In addition CT may protect against Ca^{2+} loss from the skeleton during such periods of calcium stress as pregnancy and lactation and prolonged calcium deprivation.

Subcutaneous injections of CT inhibit the 24-hour food intake of rats and rhesus monkeys. In humans a significant reduction in body weight is observed 24 to 36 hours following a single subcutaneous injection of CT. Intracerebroventricular injections of CT in the rat are also inhibitory to feeding. These results suggest that CT may have a physiologically relevant action on the CNS (Chapter 21). It is speculated that endogenous calcitonin is involved in the regulation of feeding and appetite, possibly under specialized circumstances as during infancy, lactation, or calcium-specific hunger [20]. Whether the endogenous CT would be derived from the parafollicular cells, in response to postprandial hypercalcemia, or from CT-secreting neurons within the CNS, which monitor the Ca^{2+} directly or are activated by peripheral afferents that monitor systemic Ca^{2+} levels, is unclear.

Calcitonin plays no direct role in the regulation of vitamin D metabolism. Indirectly, however, lowering of plasma Ca^{2+} levels would result in the release of PTH which would activate production and secretion of kidney vitamin D metabolites.

Because it is composed almost entirely of CT-secreting cells, the ultimobranchial gland of nonmammalian vertebrates is a rich source of calcitonin. Isolated cells from the fish ultimobranchial gland have been used in vitro for studies on CT secretion. Secretin, glucagon, and pentagastrin are stimulatory to CT secretion and, in combination, secretin and pentagastrin or secretin and glucagon have a synergistic effect on CT secretion from isolated teleost ultimobranchial cells [43].

Cyclostomes apparently lack ultimobranchial glands. In elasmobranchs and teleost fishes, ultimobranchial glands are present and contain calcitonin. Calcitonin of elasmobranchs or some other origin is, however, without effect on serum calcium levels in sharks. Although elasmobranchs are cartilaginous, they are believed to be derived from a bony ancestor. Therefore CT may be an old hormone which has been retained during the evolution of the cartilaginous elasmobranchs and the bony fishes from their primitive bony ancestors [39]. A number of studies have suggested that calcitonin also does not cause a hypocalcemic effect in teleosts. It has been suggested that CT may transport Ca^{2+} across gill membranes and prevent exposure to the high concentrations of Ca^{2+} present in the marine environment [38]. Indeed, CT administered to stickleback fish (*Gasterosteus aculeatus*) maintained in calcium-deficient water induces a marked decrease in blood calcium. This finding may indicate that previous studies failed to demonstrate an effect of CT because endogenous plasma Ca^{2+} levels were strongly buffered by exogenous sources of the cation [49].

In the chick CT is localized exclusively to the ultimobranchial glands, but in some birds (e.g., pigeon, *Columba livia*) the hormone is also localized to C cells of the thyroid gland. In the pigeon CT may function, as in mammals, to counteract hypercalcemia.

VITAMIN D

Historically, vitamin D is the name applied to two fat-soluble substances, cholecalciferol and ergocalciferol, that possess the common ability to prevent or cure rickets. Rickets (osteomalacia in adults) develops from a failure of the bones to ossify properly in the child, and it was originally believed that the disease was due to a lack of sunshine or some dietary factor. There is some truth in these early theories. Vitamins are defined as organic dietary constituents necessary for life and development but which do not act as dietary energy sources. In that respect it has been argued that the term vitamin D is a misnomer because normally the active form of vitamin D is produced within the body from dietary substrates or endogenous substances [33]. It is now universally accepted that vitamin D is a precursor of one or more steroid-like hormones produced by specific tissues within the body. These vitamin D metabolites mediate their actions on a number of target tissues, and in the absence of the hormones bones fail to mineralize.

Source, Synthesis, Chemistry, and Metabolism

In 1924 it was discovered that in animals prior irradiation of certain dietary foodstuffs was as effective in curing rickets as direct irradiation of the animal itself. Vitamin D_3 (cholecalciferol) is actually produced in the skin of humans by the action of ultraviolet light on a precursor molecule, 7-dehydrocholesterol (an intermediate in the biosynthesis of cholesterol). Actually 7-dehydrocholesterol is first converted to a so-called previtamin D_3, which subsequently equilibrates in the skin to form cholecalciferol through a temperature-dependent thermal isomerization (Fig. 9.6). From the skin, cholecalciferol is transported by a vitamin-D binding protein (transcalciferin) into the general circulation. Under continuous exposure to the sun, previtamin D_3 also photoisomerizes to lumisterol and tachysterol which are biologically inert. Because vitamin-D binding protein has no strong affinity for these products, they are not translocated into the circulation but instead remain in the skin. Within the skin these photoisomers are in a quasi-stationary state and may serve as reserve substrates for photoconversion back to previtamin D_3 when the latter substance is converted to vitamin D_3 [28].

Rickets, a vitamin D-deficiency disease, may therefore develop if the skin does not receive adequate irradiation. The disease is now a rarity in most countries because irradiated foods provide an adequate supply of the vitamin. Ergosterol is a provitamin for vitamin D_2 (ergocalciferol), and both differ from 7-dehydrocholesterol and vitamin D_3, respectively, because they possess a double bond between

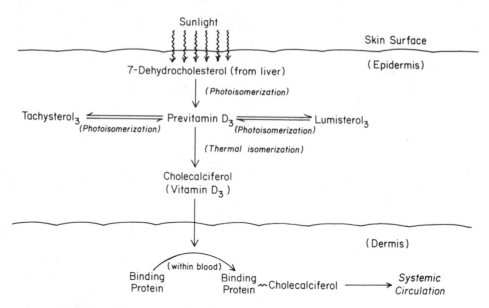

Figure 9.6 Photic stimulation of integumental cholecalciferol (vitamin D₃) formation and subsequent transfer to the general circulation by a cholecalciferol-binding protein.

C22 and C23 and a methyl group at the C24 position. Vitamin D_2 is the antirachitic principle of irradiated foodstuffs. Although vitamin D_3 is the normal physiologically relevant antirachitic substrate, vitamin D_2 is equally effective as a vitamin D in some species, including humans.

Actually, cholecalciferol is without biological activity at physiological concentrations. Cholecalciferol must first be converted to 25-hydroxyvitamin D_3 (25-OH-D_3, 25-hydroxycholecalciferol) in the liver (Fig. 9.7). The liver appears to be the major site of 25-hydroxylation in mammals [15]. In the chicken, however, the 25-hydroxylase enzyme exists in extraheptic sites such as intestine and kidney. Although this steroid is the major circulating metabolite of cholecalciferol, it must undergo at least one other chemical modification before it can function as a hormone. The 25-OH-D_3 produced in the liver then circulates to the kidney where it is converted by a mitochondrial 1α-hydroxylase to 1α,25-(OH)₂D_3 (1α,25-dihydroxycholecalciferol, 1,25-(OH)₂D_3), the hormonal form of cholecalciferol [31]. The exclusive synthesis in the kidney of 1,25-(OH)₂D_3 was demonstrated by the failure of nephrectomized rats given radioactive 25-OH-D_3 to produce radiolabeled 1,25-(OH)₂D_3. Nephrectomized animals do not show physiological responses to 25-OH-D_3, whereas physiological responses on gut and bone, whether the kidneys are present or not, are produced by 1,25-(OH)₂D_3. Chick kidney homogenates as well as isolated renal mitochondria convert 25-OH-D_3 to the active hormone. The 1,25-(OH)₂D_3 product was originally detected in chick intestinal chromatin, one of its now recognized sites of action [25]. 1,25-(OH)₂D_3 functions in the classical sense as a hormone because it must be carried by the blood from its site of synthesis to its target cells. Cholecalciferol and its hydroxylated metabolite, 25-OH-D_3, and other hydroxylated

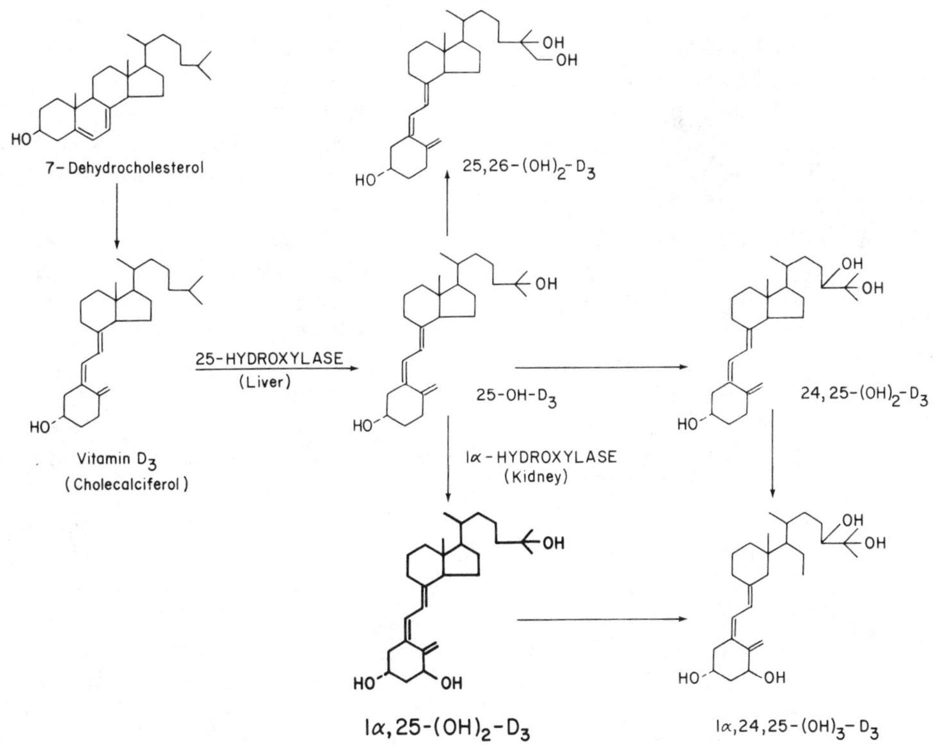

Figure 9.7   Sequential steps in the biosynthesis of vitamin D.

metabolites are bound to a plasma protein, originally referred to in the human as transcalciferin or calciferol-binding protein.

Another enzyme present in kidney mitochondria and possibly other extrarenal sites, 25-hydroxyvitamin D_3-24 hydroxylase, produces 24,25-$(OH)_2D_3$ (Fig. 9.7) which is rather inactive biologically in mammals [16]. A trihydroxylated derivative of vitamin D_3, 1,24,25-trihydroxyvitamin D_3 (1,24-25-$(OH)_3D_3$), has also been isolated from the plasma, but it too is inactive biologically (Fig. 9.7). 25,26-Dihydroxyvitamin D has also been isolated from the blood of humans and some animals receiving pharmacological doses of cholecalciferol. The origin and possible significance of this metabolite is unknown and the physiological importance of the other cholecalciferol metabolites is also unclear. Pregnant anephric female rats synthesize 1,25-$(OH)_2D_3$, and conversion of 25-OH-D_3 to 1,25-$(OH)_2D_3$ apparently takes place in the fetal placental unit of the rat [46]. The physiological significance, if any, of the placental synthesis of 1,25-$(OH)_2D_3$ is unknown.

Regulation of Vitamin D Metabolism

If a kidney 1α-hydroxylase is the key enzyme in 1,25-$(OH)_2D_3$ biosynthesis, it might be expected to be tightly regulated by endocrine or other factors released under conditions of hypocalcemia. Indeed, the production of 1,25-$(OH)_2D_3$ is markedly stimulated in animals on low calcium diets and suppressed in animals given high calcium diets. Thus, there is a strict inverse relationship between the serum Ca^{2+} level and the ability of animals to produce $1,25\text{-}(OH)_2D_3$. Conversely, whenever $1,25\text{-}(OH)_2D_3$ synthesis is suppressed, $24,25\text{-}(OH)_2D_3$ synthesis is stimulated. There is no evidence, however, that hepatic 25-OHase activity is regulated by a feedback control mechanism. Removal of the parathyroid glands eliminates the hypocalcemic stimulation of $1,25\text{-}(OH)_2D_3$ production and $24,25\text{-}(OH)_2D_3$ is produced. Conversely, PTH restores the ability of hypocalcemic animals to make $1,25\text{-}(OH)_2D_3$ and suppresses the production of $24,25\text{-}(OH)_2D_3$. In vitamin D-deficient animals there is an increase in renal 1α-OHase activity, whereas administration of vitamin D causes a dramatic disappearance of this enzyme. A direct effect of PTH on renal tubular production of $1,25\text{-}(OH)_2D_3$ has been demonstrated. Suppression of renal 1α-OHase activity is correlated with increased 24-OHase activity.

Phosphorus appears to also play an important role in the regulation of $1,25\text{-}(OH)_2D_3$ production. For example, thyroparathyroidectomized rats maintained on a low phosphorus high calcium diet also synthesize $1,25\text{-}(OH)_2D_3$ from $25\text{-}OH\text{-}D_3$. The intracellular concentration of phosphorus may therefore be an important local regulator of renal $1,25\text{-}(OH)_2D_3$ biosynthesis.

The feedback mechanism regulating $1,25\text{-}(OH)_2D_3$ production can be summarized as follows (Fig. 9.8): Hypocalcemia is stimulatory to PTH secretion from the parathyroids. PTH, acting directly or indirectly, stimulates renal cortical 1α-OHase activity, $1,25\text{-}(OH)_2D_3$ then stimulates Ca^{2+} absorption from the gut, increases release of Ca^{2+} from the bone, and stimulates Ca^{2+} reabsorption from the kidney. The increasing levels of Ca^{2+} then feed back to inhibit further synthesis of PTH. In the absence of further stimulation of 1α-OHase production 24-OHase activity is increased and any available $25\text{-}(OH)_2D_3$ is converted to the inactive me-

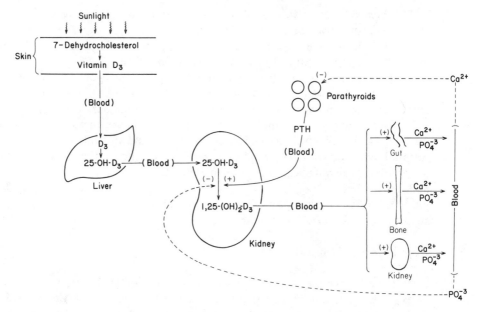

Figure 9.8 Feedback control of vitamin D biosynthesis [22].

tabolite, 24,25-(OH)$_2$D$_3$ (Fig. 9.7). Besides its effect on renal 1,25-(OH)$_2$D$_3$ production, PTH stimulates renal excretion of phosphate. Low plasma levels of phosphate are directly stimulatory to renal 1α-OHase activity and 1,25-(OH)$_2$D$_3$ production, whereas elevated levels of phosphate are inhibitory to production of the hormone. Parathyroid gland cells possess 1,25-(OH)$_2$D$_3$ receptors and there is evidence that 1,25-(OH)$_2$D$_3$ may feed back to this gland to inhibit PTH production.

Physiological Roles

In the following discussion the term vitamin D is sometimes used to refer to 1,25-(OH)$_2$D$_3$ or other possible active metabolites of cholecalciferol, because a particular physiological response might be mediated in some species by any one of a number of active substances. The role of vitamin D in Ca^{2+} absorption from the gut is well understood. Bone is another target tissue of the hormone, but its action on the skeletal system is not well characterized. Even less information is available on the kidney tubule as a possible target tissue of the actions of vitamin D.

Intestine. Calcium absorption from the intestine is the best documented action of vitamin D. The hormone also causes translocation of phosphate across the gut epithelium. Both processes require metabolic energy and are therefore active transport processes. Vitamin D may alter properties of the microvillar surface to allow entry of these ions into the mucosal cells. Transport of Ca^{2+} throughout the small and large intestines, particularly the duodenum, is improved by vitamin D.

Bone. In the absence of sunlight or a dietary source of vitamin D precursors rickets develops. Although vitamin D is necessary for proper bone growth, it seems a paradox that vitamin D also causes demineralization to provide Ca^{2+}, and possibly phosphorus, to maintain the critical plasma levels of these ions. The demineralization process may, however, be necessary to provide Ca^{2+} and phosphorus for accretion of new bone. The mechanisms by which vitamin D affects bone demineralization and bone growth are unknown.

Kidney. There is some evidence to suggest that 1,25-(OH)$_2$D$_3$ stimulates tubular reabsorption of Ca^{2+} in the kidney. In addition there are data supporting a direct role of the hormone on proximal tubular retention of phosphate. Because PTH causes phosphaturia and 1,25-(OH)$_2$D$_3$ production, feedback inhibition of parathyroid PTH release by the steroid might favor phosphate retention. A specific 1,25-(OH)$_2$D$_3$ receptor has been isolated from rat kidney cytosol [9]. A renal calcium binding protein has also been demonstrated and may facilitate tubular uptake of Ca^{2+} by the kidney as it does in the intestine.

Pregnancy. A hypophysial factor, probably prolactin, causes a marked suppression of plasma transcalciferin [6]. During chronic hyperprolactinemia (pregnancy and lactation) a similar decrease in this binding protein occurs. Androgens, on the other hand, elevate the plasma levels of this protein. It is interesting that PRL, which may regulate the concentration of transcalciferin, is also regulated in turn by 1,25-(OH)$_2$D$_3$, as shall be discussed.

Other putative roles. A number of tissues possess specific 1,25-(OH)$_2$D$_3$ receptors: skin, mammary gland, placenta, avian shell gland, and such peptide-secreting endocrine tissues as parathyroid, pituitary, pancreas, and even the brain [26, 44]. The parathyroid glands might be expected to represent a site for $1,25\text{-}(OH)_2D_3$ feedback inhibition of parathormone secretion. There is evidence that insulin is required for optimal $1,25\text{-}(OH)_2D_3$ production and prolactin and somatotropin also appear to stimulate production of the hormone. These endocrine glands may therefore represent additional sites for negative feedback inhibition by $1,25\text{-}(OH)_2D_3$. Other tissues studied that lack $1,25\text{-}(OH)_2D_3$ receptors are liver, spleen, muscle, and lung.

The synthesis of $1,25\text{-}(OH)_2D_3$ during egg laying in the Japanese quail (*Coturnix coturnix japonica*) provides an excellent model for studying the psychological and biochemical control of the renal-vitamin D endocrine system [29]. Enzyme studies of kidneys taken from birds with or without an egg in the oviduct reveal that ovulation results in an enhanced production of $1,25\text{-}(OH)_2D_3$, which is considered the active hormonal form of the steroid. Synthesis of this hormone is enhanced during the 24 hours following ovulation, even as early as 6 hours after ovulation, a time before any calcification of the egg shell begins. If no subsequent ovulation occurs following oviposition (egg-laying), $1,25\text{-}(OH)_2D_3$ production decreases rapidly within the following 6 hours (Fig. 9.9). In these studies all birds with an egg in the oviduct had undergone an ovulation during the 24-hour cycle immediately prior to that being examined. Birds with an egg in the oviduct which had not ovulated during the previous 24 hours were not studied. One cannot conclude whether the renal 1α-hydroxylase activity arose before or after ovulation because the ovulatory period examined was the first such event during the preceding 24 hours or more. But the data do demonstrate that the enzyme level remains continuously and steadily elevated when the bird is undergoing consecutive ovulations. Similar data are now available from studies on the chicken.

These are the first studies to reveal the acute control over $1,25\text{-}(OH)_2D_3$ production during a specific physiological state of an animal. It is known that calcium, inorganic phosphate, and parathyroid hormone directly affect $1,25\text{-}(OH)_2D_3$ bio-

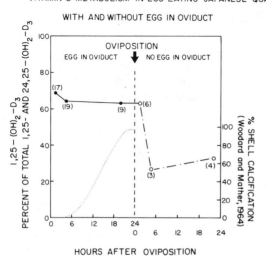

Figure 9.9 In vitro renal production of $1,25\text{-}(OH)_2D_3$, expressed as a percent of total $1,25\text{-}$ and $24,25\text{-}(OH)_2D_3$ biosynthesis, at different periods (1 to 3, 3 to 6, and 18 to 24 hours) after oviposition in Japanese quail with (—) and without (— · —) an egg in oviduct. Ovulation, when it occurs, is within 30 minutes after oviposition. If oviposition is not followed immediately by ovulation (at right), $1,25\text{-}(OH)_2D_3$ production, although still enhanced 1 to 3 hours after oviposition, falls rapidly and significantly. Eggshell calcification rate is plotted on left side of figure (· · · · ·). Number in parentheses represents number of birds contributing data to mean value. (From Kenny, [29], with permission.)

synthesis [16]. These results in quail suggest the possibility that gonadotropic hormones or their target organ hormones might also affect hormone production, as it was shown that estradiol stimulates $1,25\text{-}(OH)_2D_3$ synthesis [5]. Whether the renal response to estradiol is direct or indirect remains unclear. Similar results were obtained in the bullfrog and the rat, thus demonstrating the estrogen influence on the renal-vitamin D system is not restricted to those vertebrate species that produce calcified eggs.

There is evidence, at least in birds, that $24,25\text{-}(OH)_2D_3$ may serve a hormonal role in addition to serving as a pathway for catabolism. If chicks are raised to sexual maturity from hatching with $1,25\text{-}(OH)_2D_3$ as the sole vitamin D metabolite, fertile eggs appear to develop normally but fail to hatch [37]. In hens receiving only $25\text{-}OH\text{-}D_3$, embryonic development and hatchability are normal. $25\text{-}OH\text{-}D_3$ or some unknown metabolite thereof may be responsible for normal growth in the chick. If the requirement is specific for $25\text{-}OH\text{-}D_3$, this may represent a phylogenetically important role for this metabolite in some species [3]. It is necessary to determine the possible role of this and other vitamin D metabolites in early growth of humans and other vertebrates.

Although the role of $1,25\text{-}(OH)_2D_3$ in mammals and birds is well documented, the possible role of the hormone or related metabolites in other vertebrates is unknown. Teleost fishes synthesize cholecalciferol apparently without the aid of sunlight, and the livers of such animals are a well-known source of precursor metabolites for $1,25\text{-}(OH)_2D_3$ production in humans. Frogs and other amphibians are reported to be susceptible to vitamin D deficiency. The availability of Ca^{2+} and phosphate in aquatic environments could eliminate the need for vitamin D in some aquatic vertebrates.

A number of species of plants throughout the world cause severe calcinosis in domestic animals when ingested as part of their forage. A calcinogenic factor extracted from the leaves of *Solanum malacoxylon* has been found to be $1,25\text{-}(OH)_2D_3$ glycoside. After ingestion, endogenous glycosidases or intestinal microbes hydrolyze the glycoside to the hormonally active form. The reason for the existence of such a calcinogenic factor is unclear, but it and other related substances may function in mineral metabolism in plants [48].

HORMONE MECHANISMS OF ACTION IN CALCIUM HOMEOSTASIS

There is little doubt that parathormone actions on bone and the renal cortex involve increases in cyclic AMP [1]. The mechanism by which CT inhibits the action of PTH on bone is, however, not well understood. Although the mechanism of action of vitamin D in the gut is well defined, its actions on other tissues are not clearly understood.

Parathormone

Because the renal cortex is a major site of PTH action, this tissue has provided the major source of information on the mechanism of action of PTH. [^{3}H]-labeled PTH is localized preferentially to cells of the proximal tubules of the kidney cortex

[44]. Renal cortical membranes bind PTH and respond by increasing the production of cyclic AMP. Bovine PTH is equipotent to hPTH in stimulating human renal cortical tissue. Human PTH$^{1-34}$ is a full agonist in that it can produce a maximal effect but has approximately 1/10 the potency of the parent molecule (hPTH 1–84). Deletion of the two amino terminal residues completely abolishes the activity of PTH, thus demonstrating the importance of the N-terminus for biological activity of the hormone [17].

There is a remarkable dependency of PTH on vitamin D for mobilization of Ca^{2+} from bone in vivo. In rats on a vitamin D-deficient, low Ca^{2+} diet serum Ca^{2+} levels drop to very low values in spite of secondary hyperparathyroidism, and there is no histological evidence of enhanced bone resorption. It appears, therefore, that PTH and vitamin D act in concert to effect mobilization of bone mineral. PTH stimulates adenylate cyclase activity in particulate bone cell fractions from vitamin D-deficient and normal rats. The data suggest that the cause of skeletal refractoriness to PTH in vitamin D-deficient animals is not a defective activation of adenylate cyclase. Most likely the vitamin D requirement for PTH action is related to later steps in the biochemical events leading to bone cell activation. Vitamin D appears to be permissive to the actions of PTH, possibly by one or more mechanisms described for the actions of steroid hormones (Fig. 4.14).

Calcitonin

The entire 32 amino acid sequence appears to be required for biological activity. Seven of the nine common residues of the salmon CT's are at the N-terminal end of the molecule and are probably intimately involved in biological activity. Cleavage of the 1–7 disulfide bond in the hormone or oxidation of the methionine at 8 in the human CT molecule destroys biological activity of the hormones. The C-terminal prolinamide is also essential for activity. When studied in the rat, piscine (salmon, eel) calcitonins show markedly enhanced biological activities compared to calcitonins from other species. The high biological effectiveness of salmon CT relative to that of mammals may be due to a longer half-life in vivo, due to resistance of the hormone to degradation by plasma or tissue enzymes.

Receptors for CT are present in skeletal tissue, kidney, and testicular Leydig cells. The apparent affinities of the several calcitonin analogs for specific receptors in vitro parallel closely the biological activity of those analogs in vivo. Human CT has no greater relative potency when tested against receptors from human tissue than for receptors from rat tissues. Thus, in contrast to the marked evolutionary changes in CT structure, there is no evidence suggesting phylogenetic modification in the nature of the CT receptor.

Vitamin D

As for steroid hormones, vitamin D interacts with target tissue nuclear receptors to activate transcriptional and translational processes [24, 25, 26]. In this regard the action of the hormone on the intestine has been well characterized, whereas the effects of 1,25-$(OH)_2D_3$ on bone, kidney, and other tissues is less well understood (Fig. 9.10). There is a lag period of some 2 hours before the effects of the hormone can be noted, suggesting that the induction of new proteins is a prerequisite for the

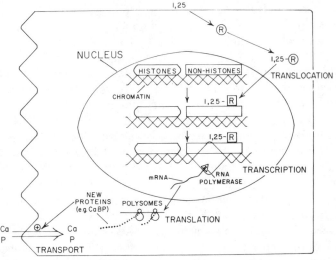

Model for early events in the interaction of 1,25-(OH)$_2$D$_3$ with the intestinal cell.

Figure 9.10 Model for early events in the interaction of 1,25-(OH)$_2$D$_3$ with the intestinal cell. (Reprinted, by permission of *The New England Journal of Medicine*, Haussler et al., [25], vol. 297, pp. 974–983, 1041–1050, 1977.)

actions of the hormone. The hormone is bound to high affinity cytosolic receptors which are then transported to the nucleus where interaction with specific sites on the nuclear chromatin allows activation of specific genes coding for mRNA production. The mRNA's then act as the templates for protein synthesis. Inhibitors of mRNA synthesis (actinomycin and ∂-amanitin) and protein synthesis (cycloheximide) block the action of vitamin D on intestinal absorption of Ca^{2+}. A number of proteins are synthesized within intestinal mucosal cells in response to vitamin D. One of these is a Ca^{2+}-binding (transport) protein (CaBP). This protein may enhance the movement of Ca^{2+} from the brush border into the cytoplasm.

Receptors for 1,25-(OH)$_2$D$_3$ are present in bone, and vitamin D causes a large (100-fold) increase in immunoreactive CaBP in chick bone. 1,25-(OH)$_2$D$_3$ stimulates alkaline phosphatase activity of osteoblastlike bone tumor cells in tissue culture. In view of the postulated role of the enzyme in calcification, these observations suggest a direct involvement of vitamin D in bone mineralization [34]. There is also evidence that the action of vitamin D on the kidney may involve synthesis of a Ca^{2+}-binding protein: A vitamin D-dependent CaBP has been localized immunohistochemically in distal tubules of avian and mammalian kidneys. Autoradiographic studies with 1,25-(OH)$_2$D$_3$ also reveal that the hormone is preferentially localized to cells of the distal tubules [44]. Nuclear receptors for 1,25-(OH)$_2$D$_3$ are also present in cells of the pars distalis of the pituitary, and it has been reported that the hormone may regulate prolactin production.

HORMONE INTEGRATION IN CALCIUM HOMEOSTASIS

Isolated bone cell populations of osteoblasts and osteoclasts have been obtained and the effects of PTH, CT, and vitamin D on these cells studied [51]. PTH and 1,25-(OH)$_2$D$_3$ stimulate acid phosphatase activity and hyaluronate synthesis within

osteoclasts and decrease alkaline phosphatase, citrate decarboxylation, and collagen synthesis in osteoblasts. Calcitonin inhibits the actions of the two hormones
on osteoclasts but not on osteoblasts. PTH, but not vitamin D, mediates its effects
through cyclic AMP production. Although vitamin D and PTH activate similar
cellular processes, they do so through separate receptors, and the action of either
hormone in vitro does not require the presence of the other. These results demonstrate that the actions of PTH and vitamin D elevate serum calcium levels by enhancing the bone-resorbing activities of the osteoclasts, while inhibiting concomitantly the bone-building activities of the osteoblasts. Calcitonin mediates its serum
Ca^{2+} lowering effect by preferentially inhibiting osteoclastic (bone-resorbing) activity without disturbing the mineralization (bone-building) activity of osteoblasts
(Fig. 9.11).

The long-term actions of PTH and CT on stimulation of osteocytes and osteoclasts in the process of bone demineralization and mineralization have been described. Bone also serves as a Ca^{2+} reservoir for the rapid uptake and release of
Ca^{2+} during daily plasma Ca^{2+} fluctuations. A layer of osteoblasts is separated from
the underlying layers of osteocytes by a *bone fluid compartment*, a so-called bone
lining cell/osteocyte unit. Calcium stored in the bone fluid compartment is present
in a labile, metastable form, which is kept from being transferred to hydroxyapatite
crystals. The CT secreted in response to food entering the digestive tract causes the
movement of serum Ca^{2+} into the bone mineral compartment. This labile Ca^{2+} then
returns to the extracellular compartment as postprandial plasma Ca^{2+} levels decline. By this process Ca^{2+} levels are maintained during periods of fasting. The re-

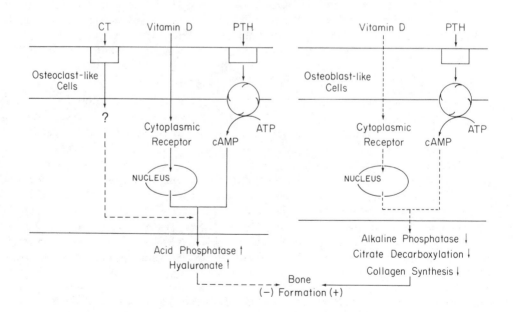

Figure 9.11 PTH, vitamin D, and calcitonin effects on osteoblastlike and osteoclast-
like cells maintained in culture. The positive (—) and negative (-----) actions of the hormones on increased (↑) or decreased (↓) cellular synthetic processes are indicated [51].

turn of Ca^{2+} to the ECF would be inhibitory to PTH release, and this might be an effective safeguard against bone resorptive activity during fasting [45].

Corpuscles of Stannius

In teleosts a pair of glands referred to as *Stannius corpuscles* are intimately attached to the kidneys. These glands may be involved in the endocrine control of the plasma electrolyte concentrations. The corpuscles contain two cell types, one which appears to be engaged in the synthesis of a hypocalcemic hormone, hypocalcin, and the other a hormone which may control plasma sodium levels. Histochemical and ultra-structural data indicate that the gland cells probably produce glycoproteins [50]. The secretory activity of the cells of the Stannius corpuscles appears to be directly affected by plasma ion levels, particularly Ca^{2+} [2]. Removal of the Stannius corpuscles leads to a rise in blood Ca^{2+} levels and a decrease in inorganic phosphate. Stanniectomy also perturbs the Na^+ and K^+ equilibrium of the body fluids. The vascular connections between the Stannius corpuscles and the kidneys suggest that the kidneys may be the target organs of the corpuscular endocrine substances (Figs. 9.12 and 9.13). Present knowledge of the calcium-regulating endocrine system of vertebrates (Table 9.1) and the effects of hormones in members of each vertebrate class (Table 9.2) are summarized [39].

PATHOPHYSIOLOGY OF CALCIUM HOMEOSTASIS

Decreased or increased production of PTH leads to hypocalcemic or hypercalcemic states, respectively. Because an important role of PTH is to enhance production of $1,25\text{-}(OH)_2D_3$, the etiology of either calcemic state is most directly related to decreased or increased levels of this steroid hormone. Calcium ions play a critical role in nerve and muscle excitability. Alterations in extracellular Ca^{2+} concentrations may therefore affect neural transmission and contractility of cardiac and skeletal muscle, thus leading to serious clinical problems.

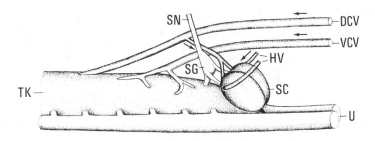

Figure 9.12 Diagrammatic lateral view of the caudal region of the trunk kidneys (TK): SC, Stannius corpuscles; SN, sympathetic nerve; SG, sympathetic ganglion, sending two nerve branches to the Stannius corpuscles and a major nerve to the kidneys; U, ureter; DCV, dorso-caudal vein; VCV, ventro-caudal vein; HV, vein from the hypaxial musculature; arrows, direction of blood flow. The venous connections between Stannius corpuscles and kidneys are not shown. (From Wendelaar Bonga, Greren, and Veenhuis, [50], with permission.)

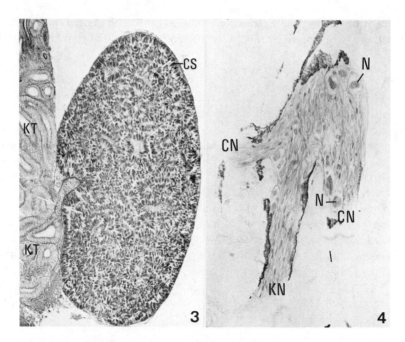

Figure 9.13 Paraldehyde fuchsin-stained section of a Stannius corpuscle (SC), showing its close topographical relation to the kidney: KT, kidney tubules, arrows, small vein running from corpuscle to kidney. 120×. (From Wendelaar Bonga, Greren, and Veenhuis, [50], with permission.)

Hypoparathyroidism

Hypoparathyroid patients display hypocalcemia as their major clinical symptom. Part of this hypocalcemia is caused by a partial deficiency of $1,25\text{-}(OH)_2D_3$ in the blood. The hyperphosphatemia resulting from PTH deficiency might also suppress $1,25\text{-}(OH)_2D_3$ production. Restoration of normocalcemia may be attained by treatment with $1,25\text{-}(OH)_2D_3$ or related metabolites. Tetany and convulsions are the most serious complications of the hypoparathyroid state. Latent tetany may be de-

TABLE 9.1 Distribution of Calcium Regulating Endocrine System in Vertebrates. ?, Not known yet; +, Present; −, Absent; ±, Absent in some species; (−), Definitive studies lacking.[a]

Vertebrates	Vitamin D metabolizing system	Parathyroids	Pituitary gland	Ovary	Calcitonin producing tissues	Stannius corpuscles
Cyclostomes	?	−	+	+	(−)	(−)
Elasmobranchs	?	−	+	+	+	(−)
Teleosts	+	−	+	+	+	+
Lungfishes	+	−	+	+	+	(−)
Amphibians	+	±	+	+	+	(−)
Reptiles	+	+	+	+	+	(−)
Birds	+	+	+	+	+	(−)
Mammals	+	+	+	+	+	(−)

[a]From [39], with permission.

TABLE 9.2 Effects of Calcium Regulating Principles in Vertebrates. +, Positive effects observed; −, No effect; ±, Mixed reports; (+), More work needed to confirm; ?, No clear studies performed.[a]

| Vertebrates | Hypercalcemic principles | | | | Hypocalcemic principles | |
	PTH	Pituitary principles	Estrogen	Vitamin D	Calcitonin	Stannius corpuscles principles
Cyclostomes	−	?	+	?	−	?
Elasmobranchs	−	?	+	?	−	?
Teleosts	−	+	+	?	±	+
Lungfishes	−	?	+	?	−	?
Amphibians	+	(+)	+	(+)	±	?
Reptiles	+	?	+	?	−	?
Birds	+	(+)	+	+	±	?
Mammals	+	(+)	+	+	±	?

[a]From [39], with permission.

tected by tapping over the facial nerves, which results in a contraction of the facial muscles (Chvostek's sign), or by producing carpal (wrist) spasm (Trousseau's sign) following occlusion of arterial blood supply to the forearm as often happens when applying a sphygmomanometer to the arm.

Hyperparathyroidism

Patients with primary hyperparathyroidism have moderate to severe hypercalcemia and elevated plasma 1,25-$(OH)_2D_3$ levels. The pathology of primary hyperparathyroidism may involve *neoplasia* or *hyperplasia*. Primary hyperparathyroidism usually results from a benign adenoma of one of the parathyroids. Hyperparathyroidism due to primary hyperplasia, on the other hand, involves overactivity of all the parathyroid glands. Secondary hyperparathyroidism often results from a peripheral defect of PTH action; the resulting hypocalcemia is the stimulus to enhanced parathyroid chief cell activity.

Pseudohypoparathyroidism

In this disorder, although Ca^{2+} levels are depressed, suggestive of PTH deficiency, the levels of the hormone may actually be increased above normal. The defect responsible in one type of pseudohypoparathyroidism appears to be related to a failure in generation of cyclic AMP. The pathology may be specifically related to a defect in a receptor-cyclase coupling protein necessary for transduction of signal between PTH receptor and adenylate cyclase [19]. In some types of pseudohypoparathyroidism end-organ resistance to PTH may result in hyperphosphatemia, which is inhibitory to 1,25-$(OH)_2D_3$ production. There may also be a refractoriness of renal 1α-hydroxylase to PTH action.

Osteomalacia

This disorder is characterized by a failure of normal mineralization of bone in the adult. (In children the disease is referred to as rickets.) This undermineralization of cartilage and bone results in retardation of growth and development of characteristic skeletal deformities. Rickets and osteomalacia encompass a group of diseases that have similar skeletal defects but diverse causes [22]. Osteomalacia is classified as vitamin D-responsive or vitamin D-resistant. The vitamin D-responsive disorders may be due to a deficiency in dietary intake of vitamin D precursors (vitamin D-deficiency rickets), inadequate exposure to sunlight, or intestinal malabsorption of Ca^{2+}. Several unusual forms of vitamin D-resistant rickets have been described which involve end-organ hyposensitivity (pseudovitamin D deficiency) to biologically active vitamin D. In one case this probably involved intestinal hyposensitivity to the hormone and was of congenital origin [47]. The vitamin D-resistant disorders result from diverse etiologies, such as familial or acquired renal-tubular phosphate wasting, defective collagen matrix formation, and specific hereditary defects in the metabolic transformation of vitamin D to its active form, probably due to failure of 1-hydroxylation. The etiological basis of one type of osteomalacia may involve a defective nuclear uptake of vitamin D [18]. The oral administration of 1,25-$(OH)_2D_3$, although effective in the treatment of some vitamin D-resistant syndromes, may cause hypercalcemia due to the high transient local concentrations of the hormone in the small intestine. A novel alternative method of providing vitamin D to the patient may be through the topical application of 1,25-$(OH)_2$-7-dehydrocholesterol combined with phototherapy. Cutaneous generation of 1,25-$(OH)_2D_3$ results, which may provide a more prolonged release and sustained stimulation of intestinal Ca^{2+} absorption [27].

Paget's Disease

This disease, which is often familial and affects mainly people of Western European or Mediterranean origin, is characterized by the presence of excessive numbers of osteoclasts, which leads to structurally weakened bone tissue. Although susceptibility to Paget's disease is believed to be transmitted by a simple autosomal Mendelian dominant gene, the etiology remains elusive. Osteoclasts from pagetic bone may be enlarged and contain greatly increased numbers of nuclei. Viruslike inclusions have been noted in the nuclei of some pagetic osteoclasts. Certain individuals may be born with the genetic susceptibility to osteoclastic invasion by a virus organism. The expression of the abnormality is, however, usually only manifested later in life. Presently the only effective treatment for Paget's disease involves the use of calcitonin.

Osteoporosis

The pathogenesis of osteoporosis (decrease in bone density) that occurs after menopause is related to a decrease in gonadal steroids. Common sites of fracture among postmenopausal females are the vertebrae, forearm, and hip. The incidence of such fractures among males of similar age is much less, whereas in younger adults there is little difference in incidence between the sexes. On this basis the prevention of such fractures might be realized if estrogen treatment is continued after menopause. Virtually all the available evidence indicates that the use of estrogens lowers the risk of postmenopausal fractures, and as such they may be considered a benefit of long-term estrogen use. In elderly people with osteoporosis there is not only reduced

$1,25\text{-}(OH)_2D_3$ secretion but also parathormone and calcitonin plasma levels are diminished. Whether these phenomena are specific characteristics of osteoporosis or are just endocrine changes common to all aging persons is unclear. There is evidence that calcitonin alone or in combination with $1,25\text{-}(OH)_2D_3$ is effective in enhancing the bone mineral content of postmenopausal and other elderly osteoporotic patients.

REFERENCES

[1] AGUS, Z. S., A. WASSERSTEIN, and S. GOLDFARB. 1981. PTH, calcitonin, cyclic nucleotides and the kidney. *Ann. Rev. Physiol.* 43:583–95.

[2] AIDA, K., R. S. NISHIOKA, and H. A. BERN. 1980. Degranulation of the Stannius corpuscles of coho salmon (*Oncorhynchus kisutch*) in response to ionic changes *in vitro*. *Gen. Comp. Endocrinol.* 41:305–13.

[3] AMEENUDDIN, S., M. SUNDE, H. F. DeLUCA, N. IKEKAWA, and Y. KOBAYASHI. 1982. 24-Hydroxylation of 25-hydroxyvitamin D_3: is it required for embryonic development in chicks? *Science* 217:451–52.

[4] AUSTIN, L. A., and H. HEATH III. 1981. Calcitonin: physiology and pathophysiology. *New Engl. J. Med.* 304:269–78.

[5] BAKSI, S. N., and A. D. KENNY. 1978. Vitamin D metabolism in Japanese quail: gonadal hormones and dietary calcium effects. *Am. J. Physiol.* 2:622–28.

[6] BOUILLON, R., G. VANDOREN, H. VAN BAELEN, and P. DeMOOR. 1978. Immunochemical measurement of the vitamin D-binding protein in rat serum. *Endocrinology* 102:1710–15.

[7] BREWER, H. B., T. FAIRWELL, W. RITTEL, T. LITTLEDIKE, and C. D. ARNAUD. 1974. Recent studies on the chemistry of human, bovine, and porcine parathyroid hormones. *Am. J. Med.* 56:759–66.

[8] BROWN, E. M., D. G. GARDNER, M. F. BRENNAN, S. J. MARX, A. M. SPEGEL, M. F. ATTIE, R. W. DOWNS, JR., J. L. DOPPMAN, and G. D. AURBACH. 1979. Calcium regulated parathyroid hormone release in primary hyperthyroidism. *Am. J. Med.* 66:923–31.

[9] CHANDLER, J. S., J. W. PIKE, and M. R. HAUSSLER. 1979. 1,25-Dihydroxyvitamin D_3 receptors in rat kidney cytosol. *Biochem. Biophys. Res. Commun.* 90:1057–63.

[10] CLARK, N. B. 1972. Calcium regulation in reptiles. *Gen. Comp. Endocrinol.* 3:430–40.

[11] CLARK, N. B., and Y. SASAYAMA. 1981. The role of parathyroid hormone on renal excretion of calcium and phosphate in the Japanese quail. *Gen. Comp. Endocrinol.* 45:234–41.

[12] COOPER, C. W., R. M. BOLMAN III, W. M. LINEHAN, and S. A. WELLS, JR. 1978. Interrelationships between calcium, calcemic hormones, and gastrointestinal hormones. *Rec. Prog. Horm. Res.* 34:259–83.

[13] COPP, D. H. 1969. Review. Endocrine control of calcium homeostasis. *J. Endocrinol.* 43:137–61.

[14] DEFTOS, L. J., M. H. WEISMAN, G. W. WILLIAMS, D. B. KARPF, A. M. FRUMAR, B. J. DAVIDSON, J. G. PARTHEMORE, and H. L. JUDD. 1980. Influence of age and sex on plasma calcitonin in human beings. *New Engl. J. Med.* 302:1351–53.

[15] DeLUCA, H. F. 1976. Recent advances in our understanding of the metabolism of vitamin D and its regulation. *Clin. Endocrinol.* 5 (Suppl.):97s–108s.

[16] DeLUCA, H. F. 1978. Vitamin D and calcium transport. *Ann. New York Acad. Sci.* 307: 356–76.

[17] DRAPER, M. W. 1982. The structure of parathyroid hormone: its effects on biological action. *Mineral Electrolyte Metab.* 8:159–72.

[18] EMIL, C., U. A. LIBERMAN, J. F. ROSEN, and S. J. MARX. 1981. A cellular defect in hereditary vitamin-D-dependent rickets type II; defective nuclear uptake of 1,25-dihydroxyvitamin D in cultured skin fibroblasts. *New Engl. J. Med.* 304:1588–91.

[19] FARFEL, Z., and H. R. BOURNE. 1982. Pseudohypoparathyroidism: mutation affecting adenylate cyclase. *Mineral Electrolyte Metab.* 8:227–36.

[20] FREED, W. J., M. J. PERLOW, and R. J. WYATT. 1979. Calcitonin: inhibitory effect on eating. *Science* 206:850–52.

[21] HABENER, J. F., and J. T. POTTS, JR. 1976. Chemistry, biosynthesis, secretion, and metabolism of parathyroid hormone. In *Handbook of physiology*, sect. 7, Endocrinology, R. O. Greep and E. B. Astwood, vol. 7, pp. 313–42, ed. G. D. Aurbach, Washington, D.C.: Amer. Physiol. Soc.

[22] HABENER, J. F., and J. E. MAHAFFEY. 1978. Osteomalacia and disorders of vitamin D metabolism. *Ann. Rev. Med.* 29:327–42.

[23] HABENER, J. F., and J. T. POTTS, JR. 1978. Biosynthesis of parathyroid hormone. *New Engl. J. Med.* 299:580–85, 635–44.

[24] HAUSSLER, M. R., and T. A. McCAIN. 1977. Basic and clinical concepts related to vitamin D metabolism and action. *New Engl. J. Med.* 297:974–83, 1041–50.

[25] HAUSSLER, M. R., M. R. HUGHES, T. A. McCAIN, and J. W. PIKE. 1977. 1,25-Dihydroxyvitamin D: molecular mechanism, physiological regulation and clinical implications. In *Molecular endocrinology*, eds. I. MacIntyre and M. Szelke, pp. 101–16. New York: Elsevier North-Holland, Inc.

[26] HAUSSLER, M. R., J. W. PIKE, J. S. CHANDLER, S. C. MANOLAGAS, and L. J. DEFTOS. 1981. Molecular action of $1,25-(OH)_2D_3$: new cultured cell models. *Ann. New York Acad. Sci.* 372:502–17.

[27] HOLICK, M. F., M. USKOKOVIC, J. W. HENLEY, J. MacLAUGHLIN, S. A. HOLLICK, and J. T. POTTS, JR. 1980. The photoproduction of $1\alpha,25$-dihydroxyvitamin D_3 in the skin. *New Engl. J. Med.* 303:349–54.

[28] HOLICK, M. F., J. A. MacLAUGHLIN, and S. H. DOPPELT. 1981. Regulation of cutaneous previtamin D_3 photosynthesis in man: skin pigment is not an essential regulator. *Science* 211:590–93.

[29] KENNY, A. D. 1976. Vitamin D metabolism: physiological regulation in egg-laying Japanese quail. *Amer. J. Physiol.* 230:1609–15.

[30] LATMAN, N. S. 1980. Pituitary stimulation of parathyroid hormone secretion: evidence in cattle for a parathyroid stimulating hormone. *J. Exp. Zool.* 212:313–22.

[31] LAWSON, D. E. M., and M. DAVIE. 1979. Aspects of the metabolism and function of vitamin D. *Vitamin Horm.* 37:1–67.

[32] LeDOUARAIN, N. M., and C. LeLIEVRE. 1970. Démonstration de l'origine neurales des cellules à calcitonine du corps ultimobranchial chez l'embryon de poulet. *Compt. Rend.* 270:2857–60.

[33] LOOMIS, W. F. 1970. Rickets. *Sci. Amer.* 223:77–91.

[34] MANOLAGAS, S. C., D. W. BURTON, and L. J. DEFTOS. 1981. 1,25-Dihydroxyvitamin D_3 stimulates the alkaline phosphatase activity of osteoblast-like cells. *J. Biol. Chem.* 256:7115–17.

[35] MUNSON, P. L. 1976. Physiology and pharmacology of thyrocalcitonin. In *Handbook of physiology*, sect. 7, Endocrinology, eds. R. O. Greep and E. B. Astwood. vol. 7, pp. 443–64, ed. G. D. Aurbach, Washington, D.C.: Amer. Physiol. Soc.

[36] MUNSON, P. L., and P. F. HIRSCH. 1966. Thyrocalcitonin: newly recognized thyroid hormone concerned with metabolism of bone. *Clin. Orthoped.* 49:209–32.

[37] NORMAN, A. W., W. L. HENRY, and H. H. MALLUCHE. 1980. 24R,25-dihydroxyvitamin D_3 and 1α,25-dihydroxyvitamin D_3 are both indispensable for calcium and phosphorus homeostasis. *Life Sciences* 27:229–37.

[38] PANG, P. K. T. 1973. Endocrine control of calcium metabolism in teleosts. *Amer. Zool.* 13:775–92.

[39] PANG, P. K. T., A. D. KENNY, and C. OGURO. 1980. Evolution of endocrine control of calcium regulation. In *Evolution of the vertebrate endocrine systems*, eds. P. K. T. Pang and A. Epple, pp. 323–56. Lubbock, Texas: Texas Tech. Univ. Press.

[40] PANG, P. K. T., T. E. TENNER, JR., J. A. YEE, M. YANG, and H. F. JANSSEN. 1980. Hypotensive action of parathyroid hormone preparations on rats and dogs. *Proc. Natl. Acad. Sci. USA* 77:675–78.

[41] PARFITT, A. M. 1976. The actions of parathyroid hormone on bone: relation to bone remodeling and turnover, calcium homeostasis, and metabolic bone diseases. *Metabolism* 25:909–44.

[42] POTTS, J. T., JR., and G. D. AURBACH. 1976. Chemistry of the calcitonins. In *Handbook of physiology*, sect. 7, Endocrinology, eds. R. O. Greep and E. B. Astwood. vol. 7, pp. 423–30, ed. G. D. Aurbach. Washington, D.C.: Amer. Physiol. Soc.

[43] ROOS, B. A., and L. J. DEFTOS. 1976. Regulation of calcitonin secretion *in vitro*. *Clin. Endocrinol.* 5 (Suppl.):217s–22s.

[44] STUMPF, W. E., M. SAR, R. NARBARTZ, F. A. REED, H. F. DELUCA, and Y. TANAKA. 1980. Cellular and subcellular localization of 1,25-$(OH)_2$-vitamin D_3 in rat kidney: comparison with localization of parathyroid hormone and estradiol. *Proc. Natl. Acad. Sci. USA* 77:1149–53.

[45] TALMAGE, R. V., S. A. GRUBB, H. NORIMATSU, and C. J. VANDERWIEL. 1980. Evidence for an important physiological role for calcitonin. *Proc. Natl. Acad. Sci. USA* 77:609–13.

[46] TANAKA, Y., B. HALLORAN, H. K. SCHNOES, and H. F. DELUCA. 1979. *In vitro* production of 1,25-dehydroxyvitamin D_3 by rat placental tissue. *Proc. Natl. Acad. Sci. USA* 76:5033–35.

[47] TSUCHIYA, Y., N. MATSUO, H. CHO, M. KUMAGAI, A. YASAKA, T. SUDA, H. ORIMO, and M. SHIRAKI. 1980. An unusual form of vitamin D-dependent rickets in a child: alopecia and marked end-organ hyposensitivity to biologically active vitamin D. *J. Clin. Endocrinol. Metab.* 51:685–90.

[48] WASSERMAN, R. H., J. D. HENION, M. R. HAUSSLER, and T. A. McCAIN. 1976. Calcinogenic factor in *Solanum malacoxylon;* evidence that it is 1,25-dihydroxyvitamin D_3-glycoside. *Science* 194:853–54.

[49] WENDELAAR BONGA, S. E. 1981. Effect of synthetic calcitonin on protein-bound and free plasma calcium in the teleost *Gasterosteus aculeatus*. *Gen. Comp. Endocrinol.* 43:123–26.

[50] WENDELAAR BONGA, S. E., J. A. GREVEN, and M. VEENHUIS. 1977. Vascularization, innervation, and ultrastructure of the endocrine cell types of *Stannius* corpuscles in the teleost *Gasterosteus aculeatus*. *J. Morphol.* 153:225–43.

[51] WONG, G. L., R. A. LUBEN, and D. V. COHN. 1977. 1,25-Dihydroxycholecalciferol and parahormone: effects on isolated osteoclast-like and osteoblast-like cells. *Science* 197:663–65.

10

Gastrointestinal Hormones

INTRODUCTION

The first hormone to be discovered was *secretin*, a chemical messenger released from the epithelium of the small intestine in response to acid released from the stomach [3]. The gut is the source of many hormones; the gastrointestinal mucosa may be considered the largest endocrine organ. Elucidation of the chemical nature of the gut hormones has been difficult because the endocrine-secreting cells are distributed individually throughout the gut epithelium. Thus, an easy source of the hormones is not readily available for chemical identification. Their specific cellular distribution has, however, been determined precisely in a number of species by immunocytochemical methods.

Of the known gastrointestinal (GI) peptides four function as hormones: gastrin, secretin, cholecystokinin (CCK), and gastric inhibitory peptide (GIP). Other candidate hormones [5] will probably derive full hormonal status after further studies [28, 39]. One of the major problems confronting the endocrinologist is to determine whether the experimentally determined biological effects of the hormones are indeed indicative of such a physiological function. Many GI hormones fall into families of related hormones which share overlapping structures. Thus, members of the same hormonal family evoke similar target tissue responses, which confuses any issue relating to their individual putative physiological roles.

The actions of the GI hormones are primarily concerned with the digestion and movement of food products along the GI tract. They release the
enzymes necessary to split the specific food substrates, such as proteins,
carbohydrates, and fats, into their simpler components, amino acids,
sugars, and fatty acids (FFA's), respectively. The GI hormones also enhance
the activity of enzymes by stimulating the secretion of acid, which provides
the pH optimum for enzymatic action. Stimulation of secretion of bile salts
provides the medium in which fats can become emulsified by increasing
the surface area for enzyme activity. Thus, a major role of the GI hormones
is to facilitate the conversion of food substrates into molecular forms that
can then gain access into the bloodstream. A number of reviews on the
endocrinology of GI function are available [12, 14, 19, 28, 39].

GASTROINTESTINAL TRACT STRUCTURE AND FUNCTION

In order to appreciate the roles and actions of hormones on digestive processes it
is necessary to review briefly the structure and function of the GI tract [18]. Food
enters the mouth, is mixed with saliva, passes down the esophagus, and enters the
stomach through the lower esophageal sphincter. The emulsified, partly digested
food is then released as a bolus of *chyme* through the pyloric sphincter into the
duodenum, the initial segment of the small intestine (small bowel). The food continues
through the jejunal (*jejunum*) and ileal (*ileum*) segments of the small intestine to enter
the large intestine (colon) where the undigested components of the food comprising
the stool are dehydrated before defecation from the anus.

Food is propelled distally along the GI tract because of peristaltic contractions
of the gut. Peristalsis results from the rhythmic contractions and relaxations of the
longitudinal and circular layers of muscle that comprise part of the wall of the gut.
Muscle contraction and relaxation are controlled by neurons of the parasympathetic
and sympathetic components of the autonomic nervous system. These *extrinsic nerve
fibers* innervate *intrinsic neurons* of the *myenteric plexus of Auerbach*, which are
found between the circular and longitudinal muscle layers. Other intrinsic neurons
of the gut form the *submucosal plexus of Meissner*, which regulates the activity of
muscles responsible for movements of the villi.

The pancreas plays an important role in gastrointestinal function. The islets
of Langerhans (the endocrine pancreas) are the source of insulin and glucagon, two
hormones important in the control of carbohydrate metabolism (Chapter 11). The
exocrine pancreas is composed of the *acinar cells* which are the source of a variety
of enzymes essential to digestion of foodstuffs arriving in the small intestine. The
pancreatic duct provides an exit for the release and delivery of these enzymes to the
small intestine. Certain ductule cells lining this excretory passageway provide water
and electrolytes (i.e., bicarbonate ion) which are also important to digestive processes.

The gallbladder is a pear-shaped hollow organ which serves as a reservoir for
bile salts excreted by the liver. Contraction of the smooth muscles of the walls of
the gallbladder discharges the *bile salts* into the common bile duct, which then con-

nects with the pancreatic duct leading to the opening into the small intestine. The bile salts are necessary for emulsification of fats within the intestine.

In the mouth starch is acted on by *ptyalin*, an *α-amylase* present within the saliva. The saliva is secreted from the salivary (parotid, sublingual, submaxillary) glands. Because the optimal pH for α-amylase is 6.7, the action of the enzyme is subsequently inhibited by the acidic environment of the stomach. In the small intestine an α-amylase secreted by the *exocrine pancreas* acts on the various polysaccharides present in the partly digested food. Other enzymes localized within the luminal surface of the mucosa further hydrolyze sugars to glucose. Glucose and other hexoses and pentoses are rapidly absorbed across the wall of the duodenum and ileum to enter the bloodstream.

Protein digestion begins in the stomach where enzymes, *pepsins*, cleave particular peptide linkages. The pepsins are released from the chief cells of the body of the stomach as precursor (proenzyme) molecules, *pepsinogens*, which are activated by gastric hydrochloric acid released from *parietal* or *oxyntic* (Greek: to make sour, acid) *cells* of the gastric glands. The actions of the pepsins are terminated in the alkaline pancreatic juice of the duodenum. In the small intestine the shorter peptides are formed by the action of protein-splitting enzymes, *trypsin* and *chymotrypsin*, released from the pancreas. Other enzymes—pancreatic carboxypeptidases, intestinal aminopeptidases, and dipeptidases—split the smaller peptides to free amino acids. These amino acids are actively transported across the intestinal lumen and enter the bloodstream.

The digestion of fats begins in the intestine. Free fatty acids are liberated by the enzymatic actions of *pancreatic lipase* on dietary triglycerides. This enzyme acts on facts that have been emulsified by the detergent action of *bile salts* released into the intestinal lumen following contraction of the gallbladder. Small *micelles* consisting of lipids and bile salts provide the reactive surface for *lipase* activity. The FFA's and monoglycerides within the micelles are released to enter the mucosal cells by passive diffusion; they may pass directly into the portal blood or become reesterified to triglycerides within the mucosal cells and enter into the lymphatics.

SOURCE AND CHEMISTRY OF THE GASTROINTESTINAL HORMONES

The gastrointestinal hormones are synthesized within a system of clear cells (enterochromaffin, argyrophil, or argentaffin cells) so called because they are selectively stained by certain silver salts. These clear cells, scattered within the gastrointestinal tract mucosa from the stomach through the colon [41], are often referred to as the diffuse or dispersed endocrine system (DES) [33], or, with the pancreatic hormones, as the gastroenteropancreatic hormones [32]. This diffuse distribution prevents the endocrinologist from removing surgically the source of any one hormone as is done for many endocrine glands. It is suggested that the distribution of endocrine cells throughout extensive areas of mucosa "ensures that hormone release is regulated by an integrated sampling of mixed luminal contents rather than by a specific stimulus that might exist transiently at only one point" [19]. One surface of each of the endocrine cells often reaches the lumen, thus providing a receptive surface for metabolite recognition.

TABLE 10.1 Localization of Hormones in Endocrine Cells and Neurons of the Gastrointestinal Tract[a]

Hormone	Endocrine cell		Neuron
	Stomach-intestine	Pancreas	
Glucagon	A	A	−
Insulin	—	B	−
Somatostatin	D	D	+
VIP	D_1	D_1	+
Substance P (+ serotonin)	EC_1	EC	+
Motilin	EC_2		
Gastrin (antrum)	Ga	G	+
(intestine)	GI		
CCK-pancreozymin	I		+
C-terminal tetrapeptide			
(of gastrin or CCK)	TG		
GIP	K		−
GLI	L		−
Neurotensin	N		+
Bombesin (?)	P	P	+
Pancreatic polypeptide	PP	PP	−
Secretin	S		−

[a] From Said, S. I. "Peptides Common to the Nervous System and the Gastrointestinal Tract", in *Frontiers in Neuroendocrinology*, vol. 6, pp. 293--331, © 1980 Raven Press, New York, with permission.

The endocrine cells of the gut and pancreas have been classified as deriving from certain cell types, designated, for example, as D (somatostatin), G (gastrin), or S (secretin) (Table 10.1). A tenet of neuroendocrinology has been the "one hormone, one cell" concept. In the gut and elsewhere, a peptide hormone (e.g., substance P or calcitonin) and the biogenic amine, serotonin (5-HT), are often found within the same cell. The physiological significance of two biologically active moieties within the same cell is unclear. By immunocytochemical methods, two structurally unrelated peptide hormones have also been found within a single cell. It is possible, however, that one of the hormones may exist as a component of the precursor molecule of the other physiologically relevant hormone. Also, the immunoreactivity may only indicate cross-reacting sequences present in an undiscovered molecular variant of a known hormone [41].

Based on their homology of structure, the gut hormones can be conveniently grouped into two families. The *gastrin family* comprises the gastrins and the cholecysto-kinins. The *secretin family* consists of secretin, glucagon, vasoactive intestinal poly-peptide (VIP), and gastric inhibitory peptide (GIP). There may be molecular hetero-geneity of a particular hormone: The hormone may exist in a number of molecular forms of variable length with differing biological potencies. Only one of these peptides is considered to be the physiological messenger and it constitutes the principal form stored within the secretory granules of the cell. Molecular forms larger than the principal form may be conceived as biosynthetic precursors (prohormones) which may escape and be detected in the circulation. Molecular forms smaller than the prin-cipal form probably represent postsecretory degradation products [36].

GASTRIN (G–17)   (pyro)Glu–Gly–Pro–Trp–Leu–Glu–Glu–Glu–Glu–Glu–Ala–Tyr–Gly–Trp–Met–Asp–Phe–NH₂

$$\quad\quad\quad\quad\quad\quad\quad\quad\quad\quad\quad\quad\quad\quad\quad\quad\quad | \;—\;—\;—\;—\;—\;—$$

$$SO_3H$$

CHOLECYSTOKININ   Lys–Ala–Pro–Ser–Gly–Arg–Val–Ser–Met–Ile–Lys–Asn–Leu–Gln–Ser–Leu–Asp–

Pro–Ser–His–Arg–Ile–Ser–Asp–Arg–Asp–Tyr–Met–Gly–Trp–Met–Asp–Phe–NH₂

$$\quad\quad\quad\quad\quad\quad\quad\quad\quad\quad\quad\quad\quad\quad | \;—\;—\;—\;—\;—\;—$$

$$SO_3H$$

```
        18  19   20   21 22 23   24 25   26  27   28  29  30  31  32  33
```

Figure 10.1 Amino acid sequences of human G–17 gastrin and cholecystokinin (CCK). Identical C-terminal pentapeptide sequences are indicated.

The Gastrin Family of Hormones

The C-terminal five amino acid sequences of gastrin and CCK are identical (Fig. 10.1). Because the biologically active site of these peptides is this pentapeptide sequence, the overlapping actions of one hormone on target tissues of the other hormone are explained. The minimal active fragment of these peptides is actually the C-terminal tetrapeptide. Pentagastrin, which exhibits full agonistic activity, is often used in physiological studies where the actions of gastrin are to be determined (Fig. 10.2). The NH₂-terminal component of gastrin and CCK influences the potency of the hormones, and may also be responsible in part for providing target cell specificity. Note that there are sulfated tyrosyl residues at the 6 and 7 (numbering from the C-terminal end) positions of gastrin and CCK, respectively. Gastrin is found in nonsulfated and sulfated forms. Sulfated gastrin is usually more active on target cells than the nonsulfated form. For example, desulfated gastrin and CCK are less potent than their sulfated counterparts in stimulating gallbladder smooth muscle contraction [36].

Gastrin circulates in most mammalian species in at least three molecular forms (Table 10.2). A macromolecular form of gastrin called big-big gastrin (component I) apparently does not circulate, as earlier reported, but could exist as an early intracellular biosynthetic precursor for one or more of the gastrins [36]. It is believed that component I serves as a *preprogastrin* for gastrin-34 (big gastrin, component II) which may in some cells function as a hormone or *progastrin*. Component III, gastrin-17, may be the physiologically relevant form of the hormone secreted by some cells, and component IV (mini-gastrin, gastrin-14) is considered to be an extracellular degradation product of component III.

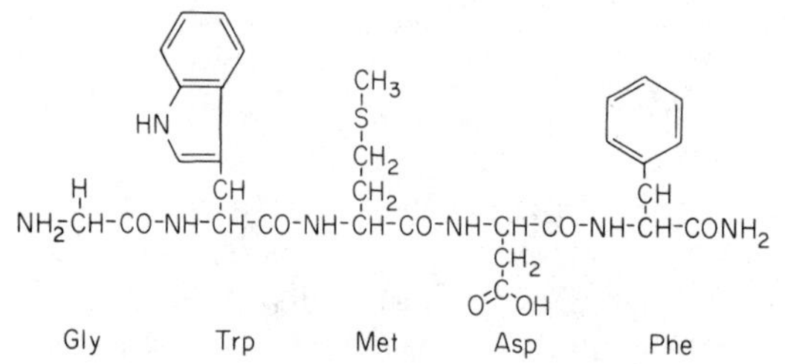

Pentagastrin

Figure 10.2 Structure of pentagastrin.

TABLE 10.2 Amino Acid Sequences Of Human Gastrin Components

Component[a]	Sequence
I Gastrin (big big gastrin)	Unknown structure, but contains G-17 at its COOH-terminus
II Gastrin₃₄ (big gastrin)	(pyro)Glu-Leu-Gly-Pro-Gln-Gly-His-Pro-Ser-Leu-Val-Ala-Asp-Pro-Ser-Lys-Lys- Gln-Gly-Pro-Trp-Leu-Glu-Glu-Glu-Glu-Glu-Ala-Tyr-Gly-Trp-Met-Asp-Phe-NH₂ <div align="right">| SO₃H</div>
III Gastrin₁₇ (little gastrin)	(pyro)Glu-Gly-Pro-Trp-Leu-Glu-Glu-Glu-Glu-Glu-Ala-Tyr-Gly-Trp-Met-Asp-Phe-NH₂ <div align="right">| SO₃H</div>
IV Gastrin₁₄ (mini-gastrin)	Trp-Leu-Glu-Glu-Glu-Glu-Glu-Ala-Tyr-Gly-Trp-Met-Asp-Phe-NH₂ <div align="right">| SO₃H</div>

[a]Gastrin-34, G-17, and G-14 also exist without a sulfate ester at their tyrosyl residue.

The Secretin Family of Hormones

Secretin is similar to glucagon in structure: 14 of the 27 amino acids of secretin are similar to those found in glucagon, which is 29 amino acids in length. Glucagon is found in the small intestine, but the significance of this *enteroglucagon* is uncertain. Most of the entire sequence of each of the peptides is required for their biological actions on their respective target tissues. The structures of GIP and VIP possess many amino acids in common with those found in glucagon and secretin (Fig. 10.3). The hormones of the secretin family lack a well-defined function site where, as in the melanotropins, particular amino acids have been conserved within the individual peptides (Fig. 8.1).

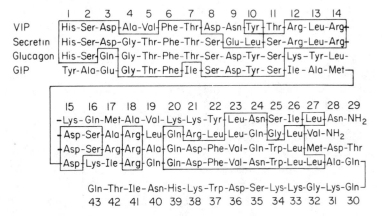

Figure 10.3 Amino acid sequences of porcine peptides of the secretin family. Boxed areas indicate identical amino acid sequences between peptides. (Modified from McGuigan [28], with permission.)

TABLE 10.3 Candidate Hormones Of The Gut

Hormone	
Substance P	^{1}Arg-^{2}Pro-^{3}Lys-^{4}Pro-^{5}Gln-^{6}Gln-^{7}Phe-^{8}Phe-^{9}Gly-^{10}Leu-^{11}Met-^{12}NH$_2$
Somatostatin	^{1}Ala-^{2}Gly-^{3}Cys-^{4}Lys-^{5}Asn-^{6}Phe-^{7}Phe-^{8}Trp-^{9}Lys-^{10}Thr-^{11}Phe-^{12}Thr-^{13}Ser-^{14}Cys-
Motilin	^{1}Phe-^{2}Val-^{3}Pro-^{4}Ile-^{5}Phe-^{6}Thr-^{7}Tyr-^{8}Gly-^{9}Glu-^{10}Leu-^{11}Glu-^{12}Arg-^{13}Met-^{14}Glu-^{15}Gly-^{16}Lys- ^{17}Glu-^{18}Arg-^{19}Asn-^{20}Lys-^{21}Gly-^{22}Glu
Neurotensin	^{1}(pyro)Glu-^{2}Leu-^{3}Tyr-^{4}Glu-^{5}Asn-^{6}Lys-^{7}Pro-^{8}Arg-^{9}Arg-^{10}Pro-^{11}Tyr-^{12}Ile-^{13}Leu

Other Candidate Hormones

The other putative hormones of the GI tract are motilin, somatostatin, substance P, neurotensin, and gastrin-releasing peptide. The formulae of these peptides are provided; they bear no structural similarity to each other or to the other GI hormones (Table 10.3). These peptides are localized in varying numbers to immunocytochemically characterized cells of the gastrointestinal mucosa. Other physiologically active peptides are also present within the GI tract and may also obtain hormone status. These include chymodenin, bulbogastrone, urogastrone, enteroglucagon, villikinin, the enkephalins, and possibly other endorphins [12, 15].

PHYSIOLOGICAL ROLES OF THE GASTROINTESTINAL HORMONES

A major role of the GI hormones is to stimulate the secretion of enzymes necessary to degrade complex food substrates into their simpler molecular components so that these smaller molecules can cross the luminal mucosal cells into the bloodstream. GI hormones also stimulate the secretion of acid or base to provide the optimal pH conditions for enzyme activity. By their actions on smooth muscle, the GI hormones move the food distally down the GI tract to the colon. They stimulate release of hormones from the pancreatic islets which then aid in cellular utilization of metabolic substrates after reaching the bloodstream. The GI hormones may even provide satiety signals to the brain to affect eating behavior (Chapter 20).

Each of the GI hormones has a bewildering number of known biological actions of questionable physiological significance. Because many of the hormones are related in structure, they can exhibit overlapping actions when studied experimentally. Gastrin and CCK are partially similar in structure: They both stimulate gastric acid and pancreatic enzyme secretion. It is likely, however, that each hormone is delivered by specific circulatory routes to its own target tissues. This would then provide the mechanism for the necessary specificity of their actions. More disconcerting is the observation that some of the GI hormones unrelated in structure have similar physiological effects. This may be because their actions are indirect, that is, mediated through effects on the release of one or more other hormones. The known physiological roles and effects of the GI hormones are shown (Table 10.4). The release of each of the gastrointestinal hormones is in response to chemical stimuli, such as hydrogen ions, certain amino acids, FFA's, and sugars. It is believed that receptors are present on the surface of the hormone-secreting cells which is in open communication with the lumen of the GI tract (Fig. 10.4).

Gastrin

Although the existence of an antral hormone controlling gastric acid secretion was postulated as early as 1905, the hormone gastrin was not isolated until 1964. The antral mucosa of the stomach is the richest source of gastrin in all investigated species; although the peptide is also present in G cells of the duodenal mucosa, contrary to some reports, it may not be present within the pancreatic islets. In the antrum and small intestine the apical pole of the cell, which possesses numerous villi, is in contact with the gastric lumen. Gastrin is present in the gastric juice, which has aroused speculation that gastrin might be released from the luminal surface (as a lumone) as well as from the basal surface. Electrical stimulation of the vagus nerve of the cat causes a minor increase in circulating gastrin, whereas a much greater amount can be detected in the gastric juice.

Food is the primary physiological stimulus of gastrin secretion. Peptide fragments, amino acids, and to a lesser extent FFA's are also stimulatory to gastrin secre-

TABLE 10.4 Physiological Roles Or Effects Of The GI Hormones And Candidate Hormones Within The GI Tract[a]

Hormone	Physiological roles
Gastrin	Increases gastric acid secretion, gastrointestinal growth, and antral motility
Secretin	Increases pancreatic and biliary bicarbonate secretion, potentiates CCK-stimulated pancreatic enzyme secretion
CCK	Stimulates gallbladder contraction and pancreatic enzyme secretion; potentiates gastric emptying, stimulates growth of the exocrine pancreas
GIP	Inhibits gastric acid secretion, stimulates insulin release
Chymodenin	Stimulates chymotrypsin release from the exocrine pancreas
Somatostatin	Inhibits antral gastrin secretion
VIP	Stimulates smooth muscle relaxation, increases blood flow and intestinal secretion
Gastrin releasing peptide	Stimulates gastrin secretion, gallbladder contraction, pancreatic enzyme secretion, and gastrointestinal motility; inhibits gastric acid secretion
Bulbogastrone	Inhibits gastric acid secretion
Urogastrone	Inhibits gastric acid secretion, stimulates oxyntic gland growth
Enteroglucagon	Unknown
Villikinin	Stimulates villous movement and lymph flow
Enkephalins	Unknown (neuromodulator?)
Neurotensin	Unknown (neuromodulator?)
Substance P	Unknown, possibly modulates gut motility and mucosal secretions
Motilin	Increases gastrointestinal motility

[a]Taken in part from [19].

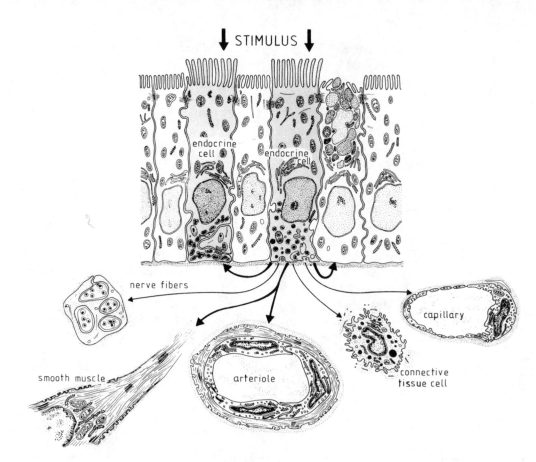

Figure 10.4 Schematic drawing indicating the possible functional actions of entero-endocrine cells. The stimulus from the intestinal lumen acts on the receptors of the brush border membrane, resulting in a release of hormones by exocytosis. The peptide hormones may exert their effect on the following (a) adjacent epithelial cells, nerve fibers, nerve cells, smooth muscle, and connective tissue cells of the lamina propria; (b) cells of the whole organism. Method (a) is described as paracrine; method (b) is referred to as endocrine. (From Grube and Forssmann, [16], with permission.)

tion, but sugars are without such an effect. Gastrin secretion is under autonomic control. For example, in some species the vagus nerve stimulates gastrin secretion in anticipation of the ingestion of food or through activation of local neural reflexes following distension of the stomach after food intake. Somatostatin- and VIP-secreting cells are found in close association with antral gastrin-secreting cells and may function in an inhibitory role by a paracrine mechanism.

One physiological function of gastrin is to stimulate hydrochloric acid and pepsinogen secretion within the fundus of the stomach; the activated enzyme then initiates the digestion of proteins. Gastrin is the most potent gastric acid secretagogue known; there is evidence obtained from the use of isolated parietal cells that gastrin has a direct stimulatory action on these cells. Thus, gastrin may not stimulate pepsinogen secretion directly but rather indirectly through release of HCl. In other words, the hydrogen ions from the acid are stimulatory to pepsinogen secretion from the chief cells (Fig. 10.5).

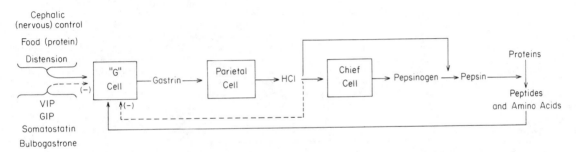

Figure 10.5 Neuroendocrine integration of gastric acid secretion.

The gastrin present within the antrum is the small (G–17) form of the molecule. The cell responsible for gastrin production in the duodenum contains the larger (G–34) form of the peptide. These two cells therefore contain different molecular forms of the peptide, which supports the observation that the two cells are ultrastructurally distinguishable. It is possible that these two circulating forms of gastrin have selective actions on different target cells. It is also possible that a particular molecular form of gastrin may be less susceptible to enzyme degradation.

Starvation or total parenteral (venous) nutrition dramatically reduces the levels of both antral and serum gastrin. This suggests that the secretion of gastrin is acutely dependent on the presence of food in the gut. If rats are fed totally by vein, tissue sensitivity to the trophic action of gastrin becomes diminished. This loss of sensitivity can be prevented by the concomitant infusion of pentagastrin. The pancreas and colonic mucosa as well as the duodenal and oxyntic gland mucosa undergo atrophy in the antrectomized rat, but these deleterious effects can be reversed by supplying gastrin exogenously. These observations suggest that endogenous gastrin is an important regulator of pancreatic, duodenal, and colonic mucosal growth in addition to its effect on oxyntic gland mucosal growth [5].

The following biological effects are ascribed to gastrin: stimulation of lower esophageal sphincter pressure; relaxation of the pyloric sphincter; stimulation of pancreatic enzyme secretion; enhancement of motor activity in the intestine; and moderate stimulation of pancreatic bicarbonate and water secretion. Recently the common C-terminal tetrapeptide amide, Try-Met-Asp-Phe-NH$_2$, which is shared by gastrin and CCK, was discovered in the pituitary stalk and in the hypothalamus [36]. Pentagastrin infusions into humans increase plasma concentrations of somatotropin but are without such an effect on prolactin secretion. This may suggest a potential role for the gastrin tetrapeptide as a local neurotransmitter in the hypothalamic-pituitary system [8]. This peptide may be the yet unidentified somatotropin-releasing factor. It is also possible that larger molecular forms of gastrin or CCK may have a somatotropin-releasing role in a hormonal gut-hypophysial axis [8].

Secretin

Secretin is one of many peptide hormones of the small intestine. The tissue concentration of secretin diminishes from duodenum to ileum. Secretinlike immunoreactivity is localized to the granular S cells, which are present between the crypts and villi of the mucosa of the small intestine where maximum concentrations of the hormone have

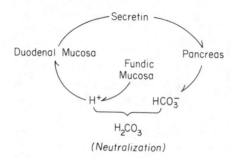

Figure 10.6 Homeostatic closed-loop endocrine mechanism of small intestine pH control.

also been extracted. Acidification of the duodenal mucosa, resulting from HCl arriving in the duodenum from the stomach, is the normal stimulus for secretin secretion. At a pH above 4.5, secretin is not released in sufficient amounts to stimulate pancreatic bicarbonate secretion [35] and continued release of secretin is pH dependent. Nevertheless, it has been difficult to demonstrate increases in plasma secretin levels after a meal. Because a secretin response (increased pancreatic secretion of water and bicarbonate) is observed in humans and dogs after injestion of meat, a small amount of secretin (insufficiently large to be detected by radioimmunoassay) may be released from the duodenum and may interact with CCK to stimulate bicarbonate secretion [35]. There is an endocrine closed-loop type of relationship governing secretin and HCO_3^- release. Secretin stimulates pancreatic secretion of HCO_3^- into the duodenum; the HCO_3^- neutralizes the H^+ from the stomach, which raises the pH, hence decreasing the release of secretin, which removes any further stimulus to bicarbonate secretion (Fig. 10.6).

The clearly defined roles of secretin are to stimulate pancreatic bicarbonate secretion and to potentiate CCK-stimulated pancreatic enzyme secretion. The numerous other physiological actions of secretin may only be pharmacological in nature and may relate to similarities in structure to glucagon, VIP, and GIP, the other members of the secretin family of hormones.

Cholecystokinin (CCK)

The presence of a hormone in the duodenal mucosa which is liberated by food (particularly FFA's) and causes contraction and emptying of the gallbladder was discovered by Ivy and Oldberg in 1928 and named *cholecystokinin* (CCK). Another hormone from the same source which stimulated the release of pancreatic enzymes and also contracted the gallbladder was named *pancreozymin* (PZ). It was subsequently established that CCK and PZ were the same hormone. Although this hormone is often referred to as CCK-PZ, CCK is the more common designation [30]. CCK is a polypeptide hormone of 33 amino acid residues, but the peptide also exists in a larger form of 39 amino acids in length. The carboxy-terminal five amino acids of CCK are identical to those in gastrin (Fig. 10.1). The seventh amino acid from the carboxy-terminus is sulfated, which is necessary for the normal physiological activity of the molecule. The shorter C-terminal decapeptide portion of the CCK molecule is actually more than 10 times as potent as the intact hormone.

Cholecystokinin is immunocytochemically localized to the I cells of the duodenal, jejunal, and ileal mucosa. Cholecystokinin is released by L-isomers of amino acids, hydrochloric acid, and certain fatty acids. Entry of high levels of hydrogen ion into the duodenum results in gallbladder contraction, a specific biological response attributed to circulating CCK. The other recognized physiological roles of CCK are stimulation of pancreatic enzyme secretion, inhibition of gastric emptying, and potentiation of secretin-induced pancreatic bicarbonate secretion. CCK also appears to be a physiological regulator of the growth of the exocrine pancreas. Although the peptide shares structural similarity with gastrin, which has a trophic growth effect on the gastrointestinal mucosa, CCK is without such an effect. Most exciting is the discovery that CCK, or related peptide, may function as a satiety hormone (Chapter 21) [29]. A CCK-related peptide is also present within the brain where it may subserve a number of physiological functions as a neuroregulator.

Gastric Inhibitory Peptide (GIP)

As early as 1886 it was demonstrated that the presence of fats in a meal inhibited gastric emptying in humans. Fat ingestion was later shown to inhibit gastric acid secretion. Crude intestinal extracts duplicated the actions of fat on gastric acid secretion and motility. The active principle was referred to as *enterogastrone*. Although a number of gut hormones exhibit enterogastronelike activity, only one, gastric inhibitory peptide (GIP), is considered to play such a physiological role [19]. This 43-amino acid peptide, which bears structural similarity to other members of the secretin family of hormones (Fig. 10.3), is localized to certain K cells of the duodenum and jejunum of humans and dogs [4].

In addition to its inhibitory effects on gastric acid secretion GIP is insulinotropic, potentiating insulin release in response to an intravenous infusion of glucose, a response which in humans improves glucose tolerance. GIP has therefore been referred to as the glucose-dependent insulinotropic peptide. Oral glucose ingestion in humans produces a sustained increase in serum GIP levels capable of stimulating insulin release. Indeed, glucose ingestion induces a greater insulin release than intravenous administration of the same amount of glucose. The insulinotropic action of GIP appears to be specifically dependent on concomitant glucose administration as fat ingestion increases serum GIP levels but not serum insulin concentrations [28]. Like glucagon and VIP, GIP is a potent stimulator of intestinal juice from the duodenal glands of Brunner (Brunner's glands, located in the vicinity of the pyloric sphincter), but this may not be a physiological function of the hormone.

Vasoactive Intestinal Peptide (VIP)

This peptide, first isolated from the pig intestine, contains 28 amino acid residues and is structurally related to secretin, glucagon, and GIP [31, 37]. Immunohistochemical studies reveal that the peptide is diffusely distributed throughout the entire length of the mammalian and avian intestinal tract (esophagus through the colon). The greatest number of VIP-immunoreactive cells are found in the small intestine, particularly the jejunum, ileum, and also in the colon. VIP was named for its potent vasodilator and hypotensive effects [37]. It relaxes a variety of smooth muscles and antagonizes the effects of smooth muscle constrictor agents. VIP inhibits histamine and pentagastrin-stimulated gastric acid secretion. Electrolyte and water secretion by the pancreas are

Physiological Roles of the Gastrointestinal Hormones

stimulated and bile flow is increased. VIP stimulates lipolysis, glycogenolysis, and insulin secretion, but because these actions are shared by some other members of the secretin family of hormones, these observed effects of VIP may be pharmacological rather than physiological in nature. In addition the presence of this peptide in nerve cells (Chapter 21) and the absence of a meal-induced change in VIP plasma concentrations further argue against its role as a humoral gastroenteropancreatic hormone. The selective localization of VIP within neurons in the CNS and autonomic nervous system, especially in the superior and inferior mesenteric ganglia, the submucosal (Meissner's) and myenteric (Auerbach's) plexuses of the intestinal wall, the cerebrovascular nerves, and nerves in the female and male genito-urinary tracts, suggests that its role may be restricted to that of a neurohormone acting by a neurocrine or paracrine mechanism in a variety of organs including the GI tract (Fig. 10.7).

Substance P (SP)

Stimulation of the abdominal vagal nerve releases a substance whose actions on smooth muscle motor activity are not blocked by atropine. This substance therefore is not acetylcholine. This peptide consists of 11 amino acid residues (Table 10.3) and

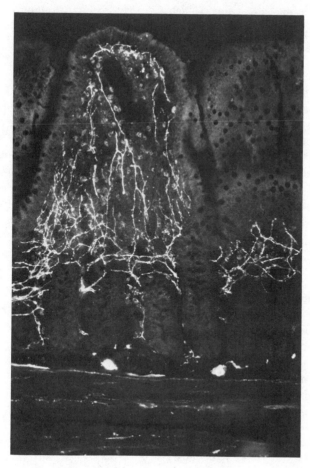

Figure 10.7 Immunoreactive VIP nerve plexus in small intestine of the rat. (Reprinted with permission from T. Hökfelt, R. Elde, O. Johansson, A. Ljungdahl, M. Schulzberg, K. Fuxe, M. Goldstein, G. Nilsson, B. Pernow, L. Terenius, D. Ganten, S. L. Jeffcoate, J. Rehfeld, and S. I. Said. 1978. [17] Distribution of peptide-containing neurons. In: *Psychopharmacology: a generation of progress*, M. A. Lipton, A. DiMascio and K. F. Killam (eds.), pp. 39–66. New York: Raven Press.

is called substance P (SP) in reference to an early preparation of active gut extract [46]. This was the first neuropeptide to be found both in the brain and gut. SP is found localized within nerve fibers in all areas of the gut wall, including the two muscle layers, the myenteric and submucosal plexuses, the mucosa, and the submucosa. Substance P is also distributed widely but selectively within the brain and spinal column; it is structurally related to a number of peptides present within the skins of anuran amphibians (Fig. 21.8).

Somatostatin

This tetradecapeptide (Table 10.3), referred to as somatostatin to describe its putative role as an STH release-inhibiting hormone, is also localized to specialized D cells of the gastrointestinal mucosa. Highest concentrations of this peptide are localized to the gastric antrum with progressively decreasing levels found within the small intestine and colon. Somatostatin-producing cells have long cytoplasmic processes that terminate on other cell types (Fig. 10.8), including the gastrin-producing and hydrochloric acid-producing cells [25]. The release of gastrin and hydrochloric acid, re-

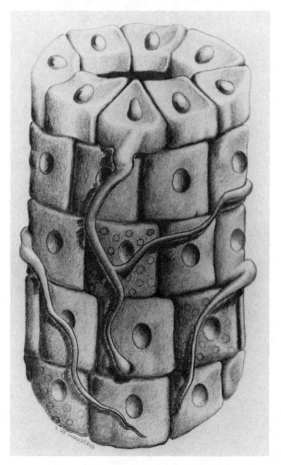

Figure 10.8 Schematic drawing showing a three-dimensional arrangement of the somatostatin cells and their processes in an antral gland. (From Larsson, et al., [25], with permission. *Science* 205:1393–94, 1979. Copyright 1979 by the American Association for the Advancement of Science.)

Physiological Roles of the Gastrointestinal Hormones

spectively, from these cells is inhibited by somatostatin. It is believed that somatostatin cells control the functions of these cells through the local release of the peptide via cytoplasmic processes. This may represent a paracrine mechanism of control. Somatostatin is also localized to D cells of the pancreatic islets and may regulate glucagon and insulin secretion (Chapter 11). The observation that long processes may emanate from other endocrine cells of the gut epithelium suggests that other GI hormones may function by a paracrine mode of control [25].

Gastrin-Releasing Peptide

Bombesin is a tetrapeptide originally isolated from frog skin. Bombesinlike immunoreactivity was subsequently localized to both the mammalian brain and GI tract. Bombesin was shown to act within the brain to inhibit gastric acid secretion in the stomach. Recently a 27-amino acid gastrin-releasing peptide (GRP) was isolated from the porcine gut which has a C-terminal decapeptide sequence identical to the C-terminal decapeptide of frog skin bombesin except for a Gln/His interchange at position 7 (Fig. 10.9) [27]. The C-terminal octapeptide fragment of GRP retains full biological activity as does the C-terminal bombesin octapeptide, suggesting that the previously demonstrated effects of bombesin in the mammal are mediated through a GRP receptor. Gastrointestinal GRP activity appears to be in structures other than endocrine cells; the peptide may be localized to intrinsic neurons of the gut. GRP can therefore be added to the growing list of peptides (substance P, neurotensin, CCK, VIP, somatostatin, endorphins) that are present in endocrine cells and in central and peripheral neurons.

Because GRP and bombesin are structurally related and exhibit similar biological activities, it is likely that GRP is the mammalian equivalent of bombesin [44]. The bombesinlike activity found in the mammalian brain is due likely to GRP. In the brain GRP may subserve a role in the CNS regulation of gastric acid secretion (Chapter 21). Does GRP of gastrointestinal tract origin perform a similar function? Synthetic porcine GRP is a potent stimulus to gastrin release when injected intracisternally but much less potent when injected intravenously. Thus, it might be inferred that GRP acts on some as yet undetermined CNS site to inhibit gastric acid secretion. It is possible that the stimulus to gastrin release is indirect and is in response to an elevated pH, resulting from diminished gastric acid secretion.

Motilin

Motilin is a candidate peptide hormone containing 22 amino acid residues (Table 10.3), which bears no structural similarity to any other known GI hormone [15]. Al-

Bombesin
```
 1    2    3    4    5    6    7    8    9   10   11   12   13   14
pGlu-Gln-Arg-Leu-Gly-Asn-Gln-Trp-Ala-Val-Gly-His-Leu-Met-NH2
```

Gastrin-Releasing Peptide
```
 1    2    3    4    5    6    7    8    9   10   11   12   13   14   15   16   17   18   19   20   21   22   23   24   25   26   27
Ala-Pro-Val-Ser-Val-Gly-Gly-Gly-Thr-Val-Leu-Ala-Lys-Met-Tyr-Pro-Arg-Gly-Asn-His-Trp-Ala-Val-Gly-His-Leu-Met-NH2
```

Figure 10.9 Primary structures of bombesin and porcine gastrin releasing peptide (GRP).

though motilin was believed to be localized to certain enterochromaffin (EC_2) cells, it is now believed to be confined to a population of nonenterochromaffin cells of unclarified nature distributed mainly throughout the duodenum and jejunum. The peptide was named for its ability to stimulate gastric motor activity. The potent actions of motilin on gastrointestinal motility and emptying of chyme into the small intestine suggest a possible physiological role for the peptide. The stimulus for secretion of motilin remains unclear but may be in response to duodenal alkalinization.

Other Putative GI Hormones

A number of other biologically active peptides are also distributed throughout the gastrointestinal mucosa. They too, in a sense, can be considered candidate hormones. Considering the size of the GI tract, it is not surprising that a great number of hormones are distributed throughout this complex organ.

Chymodenin. This biologically active peptide was isolated from porcine duodenal extracts and has a molecular weight of about 5000 [1, 2]. Its primary structure has not been determined. Chymodenin stimulates the release of pancreatic juice rich in chymotrypsin without much effect on the output of the other pancreatic enzymes. Enzyme-specific secretion is produced by chymodenin both in situ and in vitro, demonstrating the direct action of the peptide on the pancreas. This unique action of chymodenin shows that the secretion of individual pancreatic enzymes could be controlled by specific hormonal substances. Because the digestive enzymes are considered to be packaged together in granules (zymogen) within secretory cells, it is not clear how hormonal stimuli could effect the release of one particular enzyme from the constellation of enzymes present within the granules of the pancreatic acinar cells. A heterogeneous population of acinar cells, each specializing in the release of a particular enzyme, could account for such a specific enzyme secretory response. There is, however, no evidence to support such a hypothesis.

Bulbogastrone. Acidification of the duodenal bulb (area of duodenum just beyond the pylorus) inhibits the gastric acid secretion response to a test meal in certain experimental animals. This secretory response derives specifically from the duodenal bulb because acid perfusion of the postbulbar duodenum has much less effect on gastric acid secretion. Acidification of bulbar pouches reduces effectively acid secretion from vagally innervated and vagally denervated gastric pouches, suggesting that inhibition of gastric acid secretion is not mediated by a vagal pathway. Intramural (within the intestinal wall) reflex routes are also not involved as transection of the pylorus does not abolish the inhibition of acid secretion stimulated by duodenal acidification. The existence of a humoral agent mediating inhibition of gastric secretion is further supported by the observation that extracts of the duodenal bulb inhibit acid secretion. These extracts do not exhibit activities of the other GI hormones; because relatively large doses of secretin and CCK are required to inhibit gastric acid secretion, secretin and CCK may be ruled out as the humoral messengers involved in the response. Bulbogastrone, the name given to this hypothetical factor, interferes with the stimulatory action of gastrin but not acetylcholine on the oxyntic glands. Thus bulbogastrone, with secretin and GIP, may provide an additional mechanism of regulating gastric acid secretion (Fig. 10.5). The chemical nature and cellular localization of this putative humoral factor is undetermined.

Urogastrone. Pregnancy causes an improvement in the symptoms of duodenal ulceration. Extracts of urine from pregnant and nonpregnant women as well as those from men afford protection against experimentally induced ulceration in dogs. These extracts cause inhibition of gastric acid secretion and also promote fibroblastic proliferation and epithelization of the mucosa. Purification of urine led to the isolation of two fractions, the *beta* and *gamma* urogastrones, which had different physical properties but the same biological potency. The structure of β-urogastrone consists of a single polypeptide chain of 53 residues with three internal disulfide bonds, whereas γ-urogastrone lacks the C-terminal arginine residue. Although urogastrone is structurally different from other known gastrointestinal peptides, it is strikingly similar to mouse epidermal growth factor, EGF (Fig. 10.10). Mouse EGF (Fig. 12.5) is a powerful epithelial mitogen and urogastrone is equipotent in activity; both peptides are also equally potent in suppressing gastric acid secretion in a number of animals. At present urogastrone is considered the human hormonal equivalent of mEGF [13].

Immunochemical studies have localized urogastronelike material to the submaxillary glands, to Brunner's glands of the small intestine, and to saliva and gastric juice. Studies in ulcer patients confirmed the ability of urogastrone to suppress basal gastric acid secretion, and acid secretion in response to pentagastrin could also be partially blocked. The action of the peptide is specific as salivary, pancreatic, and bile secretions are not affected similarly by any doses of the peptide. Mouse EGF has a trophic effect on the oxyntic gland mucosa, but, unlike the effects of gastrin, has no such trophic effects on duodenal or colonic mucosa. Secretin inhibits the trophic effects of pentagastrin on the oxyntic mucosa but not that of mEGF; the

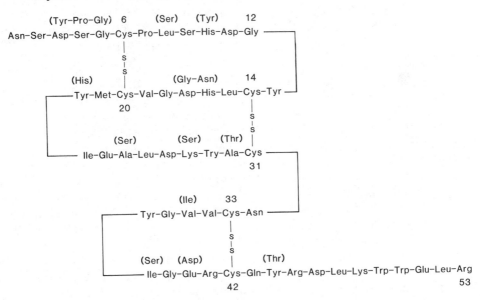

Figure 10.10 Amino acid sequence of human β-urogastrone. Positional amino acid differences between β-urogastrone and mouse EGF are shown in parentheses [13].

trophic action of mEGF is thus not mediated through increased serum gastrin levels [21].

Enteroglucagon (Glucagon). The structure and biological actions of pancreatic glucagon are well documented (Chapter 11). In addition glucagonlike substances are present within the gastrointestinal mucosa. Extracts of the pig gastrointestinal mucosa have yielded two polypeptides with glucagonlike activity. One has the same molecular weight (3500) and biological activities as glucagon and may therefore be identical to the pancreatic hormone. Cells indistinguishable from pancreatic A cells have been identified in the fundic region of the stomach in dogs. On this basis this polypeptide is referred to as *gut glucagon* or *enteroglucagon*. The other polypeptide (2900 MW), which is chemically distinct and has less biological activity than pancreatic glucagon, is referred to as *glucagonlike immunoreactivity* (GLI), or *enteroglucagonoid* [35].

Because enteroglucagon is apparently identical to pancreatic glucagon and enteroglucagonoid has not been obtained in large enough quantities for physiological testing, the possible roles of these biologically active polypeptides are not well defined.

Villikinin. Villi are a characteristic cellular feature of the mucosa of the small intestine. The fingerlike villi exhibit a number of peculiar movements, such as contraction and relaxation and a pendular swaying, and each villus moves independently of its neighbors. It is believed that lymph flow within these structures is hastened by their movements. Villous movement is affected by mechanical and chemical stimuli, nervous stimulation, and extracts of intestinal mucosa. Villous motility of an isolated jejunal loop transplanted into the carotid-jugular circulation was shown to be stimulated by intraduodenal administration of HCl. This observation suggested that villous activity might be regulated by a humoral factor [23]. In cross-circulation experiments involving carotid-jugular anastomoses between two animals administration of HCl into one animal caused a substantial increase in villar activity in both animals. Other experiments provide evidence that acid chyme releases a substance that enters the bloodstream to stimulate villous movement. A substance that stimulates villous motility was extracted from the intestinal mucosa and named villikinin to describe its physiological action. Villikinin activity is found only in mucosa of the small intestine with highest concentrations occurring in the duodenal mucosa of a number of mammalian species, including humans. Villikinin activity increases in human urine after a meal and after intraduodenal acid administration. The substance does not exhibit actions characteristic of the other GI hormones, therefore ruling any of them out as the putative humoral messenger. Villikinin appears to be a polypeptide but little is known about its chemistry.

Enkephalins. Endorphins, the so-called opiate peptides, which include the enkephalins and β-endorphin, play important roles in CNS function (Chapter 21). Opiate receptors and enkephalins have been demonstrated in the endocrinelike cells and nerves of the digestive tract [33]. Opiate drugs, well known for their powerful actions on the gastrointestinal tract, exhibit pronounced effects on gastrointestinal motility and secretion. The opiate peptides also profoundly affect activity of the GI tract, presumably by identical mechanisms as the opiate drugs. They act as presynaptic or postsynaptic inhibitors and suppress the firing of most neurons tested. For example, opiate peptides specifically inhibit electrically induced contractions of the ileal smooth muscle by inhibiting neurotransmitter (acetylcholine) release. Opiate peptides are potent inhibitors of bicarbonate and protein secretion from the pancreas, suggesting that they affect the secretory mechanisms common to CCK and secretin on pancreatic secretion. Because opiates are known to suppress the release of acetylcholine in every tissue tested the action of opiate peptides on pancreatic secretion may be attributed to inhibition of cholinergic activity that may also be involved in the action of the secretin and CCK on pancreatic bicarbonate and enzyme secretion. One may conclude that the major roles of endorphins in the GI tract are to act as neuromodulators of autonomic nervous system actions on gastrointestinal motility and secretion.

Neurotensin.   The tridecapeptide neurotensin (NT) was discovered and isolated from the bovine hypothalamus and subsequently found by radioimmunoassay to be also present in the gastrointestinal tract (Table 10.3). Neurotensin (or a neuro-tensinlike peptide) is present in discrete (N) cells rather specifically localized in the ileal mucosa of various birds and mammals. The NT-immunoreactive cells are situated in the upper two-thirds of the villi and appear to communicate with the intestinal lumen by means of microvilli. The neurotensin cells are distinct from the argentaffin cells of the gut. The morphological features of the NT-containing cells, which have microvilli and secretory granules located at the vascular pole, suggest that they may be sensitive to changes in the gut lumen. This sensitivity may provide the stimulus for the release of the peptide into the circulation [33]. The possible function of neuro-tensin in gastrointestinal function is unknown.

AUTONOMIC NERVOUS SYSTEM CONTROL OF GI FUNCTION

Although hormones play a dominant role in the control of gastrointestinal function, the autonomic nervous system subserves a similar function. "Acting singly and in concert, neural and hormonal mechanisms control the transverse flow of materials across the mucosa and the axial flow of digesta within the lumen" [26]. In addition, "The overlap of neural and endocrine segments, and the continuously changing character and location of intraluminal stimuli, engender the simultaneous release of several hormones whose interplay on digestive target tissues may be augmentatory or inhibitory. The fusion of their effects determines the orderly progress and digestion of food."

The initial phase of neural control of gastrointestinal function is regulated centrally by the anticipation of food, the so-called cephalic phase. Subsequently local neural and hormonal mechanisms are activated within the GI tract by mechanical and chemical stimuli derived from ingested food substrates. The stomach and small intestine are richly innervated by intrinsic and extrinsic nerves [11]. The intrinsic nerves comprise various plexuses that lie between the longitudinal and circular smooth muscle layers of the gut (Auerbach's plexus) and beneath the submucosal muscle layer (Meissner's plexus). These plexuses are innervated by extrinsic nerves derived mainly from the vagus nerve. Axons from neurons within the plexuses synapse with muscle fibers and glandular elements of the gut. Parasympathetic cholinergic (acetylcholine) and sympathetic adrenergic (norepinephrine) neurons affect smooth muscle motor activity and mucosal glandular secretion. Acetylcholine, for example, is a potent stimulus to gastric acid secretion. The intrinsic neurons of the gut contain a number of neurohormones such as VIP, substance P, and somatostatin.

GASTROINTESTINAL HORMONE MECHANISMS OF ACTION

Like other peptide hormones, the GI hormones interact with cell membrane receptors to stimulate or inhibit cyclic nucleotide production. Members of the secretin family (secretin, glucagon, VIP, and GIP) of hormones activate adenylate cyclase, which results in an elevation of intracellular levels of target tissue cyclic AMP. Smooth muscles of the GI tract contract or relax in response to GI hormones. As for other smooth muscle of the respiratory tract or the genito-urinary tract, muscle contraction is correlated with intracellular increases in cyclic GMP; muscle relaxation is correlated with intracellular elevations of cyclic AMP (Chapter 14). Stimulation of gastrointestinal secretions (e.g., HCl, pepsinogen, secretion from Brunner's glands) is, as for most secretory processes, regulated by intracellular increases in cyclic AMP. Although gastrin is a potent secretogogue of gastric acid secretion, acetylcholine and histamine are also stimulatory to gastrin secretion. The cholinergic neural pathways involved in gastrin and HCl secretion are unresolved. Histamine (Fig. 6.11) is present in large amounts in the oxyntic mucosa of humans and other mammals [42]. The cellular source of histamine in the gastric mucosa is not known. In addition to gastrin and acetylcholine receptors parietal cells possess histamine (H_2) receptors. The actions of histamine are mediated through cAMP. Although gastrin and acetylcholine also stimulate parietal cell HCl secretion and potentiate the actions of each other and histamine, their actions do not involve cAMP [10].

Pancreatic acinar cells possess two distinct classes of receptors coupled to different membrane nucleotide cyclases. cAMP and cGMP mechanisms may be involved in the process of acinar cell enzyme secretion [10]. Secretin (and VIP in some species) elevates pancreatic cAMP levels and stimulates amylase secretion. Cholecystokinin (and related structures) also stimulates pancreatic amylase secretion and appears to do so by mobilizing cellular calcium and elevating cGMP. Because the release of cellular Ca^{2+} precedes the elevation in cGMP, it is possible that the Ca^{2+} is stimulatory to guanylate cyclase activity and cGMP production. Secretogogues that increase Ca^{2+} efflux and cyclic AMP also cause depolarization of acinar cells. Acinar cells within the same acinus are electrically coupled; this coupling may provide a mechanism for amplifying the response of acinar cells to low concentrations of secretogogues. The potentiation of the action of CCK by secretin on acinar enzyme secretion may result because the mechanism of action of each secretogogue is different and not funneled through one cyclic nucleotide (Fig. 10.11). Because CCK potentiates the action of secretin on bicarbonate release by pancreatic ductule cells, a similar mechanism of action involving cAMP and cGMP may be involved in pancreatic fluid secretion (Fig. 10.11).

The mucosal gastrin receptor has been characterized [45]. Specific gastrin binding is present in the oxyntic gland and duodenal mucosa but is absent from the antral mucosa, liver, spleen, and kidney. Fasting decreases the circulating level of gastrin

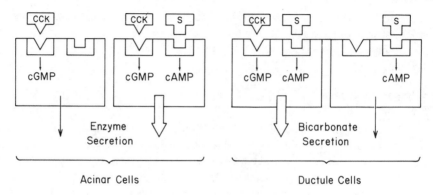

Figure 10.11 Hypothetical model for the role of CCK and secretin (S) and cyclic nucleotides on pancreatic enzyme and bicarbonate secretion.

and the number of gastrin binding sites, whereas refeeding increases the plasma gastrin levels and restores the receptor number to normal. Treatment of fasted animals with pentagastrin prevents the decrease in receptor number. Thus, gastric mucosal receptors are autoregulated, that is, their number is influenced by the availability of gastrin; they exhibit up-regulation in response to the hormone (Chapter 4).

Gastrin stimulates RNA, DNA, and protein synthesis along the entire length of the gut with the exception of the esophagus and antrum. The pancreas is also a target for the trophic action of gastrin. These trophic effects are direct actions of gastrin and are not mediated through the action of another hormone. These observations suggest that increased food intake increases circulating levels of gastrin which then increase gastrointestinal receptor numbers. This allows an enhanced trophic response to the hormone, which enables the GI tract to utilize better the increased metabolic substrates available [20, 22].

SUMMARY OF THE NEUROENDOCRINE CONTROL OF GI FUNCTION

A summary of what is known about the role of GI hormones in gastrointestinal tract function is provided (Table 10.4). Food is taken into the mouth where ptyalin (salivary α-amylase) initiates digestion of starch. Food in the mouth is responsible for a reflex (cephalic) stimulation of gastric acid secretion. The food then transverses the esophagus to enter into the stomach through the gastroesophageal junction. Local reflex stimuli, resulting from distension of the stomach and from partially digested food products, particularly peptides and amino acids, are stimulatory to gastric acid secretion. Gastrin is the major humoral stimulus to hydrochloric acid secretion from the parietal cells of the gastric mucosa. Gastrin is also indirectly stimulatory to pepsinogen secretion from the chief cells of the mucosa of the body of the stomach. The pepsinogen is acted upon by HCl and split into the active enzyme, pepsin. Increased gastric acid secretion then becomes inhibitory to further gastrin secretion. Gastrin and local reflex stimulation may then relax the pyloric sphincter and allow a bolus of food (chyme) to enter the first segment of the small intestine, the duodenum. The acid present in the chyme is stimulatory to secretin release from cells present within the duodenal mucosa. This bloodborne messenger then travels to the exocrine pancreas to cause water and bicarbonate release. These secretory products neutralize the acid present within the small intestine. Fats and proteins in the chyme stimulate the secretion of CCK from cells within the duodenal, jejunal, and ileal mucosa. CCK is carried by the blood to the exocrine pancreas and stimulates the acinar cells to release pancreatic enzymes: α-amylase, trypsin, chymotrypsin, and pancreatic lipase. Proteases split proteins and partially degraded proteins into their constituent amino acids. CCK also contracts the gallbladder, thus releasing bile salts into the intestinal lumen. These salts emulsify the fats into smaller globules and the fats are enzymatically degraded by pancreatic lipase into FFA's and monoglycerides. Starch and its partially degraded components, oligopolysaccharides, are further degraded by pancreatic α-amylase into glucose. Glucose is stimulatory to GIP secretion and possibly enteroglucagon secretion from cells of the intestinal mucosa. These humoral messengers may then stimulate the release of insulin from beta cells of the pancreatic islets. By the action of insulin on the liver, the glucose now within the portal vein is taken up into the liver cells where it may be formed into starch and stored (Fig. 10.12).

GIP and possibly other hormones (bulbogastrone) of the small intestine, released in response to gastric acid, glucose, fats, and protein products, may provide feedback to the stomach to inhibit further secretion of gastric acid. Certain intrinsic neurons and other neuronlike cells within the intestinal lining contain peptide hormones such as somatostatin, VIP, substance P, and others. These neuropeptides acting by neurocrine or paracrine mechanisms control local secretory events and smooth muscle activity. The autonomic nervous system, particularly through its cholinergic component, plays an equally important augmentary role in the movement and digestion of foods within the GI tract [40].

PATHOPHYSIOLOGY

There are two well-documented examples of direct involvement by gastrointestinal hormones in abnormal clinical conditions. Most endocrine tumors of the gastrointestinal system originate in the pancreatic islets. Although these tumors secrete hormones that are normally produced there (e.g., glucagon and insulin), these tumors may also secrete VIP or gastrin. Vasoactive intestinal peptide stimulates intestinal water secretion, and tumors consisting of VIP-secreting cells (VIPomas) are responsible for *pancreatic cholera* or the *watery diarrhea syndrome*. Patients with the Zollinger-Ellison syndrome (gastrinoma) have high circulating gastrin levels of tumor origin. The overproduction of gastric acid usually results in severe duodenal ulcer formation.

Regulation of the lower esophageal sphincter (LES), which is important in preventing the reflux of gastric contents, may be regulated by one or more GI hormones. Gastrin and motilin can contract the LES, whereas VIP is particularly potent as an inhibitor of LES tone. *Achalasia* is a condition where food accumulates in the esophagus because the gastroesophageal junction fails to relax. There is evidence that the smooth muscle of this junction is hypersensitive to normal circulating levels of gastrin, which could account for the prolonged contraction characteristic of this condition.

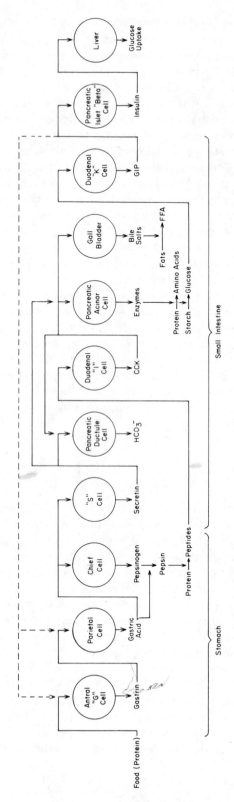

Figure 10.12 Summary scheme of hormone-metabolite control of GI function. Solid lines indicate stimulatory influences, dashed lines represent inhibitory stimuli.

Gastroesophageal reflux, on the other hand, is due to abnormal relaxation of the sphincter, and it is claimed that in some patients with this condition gastrin levels are low. The available data, however, are controversial [39].

GIP-containing cells are reported to be most numerous in duodenal samples from patients with low gastric secretory activity and less numerous in patients with duodenal ulcer disease. These observations correlate well with the proposed role of this hormone in the inhibition of gastric acid secretion. Two different types of the Zollinger-Ellison syndrome may exist, one (type I) which is due to a hyperplasia of the antral G cells and one (type II) due to gastrinoma of the pancreatic islets. There is evidence for antral G-cell hyperplasia in certain patients having hypergastrinemia without gastrinoma.

A number of GI hormones have proven useful in clinical practice [39]. Gastrin is used for testing the potential for gastric acid secretion. Pentagastrin, which is commercially relatively inexpensive, is usually used in these studies. CCK is used in the evaluation of gallbladder function; this hormone is also used to test for pancreatic exocrine function. Secretin has been used in the treatment of duodenal ulcer because it is inhibitory to gastric acid secretion and stimulatory to pancreatic bicarbonate ion secretion. Secretin and glucagon stimulate tumor gastrin release (in contrast to their inhibitory effects on antral release of the hormone) and are used in the diagnosis of the Zollinger-Ellison syndrome.

EVOLUTIONARY RELATIONSHIPS OF THE GUT HORMONES

The gut hormones are localized to specific cells distributed throughout the GI tract. Most interesting, however, is that many of the gut hormones are also found in a variety of other tissues, including the pancreas, pituitary, in neurons of the central and peripheral nervous systems, and in the skin of some vertebrates [38]. Within each of these tissues they regulate specific functions. In the hypothalamus of the brain somatostatin regulates pituitary release of growth hormone; in the pancreas this peptide may regulate insulin and glucagon secretion and in the antrum of the stomach somatostatin apparently regulates gastrin secretion.

The skin of anuran amphibians contains a number of biologically active peptides. Two of these peptides from related species of frogs, cerulein and phyllocerulein (Fig. 10.13), contain the C-terminal pentapeptide sequence found in gastrin and CCK

Gastrin$_{(17)}$ (pyro)Glu-Gly-Pro-Trp-Leu-Glu-Glu-Glu-Glu-Glu-Ala-Tyr(SO_3H)-Gly-Trp-Met-Asp-Phe·NH$_2$

CCK$_{(17-33)}$ -Asp-Pro-Ser-His-Arg-Ile-Ser-Asp-Arg-Asp-Tyr(SO_3H)-Met-Gly-Trp-Met-Asp-Phe·NH$_2$

Cerulein   (pyro)Glu-Gln-Asp-Tyr(SO_3H)-Thr-Gly-Trp-Met-Asp-Phe·NH$_2$

Phyllocerulein   (pyro)Glu-Glu-Tyr(SO_3H)-Thr-Gly-Trp-Met-Asp-Phe·NH$_2$

Figure 10.13 CCK-gastrin family of peptides.

[6, 7]. A peptide containing the C-terminal octapeptide of CCK has been found within the brain of sheep. These structurally related peptides would be expected to have been derived from a common ancestral molecule by gene duplication and divergence. A CCK-related peptide has been found in the brain and gut of cyclostomes and representatives of the agnathans, the oldest of the vertebrates. Immunoreactive gastrin has even been discovered in gut extracts of certain molluscan species [34, 43] and also in ganglia of an insect [24]. Other hormones of the gut and brain are also related to peptides found in the skin of amphibians and in glands of mollusks [9].

Members of the secretin family of peptides are similar in structure, again suggesting that they are related by a common ancestry. The genes that coded for the ancestral member of this group of peptides probably underwent duplication, thus producing one or more daughter genes. These genes, through independent mutations, diverged to yield distinct but related peptide hormones (Fig. 21.12).

REFERENCES

[1] ADELSON, J. W., and S. S. ROTHMAN. 1974. Selective pancreatic enzyme secretion due to a new peptide called chymodenin. *Science* 183:1087–89.

[2] ADELSON, J. W. 1975. Chymodenin, a duodenal peptide: specific stimulation of chymotrypsinogen secretion. *Amer. J. Physiol.* 229:1680–85.

[3] BAYLISS, W. M., and E. H. STARLING. 1902. The mechanism of pancreatic secretion. *J. Physiol.* 28:325–53.

[4] BROWN, J. C., J. R. DRYBURGH, S. A. ROSS, and J. DUPRE. 1975. Identification and actions of gastric inhibitory polypeptide. *Rec. Prog. Horm. Res.* 31:487–532.

[5] DEMBINSKI, A. B., and L. R. JOHNSON. 1979. Growth of pancreas and gastrointestinal mucosa in antrectomized and gastrin-treated rats. *Endocrinology* 105:769–73.

[6] DOCKRAY, G. J. 1979a. Evolutionary relationships of the gut hormones. *Fed. Proc.* 38: 2295–2301.

[7] DOCKRAY, G. J. 1979b. Comparative biochemistry and physiology of gut hormones. *Ann. Rev. Physiol.* 41:83–95.

[8] DOMSCHKE, W., G. LUX, and S. DOMSCHKE. 1980. Growth hormone secretion and pentagastrin. *New Engl. J. Med.* 303:458.

[9] FALKMER, S., R. E. CARRAWAY, M. EL-SALHY, S. O. EMDIN, L. GRIMELIUS, J. F. REHFELD, M. REINECKE, and T. W. SCHWARTZ. 1981. Phylogeny of the gastroenteropancreatic neuroendocrine system: a review. In *Cellular basis of chemical messengers in the digestive system*, eds. M. I. Grossman, M. A. B. Brazier, and J. Lechago, pp. 21–42. New York: Academic Press, Inc.

[10] GARDNER, J. D. 1980. Regulation of pancreatic exocrine function in vitro: initial steps in the actions of secretogogues. *Ann. Rev. Physiol.* 4:55–66.

[11] GERSHON, M. D. 1981. The enteric nervous system. *Ann. Rev. Neurosci.* 4:227–72.

[12] GLASS, G. B. J., ed. 1980. *Gastrointestinal hormones.* New York: Raven Press.

[13] GREGORY, H. 1980. Urogastrone: isolation, structure, and basic functions. In *Gastrointestinal hormones*, ed. G. B. J. Glass, pp. 397–409. New York: Raven Press.

[14] GROSSMAN, M. I. 1979. Neural and hormonal regulation of gastrointestinal function: an overview. *Ann. Rev. Physiol.* 41:27–33.

[15] GROSSMAN, M. I., J. W. ADELSON, S. S. ROTHMAN, J. C. BROWN, S. I. SAID, T. M. LIN, R. E. CHANCE, E. L. GERRING, H. GREGORY, G. B. J. GLASS, S. ANDERSON, E. S. NASSET, H. SASAKI, G. R. FALOONA, R. H. UNGER, M. CREUTZFELDT, E. KOKAS, and J. C. THOMPSON. 1974. Candidate hormones of the gut. *Gastroenterology* 67:730–55.

[16] GRUBE, D., and W. G. FORSSMANN. 1979. Morphology and function of the entero-endocrine cells. *Horm. Metab. Res.* 11:589–606.

[17] HÖKFELT, T., R. ELDE, O. JOHANSSON, A. LJUNGDAHL, M. SCHULZBERG, K. FUXE, M. GOLDSTEIN, G. NILSSON, B. PERNOW, L. TERENIUS, D. GANTEN, S. L. JEFFCOATE, J. REHFELD, and S. I. SAID. 1978. Distribution of peptide-containing neurons. In *Psychopharmacology: a generation of progress*, eds. M. A. Lipton, A. DiMascio, and K. F. Killam, pp. 39–66. New York: Raven Press.

[18] JOHNSON, L. R., ed. 1977a. *Gastrointestinal physiology*. St. Louis, Mo.: The C. V. Mosby Company.

[19] JOHNSON, L. R., ed. 1977b. Gastrointestinal hormones and their functions. *Ann. Rev. Physiol.* 39:135–58.

[20] JOHNSON, L. R., ed. 1979. Regulation of gastrointestinal mucosal growth. *World J. Surg.* 3:477–87.

[21] JOHNSON, L. R., ed. 1981. Regulation of gastrointestinal growth. In *Physiology of the gastrointestinal tract*, ed. L. R. Johnson, pp. 169–96. New York: Raven Press.

[22] JOHNSON, L. R., and P. D. GUTHRIE. 1980. Stimulation of rat oxyntic gland mucosal growth by epidermal growth factor. *Amer. J. Physiol.* 238:G45–G49.

[23] KOKAS, E., J. J. PISANO, and B. CREPPS. 1980. Villikinin: characterization and function. In *Gastrointestinal hormones*, ed. G. B. J. Glass, pp. 899–910. New York: Raven Press.

[24] KRAMER, K. J., R. D. SPEIRS, and C. N. CHILDS. 1977. Immunochemical evidence for a gastrin-like peptide in insect neuroendocrine system. *Gen. Comp. Endocrinol.* 32:423–26.

[25] LARSSON, L. I., N. GOLTERMANN, L. DE MAGISTRIS, J. F. REHFELD, and T. W. SCHWARTZ. 1979. Somatostatin cell processes or pathways for paracrine secretion. *Science* 205:1393–94.

[26] MAKHLOUF, G. M. 1974. The neuroendocrine design of the gut. *Gastroenterology* 67:159–84.

[27] MCDONALD, T. J., H. JÖRNVALL, G. NILSSON, M. VAGNE, M. GHATIC, S. R. BLOOM and V. MUTT. 1979. Characterization of gastrin releasing peptide from porcine non-antral gastric tissue. *Biochem. Biophys. Res. Commun.* 90:227–33.

[28] MCGUIGAN, J. E. 1978. Gastrointestinal hormones. *Ann. Rev. Med.* 29:307–18.

[29] MORLEY, J. E. 1982. The ascent of cholecystokinin (CCK)-from gut to brain. *Life Sciences* 30:479–93.

[30] MUTT, V. 1980. Cholecystokinin: isolation, structure, and functions. In *Gastrointestinal hormones*, ed. G. B. J. Glass, pp. 169–221. New York: Raven Press.

[31] MUTT, V., and S. I. SAID. 1974. Structure of the porcine vasoactive intestinal octacosapeptide. The amino acid sequence. Use of kallikrein in its determination. *Eur. J. Biochem.* 42:581–89.

[32] PEARSE, A. G. E. 1981. The diffuse neuroendocrine system: falsification and verification of a concept. In *Cellular basis of chemical messengers in the digestive system*, eds. M. I. Grossman, M. A. B. Brazier, and J. Lechago, pp. 13–19. New York: Academic Press, Inc.

[33] POLAK, J. M., and S. R. BLOOM. 1980. Neural and cellular origin of gastrointestinal hormonal peptides in health and disease. In *Gastrointestinal hormones*, ed. G. B. J. Glass, pp. 19–51. New York: Raven Press.

[34] PRICE, D. A., and M. J. GREENBERG. 1977. Structure of a molluscan cardioexcitatory neuropeptide. *Science* 197:670–71.

[35] RAYFORD, P. L., T. A. MILLER, and J. C. THOMPSON. 1976. Secretin, cholecystokinin and newer gastrointestinal hormones. *N. Engl. J. Med.* 295:1093–1101, 1157–64.

[36] REHFELD, J. F. 1979. Gastrointestinal hormones. *Intern. Rev. Physiol.* 19:291–321.

[37] SAID, S. I. 1980a. Vasoactive intestinal peptide (VIP): isolation, distribution, biological actions, structure-function relationships, and possible functions. In *Gastrointestinal hormones*, ed. G. B. J. Glass, pp. 245–73. New York: Raven Press.

[38] SAID, S. I. 1908b. Peptides common to the nervous system and the gastrointestinal tract. *Front. Neuroendocrinol.* 6:293–331.

[39] SAID, S. I., and A. M. ZFASS. 1978. Gastrointestinal hormones. *Disease-A-Month* 24:1–40.

[40] SINGH, M., and P. D. WEBSTER. 1978. Neurohormonal control of pancreatic secretion. *Gastroenterology* 74:294–309.

[41] SOLCIA, E., C. CAPELLA, R. BUFFA, B. FRIGERIO, L. USELLINI, and R. FIOCCA. 1980. Morphological and functional classification of endocrine cells and related growths in the gastrointestinal tract. In *Gastrointestinal hormones*, ed. G. B. J. Glass, pp. 1–17. New York: Raven Press.

[42] SOLL, A. H., and J. H. WALSH. 1979. Regulation of gastric acid secretion. *Ann. Rev. Physiol.* 41:35–53.

[43] STRAUS, E., R. S. YALOW, and H. GAINER. 1975. Molluscan gastrin: concentration and molecular forms. *Science* 190:687–88.

[44] TACHÉ, Y., W. MARKI, J. RIVIER, W. VALE, and M. BROWN. 1981. Central nervous system inhibition of gastric secretion in the rat by gastrin-releasing peptide, a mammalian bombesin. *Gastroenterology* 81:298–302.

[45] TAKEUCHI, K., G. R. SPEIR, and L. R. JOHNSON. 1980. Muscosal gastrin receptor. III. Regulation by gastrin. *Amer. J. Physiol.* 238:G135–G140.

[46] VON EULER, U. S., and J. H. GADDUM. 1931. An unidentified depressor substance in certain tissue extracts. *J. Physiol.* 192:74–87.

11

PANCREATIC HORMONES
AND METABOLIC REGULATION

INTRODUCTION

In 1889 Von Mering and Minkowski noted that total pancreatectomy in dogs resulted in severe and fatal diabetes. Subsequent experimenters using a large variety of animal species observed also that polyuria and glycosuria (characteristic symptoms of diabetes mellitus) and death always followed removal of the pancreas. It was then noted that after ligation of the pancreatic ducts in rabbits the acinar component of the gland atrophied but the islets remained normal; the animals did not become hyperglycemic as they did after total pancreatectomy. From these and other observations, it was concluded that the islets of Langerhans rather than the pancreatic acinar cells are essential in the control of carbohydrate metabolism.

Two mechanisms of control were suggested: The blood was modified while passing through the islet tissue and the islets might produce an internal secretion. Extracts from the ligated pancreas of dogs, which consisted mainly of islet tissue, were shown to reduce blood sugar levels of diabetic dogs. Banting and Best [2] provided convincing evidence that, indeed, the pancreatic islets produced an internal secretion, a hormone, which was responsible for the control of blood glucose levels. In 1926 insulin was obtained in crystalline form and in 1954 Sanger determined the primary structure of this hormone, a discovery which was awarded a Nobel Prize [35]. The physiological roles and chemistry of the other major pancreatic hormone concerned with carbohydrate metabolism, glucagon, have also been elucidated. More recently it has been discovered that the pancreas is the source of other hormones (e.g., somatostatin and pancreatic polypeptide) also concerned with nutrient homeostasis.

The endocrine roles of the pancreas are to maintain a constant blood glucose level and to facilitate cellular storage of foodstuffs following a meal, and to provide for the mobilization of these depot metabolic substrates during periods of fasting. The underproduction or overproduction of insulin or glucagon can therefore profoundly affect the storage and utilization of carbohydrates, fats, and proteins within the liver, adipose tissue, and muscle, thus severely affecting cellular metabolic processes. Of all the described endocrinopathies, diabetes mellitus is by far the most common.

THE ENDOCRINE PANCREAS

The endocrine pancreas, which consists of islets of tissue (Fig. 11.1) dispersed among the much larger mass of the exocrine pancreas, was first described by Langerhans in 1869 in his doctoral dissertation. There are approximately 1 to 2 million islets in a normal human pancreas, but they represent only about 1% to 2% of pancreatic tissue. Two main cell types can be visualized by most histological methods: The α cells are the source of glucagon and the more prevalent β cells are the source of insulin. The following cells are present in much smaller numbers: D cells, the source of pancreatic somatostatin (SS) and F cells, the source of pancreatic polypeptide (PP). Several lines of evidence point to the β cell as the source of insulin. Fluorescent-labeled antibodies

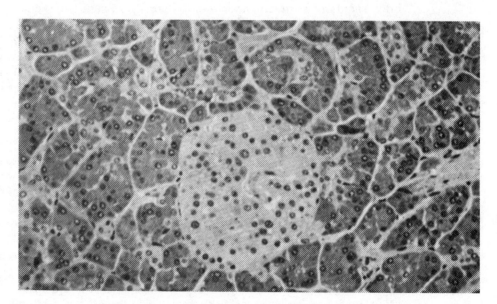

Figure 11.1 Photomicrograph of a human pancreatic islet.

to insulin localize to the β cells, and alloxan, a drug which specifically destroys the β cells, causes diabetes mellitus. In addition stimuli which increase insulin secretion cause β-cell degranulation.

In humans the pancreas arises during the fifth week of gestation from two diverticula of the duodenum close to the hepatic diverticulum. The two primordia then fuse and the duct of the ventral diverticulum becomes the main pancreatic duct leading to the opening into the duodenum. Initially, each primordium consists of a network of anastomosing tubules lined by a single layer of cells. These cells differentiate into the individual acini which constitute the functional units of pancreatic enzyme secretion. It is believed the islet cells derive from the embryonic pancreatic ducts which are endodermal in origin, but it has also been argued that they are derived from the neural ectoderm.

Although much information has accumulated relative to the endocrine role of the pancreatic islets, it is not clear why the pancreatic cells are disseminated in discrete clusters within the exocrine gland in most higher vertebrates. There is evidence, however, that the *peri-insular acini* differ both in their cytological features and secretory activity from the remaining exocrine pancreas. There is also evidence for the preferential release of certain enzymes from the exocrine pancreas in response to certain intragastroduodenal nutrients. It is hypothesized, therefore, that the coordination of particular exocrine gland enzyme secretions may be regulated by hormones deriving from the pancreatic islets. Evidence indicates that acinar amylase mRNA levels progressively decrease in rats rendered diabetic. Insulin reverses this effect in the pancreatic acinar cells by inducing a selective increase in amylase mRNA synthesis [26]. Through a paracrine action on amylase production within adjacent acinar cells, insulin may indirectly control the degradation of starch within the gut and thus control the availability of glucose for absorption into the animal.

Glucose homeostasis involves a push-pull system that controls glucose flux into and out of the extracellular space [42]. By their actions on the liver, adipose tissue, and muscle, insulin and glucagon maintain a balance of glucose production and utilization that requires "a coordinated relationship of the glucagon-producing α cells and the insulin-secreting β cells under the guidance of a perceptive glucose sensor" [43]. The individual insulin cells, glucagon cells, and somatostatin cells are believed to be arranged within the pancreas in such a manner as to accomplish this feat. In humans and rats, the generalized arrangement of the cellular subtypes of the pancreatic islets is demonstrated (Fig. 11.2). Endocrine cells are arranged as cords among the capillary channels within the islets [42, 43]. These plasma membrane specializations are known to permit electrical conductivity between cells as well as the passage of low molecular weight substances from one cell to another. There is evidence that depolarization of one islet cell may lead to the concomitant depolarization of other islet cells. Thus, it is possible that hormone secretion from the pancreatic islets may involve the functional integration of a number of secretory units. It may be significant that the α and D cells contact other cell types, whereas the β cells mainly contact other β cells. The membranes of these three cell types may make close contact with each other by way of tight junctions. Gap junctions have been demonstrated between β cells as well as between α and β cells. The peripheral tricellular zone of the islets is innervated by autonomic afferent nerves and is particularly well vascularized.

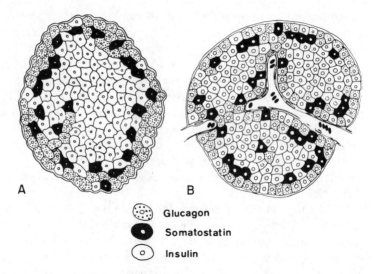

A   B

:o: Glucagon

● Somatostatin

○ Insulin

Figure 11.2 (A) Schematic representation of the number and distribution of insulin-, glucagon-, and somatostatin-containing cells in the normal rat islet. Note the characteristic position of most glucagon- and somatostatin-containing cells at the periphery of the islet, surrounding the centrally located insulin-containing cells. Cell types in the islet for which a characteristic function and morphology is not defined are intentionally omitted. (B) Schematic representation of the number and distribution of insulin-, glucagon-, and somatostatin-containing cells in the normal human islet. Large vascular channels penetrate the islet and are followed by glucagon- and soma-tostatin-containing cells. This pattern divides the total islet mass into smaller sub-units, each of which contains a center formed mainly of insulin cells and surrounded by glucagon and somatostatin cells. Cell types for which a definite function and mor-phology have not been determined are intentionally omitted. (From Unger et al., [42], with permission of Academic Press, New York.)

INTERMEDIARY METABOLISM

In order to appreciate fully the physiological roles of the pancreatic hormones and the consequences of underproduction or overproduction of these hormones, one should review the general outline of carbohydrate metabolism and the relationships of lipid and protein metabolism to glucose production. The consequences of an excess or deficiency of insulin, for example, are hypoglycemia or hyperglycemia, respectively, which result from metabolic defects in glucose metabolism.

As discussed earlier (Chapter 10), the gastrointestinal hormones promote the movement of foodstuffs through the GI tract and provide the chemical environment and enzymes necessary for their degradation into less complex metabolic substrates. These molecular products (e.g., monosaccharides, free fatty acids (FFA's), and amino acids) then traverse the luminal lining of the gut and enter the hepatic portal vein and/or the lymphatic system. Most venous outflow of the abdominal gastrointestinal organs passes through the liver before reaching the hepatic veins to be carried to other parts of the body.

The normal fasting level of glucose in the peripheral venous blood of humans is 60 to 80 mg/dl. The movement of glucose into hepatic cells is by facilitated diffusion in response to the concentration gradient, which results from the intracellular concentration of the monosaccharide. Once within the hepatocyte, glucose may move in a pathway toward glycogen formation (glycogenesis) or it may be catabolized through the glycolytic (Embden-Meyerhoff) pathway to pyruvic acid. An alternate pathway for glucose catabolism which is prominent in certain cells (e.g., adrenal steroidogenic cells) is the *direct oxidative pathway*, or *hexose monophosphate shunt* (HMP). The HMP pathway provides pentoses which are essential components of nucleic acids and nucleotides. This pathway also provides $NADPH_2$ which is important in many reductive biosynthetic processes such as fatty acid and steroid hormone synthesis. Intracellular glucose is first converted to glucose-6-PO_4 by the enzyme *glucokinase* (Fig. 11.3). Depending on the particular hormonal status of the hepatocyte, the glucose-6-PO_4 may be converted to glucose-1-PO_4 by phosphoglucomutase and then combined with uridine diphosphate to form uridine diphosphoglucose (UDPG). Through the action of the enzyme *glycogen synthetase*, the glucose moiety is transferred to already existing glycogen polymers through a glycosidic linkage.

Hormonal stimulation of hepatic *phosphorylase* may subsequently cleave the glycogen polymer into monomeric glucose-1-PO_4 units. The glucose-1-PO_4 produced through *glycogenolysis* is converted to glucose-6-PO_4. The glucose-6-PO_4 can then follow one of two pathways: It may be converted to glucose through the action of glucose-6-phosphatase (an enzyme specific to liver and kidney) and released from the cell or it may be metabolized through a number of enzymatic steps to pyruvic acid.

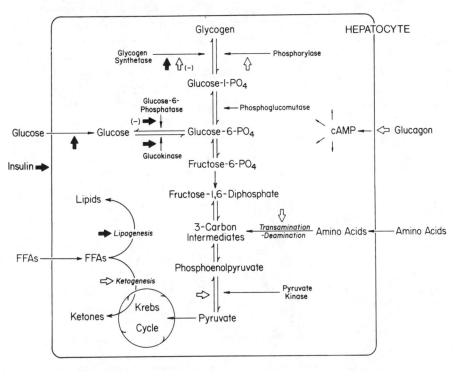

Figure 11.3 General scheme of hormonal regulation of hepatic carbohydrate metabolism. The more prominent actions of insulin (solid arrows) and glucagon (open arrows) are indicated.

Intermediary Metabolism

Pyruvic acid is then converted to acetyl-CoA which can enter into the *Krebs* (*citric acid*) *cycle* or be utilized in fat synthesis (*lipogenesis*).

Glycogen formation and deposition within hepatic cells provides an important storage form of readily utilizable carbohydrate for energy production through the glycolytic pathway and the citric acid cycle. Similar depositions of glycogen are found within skeletal muscle cells and other cells (e.g., sperm cells) that require immediate sources of this substrate for energy production. Hormones play key roles in the conversion of these metabolites into more readily available and utilizable energy substrates.

Molecular interconversion between carbohydrates, proteins, and fats provides the intermediates for utilization within the Embden-Meyerhoff pathway and the citric acid cycle. For example, glycerol derived from the breakdown of fats (lipolysis) can enter the glycolytic pathway; *deamination* of amino acids or *transamination* between certain amino acids and keto acids may provide intermediates, such as pyruvic acid or α-ketoglutaric acid, that can be utilized within the glycolytic pathway or citric acid cycle, respectively (Fig. 11.4). Utilization of noncarbohydrate substrates, such as amino acids, provides a glucose-sparing action, and the molecules may also be employed directly in glucose formation (*gluconeogenesis*).

Free fatty acids (FFA's) absorbed from the gut may be reformed within mucosal cells into monoglycerides, diglycerides, or triglycerides and complexed with phospholipids and proteins within these cells into small micelles referred to as *chylomicrons*. These particles circulate initially within the lymphatic ducts and are then delivered to the blood vascular system. Through the action of the enzyme *lipoprotein lipase* localized within the endothelium of the capillaries, the chylomicrons are cleared from the circulation. The released FFA's are then taken up by adipose cells to be reesterified into triglycerides. Most of the glycerol required for fat synthesis is derived from the glycolytic metabolism of glucose within adipocytes. Within these cells the fats are stored in the form of one or more large fat globules. Through the initial action of *triglyceride lipases* and the subsequent action of diglyceride and monoglyceride

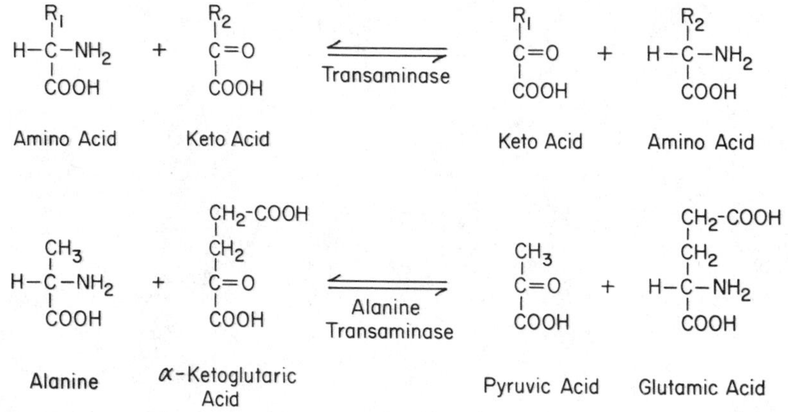

Figure 11.4 General (A) and specific (B) scheme of amino acid-keto acid transamination.

lipases, these fats are converted back to FFA's and glycerol and released into the bloodstream.

Within the liver the glycerol liberated by fat breakdown (lipolysis) within adipocytes is converted to phosphoglyceraldehyde and utilized within the glycolytic pathway by catabolism to pyruvic acid or by conversion through glucogenic processes to glucose. The FFA's are broken down by β-oxidation within mitochondria to acetyl-CoA. The acetyl-CoA is then utilized within the Krebs cycle, another example of a glucose-sparing mechanism. Free fatty acids are also derived de novo from acetyl-CoA through a lipogenic pathway present in many cells. Fatty acid synthesis stops in most cells when the chain is 16 carbon atoms long. Within fat cells the FFA's are combined with glycerol to form neutral fats. Fatty acids are also combined with phosphoric acid and other cellular components to form phospholipids, which may comprise important structural elements of cell membranes or other organelles.

Amino acids derived from the breakdown of proteins within the digestive tract are actively transported across the intestinal mucosal cells and delivered to the liver where they are utilized after deamination or transamination processes in carbohydrate metabolism (Fig. 11.4). They also pass through the liver to the general circulation to be used by other cells as energy substrates, or they can be employed as building blocks in protein synthesis, particularly in muscle cells. The entrance of amino acids into cells involves an active transport mechanism that is stimulated by insulin and other growth hormones.

INSULIN

Insulin is one of a number of hormones that are required for normal growth and development (Chapter 12). In addition it is the only hormone that directly lowers blood glucose levels. Most other hormones, if they have an effect on glucose metabolism, tend to elevate blood levels of the sugar. Knowledge of the chemistry and biological actions of insulin is therefore imperative for an understanding of the normal and abnormal physiology of carbohydrate metabolism.

Synthesis, Chemistry, and Metabolism

Insulin is a polypeptide consisting of an A and B-chain of 21 and 30 amino acids, respectively. The two chains of the dimer are linked through a pair of disulfide bonds; an intrachain disulfide bond connects the sixth and eleventh amino acids within the A chain. There are minor differences in the primary structure of insulin from different vertebrate species. In mammals these differences most often are restricted to the 8, 9, and 10 positions within the intrachain disulfide bond of the A chain and to position 30 of the B chain (Fig. 11.5). Although these differences do not alter considerably the biological potency of the mammalian insulins utilized in replacement therapy for diabetes mellitus, they are sufficient to make insulin antigenic in some patients. Individuals who become resistant to insulin from one species of animal usually respond to insulin from another source.

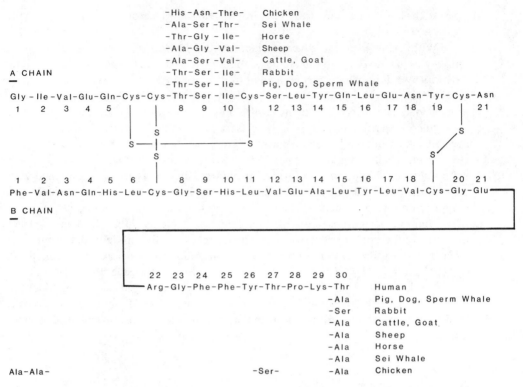

Figure 11.5 Comparative primary structures of the vertebrate insulins.

Insulin is synthesized from a *proinsulin* molecule where the two chains are united by a connecting peptide usually consisting in the human of 31 amino acids not counting the pair of basic residues at the sites of cleavage (Fig. 11.6). Studies on the translation of insulin mRNA have demonstrated that proinsulin is itself derived from a *preproinsulin* precursor [40]. After removal of a C-terminal 23 amino acid sequence, the proinsulin structure folds onto itself to provide disulfide linkages between the two presumptive individual chains. Enzymatic action then cleaves the connecting peptide to yield the definitive hormonal product (Fig. 11.6). Under conditions of excessive stimulation, proinsulin is also secreted by vesicular exocytosis with insulin from the β cells. Because of its slower disappearance rate, proinsulin may constitute up to 50% of the insulinlike material in the blood in the basal state.

Insulin is complexed with zinc within the β cell of the pancreas and in some species in the form of rhombic crystals within the secretory vesicles. Insulin is normally degraded within the liver and kidneys, having a half-life of about 5 minutes in the human. The major enzyme responsible for insulin degradation is *hepatic glutathione insulin dehydrogenase* which disrupts the hormone into its individual A and B chains. The transhydrogenase acts in conjunction with *glutathione*, a cysteine-containing tripeptide, that acts as a cofactor for the transhydrogenase and reduces the individual half-cystine moieties of the interchain disulfide bonds.

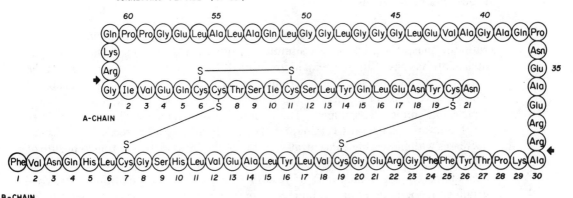

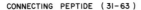

Figure 11.6 Primary structure of porcine proinsulin.

Physiological Roles

In response to elevated glucose levels insulin is promptly released from the pancreatic islets. Insulin interacts with plasmalemmal receptors of a number of different cell types. Most important are the actions of insulin on hepatic cells, muscle cells, and adipose tissue cells. In each case the effect of insulin is to enhance the uptake of glucose into the cells where it is stored as glycogen or used as an energy substrate in the synthesis of proteins or fats.

Within the liver insulin activates glycogen synthetase, which produces a direct flow of glucose toward glycogen formation. Glucokinase activity is enhanced, which provides a pool of glucose-6-PO_4 which is then converted to glucose-1-PO_4 and to uridine diphosphoglucose. Conversion of intracellular glucose to glucose-6-PO_4 prevents glucose release from hepatocytes, and extracellular glucose preferentially moves into these cells in the direction of its concentration gradient (Fig. 11.3).

In fat cells insulin-stimulated glucose uptake results in enhanced catabolism of the sugar to glycerol. Insulin activation of endothelial cell *lipoprotein lipase* results in the release of free fatty acids from chylomicrons. These fatty acids are transported into fat cells where they combine with glycerol to form triglycerides and are added to the lipid droplets within the fat cells.

Insulin stimulates the active transport of glucose and amino acids into muscle cells and, by an unknown mechanism, protein synthesis is enhanced. Glycolysis and oxidative phosphorylation of glucose derivatives provide the energy required for such metabolic activity.

Insulin plays an important role in potassium homeostasis. Insulin is stimulatory to K^+ uptake by cells and at excessively high concentrations causes extracellular hypokalemia. Low levels of insulin appear to have a permissive effect in the cellular uptake of potassium. Infusion of somatostatin, which reduces fasting insulin levels, is associated with an increase in basal serum K^+ concentration in the human.

Mechanisms of Action

Although most peptide hormones mediate their effects through an initial interaction with the plasma membrane to stimulate production of a cyclic nucleotide, the immediate actions of insulin remain unclarified. Insulin receptors are present on the outer plasma membrane of most vertebrate cells studied. The active site of insulin is considered a domain formed by the folding of the A and B chains into a three-dimensional molecular complex. The interaction of insulin with its receptors may involve negative cooperativity (Chapter 4) where the affinity of the receptor for insulin decreases with increasing concentrations of bound hormone. In addition exposure of cells, either in vivo or in vitro, to high concentrations of insulin results in a decrease in the number (down regulation) of insulin receptors. Under conditions of hypo-insulinemia the number of insulin receptors is increased, whereas administration of insulin to normal or diabetic animals decreases the number of binding sites. The full biological effects of insulin are manifested when less than 10% of the total plasma membrane receptors are occupied.

The mechanism of induced down regulation by insulin of its receptors does not occur by the simple acceleration of receptor internalization and degradation. One or more steps subsequent to insulin-receptor interaction are necessary as several agents (insulin "mimics") that do not interact with the insulin receptor per se also decrease the number of insulin binding sites. The effects of these agents are specific for the insulin receptor, and do not affect other receptors possessed by the cells.

There is only meager evidence for a role of a cyclic nucleotide in the cellular actions of insulin. Nevertheless, it has been postulated that insulin may act by decreasing the activity of adenylate cyclase and by stimulating the production of cGMP. In some systems insulin does antagonize the cellular increase in cAMP levels in response to other hormones. However, at present there is no convincing evidence that all or any of the actions of insulin are mediated by cyclic nucleotides as intracellular messengers. It has been suggested, therefore, that insulin action may be mediated by a cyclic nucleotide-independent phosphorylation-dephosphorylation mechanism. Insulin does stimulate phosphorylation of a subunit of its own receptor, and it has been proposed that this event could be a very early step in insulin action. Phosphorylation of the plasmalemmal receptor could act as a direct signal, alter the rate of receptor-hormone internalization, modify the activity of a membrane protease which generates a peptide second messenger, *or* could initiate a cascade of phosphorylation-dephosphorylation reactions that are responsible for the effects of insulin [23, 28].

The observation that insulin (like some growth factors, e.g., NGF) is internalized is of considerable interest. It is suggested that internalization by vesicular endocytosis provides a mechanism for hormone degradation. It has been postulated that ligand-induced internalization of receptors through specialized areas of the plasma membrane is mediated by a *transglutaminase*. The action of this enzyme is hypothesized to involve cross-linking of receptors in the area of the endocytotic pits, thus facilitating aggregation and internalization of the hormone (Fig. 4.17). Transglutaminase may play a role in insulin receptor internalization and subsequent receptor loss [1]. For example, dansylcadaverine, a potent inhibitor of transglutaminase, also inhibits the process of

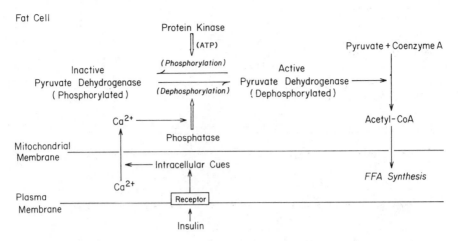

Figure 11.7 Mechanism of insulin activation of the mitochondrial pyruvate dehydrogenase complex.

ligand-induced receptor aggregation and internalization of a number of hormones. This agent effectively inhibits insulin-induced receptor loss in human fibroblasts.

The most sensitive insulin responsive system studied is the *pyruvate dehydrogenase complex* of fat cells [8]. This enzyme complex is localized within mitochondria where its activity is regulated by a cyclic nucleotide-independent phosphorylation-dephosphorylation mechanism. The enzyme is inactivated by a protein kinase in the presence of ATP as phosphate donor. Dephosphorylation by pyruvate dehydrogenase phosphatase converts the complex into an active dephosphorylated form (Fig. 11.7). Activation of the phosphatase may be by an insulin-induced mitochondrial Ca^{2+} influx. Unresolved is the means by which plasma membrane activation by insulin is in turn conveyed to such a distant site within the cell.

A major physiological role of insulin is formation of glycogen from glucose in a number of tissues. Glycogen formation is controlled by the activity of a glycogen synthetase. This enzyme is active in the dephosphorylated state and inactive in the phosphorylated state. Hepatic phosphorylase, the enzyme responsible for activating glycogenolysis, is, on the other hand, activated upon phosphorylation by action of a cyclic AMP-dependent protein kinase (Fig. 11.8). An attractive hypothesis has been that insulin mediates its action by an inhibition of the phosphorylated state of these two enzymes. Nevertheless, in both muscle and liver it has been shown that insulin acts to regulate glycogen synthetase by a mechanism not directly related to tissue cyclic AMP concentration. It has also been suggested, at least in adipose tissue cells, that the glucose-6-PO₄ may bind to glycogen synthetase and, by altering the conformation of the enzyme, make it a better substrate for the action of glycogen synthetase phosphatase. It could be further hypothesized that insulin activation of glucokinase would provide the substrate glucose-6-PO₄ necessary to activate glycogen synthetase phosphatase.

An important physiological role of insulin is the control of protein synthesis in muscle. Insulin stimulates the active transport of glucose and amino acids into muscle

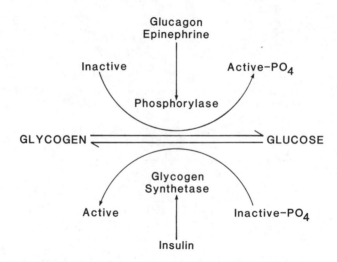

Figure 11.8 General scheme for the control of glycogen synthesis and degradation.

and promotes muscle protein synthesis in the absence of concomitant sugar or amino acid transport. Although muscle RNA synthesis can be inhibited by actinomycin D, insulin is still capable of increasing protein synthesis, suggesting that insulin acts at a site distal to the synthesis of mRNA. A cell-free system from skeletal muscle of diabetic rats is less efficient in synthesizing proteins than the same system from normal rats. This defect was found to reside in the ribosomes, not in other cytoplasmic protein factors, obtained from diabetic animals and could be corrected by injecting insulin into diabetic animals prior to isolating the ribosomes. When RNA synthesis was inhibited in diabetic rats prior to insulin injection, the hormone still corrected the defect in the ribosomes. However, when diabetic animals were given an inhibitor of protein synthesis prior to receiving insulin, the defect in the ribosomes could not be corrected. Messenger RNA apparently is synthesized or already present in a normal quantity in diabetic animals. However, ribosomes from diabetic animals may lack a factor necessary for the binding or translation of mRNA; insulin must stimulate the synthesis of this factor (translation factor) which is apparently a protein [5]. The translation factor may be a cytoplasmic protein which modifies the function of ribosomes or it may be a part of the ribosome itself, a ribosomal protein.

GLUCAGON

A second important pancreatic hormone which regulates glucose homeostasis was discovered by Kimball and Murlin [24]. Numerous workers had noted that injections of pancreatic extracts into diabetic animals produced a transient hyperglycemia before the hypoglycemic effects of the extracts were observed. Collins and Murlin [7] suggested that besides insulin the extracts might contain a physiologically relevant hyperglycemic factor, which they named glucagon. Glucagon is essential for the complete metabolic syndrome of severe diabetes, previously attributed entirely to the direct consequences of insulin deficiency [44, 45].

Synthesis, Chemistry, and Metabolism

Mammalian pancreatic glucagon is a single-chain polypeptide of 29 amino acid residues which bears a striking structural similarity to secretin, gastric inhibitory peptide (GIP), and vasoactive intestinal peptide (VIP) (Fig. 10.3). Studies on the biosynthesis of pancreatic glucagon indicate that glucagon is derived from a large precursor (preprohormone) which then undergoes a number of posttranslational modifications to yield the definitive hormone [40]. The amino acid sequences of glucagons derived from a number of mammalian species (bovine, ovine, rabbit, rat) including the human are identical (Fig. 11.9). Glucagons from the turkey and the chicken are identical and differ from mammalian glucagons by substitution of the penultimate asparagine (position 28) by serine. Duck glucagon differs from human glucagon by two residues: The asparagine at position 28 is again replaced by serine and the serine at position 16 is substituted by threonine. Such a high degree of structural conservation within the glucagons from these species strongly suggests that the integrity of most of the molecule is necessary for its biological activity.

Physiological Roles

The classical experiments of Foà demonstrated conclusively the role of glucagon in glucose homeostasis [17, 18]. In cross-circulation experiments, the pancreatoduodenal vein of one dog (A) was anastomosed to a femoral vein of a second dog (B) and a return flow was established between a femoral artery of dog B and a femoral vein of dog A. Reduction of plasma blood glucose levels in dog A by insulin resulted in an elevation of blood glucose levels in dog B. Conversely, when hyperglycemia was induced in dog A by administration of glucagon or glucose, a rapid hypoglycemia developed in dog B. These results demonstrated that a reduction or an elevation of blood glucose in dog A was the stimulus to glucagon or insulin secretion, respectively, in dog B. From these experiments, the importance of pancreatic glucagon, with insulin, in the control of blood glucose levels was elucidated. Subsequent experiments showed that glucagon had a direct effect on glycogenolysis and gluconeogenesis in the isolated perfused liver.

The biological actions of glucagon are essentially the opposite of those of insulin (Fig. 11.3). Glucagon stimulates hepatic glucose release through a glycogenolytic action or through gluconeogenesis. The glycogenolytic action is particularly important in maintaining the short-term levels of blood glucose in well-fed animals that have available stores of liver glycogen. Under conditions of prolonged fasting, exercise, or during neonatal life, the gluconeogenic actions of glucagon are crucial to the maintenance of glucose homeostasis.

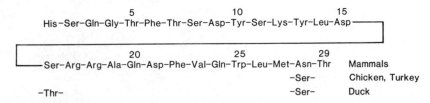

Figure 11.9 Primary structure of mammalian glucagon and related structures of avian glucagons.

Glucagon at physiological levels stimulates the conversion of amino acids to glucose within the liver. This gluconeogenic action of the hormone appears to be an intrahepatic mechanism rather than a result of stimulation of membrane transport of amino acids. Glucagon also promotes the conversion of amino acids and glycerol into glucose, apparently by affecting the enzymes in the gluconeogenic and glycolytic pathways in the liver (Fig. 11.3).

Glucagon has a lipolytic action on adipose tissue: The FFA's and glycerol liberated from fat cells are utilized to a minor extent within the hepatocyte in gluconeogenesis. Insulin is such a potent inhibitor of fat cell lipolysis that the actions of glucagon may be manifested only when insulin concentrations are low. The ability of administered glucagon to stimulate lipolysis has nevertheless been demonstrated in the human diabetic.

Mechanisms of Action

The major target tissues of glucagon are liver and adipose tissue. Cardiac muscle may also be a site of action under certain conditions. The actions of the hormone are at the level of the plasma membrane to stimulate adenylate cyclase production of cyclic AMP; this initial action of the hormone is followed by activation of a cAMP-dependent protein kinase and subsequent substrate phosphorylation. The actions of

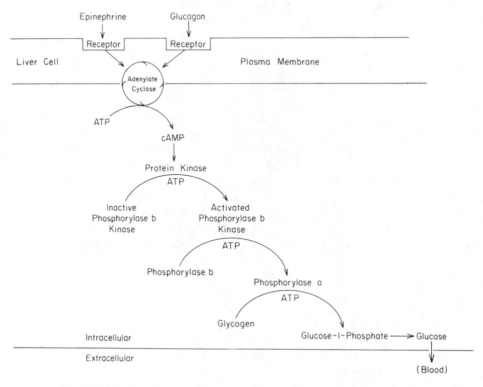

Figure 11.10 Glucagon activation of hepatic adenylate cyclase and the subsequent events in glucose formation.

glucagon on the hepatocyte are similar to those of epinephrine but each hormone mediates its effects through separate receptors (Chapter 14). In the hepatocyte a cascade of protein (enzyme) phosphorylations eventually results in the release of individual glucose units from the glycogen polymer (Fig. 11.10). Conversion of inactive (dephosphophosphorylase) phosphorylase to the active enzyme is the final key step in this cascade phenomenon. At the same time phosphorylation of glycogen synthetase apparently inactivates this enzyme (Fig. 11.8). Glucagon also stimulates gluconeogenesis within the hepatocyte; again its action is mediated through the intracellular messenger cAMP. The actions of the cyclic nucleotide block the flow of carbohydrate substrates from glucose-6-PO_4 to pyruvate, specifically by inhibiting enzyme activities between pyruvate and phosphoenolpyruvate. Within the hepatocyte glucagon also prevents the conversion of FFA's to ketone bodies. The control site of hepatic ketogenesis is at the level of the enzyme carnitine fatty acid transferase. This enzyme promotes the reversible coupling of long-chain fatty acids to carnitine which is required for the translocation of fatty acids into mitochondria for oxidation. Utilization of ketones for the production of ATP within mitochondria by oxidative phosphorylation provides a glucose-sparing action. Figure 11.3 summarizes the actions of glucagon on the hepatocyte.

Although glucagon is a potent lipolytic hormone, there is great species variation with respect to the sensitivity of adipose tissue to the hormone. Here, as for the hepatocyte, cAMP formation is increased in response to glucagon. In the adipocyte activation of one or more *hormone-sensitive* lipases (triglyceride, diglyceride, and monoglyceride lipases) results in the release of fatty acids and glycerol from fats. These metabolic products of lipolysis circulate to the liver where they subserve substrate roles in gluconeogenic processes. By the actions of glucagon on adipocytes and hepatocytes, plasma glucose levels are elevated; thus, under pathological conditions of pancreatic function the actions of the hormone are diabetogenic.

Modification of the NH_2-terminal or COOH-terminal regions of glucagon results in decreased potency and sometimes nearly complete loss of biological activity. Removal of the histidine from the NH_2-terminus lowers the affinity for the receptor 15-fold. Glucagon 1-21 is a full agonist, though less potent than the parent peptide. The NH_2-terminal fragment, His-Ser-Gln-Gly-Thr-Phe, is a partial agonist of hepatic adenylate cyclase. It may be feasible, therefore, to tailor the structure of the NH_2-terminal amino acid residues in a manner that will lead to a derivative which binds to the receptor but fails to stimulate adenylate cyclase activity. There is evidence that it may be possible in the near future to incorporate this fragment into the native hormone to produce a potent blocking agent of endogenous glucagon [22].

OTHER PANCREATIC PEPTIDE HORMONES

The α and β cells are the predominant cell types within the pancreas. Nevertheless, using immunocytochemical methods at least two other peptide hormone-containing cells have been demonstrated to be present within the islets. The control of insulin and glucagon secretion from the islets is much more complicated than described and may be regulated or modulated by these newly discovered pancreatic peptide hormones.

Somatostatin (SS)

Immunoreactive SS was shown by immunofluorescence to be localized to a discrete population of cells (D cells) of the endocrine pancreas. The juxtaposition of SS-containing D cells to the α and β cells of the islets is consistent with a local or paracrine role for the hormone. Somatostatin is a tetradecapeptide containing a disulfide bond (Fig. 6.6); in the pancreas the hormone is derived, as for insulin and glucagon, from a preprohormone [40]. Somatostatin has been isolated from the pancreas and found to be identical structurally to ovine and porcine hypothalamic SS. The observation that this tetradecapeptide sequence is found outside the nervous system and in different vertebrate orders supports the concept that SS may function in a variety of roles in different organs and species [37].

Somatostatinlike immunoreactivity is elevated in the arterial plasma of dogs that have received a protein meal, suggesting that SS may function as a humoral messenger in the control of gastrointestinal function. Infusions of SS, at a rate approximating the postprandial increase in endogenous plasma somatostatinlike activity, markedly lower postprandial triglyceride levels. In addition neutralization of circulating SS by antibodies to the peptide is accompanied by higher levels of plasma triglycerides. Somatostatin may, therefore, function as a splanchnic humoral hormone which regulates the movement of nutrients from the gut to the internal environment [36]. According to one hypothesis, the function of pancreatic SS may be to restrain the rate of nutrient entry into the body by inhibiting various digestive events in response to signals from enteric hormones and rising nutrient concentrations [43]. This would allow the islet hormones to coordinate the influx of nutrients from the gut with their movement from the extracellular space into the various tissues.

Pancreatic Polypeptide (PP)

A linear polypeptide consisting of 36 amino acid residues has been isolated from the human, pig, cow, sheep, and chicken pancreas (Fig. 11.11). Avian and beef pancreatic polypeptides (PP) exhibit homology at 16 of 36 amino acid residues, whereas the mammalian polypeptides only differ by two to three residues [16, 25].

The physiological functions of these pancreatic polypeptides are not clearly delineated, but some actions of the hormone in the chicken have been described [21]. In the chicken avian PP decreases liver glycogen apparently by stimulating hepatic

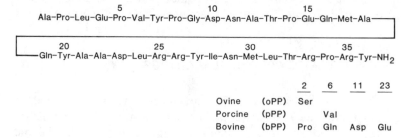

Figure 11.11 Primary structure of human pancreatic polypeptide. Variations within ovine, porcine and bovine PP sequences are shown [16].

lipogenesis. Avian PP decreases plasma glycerol and FFA's in the chicken by inhibiting adipose tissue lipolysis, apparently by reducing fat cell cyclic AMP levels [31]. In humans PP suppresses secretion of somatostatin (SS) from the gut and pancreas. Similarly, there is a postprandial rise in plasma PP in humans which can be suppressed by infusions of SS. Administration of antisera to SS in dogs increases plasma PP levels, suggesting that an inhibitory control of PP secretion by SS takes place under physiologic conditions. It was suggested, therefore, that the SS-containing D cells and PP-containing F cells control the secretory activity of each other (and probably of insulin and glucagon) within the pancreatic islets by a paracrine mechanism.

Ingestion of a protein meal is a stimulus to PP secretion in humans. Because intravenous infusions of amino acids only modestly elevate plasma PP levels, protein digestion within the GI tract is most likely the stimulus to PP secretion from the pancreatic islets. Acute hypoglycemia is a stimulus to PP secretion, whereas hyperglycemia is associated with a decrease in plasma PP levels. Vagal cholinergic innervation of the pancreas is important in the regulation of PP release. For example, secretion of PP in response to insulin-induced hypoglycemia in humans is abolished by cholinergic (atropine) blockade. Electrical stimulation of the vagus nerve increases portal levels of PP in the pig, a response that is partially inhibited by cholinergic blockade. Protein-rich meals may activate the release of some factor, possibly cholecystokinin, which enhances the release of PP, possibly in concert with vagal activation of pancreatic F cells. These observations support the belief that PP plays a role in nutrient homeostasis [16].

CONTROL OF PANCREATIC ISLET FUNCTION

Although insulin secretion from the pancreatic islets is regulated by endocrine, neural, and metabolic factors (Table 11.1), blood glucose is the most important regulator. The temporal hyperglycemia, which develops after an exogenous carbohydrate source, is stimulatory to insulin and inhibitory to glucagon secretion (Fig. 11.12A). The β cells of the pancreas must possess glucose or glucose metabolite receptors as elevated glucose concentrations are directly stimulatory to insulin secretion from pancreatic islets incubated in vitro. Mannose and fructose are also stimulatory, the latter most likely because it is converted intracellularly to glucose. Apparently the stimulatory action of glucose on insulin secretion is due to its metabolism within pancreatic islet cells as such agents as 2-deoxyglucose and mannoheptulose, which inhibit glucose catabolism, prevent insulin secretion. It is believed that some product(s) of glucose metabolism acts on the intracellular processes involved in insulin vesicular exocytosis. Although cyclic AMP is implicated in the release of insulin and Ca^{2+} uptake is required in the stimulus-secretion coupling mechanism in insulin secretion, the integrated role of these intracellular messengers is unclear [27].

The amino acids arginine and leucine as well as such keto acids as acetoacetic acid are also stimulatory to insulin secretion. Insulin is important in the utilization of these substrates in protein and fat synthesis, respectively. It is interesting to speculate that stimulation of insulin secretion by these metabolic substrates is adaptive in nature

TABLE 11.1. Stimuli Affecting Pancreatic Islet Hormone Secretion[a]

	Adrenergic α	Adrenergic β	Cholinergic	Insulin	Glucagon	PP	SS	Neurotensin	Glucose High	Glucose Low	Arginine (amino acids)
Insulin	−	+[1]	+[3]		+		−	+[4] −[5]	+		+[6]
Glucagon	+[2]	+[1]	+[3]	+			−	+[4] −[5]		+	+[6]
Somatostatin	−[2]	+[1]		−	+	−		+[4] −[5]	+		+[6]
Pancreatic polypeptide	+[1]		+[3]				−			−	+

[a]Data derived mainly from studies in mammals (particularly the rat and the dog). Inhibitory (−) or stimulatory (+) secretory responses are indicated. Adrenergic stimuli are mediated through α- or β-adrenoceptors (Chapter 14). [1]Blocked by β-adrenoceptor antagonists. [2]Blocked by α-adrenoceptor antagonists. [3]Blocked by atropine. [4]In the presence of 3 mM glucose. [5]In the presence of 23 mM glucose. [6]Blocked by neurotensin.

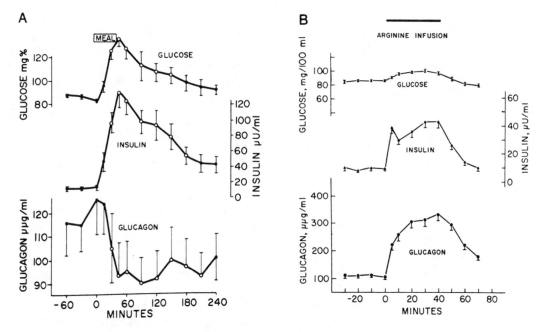

Figure 11.12 (A) The effect of a large carbohydrate meal on the plasma concentration of pancreatic glucagon, insulin, and glucose in 11 normal humans. (From Müller et al., [32], with permission.) (B) The effect of an infusion of arginine on the peripheral venous plasma levels of pancreatic glucagon, insulin, and glucose in normal humans. (Reprinted, by permission of the *New England Journal of Medicine*, from Müller, et al., [32], vol. 283, pp. 109–115, 1970.)

and the insulin released is stimulatory to their utilization in protein and fat synthesis. Orally administered glucose is a greater stimulus to insulin secretion than intravenously injected glucose. There is evidence that glucose within the GI tract is stimulatory to gastric inhibitory peptide (GIP) secretion which then, through circulation to the pancreatic islets, is stimulatory in conjunction with glucose to insulin secretion. A number of oral hypoglycemic agents—tolbutamide and other sulfonylurea derivatives as chlorpropamide—are stimulatory to insulin secretion. Most endocrine tissues undergo hypertrophy and hyperplasia after prolonged stimulation. Although the β cells become hypertropic under conditions of continued insulin secretion as do other endocrine cells, they also undergo exhaustion rather than proliferation. The cells become vacuolated under such prolonged stimulation, eventually die, and are not subsequently replaced; an irreversible diabetes mellitus results from a total loss of pancreatic β-cell function.

The pancreas receives neural innervation from the sympathetic and parasympathetic divisions of the autonomic nervous system. Secretions from the exocrine and endocrine tissues of the pancreas can be increased by parasympathetic vagal stimulation or by sympathetic stimulation. Neurotransmitters of cholinergic (acetylcholine) and adrenergic (norepinephrine) neurons directly affect pancreatic insulin secretion. Both cholinergic and adrenergic neuronal fibers can be detected in the endocrine and exocrine pancreas. Electron microscopic histochemical studies reveal that both types of neurons innervate the α and β cells of the islets. Transplantation experiments reveal, however, that the pancreatic β cells do not require an intact innervation for functioning. Similarly, unilateral or bilateral vagotomy does not result in observable effects on depression of insulin secretion due to an intravenous glucose load. Nevertheless, cholinergic drugs potentiate glucose-induced insulin release, and the insulin-releasing effect of electrical vagus stimulation increases with the blood-glucose concentration. Probably the vagal nerve modulates the responsiveness of β cells to blood sugar variations in vivo. Furthermore, nervous input to the pancreas may represent a trophic influence of importance for islet cell growth and function over an extended period, and there are some data to support such an hypothesis.

Epinephrine of adrenal chromaffin cell origin affects insulin secretion under physiological states such as stress. The effects of the catecholamine are mediated through adrenergic receptors possessed by the islet β cells: Stimulation of α-adrenergic receptors is inhibitory to insulin secretion, whereas stimulation of β-adrenergic receptors possessed by the cells is stimulatory to insulin secretion. The possible individual and integrated roles of these β-cell adrenergic receptors in the control of islet insulin secretion are unknown. However, under conditions of stress epinephrine is secreted from the adrenal medulla; its hyperglycemic effect is obviously of adaptive importance (Chapter 14). It might be advantageous if, during stress, insulin secretion is depressed so that glucose is more readily available (rather than stored as glycogen or fat) to tissues, such as the liver, muscle, and brain, that are particularly active under such conditions. Glucagon secretion, on the other hand, is stimulated by epinephrine and norepinephrine; this response provides a mechanism of activating hepatic glucose production and release.

Most amino acids stimulate (aminogenic action) the secretion of insulin and glucagon (Fig. 11.12B). The enormous structural differences within the R-chain of the active amino acids argue against a structure-activity relationship involving a receptor activation. Aminogenic insulin secretion is important, at least from a teleological viewpoint, in that the secreted insulin is available to incorporate amino acids into proteins in muscle and other tissues. The concomitant release of glucagon may serve to prevent hypoglycemia as a consequence of the insulin secretion. Aminogenic glucagon secretion is abolished whenever exogenous glucose accompanies the influx of amino acids such as occurs when carbohydrate is ingested with protein during a meal. In carnivores the release of glucagon as well as insulin in response to a protein meal would be of obvious adaptive value [45].

Insulin is directly inhibitory to glucagon secretion and, conversely, glucagon is stimulatory to insulin secretion. Somatostatin on the other hand is inhibitory to the secretion of glucagon and insulin as well as pancreatic polypeptide. It is possible that metabolic substrates, such as glucose or certain amino acids or vagal nerve afferent stimuli, regulate the secretory activity of one or more of these cells which, in turn, through the release of their hormones (glucagon, insulin, SS, or PP), reciprocally affect the secretion of each other (Fig. 11.2).

There is evidence that the pancreatic glucose sensor may be solely a component of the β cell. In response to glucose, information may be conveyed to the α cells directly by way of tight junctions or through the release of insulin, which may then interact with receptors on the α cells. In either case glucose release would be lowered by the action of insulin on its target tissues, such as liver, adipose tissue, and muscle, and additionally through its inhibition of glucagon secretion, a normally hyperglycemic action. In the absence of β cells, as in certain types of diabetes, both these effects of insulin would be lacking. Indeed, the α cell may then be hyperactive; in the juvenile diabetic (who lacks insulin) glucagon levels are elevated even in the presence of hyperglycemia. The observation that glucagon is increased relative to insulin levels in all known forms of endogenous hyperglycemia supports the view that glucagon participates in the marked hepatic overproduction of glucose that is characteristic of the insulin-deficient state [42].

Two models have generally been discussed to explain the nature of the cellular sensor responsible for regulating insulin secretion: the *fuel receptor model* and the *fuel metabolism model*. The first involves typical structure-function considerations as generally applied to hormone structures. According to the second model, the fuel molecules themselves act as stimuli or inhibitors of hormone release as a result of their metabolism within the islet cells. A third model incorporates experimental data supporting both models [29].

A number of neural or endocrine influences affect glucose homeostasis and glucose intolerance in the diabetic [14]. Somatotropin, in particular, is diabetogenic, but its exact mode of action is undetermined. STH is stimulatory to insulin secretion, but at the same time this hormone reduces the sensitivity of peripheral tissues (e.g., muscle and adipose tissues) to insulin. Acromegalics have increased circulating levels of STH and exhibit abnormal glucose tolerance due to severe insulin resistance. Somatotropin-induced insulin release may be indirect because of the developing hyperglycemia resulting from inhibition of glucose uptake by peripheral tissues. Elevated plasma glucose levels would then be stimulatory to insulin secretion; elevated insulin levels, however, would lead to down regulation of peripheral tissue insulin receptors (insulin resistance) and the vicious cycle would continue.

Glucocorticoids are increased in Cushing's syndrome (Chapter 15); the effect of these adrenal steroids is generally to increase gluconeogenesis in the liver. In addition glucocorticoids have a catabolic action on muscle and adipose tissues. The liberated amino acids and FFA's provide substrates for increased gluconeogenesis within the liver. Glucocorticoids also enhance the actions of adrenal catecholamines on their target tissues: For example, the lipolytic actions of catecholamines on adipose tissue are enhanced. All these actions of glucocorticoids are hyperglycemic and therefore are potentially diabetogenic over a prolonged period.

PANCREATIC ISLET PATHOPHYSIOLOGY

Diabetes mellitus was first described about 1500 B.C. in Egypt [30]. *Mellitus*, the Latin word for honey, characterizes the high sugar content of the urine of diabetics. The word *diabetes*, derived from the Greek for siphon, refers to the copious excretion of water that characterizes the disease. For centuries the disease was known as "the pissing evil" in England, an epithet that appropriately characterizes its most observable symptom.

Although diabetes mellitus is generally thought to result from a lack of insulin, it can, however, be considered a heterogeneous group of diseases. The juvenile-onset form of the disease does result from a deficiency of the hormone. The vast majority of diabetics who suffer from *maturity-onset diabetes*, however, generally have above normal levels of insulin and their tissues do not respond to the hormone [33]. This phenomenon, referred to as *insulin resistance*, may be due to multiple causes.

In patients with *insulin-dependent diabetes mellitus* there is a marked decrease in the number of insulin-containing β cells [4]. The pathogenesis may result from the development of islet cell surface antibodies. The cues responsible for the production of cytotoxic antibodies is not known. Autoantibodies are thought to have a role in the pathogenesis of several other endocrine-based disease states.

Juvenile-onset diabetes develops in youth; the symptoms begin rather abruptly, and control of the disease almost always requires insulin replacement therapy. There is evidence that juvenile-onset diabetes may be caused by a virus but initiation may require more than a single virus infection. The symptoms may only be manifested when sufficient damage has been caused by a number of infections such as mumps and rubella.

The circulating levels of insulin rise in individuals who have insulin resistance and pancreatic islets that function normally. Some patients treated with exogenous insulin develop antibodies to the hormone, and these proteins inhibit access of the active hormone to its receptors. Insulin resistance may also develop in individuals who produce an abnormal hormone that has decreased receptor affinity. In the abnormality of *familial hyperproinsulinemia*, for example, individuals possess elevated circulating levels of a partially cleaved proinsulin. This abnormality is inherited as an autosomal dominant and probably involves a mutation of arginine 32 of the cleavage site connecting the B chain to the C peptide [19, 20]. Another defect resulting in hyperproinsulinemia involves a mutation at the cleavage site connecting the C peptide to the A chain (Fig. 11.6). A biologically defective insulin molecule was produced in another hyperinsulinemic patient, most likely by a single point mutation (probably a single base change in the DNA), resulting in substitution of leucine for phenylalanine at position 24 or 25 of the insulin B chain. These positions are known to comprise part of the active receptor-binding region of insulin which is responsible for its biological activity [20]. The structurally defective insulin is devoid of biological activity and the abnormal hormonal variant antagonizes the action of normal insulin on its receptor.

Receptor impairment appears also to play a major role in insulin resistance [15]. This target cell abnormality may be due to defects in insulin receptor number or affinity for the hormone. There is indeed evidence that receptor concentration as well as affinity are influenced by many factors. In obese individuals, for example, insulin receptor numbers are reduced in liver, muscle, and fat, and in animals and humans this reversible defect appears to result from the hyperinsulinemia caused from overeating [15, 33]. Restriction of caloric intake ameliorates the hyperinsulinemia and enhances the binding of insulin to cells taken from such individuals. In vitro studies using human adipocytes reveal that chronic exposure of the cells to insulin results in subsequent resistance of the cells to the antilipolytic effects of the hormone.

In the absence of insulin most activities described relating to the actions of insulin are reversed. Failure to activate hepatic glycogen synthetase increases the levels of glucose-6-PO_4, and this substrate is now available for dephosphorylation by glucose-6-phosphatase to glucose. The concomitant decreased activity of glucokinase results in the loss of glucose from the hepatocytes and, more importantly, impedes the flow of glucose into the cells, thus failing to provide substrates for glycolysis and ATP production by way of the Krebs cycle. This sets up a situation within hepatocytes and all other cells where, although there are increased circulating levels of glucose, there is little intracellular glucose for ATP production. Thus, cellular famine exists in the midst of plenty. Indeed, polyphagia is a characteristic behavioral trait of these energy-starved individuals. The resulting excess of sugar in the blood leads to the excretion of large amounts of urine (polyuria), which in turn leads to dehydration and intense thirst (polydipsia).

The unavailability of glucose for lipogenesis within fat cells results in increased lipolysis; the released FFA's and glycerol are now available to liver cells as substrates for glucogenesis, which enhances the hyperglycemia, the cardinal symptom of diabetes mellitus. The FFA's released from the fats stored within the adipocytes undergo β oxidation with resultant production of acetyl-CoA. Although this high energy compound is available for entry into the Krebs cycle, the increased levels of this substrate may result in condensation of acetyl-CoA moieties into acetoacetyl-CoA. In the liver deacylase activity converts acetoacetyl-CoA to acetoacetic acid. This β-keto acid can then be converted to β-hydroxybutyric acid and acetone (Fig. 11.13). These ketones, acetoacetate and β-hydroxybutyrate, are normally used as energy substrates. If, however, the entry of acetyl-CoA into the citric acid cycle is depressed, the rate of

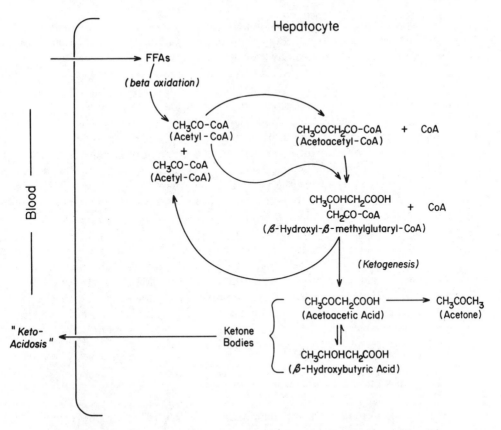

Figure 11.13 Scheme of ketone biosynthesis: the hydroxymethylglutaryl-CoA cycle.

ketone formation may exceed the tissue oxidation of these substrates. They then accumulate within the bloodstream, which is followed by an elevation of ketone bodies in the urine (ketonuria). This diabetic ketosis may result in a fatal metabolic acidosis. The urinary ketone bodies are excreted as sodium salts and large volumes of water are osmotically removed from the plasma, thus intensifying the dehydration already present due to the hyperglycemic diuresis. The loss of sodium disturbs the bicarbonate buffering system of the plasma, thus intensifying the blood acidosis. Ketones are also removed through the lungs, producing the characteristic fruity smell of the diabetic in a state of ketosis.

In the absence of insulin, amino acids and glucose cannot enter muscle cells, which results in protein catabolism. The amino acids released from muscle in the diabetic are now available through deamination and transamination for glucose formation. Utilization of amino acids in hepatic gluconeogenesis results in a *negative nitrogen balance*. The protein catabolism results in protein depletion and tissue wasting, and failure to grow is a symptom of diabetes in children. The protein depletion and accompanying hyperglycemia of the diabetic are also associated with poor resistance to infections.

Islet Cell Tumors

Because of the profound effects of pancreatic hormones on nutrient homeostasis, one should expect that malignancies or neoplasms of pancreatic islet cell function would have profound effects on carbohydrate, protein, and fat metabolism. Three neoplasms of the islets are insulinoma, glucagonoma, and somatostatinoma. Other tumors (e.g., gastrinomas, VIPomas) of unknown cellular origin within the pancreas may secrete other peptide hormones that cause dire gastrointestinal tract disturbances.

Benign and malignant insulin-secreting tumors exhibit complete autonomy of insulin release. If mild, the resulting hypoglycemia can be controlled by an increase in food intake; if severe and intractable, it can lead to convulsions and death if the tumor is not surgically removed. The excessive release of glucagon from an α-cell tumor leads to hyperglucagonemia, and the metabolic disturbances that prevail vary with the capability of the individual to secrete insulin [43]. Development of a somatostatinoma results, not unexpectedly, in hypersomatostatinemia. Patients with such tumors may exhibit a hypoinsulinemia and a hypoglucagonemia. Because somatostatin may perform a number of functions within the GI tract, it is not surprising that digestive tract functioning may also be impaired. Excessive amounts of PP are released by all VIPomas and most multiple endocrine adenomas (MEA's). Multiple endocrine neoplasia is characterized by tumors that often occur synchronously in a number of endocrine glands. One type predominantly involves the parathyroid and pituitary glands and the pancreatic islets. Table 11.2 summarizes the major pathologies of the pancreatic islets.

Exogenous Insulin Production

In the past porcine or other mammalian sources of insulin have provided the replacement therapy required by the diabetic. These nonhuman sources of insulin

TABLE 11.2 Pathophysiology Of The Endocrine Pancreas[a]

Disease	Etiology
Juvenile-onset diabetes	Viral-induced β-cell destruction
Maturity-onset diabetes	Insulin-resistant diabetes; decrease in insulin receptor number and/or affinity
Insulin-dependent diabetes	Cytotoxic autoantibodies to β cells lead to β-cell destruction
Familial hyperproinsulinemia	B-C proinsulin, mutation at the cleavage site between the B chain and the connecting (C) peptide
	A-C proinsulin, mutation at the cleavage site between the A chain and the connecting (C) peptide
	Defect in primary structure of insulin B chain at positions 24 or 25
Insulinoma	Excess insulin secretion from β-cell pancreatic tumor
Glucagonoma syndrome	Excess glucagon secretion from α-cell pancreatic tumor
Somatostatinoma	Excess somatostatin secretion from an islet D cell neoplasm
Hypoglucagonemia or isolated glucagon deficiency	Possibly due to autosomal recessive inheritance

[a] No pathological condition or tumor has been reported which solely secretes PP, although very high levels of the peptide are often found in pancreatic disease states, exocrine and endocrine.

often prove to be immunogenic in some individuals and other sources must be provided. There is hope that DNA recombinant technology will provide a plentiful supply of human insulin (Chapter 3). Two general approaches are being investigated. Sequences of DNA encoding for the A and B peptide chains of insulin have been ligated separately into the *Escherichia coli* β-galactosidase gene. The individual polypeptide chains produced by the bacterium are then released by enzymatic cleavage from the translation product and purified and recombined to form the biologically active insulin (Fig. 3.5). An alternate approach has utilized human preproinsulin DNA inserted into a plasmid which was then used to transform a strain of *E. coli*. The preproinsulin polypeptide sequence was synthesized and correctly cleaved by the bacterium. The polypeptide could then be successfully converted to an insulinlike component by tryptic digestion. This method may eventually prove feasible for the production of adequate amounts of human insulin for therapeutic purposes [6].

COMPARATIVE ENDOCRINOLOGY

Insulin, glucagon, somatostatin, and pancreatic polypeptide are present within pancreatic tissue of representatives of all vertebrate classes. Indeed, these or immunologically related peptides are present within tissues of a number of invertebrate species. The ratio of α and β cells varies between members of different vertebrate classes, possibly suggesting differences in the relative importance of these hyperglycemic or hypoglycemic factors among species. Except in cyclostomes, where experimental evidence is conflicting, insulin and glucagon generally exert hypoglycemic and hyperglycemic actions in most vertebrate species studied. Pancreatic somatostatin-containing cells are present in avian and teleost species and are therefore likely in members of all vertebrate classes.

Although endocrine pancreatic cells are dispersed as islets of tissue within the exocrine pancreas of mammals, islet tissue occurs as a compact mass of tissue devoid, or nearly so, of exocrine pancreas in teleosts and cyclostomes [10, 11]. The endocrine pancreas of teleosts, for example, consists of macroscopically visible *Brockman bodies* or *principal islets* as they are usually called [3]. Smaller accessory macroscopic or microscopic bodies are scattered throughout the body cavity. The principal islet of the anglerfish (*Lophius americanus*) is large and has been particularly useful as a source of insulin for structural analysis.

The complete covalent structure of insulin from a variety of vertebrate species has been determined [12, 13, 39]. Like many protein hormones, the molecule contains sites where amino acid substitutions appear to be tolerated (variable positions) and those which appear to be completely immutable (conservative or invariant residues). Insulin has been isolated and purified from the islet organs of a cyclostome, the hagfish *Myxine glutinosa*, a member of the earliest class of vertebrates. Hagfish insulin is structurally similar to other vertebrate insulins with respect to the following: the positions of the six half-cystine residues; the N-terminal seven residues; the C-terminal six residues of the A chain; and several shorter sequences in the B chain. Of 24 residues known to be invariant among other vertebrate insulins, 23 are identical in hagfish insulin [34].

In contrast to the conservative nature of the amino acid residues of the A and B chains of the vertebrate insulins, the amino acid moieties of the C-peptides are much more variable. Such variability would suggest that the connecting peptide plays no endocrine role even though it is secreted with insulin. The structural elements conserved within the C-peptide may play important roles in dictating the folding of the peptide chain necessary for correct disulfide bond formation as well as the specific cleavage sites of proinsulin by the converting enzymes [39].

The endocrine cells of the vertebrate pancreas have evolved from the gut; glucagon- and somatostatin-producing cells are present in the intestinal linings of humans and other mammals. It has been hypothesized that there is a close evolutionary relationship between the acinar cells and the islet β cells [38]. Primitive secretory cells of the intestinal mucosa may have released a number of digestive hydrolytic enzymes into the gut, including a protein probably resembling proinsulin. This primitive proinsulin may have had some hydrolytic activity which has since been lost. During digestion this proinsulin could have been degraded to an insulinlike fragment that found access to the blood where it enhanced the utilization of other similarly absorbed nutrients. Such a rudimentary regulatory system probably provided some selective advantage to these early organisms. With time these proteinaceous secretory products were packaged, stored, and released in response to nutrient cues as is still the case for the hormone-secreting cells of the vertebrate endocrine gastrointestinal tract. A definitive pancreatic tissue then evolved and the secretory products were delivered more directly to the circulatory system. Morphological elements of such an evolutionary scheme can be visualized in the gastrointestinal tract and pancreatic components of present-day vertebrates.

The pancreatic hormones have been demonstrated in tissues from a variety of invertebrate species. Insulin and pancreatic polypeptidelike immunoreactivity has been localized to neurons within the brain of the silkworm moth *Bombyx mori*. Insulinlike and PP-like immunoreactivity has also been found in the medial neurosecretory cells of the blowfly *Calliphora vomitoria*. In addition PP-like material isolated from the blowfly (10^6 heads) appears to bear close structural similarity to the mammalian hormone [9]. Somatostatinlike immunoreactivity has been found in the neural ganglion of the ascidian *Ciona intestinalis* and PP-like immunoreactivity in neurons of the earthworm *Lumbricus terrestris* has been discovered. Lastly, PP- and SS-like immunoreactivity have been demonstrated in the cockroach midgut. These observations indicate that each of the pancreatic peptides appeared early in evolution and that each hormone subserves a variety of physiological functions within these animals.

REFERENCES

[1] BALDWIN, D., JR., M. PRINCE, S. MARSHALL, P. DAVIES, and J. M. OLEFSKY. 1980. Regulation of insulin receptors: evidence for involvement of an endocytotic internalization pathway. *Proc. Natl. Acad. Sci. USA* 77:5975–78.

[2] BANTING, F. G., and C. H. BEST. 1922. The internal secretion of the pancreas. *J. Lab. Clin. Med.* 7:465–80.

[3] BRINN, J. E., JR. 1973. The pancreatic islets of bony fishes. *Amer. Zool.* 13:653–65.

[4] CAHILL, G. F., and H. O. McDEVITT. 1981. Insulin-dependent diabetes mellitus: the initial lesion. *New Engl. J. Med.* 304:1454–66.

[5] CASTLES, J. J. 1970. The effect of insulin on protein synthesis in muscle. *Med. Clinics of North America* 54:201–207.

[6] CHAN, S. J., J. WEISS, M. KONRAD, T. WHILE, C. BAHL, S. D. YU, D. MARKS, and D. F. STEINER. 1981. Biosynthesis and periplasmic segregation of human proinsulin in *Escherichia coli*. *Proc. Natl. Acad. Sci. USA* 78:5401–5405.

[7] COLLINS, W. S., and J. R. MURLIN. 1929. Hyperglycemia following the portal injection of insulin. *Proc. Soc. Exp. Biol. Med.* 26:485–90.

[8] CZECH, M. P. 1977. Molecular basis of insulin action. 1977. *Ann. Rev. Biochem.* 46:359–84.

[9] DUVE, H., A. THORPE, R. NEVILLE, and N. R. LAZARUS. 1981. Isolation and partial characterization of pancreatic polypeptide-like material in the brain of the blowfly *Calliphora vomitoria*. *Biochem. J.* 197:767–70.

[10] EPPLE, A., and T. L. LEWIS. 1973. Comparative histophysiology of the pancreatic islets. *Amer. Zool.* 13:567–90.

[11] EPPLE, A., and J. E. BRINN, JR. 1975. Islet histophysiology: evolutionary correlations. *Gen. Comp. Endocrinol.* 27:320–49.

[12] FALKMER, S., S. EMDIN, N. HAVU, G. LUNDGREN, M. MARQUES, Y. ÖSTBERG, D. F. STEINER, and N. W. THOMAS. 1973. Insulin in invertebrates and cyclostomes. *Amer. Zool.* 13:625–38.

[13] FALKMER, S., J. F. CUTFIELD, S. M. CUTFIELD, G. G. DODSON, J. GLIEMANN, S. GAMMELTOFT, M. MARQUES, J. D. PETERSON, D. F. STEINER, F. SUNDBY, S. O. EMDIN, N. HAVU, Y. ÖSTBERG, and L. WINBLADH. 1975. Comparative endocrinology of insulin and glucagon production. *Amer. Zool.* 15(Suppl. 1):255–70.

[14] FELIG, P., R. S. SHERWIN, V. SOMAN, J. WAHREN, R. HENDLER, L. SACCA, N. EIGLER, D. GOLDBERG, and M. WALESKY. 1979. Hormonal interactions in the regulation of blood glucose. *Rec. Prog. Horm. Res.* 35:501–32.

[15] FLIER, J. S., R. KAHN, and J. ROTH. 1979. Receptors, antireceptor antibodies and mechanisms of insulin resistance. *New Engl. J. Med.* 300:413–19.

[16] FLOYD, J. C., JR., S. S. FAJANS, S. PEK, and R. E. CHANCE. 1977. A newly recognized pancreatic polypeptide: plasma levels in health and disease. *Rec. Prog. Horm. Res.* 33:519–70.

[17] FOÀ, P. P. 1973. Glucagon: an incomplete and biased review with selected references. *Amer. Zool.* 13:613–23.

[18] FOÀ, P. P., G. GALANSINO, and G. POZZA. 1957. Glucagon, a second pancreatic hormone. *Rec. Prog. Horm. Res.* 13:473–510.

[19] GABBAY, K. H. 1980. The insulinopathies. *New Engl. J. Med.* 302:165–67.

[20] GIVEN, B. D., M. E. MAKO, H. S. TAGER, D. BALDWIN, J. MARKESE, A. H. RUBENSTEIN, J. OLEFSKY, M. KOBAYASHI, O. KOLTERMAN, and R. POUCHER. 1980. Diabetes due to secretion of an abnormal insulin. *New Engl. J. Med.* 302:129–35.

[21] HAZELWOOD, R. L., S. D. TURNER, J. R. KIMMEL, and H. G. POLLOCK. 1973. Spectrum effects of a new polypeptide (third hormone?) isolated from chicken pancreas. *Gen. Comp. Endocrinol.* 21:485–97.

[22] JOHNSON, D. G., C. U. GOEBEL, V. J. HRUBY, M. D. BREGMAN, and D. TRIVEDI. 1982. Hyperglycemia of diabetic rats decreased by a glucagon receptor antagonist. *Science* 215:1115–16.

[23] KASUGA, M., F. A. KARLSSON, and C. R. KAHN. 1982. Insulin stimulates phosphorylation of the 95,000 dalton subunit of its own receptor. *Science* 215:185–87.

[24] KIMBALL, C. P., and J. R. MURLIN. 1923. Aqueous extracts of pancreas. III. Some precipitation reaction of insulin. *J. Biol. Chem.* 58:337–46.

[25] KIMMEL, J. R., L. J. HAYDEN, and H. G. POLLOCK. 1975. Isolation and characterization of a new pancreatic polypeptide hormone. *J. Biol. Chem.* 250:9369–76.

[26] KORC, M., D. OWERBACH, C. QUINTO, and W. J. RUTTER. 1981. Pancreatic islet-acinar cell interaction: amylase messenger RNA levels are determined by insulin. *Science* 213:351–53.

[27] LACY, P. E., and M. H. GREIDER. 1979. Anatomy and ultrastructural organization of pancreatic islets. In *Endocrinology*, vol. 2, eds L. J. DeGroot, G. F. Cahill, Jr., L. Martini, D. H. Nelson, W. D. Odell, J. T. Potts, Jr., E. Steinberger, and A. I. Winegrad, pp. 907–19. New York: Grune & Stratton, Inc.

[28] LARNER, J., K. CHENG, C. SCHWARTZ, K. KIKUCHI, S. TAMURA, S. CREACY, R. DUBLER, G. GALASKO, C. PULLIN, and M. KATZ. 1982. A proteolytic mechanism for the action of insulin via oligopeptide mediator formation. *Fed. Proc.* 41:2724–29.

[29] MATSCHINSKY, F. M., A. A. PAGLIARA, W. S. ZAWALICH, and M. D. TRUS. 1979. Metabolism of pancreatic islets and regulation of insulin and glucagon secretion. In *Endocrinology*, vol. 2, eds. L. J. DeGroot, G. F. Cahill, Jr., L. Martini, D. H. Nelson, W. D. Odell, J. T. Potts, Jr., E. Steinberger, and A. I. Winegrad, pp. 935–49. New York: Grune & Stratton, Inc.

[30] MAURER, A. C. 1979. The therapy of diabetes. *Am. Scientist* 67:422–31.

[31] McCumbee, W. D., and R. L. Hazelwood. 1977. Biological evaluation of the third pancreatic hormone (APP)P hepatocyte and adipocyte effects. *Gen. Comp. Endocrinol.* 33:518–25.

[32] Müller, W. A., G. R. Faloona, E. Aguilar-Parada, and R. H. Unger. 1970. Abnormal alpha cell function in diabetes. Response to carbohydrate and protein injection. *New Engl. J. Med.* 283:109–15.

[33] Olefsky, J. M., and G. M. Reaven. 1977. Insulin binding to diabetes: relationships with plasma insulin levels and insulin sensitivity. *Diabetes* 26:680–88.

[34] Peterson, J. D., D. F. Steiner, S. O. Edmin, and S. Falkmer. 1975. The amino acid sequence of the insulin from a primitive vertebrate, the Atlantic hagfish (*Myxine glutinosa*). *J. Biol. Chem.* 250:5183–91.

[35] Sanger, F. 1959. Chemistry of insulin. *Science* 129:1340–44.

[36] Schusdziarra, V., E. Zyznar, D. Rouiller, J. C. Brown, A. Arimura, and R. H. Unger. 1980. Splanchnic somatostatin: a hormonal regulator of nutrient homeostasis. *Science* 207:530–32.

[37] Spiess, J., J. Rivier, J. Rodkey, C. Bennett, and W. Vale. 1979. Isolation and characterization of somatostatin from pigeon pancreas. *Proc. Natl. Acad. Sci. USA* 76:2974–78.

[38] Steiner, D. F., J. D. Peterson, and H. Tager. 1973. Comparative aspects of proinsulin and insulin structure and biosynthesis. *Amer. Zool.* 13:591–604.

[39] Steiner, D. F., and H. S. Tager. 1979. Biosynthesis of insulin and glucagon. In *Endocrinology*, vol. 2, eds. L. J. DeGroot, G. F. Cahill, Jr., L. Martini, D. H. Nelson, W. D. Odell, J. T. Potts, Jr., E. Steinberger, and A. I. Winegrad, pp. 921–34. New York: Grune & Stratton, Inc.

[40] Tager, H. S., C. Patzelt, R. K. Assoian, S. J. Chan, J. R. Duguid, and D. F. Steiner. 1980. Biosynthesis of islet cell hormones. *Ann. New York Acad. Sci.* 343:133–47.

[41] Unger, R. H., E. Aguilar-Parada, W. A. Muller, and A. M. Eisentraut. 1970. Studies of pancreatic alpha cell function in normal and diabetic subjects. *J. Clin. Invest.* 49:837–48.

[42] Unger, R. H., P. Raskin, C. B. Srikant, and L. Orci. 1977. Glucagon and the A cells. *Rec. Prog. Horm. Res.* 33:477–517.

[43] Unger, R. H., R. E. Dobbs, and L. Orci. 1978. Insulin glucagon, and somatostatin secretion in the regulation of metabolism. *Ann. Rev. Physiol.* 40:307–43.

[44] Unger, R. H., and L. Orci. 1981a. Glucagon and the A cell. *New Engl. J. Med.* 304:1518–24, 1575–80.

[45] ———, eds. 1981b. *Glucagon.* New York: Elsevier North-Holland, Inc.

12

GROWTH HORMONES

INTRODUCTION

A number of hormones are essential to normal body growth through their actions on bone and specialized organs such as the reproductive organs and the mammary glands. Although pituitary growth hormone (somatotropin, STH) is clearly associated with growth (Chapter 5), most of its actions are mediated indirectly through the effects of a group of polypeptide hormones, the *somatomedins*. Besides the important actions of insulin on carbohydrate and fat metabolism, this group of hormones plays an important role in growth regulation. *Prolactin*, of course, is necessary for mammary gland growth and development during the latter stage of pregnancy. *Placental lactogen* may prove to be significant in maternal and fetal growth during pregnancy. Other putative growth factors affect the growth, proliferation, and differentiation of specific cell types: nerve growth factor, erythrocyte-stimulating factor (erythropoietin), epidermal and fibroblast growth factors, platelet-derived growth factor, and a number of thymic factors (e.g., thymosin, thymopoietin, and serum thymic factor) [18].

Growth inhibiting factors, chalones, have been described. When more is known about their origin, synthesis, release, metabolism, and mechanisms of action, some of these factors may be considered as hormones. Certain steroid hormones, particularly androgens, play crucial roles in normal growth processes. Other steroid hormones, such as the glucocorticoids, and the thyroid hormones, are essential (permissive) for the growth-promoting activities of the polypeptide growth hormones. The individual roles of growth hormones and the integrated actions of the hormones in growth and development will be discussed.

GROWTH AND CELLULAR PROLIFERATION

All cells in the body are derived from a single cell, the fertilized egg. Although each cell possesses the same genetic information, there are many different kinds of cells. After repeated divisions of the egg to produce cells of a smaller, rather uniform cytoplasmic mass, the cells migrate and continue to divide to produce ultimately the embryo. During this process of cell division and subsequent tissue and organ formation it is believed that certain genes are turned on or off, a process which provides the regulatory cues for individual cell differentiation and function. In any organism certain cells are specialized to provide specific functions. Some make hemoglobin, some synthesize keratin, some produce antibodies, and others, such as the liver hepatocyte, participate in a wide spectrum of cellular activities.

There are apparently no alternative states of differentiation available to cells of any tissue type. These specialized cells are capable of only two gene-directed activities: They may differentiate for cell division by mitosis or they may differentiate for tissue function (phenotypic expression). Generally this latter option ultimately leads to the death of the cells involved. For example, cells of the basal layer of the epidermis must divide to replace cells lost from the skin surface. Once these cells leave the basal layer and migrate toward the surface of the skin they differentiate to make keratin, and their ultimate fate is to die and provide a cornified protective layer to the outer skin [6]. Some cell types can dedifferentiate and pass through a proliferative phase again. Nerve cells, in contrast, undergo an irreversible proliferative death (they cannot dedifferentiate) but not a cellular death.

Cells pass through specific stages in their life cycle [34]. The fully mature cell (e.g., skeletal muscle or nerve) is said to be in G_0 (G stands for gap) and is not committed to division (Fig. 12.1). These cells have varying life spans depending on their specific activities: Erythrocytes survive about 120 days in humans; some epithelial cells of the gut live only a few days; certain neurons in the brain may be as old as the individual. G_1 is a growth phase preparatory to S, the synthetic phase where the DNA is duplicated. The G_2 phase is not clearly defined functionally, but it is a short period (3 to 4 hours) where some protein synthesis occurs. During this time preparations are made for entry into the complex events of the next phase, mitosis (M). Fol-

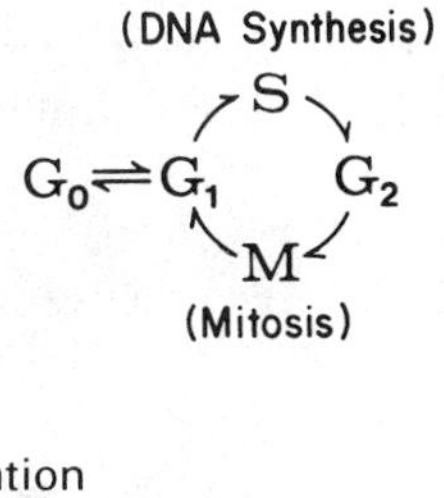

(DNA Synthesis)

$$G_0 \rightleftharpoons G_1 \quad \overset{\nearrow\ S\ \searrow}{\underset{\nwarrow\ M\ \swarrow}{}} \quad G_2$$

(Mitosis)

Figure 12.1 The mammalian cell cycle.

lowing mitosis, the daughter cells may reenter the proliferation cycle or may become resting G_0 cells.

The control point of cell division is believed to be at the transition from G_0 to G_1. Because chemical messengers affect cell division as well as differentiation, it is important to determine whether hormone effects are specific to certain phases of the cell cycle. Hormone receptors may vary in number throughout the cell cycle and thus affect the responsiveness of the cells to the actions of hormones. Cyclic nucleotides surely play important roles in cellular control mechanisms. According to the yin-yang hypothesis (Chapter 4), cyclic nucleotides may provide the stimulus for cell division or cellular differentiation (the nonmitotic state). Uncontrolled cell division is characteristic of cancer cells, and it has been claimed that some types of cancer cells contain elevated levels of cGMP. Failure of cells to divide, on the other hand, may result in loss of organ structure and function; aging of the nervous system may be one example. It is important, therefore, to understand the mechanisms by which growth-stimulating hormones affect cellular function.

SOMATOTROPIN AND THE SOMATOMEDINS

The pivotal role of pituitary growth hormone, now known as somatotropin (STH), in the control of growth has been firmly established. Congenital failure to synthesize and secrete STH leads to dwarfism; hypersecretion of STH, on the other hand, leads to gigantism if overproduction of the hormone is initiated early in life or to acromegaly if oversecretion occurs in the adult animal. Nevertheless, it was later discovered that the effects of STH on growth may be indirect and possibly mediated through other growth hormones.

Somatotropin causes growth of the epiphyseal regions of the long bones. Growth of bone can be monitored by measuring the incorporation of sulfur (^{35}S) into the epiphyseal cartilage. When bones from young animals are incubated in a medium containing normal serum and this radioactive isotope of sulfur, the sulfur is incorporated into the sulfated polysaccharides of the cartilage. However, when bones are incubated in serum from hypophysectomized animals, no incorporation of ^{35}S takes place. This was initially considered to be due to the lack of STH in the serum. When STH was added to serum from hypophysectomized animals, incorporation of the radioactive sulfur into cartilage still failed to occur. If, however, hypophysectomized animals were injected with STH some hours prior to blood collection, the serum supported the incorporation of the radioactive sulfur into bone. The conclusion was drawn that STH acts indirectly on bones by way of the production of a *sulfation factor* [37].

The sulfation factor is now known to consist of a complex of peptides collectively referred to as the *somatomedins* [43]. Injected radiolabeled STH rapidly localizes to the liver rather than to the epiphyses of the long bones. Somatomedins are secreted by the liver and possibly some other tissues in response to somatotropin stimulation. The somatomedins are not, however, stored within the liver; hence, the liver is not a source of extractable growth factors. Somatomedins are carried in the circulation by transport proteins which may decrease their clearance from the circulation and reduce their rate of tissue delivery. In humans synthesis of plasma somatomedin-binding proteins is STH dependent, but the mechanisms involved in the coordinate control of somatomedin and carrier protein production are unknown.

Somatomedin is generally used to refer to those growth factors found in the plasma that are under the control of STH, have insulinlike properties, and promote the incorporation of sulfate into cartilage (the "somatomedin hypothesis"). Five substances isolated from the plasma in pure or rather pure form fulfill these criteria: somatomedin A (SMA); somatomedin C (SMC); nonsuppressible insulinlike activity (NSILA-I and NSILA-II) or, as they are usually called, insulinlike growth factors I and II (IGF-I and IGF-II); and MSA (multiplication stimulating activity).

Certain purification procedures and the use of a variety of bioassays indicate that the somatomedins are chemically related but not identical in structure. The peptides bear some structural relationship to insulin and therefore exhibit some affinity for insulin receptors. Conversely, insulin at high concentration will bind to somatomedin receptors. The so-called nonsuppressible insulinlike activity present in the blood cannot be neutralized by antibodies against insulin. The amino acid sequence of these insulinlike growth factors, IGF-I and IGF-II, nevertheless, reveals a high degree of similarity to insulin. These polypeptides consist of 70 and 67 amino acid residues, respectively [24], and have a proinsulinlike structure with a shorter connecting peptide of 12 amino acids and an extension of eight residues at the A-chain terminus (Fig. 12.2). A close structural homology between SMC and IGF-I has also been shown.

Cells maintained in tissue culture generally require serum for growth. Because growth factors in serum are produced by certain cells in the body, and as all cells in an organism contain the same genetic information, it was postulated that some cells might grow in serum-free media by producing their own growth factors. Certain rat

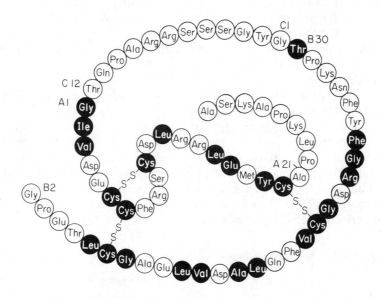

Figure 12.2 Primary structure of human IGF-I. The amino acids in black circles denote those in identical position in the A and B chain of human insulin. (From Humbel and Rinderknecht, [24], by permission.)

liver cells, for example, do not require serum for growth, and the conditioned medium from such cells has multiplication stimulating activity (MSA). MSA refers to a group of polypeptides which stimulates DNA synthesis and cell multiplication of normal fibroblasts in vitro. MSA stimulates sulfate incorporation into cartilage, binds to insulin and other somatomedin receptors, and its production is STH dependent. The primary structure of MSA from a strain of rat liver cells has been determined. The polypeptide consists of a single chain of 67 residues and displays 93% homology with human IGF-II. There are only five conservative amino acid differences between the sequences of rat MSA and human IGF-II and, on that basis, the term rat IGF-II has been proposed to refer to this polypeptide [30]. Specific receptors for MSA have been identified in four systems: human skin fibroblast, a rat liver cell line, the chick embryo fibroblast, and purified rat liver membranes.

Insulin is more potent in stimulating metabolic effects in insulin target tissues than are the somatomedins IGF-I and IGF-II. On the other hand, insulin is a less potent stimulator of cell proliferation than these growth factors. In vivo, more than 95% of the plasma somatomedins seem to be tightly bound to specific carrier proteins, and these complexes are rather impermeable to the vascular lining. Therefore, the bioavailability of serum somatomedins to the tissues is restricted to the low concentrations of free somatomedins, concentrations too small to elicit insulinlike effects in vivo. These concentrations, however, are probably high enough to allow for the growth-promoting effects of the somatomedins. The somatomedin receptors are believed to be structurally related to the insulin receptors; a generic term, isoreceptor, for these membrane components has been suggested [4].

Another peptide, referred to as somatomedin B, is stimulatory to cell proliferation and appears to be STH dependent. However, it lacks cartilage sulfation activity and does not interact with insulinlike receptors. In addition its structure is not similar to that of insulin or other insulinlike peptides (Fig. 12.3). This polypeptide, as expected, has a different spectrum of biological activity and does not compete in the MSA or the somatomedin A radioreceptor assays [33]. Depending on the strict definition of the term somatomedin B may or may not be considered a somatomedin, although it is a growth-stimulating peptide.

Somatomedins inhibit basal activity of adenylate cyclase in membrane preparations of fat cells, liver, and spleen lymphocytes of the rat and in chondrocytes of chick embryos. Hormone-stimulated adenylate cyclase enzyme activity is also inhibited by somatomedins. In human peripheral lymphocytes somatomedins inhibit basal adenylate cyclase activity and stimulate guanylate cyclase activity. It is interesting that somatomedins, like insulin, may manifest their actions through an inhibition of adenylate cyclase. Thus, a lowering of cyclic AMP concentrations and an elevation of cyclic GMP levels may be a common feature of cellular growth as affected by growth-promoting hormones.

```
              5                  10                 15                 20
 Asp-Gln-Glu-Ser-Cys-Lys-Gly-Arg-Cys-Thr-Glu-Gly-Phe-Asn-Val-Asp-Lys-Lys-Cys-Gln-Cys-Asp─┐
                                                                                           │
             25                 30                 35                 40                    │
   └─Glu-Leu-Cys-Ser-Tyr-Tyr-Gln-Ser-Asn-Cys-Thr-Cys-Tyr-Thr-Ala-Glu-Cys-Lys-Pro-Gln-Val-Thr
```

Figure 12.3 Primary structure of human somatomedin B.

Although somatomedins apparently play a significant role in fetal growth, levels of somatomedins in the circulation are reported to be low in the fetus and in early postnatal life. It has been proposed that fetal and early postnatal growth is regulated by an embryonic form of somatomedin [41]. Embryonic somatomedin production is independent of the pituitary and is said to be produced from all fetal cells. Embryonic somatomedin is present in high concentration in the fetal circulation and declines when adult somatomedins are produced. Thus, there may be hormonal forms of somatomedins that are specific to the fetus and alter with maturation, an observation that "may prove to be a general principle of fetal endocrinology" [41].

INSULIN

Although insulin plays the dominant role in the control of carbohydrate metabolism in humans and other vertebrates, it also profoundly affects growth processes in animals. Diabetic children, for example, fail to grow even though somatotropin levels are normal, whereas infants of mothers with islet hyperplasia and hyperinsulinism have increased stature. This might not be too surprising considering the structural similarities between insulin and some somatomedins. The growth-promoting actions of insulin are amply documented, and protein catabolism is accelerated in the absence of insulin. Insulin is required for the full anabolic effect of STH, an action that may be because insulin, through its action on glucose uptake by muscle, provides the energy substrates necessary for protein synthesis. However, insulin also increases the incorporation of amino acids into muscle by an action that is independent of its effects on glucose metabolism. This may result from the direct action of insulin on the transport of amino acids into cells as well as activation of ribosomal translational capacity, as protein synthesis per se is not dependent on glucose availability or RNA synthesis. Insulin stimulates the growth of immature hypophysectomized rats, but this action is manifested only when the protein-sparing action of insulin is enhanced by the concomitant feeding of a high carbohydrate diet. Similarly, insulin levels are decreased in Laron dwarfism, suggesting that insulin may play a permissive role in STH action on the generation of somatomedin by the liver.

Insulin at a high concentration, as in familial insulin resistance, stimulates general body growth through low-affinity binding to somatomedin receptors. Although there is insulin-receptor deficiency in this endocrinopathy, the number of somatomedin receptors appears to be normal. The high circulating levels of insulin thus cause acral (affecting the extremities) overgrowth as well as enlargement of the kidney and adrenal glands; these actions of insulin may result from cross-reactivity with somatomedin receptors [14].

PROLACTIN

In humans prolactin (PRL) plays an important role in milk synthesis, a function that of necessity requires development and growth of the mammary glands. Because of the close structural similarity between PRL and STH, it is not surprising that many effects of PRL are growth related and are usually involved in reproductive processes of the individual (Chapters 5, 19).

Prolactin, with estrogens and adrenal steroids, is essential for ductile branching during the prepubertal and postpubertal period to form the fully developed system of the mammary glands of the mature female. Large amounts of PRL, even in the absence of adequate amounts of estrogens (as occurs in prolactin-secreting tumors in men or postmenopausal women), are usually associated with clinically evident enlargement of the breasts [12]. Prolactin also stimulates production of somatomedins by the rat liver and could conceivably affect general body growth by an STH-like action.

Prolactin also affects directly the growth and function of the ovary and testes, in some cases by modulating the action of gonadotropins on the gonads. In nonmammalian vertebrates PRL has such growth-related actions as stimulation of tail and gill growth in amphibians. Prolactin is required for limb regeneration in the salamander and tail regeneration in lizards. Many structural changes in the skin of the salamander that are related to water drive involve the actions of PRL. Hypertrophy of the pigeon crop-sac mucosa as well as epidermal hyperplasia related to brood patch formation in the dove are regulated by PRL. Other physiological actions of this hormone are discussed in Chapters 5 and 19.

PLACENTAL LACTOGEN

During pregnancy the placenta secretes hormones which augment maternal pituitary and gonadal functions. In addition to chorionic gonadotropin and a number of steroids the placenta also synthesizes and secretes chorionic somatomammotropin. This protein hormone, although similar to somatotropin in structure, lacks significant growth-promoting activity but displays considerable lactogenic activity and is therefore referred to as placental lactogen (PL). In the human PL is found in the maternal plasma as early as the sixth week of pregnancy and reaches a concentration three orders of magnitude greater than that of STH during the second trimester [3]. Placental lactogen is synthesized within the *syncytiotrophoblastic* epithelial cells of the chorionic villi of the placenta (Chapter 19).

Placental lactogen increases sulfate uptake into cartilage in hypophysectomized rats both in vivo and in vitro, and also stimulates growth and induction of milk protein synthesis in mouse mammary explants. Development and maturation of the testes of immature and genetically dwarf mice is also stimulated by PL. All these biological actions are similar to the actions of human prolactin. Placental lactogen mimics the action of STH on most of its target tissues but is much less potent than pituitary somatotropin. The physiological significance of any of these effects is unclear. There is, for example, no evidence that PL can increase linear growth in hypopituitary dwarfs [42]. It might be expected, however, that this hormone evolved to play some specific role(s) related to pregnancy and reproductive processes. PL secretion during the second trimester of human pregnancy may supplement this action of choriogonadotropin on the corpus luteum which is diminishing [9]. In addition the primary role of PL may be to stimulate the development of the mammary glands during pregnancy without actually causing milk secretion. Pituitary prolactin then initiates milk secretion soon after parturition. It has been suggested that PL may alter the maternal metabolism so that adequate supplies of glucose, amino acids,

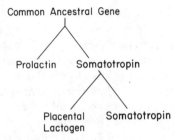

Figure 12.4 Hypothetical scheme for the evolution of somatotropin, prolactin, and placental lactogen [42].

and minerals are available to the fetus during the latter part of pregnancy, a time when fetal growth requirements are rapidly increasing.

Human placental lactogen and STH are both single-chain polypeptides containing 191 amino acid residues. Both hormones are internally cross linked through two disulfide bridges and are identical throughout 85% of their primary structures; 162 residues in each polypeptide are identical and occupy similar positions in the hormones. The high degree of structural similarity between hPL and human and ovine STH suggests that the polypeptide arose from a relatively recent duplication of an STH gene (Fig. 12.4), rather than from the more distantly related lactogenic hormones [3]. A placental lactogen immunologically similar to hPL is present in the plasma of the rhesus monkey, baboon, chinchilla, hamster, goat, cow, sheep, and a number of other mammalian species. In general the level of the placental lactogen begins to rise at or before midpregnancy and usually remains elevated until term [25].

NERVE GROWTH FACTOR

Growth and differentiation of sensory and motor components of the peripheral nervous system are enhanced by factors released from peripheral target tissues. On the other hand, an intact innervation and release of supporting substances from nerve endings are essential for normal development of the innervated target tissues. There is accumulating evidence that specific chemical messengers are important in these reciprocal actions between nerves and target tissues.

Certain mouse sarcomas induce a pathologic hypertrophy of chick embryonic sensory and sympathetic ganglia [27]. This neuronal hypertrophy depends on a humoral protein factor released by the transplanted tumors. This substance was named nerve growth factor (NGF) and its chemistry and biological roles have been well characterized [20]. NGF is also present in snake venom and in the submandibular salivary glands of adult male mice. NGF is synthesized within tubular cells of the submandibular gland and its production is androgen dependent. Salivary gland NGF levels in female mice rise during pregnancy and lactation when androgen levels are elevated. Testosterone given to female mice causes tubular cell hypertrophy and the content of salivary gland NGF rises markedly. In contrast, castration of male mice causes submandibular tubule atrophy and the salivary gland content of NGF falls dramatically. The functional significance of NGF in salivary glands, snake venom glands, and tumors is unknown.

Removal of the submaxillary glands from adult mice produces a reduction in the serum concentration of NGF in both sexes, indicating that the normal circulating levels of NGF are dependent on these glands. Evidence suggests that NGF in blood and tissues is not, however, solely derived from salivary glands but is also produced in other undefined endogenous tissues. Nerve growth factor is synthesized by a variety of normal and tumor tissues; in addition to transformed fibroblasts primary explant fibroblasts synthesize NGF. Cells of neural crest origin are also capable of synthesizing NGF, as are muscle cells. In humans normal levels of NGF do not differ between males and females. No other species, of either sex, contains the high level of the hormone found in the mouse. In other mammals the exact site(s) of synthesis and subsequent method of delivery of NGF to its putative target tissues is still obscure.

Peripheral sympathetic neurons (postganglionic neurons of the autonomic nervous system, see Chapter 14) are the primary target cells for NGF and respond to the protein throughout life. Injections of NGF antiserum in newborn mice or chick embryos cause almost complete destruction of the sympathetic nervous system (immunosympathectomy). Exposure in utero to maternal antibodies to NGF, in addition to producing immunosympathectomy, destroys peripheral nervous system sensory neurons in the dorsal root ganglia. These neurons may depend on NGF for survival during prenatal development [5]. Other dorsal root cells may manifest a temporal difference in their dependence on NGF. NGF antiserum administration to adult animals causes deleterious effects on sympathetic neurons which are reversible after antiserum treatment is stopped. Thus, it appears that an endogenous NGF is critical for sympathetic nervous system development, and NGF may function in the maintenance of sympathetic neurons throughout life.

Mouse salivary gland NGF is a molecular complex consisting of three types of polypeptide chains, designated α, β, and γ [21]. Each of these subunits consists of a pair of molecules. The β subunit is clearly a dimer of identical chains. Only the β moiety possesses nerve growth-promoting activity. NGF is synthesized as a precursor peptide, a proNGF. The individual β chains of NGF are then cleaved by the γ subunit which is an endopeptidase. The active form of NGF consists of 118 amino acid residues and includes three interchain disulfide bonds. The α subunits apparently play a role in maintaining the functional integrity of the molecular complex of NGF. It is not known whether the individual monomer subunit or the dimer complex of NGF is the active form of the hormone.

There is apparent homology between NGF and proinsulin and there are also striking similarities between the biological activities of the two molecules. Both hormones bind initially to cell membranes which results in an enhancement of a number of ensuing anabolic processes, such as RNA synthesis, polysome formation, and protein and lipid synthesis, that are characteristic of cellular growth. NGF may be viewed as a protein hormone whose structural gene may have evolved from an ancestral proinsulin gene and whose mode of action on neurons might, therefore, be somewhat similar to that of insulin on its target tissues [5]. Insulin and proinsulin can compete for the binding of NGF to a limited extent, further emphasizing the relationship of NGF to proinsulin.

After an initial interaction with the cell plasma membrane, NGF is internalized and, by retrograde axonal transport, apparently carried to the soma of the cell. Retrograde transport of NGF is specific as other proteins of similar size and charge are transported to a much lesser extent. It is interesting that insulin may be similarly internalized in its target cells to invoke its cellular effects [20]. Binding of NGF is specific to target tissue surface receptors because motor neurons which can internalize and transport tetanus toxin fail to do so with NGF. Similarly, cholinergic parasympathetic nerves, which like motor neurons are refractory to the biological actions of NGF, do not transport NGF.

Although NGF is internalized and transported to the perikaryon of individual neurons, there is no evidence that NGF reaches the nucleus or that its actions are indeed manifested intracellularly. For example, NGF injected into the cytoplasm of pheochromocytoma cells does not induce fiber outgrowth, as when added to the culture medium. Furthermore, antibodies to NGF introduced into the cytoplasm do not prevent fiber outgrowth evoked by NGF when added to the culture medium. These observations suggest that a second messenger may be required for the action of NGF at the plasma membrane [22].

An adrenomedullary clonal rat cell line responds to NGF and provides a unique model system for studying the action of the polypeptide hormone. NGF increases cAMP levels within these cells and affects quantitative changes in the rates of synthesis of existing proteins. cAMP analogs cause similar quantitative changes in these proteins. Thus, strong evidence exists that NGF mediates its effects, at least on these cells, through cAMP [13].

NGF exerts a pleiotropic effect on nerve cells which includes the synthesis of specific enzymes, tyrosine hydroxylase and dopamine β-hydroxylase, involved in adrenergic nervous transmission. The stimulation by NGF of nerve fiber outgrowth is reflected in the accumulation of large masses of neurofilaments that are found in developing axons. Neurite outgrowth in response to NGF is an RNA-independent event, which suggests that NGF may stimulate fiber outgrowth by acting in a selective fashion on protein synthesis at a stage after transcription. Ornithine decarboxylase is a key enzyme in the biosynthesis of polyamines and may serve an important regulatory role in cell division and growth. In the brain the intraventricular injection of NGF leads to a marked increase in the activity of this enzyme. Adrenal glucocorticoids appear to be required for NGF to enhance the activity of ornithine decarboxylase.

Clearly, NGF functions in the survival of peripheral sympathetic and spinal sensory neurons during defined periods of their ontogenesis. In addition NGF directs growing sympathetic nerve fibers toward their corresponding target tissues. Although it is believed that target cells innervated by the sympathetic neurons manufacture and secrete small amounts of NGF, there is no evidence for a preferential synthesis and storage of NGF by sympathetically innervated end organs. The continued availability of NGF to sympathetic neurons is nevertheless essential for neuron survival [27].

OTHER PEPTIDE GROWTH FACTORS

Other peptide growth factors have been discovered and it is likely still others will be found in the future. Although their physiological roles are unclear, these factors are important tools for the study of the growth requirements of cells maintained in tissue culture [18]. These peptides also provide important insights into evolution of hormone structure and common mechanisms of hormone action. These growth factors may eventually prove to be of immense medical importance.

Epidermal Growth Factor

Administration of partially purified nerve growth factor from mouse submaxillary glands to newborn mice results in early opening of the eyelids and precocious eruption of the teeth. A heat-stable protein, distinct from NGF, was isolated from these extracts which possessed the ability to accelerate tooth eruption and eyelid opening in neonatal mice and rats. The biological activity was subsequently found to be due to a direct stimulation of the proliferation and keratinization of epidermal tissue. Autoradiography using [³H]thymidine revealed that this *epidermal growth factor* (EGF) enhanced cell proliferation in the basal layer of the skin.

Mouse EGF consists of 53 amino acids and is conformationally restricted by three intrachain disulfide bonds (Fig. 12.5). EGF is found within the salivary gland combined with an EGF-binding protein which is an arginine esterase. This observation is interesting because NGF is also found within the submaxillary glands. NGF is associated with other proteins, and one of the subunits of this complex is also an arginine esterase, which may be similar but not identical to the EGF-binding esterase as the latter does not complex with NGF. EGF and NGF appear to be derived from inactive precursors and the biosynthesis and activation of both may be similar, perhaps under the control of the same genetic locus. This is further substantiated by the discovery that the synthesis of both peptides is androgen dependent.

Release of the peptide from the salivary glands (in mice) may be under nervous system control because α-adrenergic agonists increase serum levels of EGF, as does electrical stimulation of the superior cervical ganglia. Although mouse EGF is found in duct cells of the submaxillary glands, these glands are not the sole source of the peptide as removal of the glands does not eliminate immunoreactive EGF-like material from the blood.

In addition to effects on tooth eruption, eyelid opening, and skin proliferation in the neonate and embryo EGF stimulates growth in a number of cultured normal epithelial cells. EGF is without effect on tissues of mesodermal origin. In epithelia EGF rapidly stimulates the transport of small molecules into cells, which is followed by an increase in the rate of RNA synthesis and a conversion of preexisting ribosomes

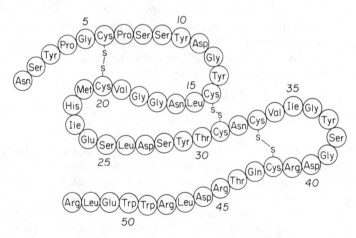

Figure 12.5 Primary structure of mouse epidermal growth factor (EGF).

into polysomes. As for most other growth factors, no clear effect of EGF on cyclic nucleotide activity has been demonstrated.

The initial action of EGF is to interact with specific plasma membrane receptors; this results in a complex program of biochemical and morphological events which ultimately result in cellular growth and proliferation. One consequence of the binding of EGF to its membrane receptor is a rapid activation of a cyclic AMP-independent phosphorylating system [8]. The mechanism by which EGF stimulates protein phosphorylation through activation of cellular protein kinase(s) is unknown. Other investigators have noted increased protein phosphorylation by growth-promoting agents; this suggests that a mitogen-sensitive phosphorylation system might be an important biochemical aspect of the control of cell proliferation.

EGF, like insulin and other growth factors, is internalized after initial binding to the plasma membrane. The significance of the internalization of EGF and its receptor in the mechanism of action of this growth factor and in the general action of other polypeptide hormones is unclear. Internalization of a hormonal ligand could, on the other hand, provide a mechanism for degradation of the hormone. Another feature of EGF and insulin is that both induce the loss of their specific receptors. This may involve a ligand-induced adsorptive pinocytosis where the hormone-receptor complex is internalized and then degraded by lysosomes (Fig. 4.17).

Some known biological effects of EGF in the mammal include the following: enhanced proliferation and differentiation (keratinization) of the epidermis; increased growth and maturation of the fetal pulmonary epithelium; stimulation of ornithine decarboxylase activity and DNA synthesis in the digestive tract; acceleration of the healing of wounds of the corneal epithelium; and phosphorylation of membrane and nuclear proteins. Human milk is mitogenic to a number of cultured cell lines, an activity neutralized by antibodies to human EGF. These observations and other experimental results identify EGF as a major growth-promoting agent in breast milk [7]. Because EGF is not entirely destroyed in the digestive tract, it might act directly on tissues of the digestive tract and may even be absorbed into the circulation to affect other tissues of the neonate. It is possible that EGF or other growth factors in the saliva may subserve other undiscovered physiological roles; most interesting is the discovery that EGF promotes plant shoot growth and possibly growth of roots. It has been hypothesized, therefore, that EGF or EGF-like substances may control plant community productivity [10]; that is, the presence of a growth factor, such as EGF, in the saliva of an herbivorous animal might provide the stimulus for plant regrowth after grazing. Many animals lick their wounds, an activity which could involve EGF.

A surprising finding is that peptic ulcer in humans undergoes remission during pregnancy, and urine contains a potent inhibitor of gastric acid secretion. This substance, *urogastrone*, consists of a single polypeptide chain of 53 residues with three disulfide bonds. It was then discovered that mouse EGF is of the same length and differs from urogastrone only in 16 of the 53 residues (Fig. 10.10). Urogastrone is a gastrointestinal peptide that is inhibitory to gastric acid (HCl) secretion directly at the level of the gastric mucosa. Urogastrone, like EGF, induces premature opening of eyes in young mice. Both peptides stimulate DNA synthesis within human fibroblasts and at submaximal concentrations their effects are additive. Binding data also reveal that they share the same receptor site on fibroblasts. Immunocytochemical studies indicate that cells of the human submandibular gland contain urogastrone-like activity. In the gastrointestinal tract urogastrone appears to be localized to cells

Other Peptide Growth Factors

of Brunner's glands. Urogastrone in the human and EGF in the mouse are known to be elevated during pregnancy. Because androgen levels are also elevated during pregnancy, it is possible that elevated levels of these peptides in the blood reflect the changing hormonal status of the female. Present evidence suggests, therefore, that urogastrone is the human hormonal equivalent of mouse EGF [23].

Fibroblast Growth Factor

Pituitary and brain extracts contain a *fibroblast growth factor* (FGF) which, in the presence of small amounts of a glucocorticoid, is able to stimulate proliferation of many cells of endodermal and mesodermal origin [17]. FGF is mitogenic for malignant adrenal cells and for normal bovine adrenal cortical cells in culture. ACTH inhibits the mitogenic effects of FGF and functions as the differentiated signal for these cells [18]. Epidermal growth factor is without effect on these cells and many other cells stimulated by FGF, thus demonstrating the difference in the mitogenic activities of these two peptides. FGF is also mitogenic for cells derived from human amniotic fluid, primate smooth muscle, primary cultures of rabbit ear chondrocytes, rabbit articular chondrocytes, and human glial cells. In contrast to its effect on mesoderm-derived cells, FGF is not mitogenic for cells which arise from embryonic ectoderm.

Ovarian granulosa cells maintained in tissue culture are highly sensitive to EGF and FGF, whereas LH and FSH are without such a mitogenic effect. Luteal cells, derived from granulosa cells by cytomorphosis, lose their sensitivity to EGF but retain their sensitivity to FGF. Thus during luteinization granulosa cells not only shift their sensitivity to gonadotropins (Chapter 18) but also to mitogens.

Nerves may release a trophic factor which is necessary for limb regeneration in some poikilothermic vertebrates. The chemical nature of the trophic principle(s) is unknown, but this factor(s) affects the mitotic rate and accumulation of blastema cells in the regenerating limb. Although this factor is not unique to nerve, it is present in nerve tissue in greater concentrations than in other tissues. This neurotrophic principle has been extracted from brain tissue and appears to be chemically and biologically similar to an FGF obtained from the pituitary gland. It induces proliferation of undifferentiated cells similar to that which takes place in a regeneration blastema. It is postulated that FGF is similar or identical to the neurotrophic factor promoting blastema formation. The primary structure of FGF is unknown.

Platelet-Derived Growth Factor

Whole blood serum is a requirement for the growth of certain cells (smooth muscle, fibroblasts, 3T3, and glial) in culture. Although there are many factors present in serum that are necessary for viability and growth of cells in culture, serum prepared from cell-free plasma has little or no mitogenic activity. This activity can, however, be restored by adding material released from blood platelets to sera. Thus, the mitogen principle in whole blood serum may be derived from platelets. This *platelet-derived growth factor* (PDGF) is released from platelets during platelet aggregation in the process of blood clot formation [40]. At sites of wounding the platelets adhere to the endothelial lining of the vessel in such a way as to plug the defect. Platelets also release one or more chemical messengers which stimulate contraction of the injured vessels to prevent further loss of blood. At sites of injury platelets release PDGF in response to thrombin. The role of PDGF at these sites may be to induce proliferation of smooth muscle cells within the arterial wall—the intima—as a component of a wound-healing process. Animals made thrombocytopenic with an antiplatelet serum fail to produce smooth muscle proliferative lesions in response to vessel injury. These lesions also fail to form in animals whose platelet function is inhibited by drugs (e.g., dipyridamole) which prevent platelet adhesion and granule release at sites of endothelial injury.

Although the structure of PDGF is undetermined, human PDGF consists of two glycopeptides, one with a molecular weight of 35,000 (PDGF-I) and the other of about 32,000 (PDGF-II). Each polypeptide consists of two subunits; it is possible that PDGF-II is derived by proteolytic cleavage of PDGF-I [1]. PDGF fulfills the biological criteria of a hormone in that it is released from a cell and acts at a low (nanomolar) concentration on particular target cells to elicit a specific response. PDGF is localized within α granules of the platelet; interaction of platelets with localized surfaces of damaged blood vessels provides for a site-specific release mechanism of PDGF to act as a local hormone. The wide distribution of smooth muscle cells throughout the body would, indeed, necessitate such a specialized mode of hormone delivery.

Atherosclerosis is recognized as a principal cause of death in the Western Hemisphere [39]. Atherosclerotic lesions are localized to the innermost layers of the artery wall—the tunica intima and tunica media. This disease process, which results from endothelial disruption due to a number of possible causes, involves smooth muscle proliferation, formation of large amounts of a collagen matrix by the proliferated smooth muscle cells, and the deposition of lipids within these cells and the surrounding connective tissue. These atherosclerotic plaques impede blood flow in affected vessels, which may lead to brain stroke, heart attack, or other complications, depending on the particular vascular bed concerned. Although PDGF serves an important role in the healing process of the vascular system, it may play a dominant part in the development of atherosclerosis. Therefore, PDGF may be used in the prevention and therapy of atherosclerosis to protect the endothelial cells from injury and to develop methods to inhibit platelet function that do not compromise concomitantly the roles of these cellular elements in blood coagulation [39].

ERYTHROPOIETIN

The circulating red cell mass in adult humans is remarkably constant. It has been estimated that a 70-kg individual has about 2.3×10^{13} red blood cells, and that, under normal conditions, they are synthesized at a rate of about 2.3×10^6 per second [16]. Exposure of individuals to high altitudes (low oxygen tension: hypoxia), however, results in increased *erythropoiesis* (Greek: *poietin*, to make), whereas hypertransfusion (hyperoxia) results in reduced erythropoiesis. The presence of an erythropoietic factor was implicated in a parabiotic experiment where subjection of one rat to hypoxia resulted in increased erythropoiesis in its parabiotic partner. Transfusion of plasma from anemic animals into normal animals causes erythropoiesis thus suggesting the existence of a humoral erythropoietic factor (*erythropoietin*, erythrocyte-stimulating factor, EP). Erythropoietin is elevated by conditions that create tissue hypoxia and decreased by conditions that create tissue hyperoxia. Agents that increase the metabolic rate and oxygen consumption, such as thyroid hormones, or pharmaceutical agents, such as dinitrophenol (an uncoupler of oxidative phosphorylation), produce a state of increased need for oxygen. Under these conditions EP is produced, which leads to increased erythropoiesis. Thus, the ratio of oxygen supply to oxygen need appears to determine the level of EP formation and, therefore, the stimulus to erythropoiesis [36].

Bilaterally nephrectomized rats, unlike intact animals, do not respond to phlebotomy (blood withdrawal) or red blood cell destruction by increased EP production. In humans EP levels are low in the serum of anephric patients, but, after successful renal transplantation, EP increases in the blood. Erythropoietic activity is detected in perfusates from isolated kidneys and is also produced by renal cell cultures in vitro. These data establish the kidney as a source of the erythropoietic factor. Erythropoietin levels are diminished after hypophysectomy and, like the somatomedins, is increased in response to somatotropin. It is also produced in response to androgen stimulation (Chapter 17). The mechanism of release of EP from the kidney is unknown, as is the nature of the receptors that sense lowered plasma levels. Current evidence suggests that the hypoxic state stimulates the release of prostaglandins from renal cortical tissues which then stimulate medullary EP-producing cells. Administration of EP antiserum to normal mice decreases erythropoiesis, providing support for the control of normal erythropoiesis by EP.

There are a number of hypotheses regarding the production and release of EP [19]. The *erythrogenin theory*, or REF theory, states that in response to hypoxia receptors of the juxtaglomerular apparatus, as well as some glomerular components, cause the release of an enzyme into the circulation. This enzyme is called renal erythropoietic factor (REF) or *erythrogenin*. At the same time, the liver releases an α-globulin, *erythropoietinogen*, into the circulation. According to this scheme, REF en-

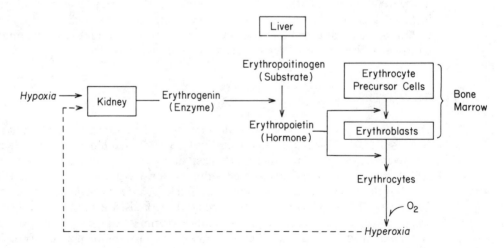

Figure 12.6 Erythrogenin theory for the biogenesis of erythropoietin.

zymatically cleaves off a portion of this protein, thus changing it into active EP which is carried to the bone marrow to act on stem cells (Fig. 12.6). The *proerythropoietin theory* states that the kidney releases a prohormone, called proerythropoietin, which is activated by a serum factor to yield *erythropoietin*. Support for either of these theories is based on the fact that a factor, extracted from the kidneys, is capable of generating EP when incubated with plasma.

Although the kidney is the primary source of EP, EP is also known to originate in other tissues. Evidence has shown that a low basal rate of erythropoiesis is maintained by both anephric patients and those with chronic renal failure. This extrarenal source of EP may be the liver; because the liver is the primary producer of fetal erythropoietin, it may maintain some degree of that function until adulthood. In the presence of intact kidneys the liver would play an insignificant role in EP production, but if the kidneys were nonfunctional or removed, the liver's role would be of greater importance. Erythropoietin is found in the plasma and urine of many mammalian species as well as in birds and fishes.

Because of a lack of adequate sources of material, the structure of EP is unknown. Plasma EP is a sialo-protein with a molecular weight of 46,000. This protein may, however, be a dimer as urinary EP has a molecular weight of 23,000 daltons. This glycoprotein contains over 25% carbohydrate, consisting of sialic acid and a number of sugars. The sialic acid residues are necessary for biological activity in vivo as in the asialo form it is cleared too rapidly by the liver.

The effects of EP are not noted until 2 to 3 days after stimulation, due to the time it takes for reticulocytes to mature. The half-life of EP, however, is only about 5 hours. This implies that a continuous supply of erythropoietin is not necessary for developing erythroblasts; all that may be needed is a priming stimulus. The role of EP is to enhance proliferation of erythrocyte precursor cells in bone marrow (or fetal liver) into erythroblasts (cells determined to become erythrocytes) and to stimulate proliferation of newly formed erythroblasts. Stimulation of RNA synthesis is the primary nuclear event in the molecular mechanism of EP action. Experiments suggest that EP has its primary effect on the cytoplasmic membrane of marrow cells to produce an active cytoplasmic protein intermediate that interacts with the nucleus to stimulate synthesis of a variety of RNA's. DNA synthesis, cell division, and maturation (hemoglobin synthesis) in the responsive cells follow. The role of cyclic nucleotides as intermediates is postulated but not clearly understood [16].

Anemia results from any of a number of events that lead to hemorrhage, hemolysis, or decreased red blood cell production by bone marrow. Some patients with rheumatoid arthritis, chronic infection, and other malignancies may become anemic because of lowered EP levels. Neuraminidase (a sialase enzyme) inactivates EP and may play a role in producing anemia in some previously mentioned conditions. Chronic renal disease with progressive loss of renal mass also results in decreased production of EP.

Polycythemia (enhanced erythrocyte proliferation) is due to several etiologic factors; in some cases an inappropriate increase in EP production is the causative factor. Because erythropoietin induces marked reticulocytosis and pronounced increases in the circulating red cell mass, EP may have potential therapeutic value in the management of certain anemias in which responsive stem cells and erythroid precursors are available but EP plasma levels are low.

THYMIC HORMONES

The thymus gland is a lobular organ which lies in the upper thorax above the heart and in front of the aorta (Fig. 12.7). In humans and other mammals the thymus begins to atrophy shortly after puberty. Removal of the gland in the adult animal usually causes no harmful effects. On this basis the thymus was considered to be an organ without a function. It is now realized that the thymus is an endocrine organ which plays a pivotal role in the development of immunological competence [28].

Thymectomy of mice immediately after birth results in a wasting disease characterized by severe depletion of white blood cells, specifically lymphocytes. Certain lymphocytes synthesize antibodies and, without such molecules, an animal cannot mount any immunological defense. In addition in the absence of antibody production an immune imbalance may contribute to the etiology of many diseases. Reimplantation of the thymus into young mice prevents the animals from developing the wasting disease; lymphocytes are produced and the animals are capable of developing an immunological response. A rather puzzling observation, however, was that the lymphocytes in animals receiving a thymus graft were of host origin. It had been thought that the thymus was the source of all the animal's lymphocytes. The results suggested that the thymus was responsible for stimulating proliferation of host lymphocytes. Was the thymus gland the source of a lymphocyte-stimulating hormone? The definitive answer came from an experiment where a thymus gland was placed in a small plastic capsule with pores so small that no thymus or other cells could escape or enter. Molecules could, however, pass freely in and out through the pores of the capsule. Young mice receiving only a plastic capsule implant developed the wast-

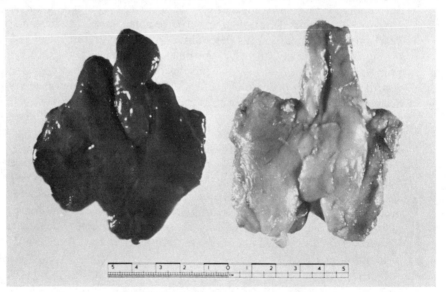

Figure 12.7 Thymus glands from a 9-year-old girl (left) and an 80-year-old man (right). Although size and shape were similar, the gland from the older person was yellow in color and fatty. (From Kendall, Johnson, and Singh. "The weight of the human thymus gland at necropsy." J. Anat. 131:485–499, 1980 [26], Cambridge University Press, London.)

ing disease. Mice receiving a capsule containing a thymus gland, on the other hand, grew and survived like normal animals and were capable of developing an immunological response. The results clearly indicated that the thymus might produce a hormone whose role was to activate lymphocytes for antibody production. An attempt to isolate such a factor from the thymus would be the next step to determine if it indeed were capable of stimulating lymphocyte antibody production.

It was eventually demonstrated that a partially purified thymus gland preparation, termed *thymosin fraction five*, could correct some of the immunological deficiencies resulting from a lack of thymic function in a number of animal models, as well as humans with primary and secondary immunodeficiency diseases [16]. This thymosin fraction induced lymphocyte differentiation and enhanced immunologic function in genetically athymic mice, adult thymectomized mice, and strains of mice with autoimmune reactions. Several thymosin fractions are active in various immunological assays, but only a few have been chemically characterized.

Generalized Roles

White blood cells (leukocytes) are produced in the bone marrow. Stem cells in this hemopoietic tissue give rise to the following white blood cell types: granulocytes (neutrophils, eosinophils, basophils), monocytes (which give rise to some macrophages), and lymphocytes. Lymphocytes may reside within the thymus gland or pass on through to compose a body of circulating T (thymus-derived) lymphocytes. Other lymphocytes of bone cell origin (B lymphocytes) establish themselves in other lymphoid tissues where they can become transformed into plasma cells which secrete antibodies.

The T lymphocytes become competent to participate in the immune response by actual passage through the thymus, where they come into contact with one or more thymic hormones, or, alternatively, they are stimulated to become immunologically competent in response to humoral factors (hormones) released by the thymus. Both processes may be components of the maturation process of T lymphocytes. The fully differentiated T cells play a variety of roles in the immune response: They function as killer cells to combat tumor cell development; they release substances (lymphokines) that affect macrophage function; and they may function as helper cells with B cells in antibody production. The lymphocytes are considered to represent a complex group of cells derived from a common origin which are related by a linear or a branching differentiation [15]. The large number of diversely differentiated lymphocytes and other white blood cells are poorly understood. The processes that determine the commitment to any one of the pathways of differentiation may be under hormonal control. Clearly, the thymus may be a key element in the complex program, culminating in the fully developed immune system. Abnormalities of thymic function may, on the other hand, be responsible for some pathologies related to the immune system. Excess activity of certain lymphocytes may lead to hyperimmune conditions or to immunological deficiencies such as agammaglobulinemia (total inability to produce antibodies). Failure of the thymus to develop is manifested in DiGeorge's syndrome, which is characterized by a seriously deficient immune system usually revealed by an abnormal reaction to vaccination.

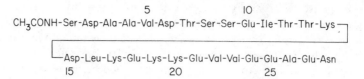

$$CH_3CONH-Ser-Asp-Ala-Ala-Val-Asp-Thr-Ser-Ser-Glu-Ile-Thr-Thr-Lys$$
$$—Asp-Leu-Lys-Glu-Lys-Lys-Glu-Val-Val-Glu-Glu-Ala-Glu-Asn$$

5   10

15   20   25

Figure 12.8 Primary structure of bovine thymosin α_1.

The Thymosins

Thymosin is generally used to designate a biologically active class of substances found within extracts of the thymus gland. Subfractionations and purification of these extracts have yielded specific thymosin polypeptides whose primary structures have been determined.

A thymosin polypeptide (thymosin α_1) was isolated from calf thymus that consists of 28 amino acid residues and is highly active in several bioassay systems (Fig. 12.8). This polypeptide is probably derived from a larger precursor molecule and appears to be identical to a similar polypeptide derived from other species (human, pig, sheep, chinchilla, and mouse) [15]. The structure of thymosin β_4 has also been reported (Fig. 12.9). This polypeptide appears to act on stem cells to form prothymocytes, whereas thymosin α_1 may act on prothymocytes to induce their differentiation to more mature T cells [15]. Thymosin β_4 is also found in high concentrations in tissues other than the thymus.

Thymosins are being used in clinical tests with children with primary immunodeficiency diseases. No undesirable side effects have been noted and significant clinical improvement has been indicated [15]. Immune modulation using thymosins is being considered in the field of immunotherapy for the treatment of cancer. Thymosins appear to trigger maturational progression of several early stages of T-cell development and to augment the capacity of certain mature T cells to respond to antigens. One action of the thymosins may be to act through cGMP to induce the expression of alloantigens on the surface of T cells as they develop their functional capacity for immunological competence.

Thymopoietin

A substance originally named thymic factor but now referred to as thymopoietin was isolated from the bovine thymus and found to induce differentiation of bone mar-

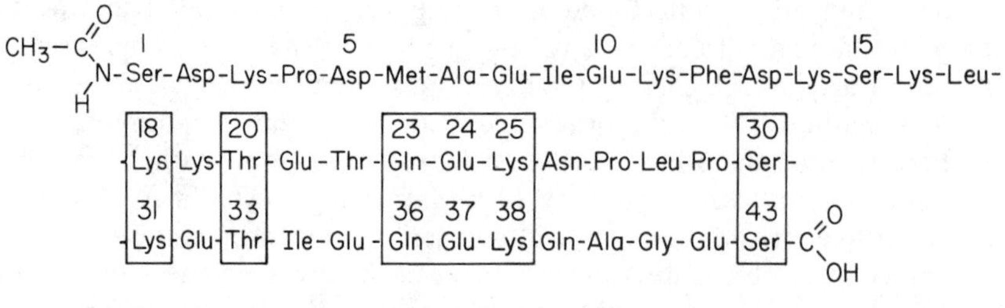

$$CH_3-C(=O)-N(H)-Ser-Asp-Lys-Pro-Asp-Met-Ala-Glu-Ile-Glu-Lys-Phe-Asp-Lys-Ser-Lys-Leu-$$

1   5   10   15

18 | 20 | 23 24 25 | 30
-Lys-Lys-Thr- Glu - Thr - Gln - Glu - Lys -Asn-Pro-Leu-Pro-Ser-

31 | 33 | 36 37 38 | 43
-Lys-Glu-Thr- Ile - Glu - Gln - Glu - Lys -Gln-Ala-Gly- Glu -Ser-C(=O)OH

Figure 12.9 Primary structure of bovine thymosin β_4. The residues 31–43 are aligned with residues 18–30 to indicate regions of internal duplication [15].

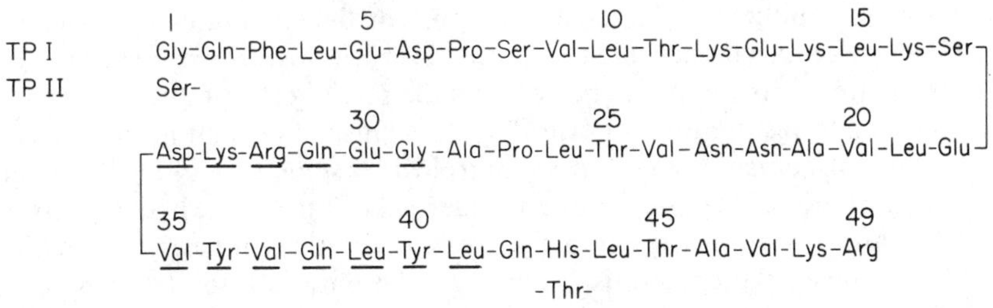

```
        |            5              10             15
TP I    Gly-Gln-Phe-Leu-Glu-Asp-Pro-Ser-Val-Leu-Thr-Lys-Glu-Lys-Leu-Lys-Ser┐
TP II   Ser-                                                                  │
                30             25             20                              │
    ┌Asp-Lys-Arg-Gln-Glu-Gly -Ala-Pro-Leu-Thr-Val -Asn-Asn-Ala-Val-Leu-Glu─┘
    │
    │ 35            40             45             49
    └Val-Tyr-Val-Gln-Leu-Tyr-Leu-Gln-His-Leu-Thr-Ala-Val-Lys-Arg
                            -Thr-
```

Figure 12.10 Primary structure of bovine thymopoietin I (TPI) and thymopoietin (TPII). The tridecapeptide sequence (underlined) is fully biologically active.

row cells to T lymphocytes. This putative hormone is composed of 49 amino acids (Fig. 12.10). Two closely related polypeptides, thymopoietin I and II, were isolated; they differ by two residues and probably represent isohormonal variants in cattle. Synthetic thymopoietin has been prepared and found to be biologically active. A synthetic tridecapeptide fragment of thymopoietin possesses the same full biological activity as the entire molecule (Fig. 12.10).

Serum Thymus Factor

A factor secreted by the thymic epithelium has been isolated from normal mouse and pig sera and named serum thymic factor (STF). This peptide normalizes a number of immune responses in athymic or thymectomized mice [2]. The nonapeptide amino acid sequence of STF has been determined (Fig. 12.11). Synthetic STF possesses all the biological activity of the natural peptide: It enhances the generation of alloantigen-reactive cytotoxic T cells in thymectomized mice, induces production of suppressor T cells in mice, and is a lymphocyte mitogen in vitro and in vivo.

Thymic Humoral Factor

Another factor has been isolated from the calf thymus which possesses a wide range of biological activities. This thymic humoral factor (THF) reestablishes the immune response in thymectomized mice and restores cellular graft versus host reactivity. THF is reported to be composed of 31 amino acid residues; its primary structure is unknown.

CHALONES

Many hormones stimulate synthetic processes within cells of their target tissues. An increase in cell function and cell size (hypertrophy) is often followed by cell proliferation (hyperplasia). As noted, growth factors are potent mitogens. Mitotic activity of the many tissues of the body is variable. Brain cells, for example, seldom divide,

Gln-Ala-Lys-Ser-Gln-Gly-Gly-Ser-Asn

Figure 12.11 Primary structure of bovine serum thymic factor (STF).

whereas epithelial cells, especially those of the epidermis or the intestinal lining, divide at a much higher rate to replace those cells lost from the surface. When epidermal cells are destroyed by tissue damage, the rate of cell production in the basal layer increases to restore the lost cells [29]. A balance of cellular mitotic activity could probably not be maintained unless controlled by some type of feedback mechanism. The critical moment in the life of an epidermal cell may be when it emerges from mitosis: It must prepare for division again or for keratin synthesis and death [6].

When the epidermis is damaged the mitotic rate of nearby cells is enhanced. It was thought that mitosis was in response to a "wound hormone." The opposite view is now favored: The epidermis normally contains a mitotic inhibitor whose loss from the damaged area permits the increase in mitotic activity of the adjacent cells. Bullough has proposed these substances be referred to as *chalones* (Greek: *chalan*, to slacken, slow down), which suggests that they act as mitotic inhibitors. A number of classic experiments have provided strong support for the chalone hypothesis [6].

A tissue-specific mitotic inhibitor has been extracted from the epidermis. This substance has been obtained from the skins of a variety of vertebrate species; it is tissue specific but not species specific. Evidence for the existence of other tissue chalones has been provided. Certain white blood cells, postmitotic granulocytes, apparently synthesize a tissue-specific inhibitor of mitosis which is released into the blood and is inhibitory to the mitotically active progranulocytes in the bone marrow. Similarly, evidence for an inhibitor of proerythrocytes in bone marrow has been provided.

Are some cancers, disease states characterized by uncontrolled mitotic activity, the result of a deficient chalone mechanism? Will injections of the tissue-specific chalone lead to restoration of cell division of the normal state? Injections of tissue-specific chalones have been used to stop and even reverse tumor growth. For example, it has been reported that granulocyte extracts inhibit granuloma growth in the rat and cause leukemic regression in humans. Skin extracts have been reported to inhibit human epidermoid tumor growth [11].

A major problem confronting research is that sufficient quantities of these putative inhibitors have not been available. Until such factors have been chemically and biologically characterized one should view much of the information as highly speculative. Nevertheless, the importance of further research toward the possible isolation and characterization of such putative chalones is clearly justified [35].

HORMONE INTERACTION IN GROWTH

Pituitary STH is essential for normal growth in humans and probably most vertebrates. Somatotropin secretion is apparently regulated by stimulating (GRF) and inhibiting (somatostatin) factors from the hypothalamus. Diverse stimuli mediate pituitary STH secretion by their initial actions within the hypothalamus (Chapter 6). It is not known if somatomedins are involved in a feedback control of STH secretion. Hypersecretion of pituitary STH may result in gigantism if it occurs during adolescent development. In the adult excess STH secretion results in acromegaly. Overproduction of STH may result from overstimulation of the pituitary by the hypothalamus or from development of pituitary tumors consisting of somatotrophs.

Somatotropin mediates its major growth-promoting activity indirectly by its action on hepatic somatomedin production. Somatomedins then affect growth through their actions on skeletal tissues and many other connective tissues and organs. Several growth hormones (e.g., prolactin, chorionic somatomammotropin, insulin) may also exert part of their growth-promoting activity through effects on hepatic somatomedin production. The structures of hPL and PRL are similar to that of STH. Somatomedin levels remain normal in hypophysectomized pregnant rats even in the absence of PRL and STH; these levels decline promptly postpartum. Thus, other STH-related factors may be important in somatomedin production during particular physiological states as pregnancy.

Somatotropin has a direct action on a number of target cells in addition to its action on hepatic somatomedin production. The physiological significance of these nonhepatic actions is unclear. These actions of STH have been described as diabetogenic in nature. For example, STH stimulates lipolysis, which provides substrates for glucose formation and thus has a sparing effect on direct glucose utilization (Chapter 11). It is difficult to rationalize this antiinsulin action of STH because the somatomedins produced by STH have insulinlike actions. The elevated glucose levels produced by STH could act as substrates for the metabolic actions of the somatomedins on their many target tissues. The direct and indirect actions of STH are depicted in Figure 12.12.

Glucocorticoids at excess levels are inhibitory to growth, apparently due to their antagonistic effect on pituitary STH secretion. Glucocorticoids may also decrease pituitary TSH secretion, which would result in decreased circulating levels of thyroid hormones. Thyroid hormones are essential for normal growth and skeletal maturation. Bone growth and epiphysial closure, for example, are delayed in hypothyroid children. In the absence of thyroid hormones STH secretion may be further decreased. Thyroid hormones also potentiate (exert a permissive action on) the actions of STH on many tissues.

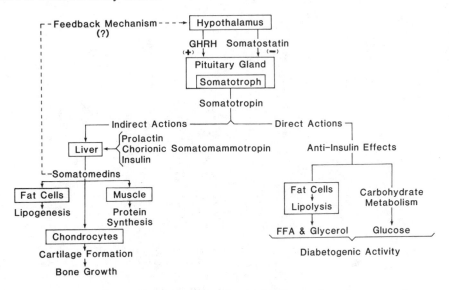

Figure 12.12 Summary scheme of the direct and indirect actions of somatotropin on growth and metabolism [43].

Hormone Interaction in Growth

Estrogens are inhibitory to growth most likely because of a blunting of the metabolic and growth-promoting effects of STH. Because somatomedin action is not altered by estrogens, it appears that these steroid hormones mediate their effects on growth indirectly by inhibiting hepatic somatomedin production. Estrogens have been used to limit stature in girls with excessive predicted height and to decrease growth activity in acromegalics [37].

Androgens exert anabolic growth effects through their actions on protein synthesis. Testosterone, dihydrotestosterone, and other androgenic metabolites affect a variety of tissue types. They cause the epiphyses to fuse (ossify) in the long bones, eventually inhibiting further linear growth. Excess androgen secretion early in adolescent development can, therefore, lead to shortened stature. Although androgens potentiate the growth-promoting action of STH, the effects of androgens are independent of somatomedin activity on cartilage and do not enhance somatomedin production. Androgens also stimulate erythropoiesis (Chapter 17).

Figure 12.12 depicts the relationship between STH and plasma levels of somatomedins. Hypopituitary dwarfs, as might be expected, have very minimal plasma levels of IGF-I and IGF-II. Although levels of IGF-I are greatly increased in acromegalics, levels of IGF-II did not differ from controls. In contrast to IGF-I, IGF-II production is STH dependent; this dependence of IGF-II, however, only becomes

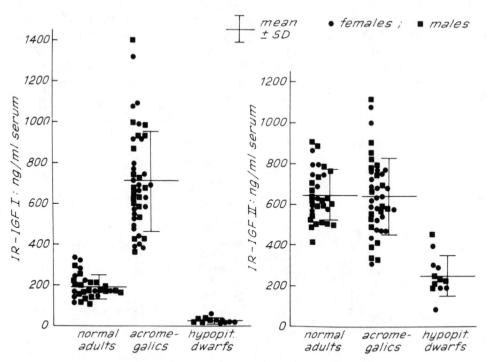

Figure 12.3 Serum immunoreactive (IR) IGF-I and II levels in normal adults, acromegalic patients, and patients with isolated growth hormone deficiency. (Reproduced from Zapf, et al., [45], from *The Journal of Clinical Investigation*, 1981, Vol. 68: 1321–1330, by copyright permission of The American Society For Clinical Investigation.)

apparent when STH levels fall below normal [45]. These results indicate that production of the two somatomedins is regulated differently.

Laron dwarfism (idiopathic short stature) is usually a familial disorder, and affected persons are generally resistant to the effects of endogenous and exogenous STH. Somatotropin from these individuals is, by chemical and biochemical criteria, similar to STH from normal individuals. The growth-promoting effects of STH are believed to be through production of somatomedins by the liver; indeed, affected individuals have decreased circulating levels of somatomedins. Laron dwarfism has, therefore, been theorized to be caused by hepatic unresponsiveness to circulating STH [14]. Because somatotropin from individuals with Laron-type dwarfism binds normally to liver receptors, the defect may relate to a postreceptor site flaw within the hepatocyte.

Dwarfism in the African pygmy has been an enigma for centuries. Although it was originally believed that the pygmy's short stature might be due to end-organ resistance to somatomedins, it has been shown that pygmies have decreased circulating levels of IGF-I (Fig. 12.14). Plasma levels of IGF-II are, in contrast to hypopituitary dwarfs, within the range found in normal adults [32]. Thus, normal serum levels of IGF-II are inadequate for promotion of normal growth in the absence of IGF-I, at least in the pygmy. The role of IGF-II in growth remains to be clarified.

As more is understood about newly discovered growth stimulants, such as the epidermal and fibroblast growth factors, other disease states related to the underproduction or overproduction of these factors will likely be documented and described. Enhanced production of platelet-derived growth factor may, for example, be an important etiological factor in atherosclerosis. Failure of renal erythropoietin

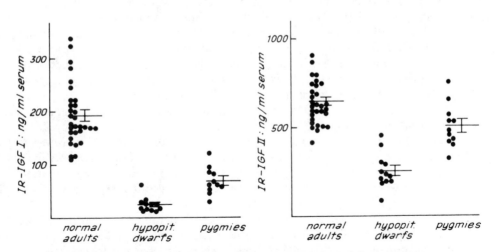

Figure 12.14 Serum concentrations of IGF-I and IGF-II in controls, hypopituitary dwarfs, and pygmies. IGF-I and IGF-II were measured in the same adult controls. Lines and bars denote means ± S.E.M. Note that only one pygmy has an IGF-I value within the lower normal range, whereas all but one have IGF-II values within the normal range. All values are corrected for cross-reactivity. (From Merimee, Zapf, and Froesch, [32], reprinted, by permission of *The New England Journal of Medicine*, vol. 305, pp. 965–968, 1981.)

production or thymic gland function may be responsible for the numerous anemias associated with deficits of the cellular elements of the blood. A large molecule that may regulate the growth of bones has been isolated from humans and other animals [31]. This skeletal growth factor may be released during bone resorption and may stimulate the synthesis of new bone.

CONCLUSIONS AND SPECULATIONS

Growth, often defined as simply an increase in size, may occur as a result of three processes: Cells may enlarge (become hypertrophic), cells may increase in number (become hyperplastic), and intercellular substances (extracellular matrix) may be produced. In living organisms these are orderly processes that require exogenous substrates as fuel and structural components of muscle, bone, adipose tissue, and other organs. Hormones are critical in making these materials available to cells and in stimulating cell division and the secretion of materials (e.g., collagen) for the extracellular framework of the body.

With few exceptions, most hormones stimulate tissue and organ growth, and in their absence target tissues atrophy. For example, in response to MSH integumental melanocytes (of the frog, *Xenopus laevis*) increase in number from as few as $10/mm^2$ of epidermis to as many as 1000 to 2000 mm^2 (Fig. 8.8). In the absence of MSH the melanocytes soon atrophy and disappear from the skin.

It is surprising how little is understood about the mechanisms of action of growth-promoting hormones. A role for cyclic AMP in the actions of these hormones has minimal evidence. It has, however, been demonstrated that somatotropins stimulate guanylate cyclase activity in a variety of tissues from the rat [44]. Conversely, adenylate cyclase of rat liver plasma membranes is increased in hypophysectomized animals; this increase in enzyme activity is subsequently lowered by administration of somatotropin. There is rapidly accumulating evidence that other growth-promoting hormones—prolactin (in mammary gland), thymosin (in thymocytes), and the somatomedins—mediate their actions through a decrease in intracellular cyclic AMP levels and/or an increase in cyclic GMP concentration.

As cAMP and cGMP play contrasting roles in the rapid responses of tissues, such as smooth muscle, to first messengers, it is possible that these cyclic nucleotides may also have similar contrasting roles in the prolonged actions of growth hormones. This view may be compatible with a generally held belief that cyclic AMP plays a role in the rapid expression of a differentiation function (e.g., melanin or keratin synthesis), whereas cyclic GMP may, in contrast, effect dedifferentiation leading to cellular proliferation.

It would seem that, at least with some somatomedins and nerve growth factor, the growth factors meet most of the criteria necessary to be considered hormones. The structures of these chemical messengers are known; the messengers are in the circulation during the period of their putative effects. In the absence of growth factors the target organs atrophy; for example, without somatomedins there is no appreciable growth (as in the pygmy).

It is unlikely that all the growth hormones have been discovered. The placenta still appears to be a source of surprises [9]. The effects of nerve growth factor appear to be restricted to sympathetic nervous system neurons and certain sensory neurons.

Table 12.1. Polypeptide Cellular Growth Factors

Factor		Source	Major physiological effects
Somatomedins		Liver	Chondrogenesis, insulinlike actions (protein synthesis, lipogenesis, glycogenesis)
A	(somatomedin-A)		Unknown
B	(somatomedin-B)		Unknown
C	(somatomedin-C)		Unknown
MSA	(multiplication stimulating activity)		Probably identical to IGF-II
IGF-I	(insulinlike growth factor-I)		Required for normal growth and attainment of stature
IGF-II	(insulinlike growth factor-II)		Unknown
Prolactin		Pituitary gland	Mammary gland development and growth
Insulin		Pancreatic islets	Anabolic effects (glycogenesis, protein synthesis, lipogenesis)
Placental lactogen		Placenta	Unknown (fetal growth?)
Nerve growth factor (NGF)		Salivary gland, other (?)	Neurite (sympathetic) orientation and growth
Epidermal growth factor (EGF)		Salivary gland, other (?)	Mitogen of epithelial cells
Fibroblast growth factor (FGF)		Unknown	Mitogen of fibroblasts and other mesenchymal-derived cells
Platelet-derived growth factor (PDGF)		Blood platelets	Vascular (intimal) smooth muscle proliferation
Erythropoietin (EP)		Kidney	Erythrocyte differentiation and production
Thymosins α_1, β_4		Thymus gland	Lymphocyte proliferation and differentiation
Thymopoietin (TP)		Thymus gland	Lymphocyte proliferation and differentiation
Serum thymic factor (STF)		Thymus gland	Lymphocyte proliferation and differentiation
Thymic humoral factor (THF)		Thymus gland	Lymphocyte proliferation and differentiation
Chalones		Diverse tissues	Inhibitors (local hormones) of cellular proliferation

It might be expected, however, that one or more factor(s) would direct the growth processes of neurons of the parasympathetic system. Little is known about chemical messengers that may be involved in fetal growth and development. Table 12.1 provides a list of growth factors (hormones); as analytical methods for detection and structural determination improve, the list should lengthen.

REFERENCES

[1] ANTONIADES, H. N. 1981. Human platelet-derived growth factor (PDGF): purification of PDGF-I and PDGF-II and separation of their reduced subunits. *Proc. Natl. Acad. Sci. USA* 78:7314–17.

[2] BACH, J. F. 1978. The thymus and its role. *Endeavor* 2:154–60.

[3] BEWLEY, T. A. 1977. The chemistry of chorionic somatomammotropin. In *Hormonal proteins and peptides*, ed. C. H. Li, pp. 61–137. New York: Academic Press, Inc.

[4] BHAUMICK, B., R. M. BALA, and M. D. HOLLENBERG. 1981. Somatomedin receptor of human placenta: solubilization photolabeling, partial purification, and comparison with insulin receptor. *Proc. Natl. Acad. Sci. USA* 78:4279–83.

[5] BRADSHAW, R. A. 1978. Nerve growth factor. *Ann. Rev. Biochem.* 47:191–216.

[6] BULLOUGH, W. S. 1975. Mitotic control in adult mammalian tissues. *Biol. Rev.* 50:99–127.

[7] CARPENTER, G. 1980. Epidermal growth factor is a major growth-promoting agent in human milk. *Science* 210:198–99.

[8] CARPENTER, G., and S. COHEN. 1979. Epidermal growth factor. *Ann. Rev. Biochem.* 48:193–216.

[9] CHATTERJEE, M., and H. N. MUNRO. 1977. Structure and biosynthesis of human placental peptide hormones. *Vit. Horm.* 35:149–208.

[10] DYER, M. I. 1980. Mammalian epidermal growth factor promotes plant growth. *Proc. Natl. Acad. Sci. USA* 77:4836–37.

[11] FINKLER, N., and P. ACKER. 1978. Chalones: a mini-review. *Mt. Sinai J. Med.* 45:258–64.

[12] FRANTZ, A. G. 1978. Prolactin. *New Engl. J. Med.* 298: 201–207.

[13] GARRELS, J. I., and D. SCHUBERT. 1979. Modulation of protein synthesis by nerve growth factor. *J. Biol. Chem.* 254:7978–85.

[14] GOLDE, D. W., N. BERSCH, S. A. KAPLAN, D. L. RIMOIN, and C. H. LI. 1980. Peripheral unresponsiveness to human growth hormone in Laron dwarfism. *New Engl. J. Med.* 303: 1156–58.

[15] GOLDSTEIN, A. L., T. L. K. LOW, G. B. THURMAN, M. M. ZATZ, N. HALL, J. CHEN, S. K. HU, P. B. NAYLER, and J. E. MCCLURE. 1981. Current status of thymosin and other hormones of the thymus gland. *Rec. Prog. Horm. Res.* 37:369–415.

[16] GOLDWASSER, E. 1975. Erythropoietin and the differentiation of red blood cells. *Fed. Proc.* 34:2285–92.

[17] GOSPODAROWICZ, D., C. R. ILL, P. J. HORNSBY, and G. N. GILL. 1977. Control of bovine adrenal cortical cell proliferation by fibroblast growth factor. Lack of effect of epidermal growth factor. *Endocrinology* 100:1080–89.

[18] GOSPODAROWICZ, D., and J. G. MORAN. 1976. Growth factors in mammalian cell culture. *Ann. Rev. Biochem.* 45:531–58.

[19] GRABER, S. E., and S. B. KRANTZ. 1978. Erythropoietin and the control of red cell production. *Ann. Rev. Med.* 29:51–66.

[20] GREENE, L. A., and E. M. SHOOTER. 1980. The nerve growth factor: biochemistry and synthesis. *Ann. Rev. Neurosci.* 3:353–402.

[21] HARPER, G. P., and H. THOENEN. 1981. Target cells, biological effects, and mechanism of action of nerve growth factor and its antibodies. *Ann. Rev. Pharmacol. Toxicol.* 21:205–29.

[22] HEUMANN, R., M. SCHWAB, and H. THOENEN. 1981. A second messenger required for nerve growth factor biological activity? *Nature* 292:838–40.

[23] HOLLENBERG, M. D. 1979. Epidermal growth factor-urogastrone, a polypeptide acquiring hormonal status. *Vit. Horm.* 37:69–110.

[24] HUMBEL, R. E., and E. RINDERKNECHT. 1979. From NSILA to IGF (1963–1977). In *Somatomedins and growth*, eds. G. Giordano, J. J. Van Wyk, and F. Minuto, pp. 61–65. London: Academic Press, Inc.

[25] KELLY, P. A., T. TSUSHIMA, R. P. C. SHIU, and H. G. FRIESEN. 1976. Lactogenic and growth

hormone-like activities in pregnancy determined by radioreceptor assays. *Endocrinology* 99:765–74.

[26] KENDALL, M. D., H. R. M. JOHNSON, and J. SINGH. 1980. The weight of the human thymus at necropsy. *J. Anat.* 131:485–99.

[27] LEVI-MONTALCINI, R., and P. CALESSANO. 1979. The nerve-growth factor. *Sci. Amer.* 240: 68–77.

[28] LEVY, R. H. 1964. The thymus hormone. *Sci. Amer.* 211(1):66–77.

[29] MARKS, F., S. BERTSCH, and J. SCHWEIZER. 1978. Homeostatic regulation of epidermal cell proliferation. *Bull. Cancer* 65:207–22.

[30] MARQUARDT, H., and G. J. TODARO. 1981. Purification and primary structure of a polypeptide with multiplication-stimulating activity from rat liver cell cultures. *J. Biol. Chem.* 256:6859–65.

[31] MAUGH, T. H. II. 1982. Human skeletal growth factor isolated. *Science* 217:819.

[32] MERIMEE, T. J., J. ZAPF, and E. R. FROESCH. 1981. Dwarfism in the pygmy. *New Engl. J. Med.* 305:965–68.

[33] NISSLEY, S. P., and M. M. RECHLER. 1978. Multiplication-stimulating activity (MSA): a somatomedin-like polypeptide. *Natl. Cancer Inst. Monogr.* 48:167–77.

[34] PARDEE, A. B., R. DUBROW, J. L. HAMLIN, and R. F. KLETZIEN. 1978. Animal cell cycle. *Ann. Rev. Biochem.* 47:715–50.

[35] PATT, L. M., and C. HOUCK. 1980. The incredible shrinking chalone. *FEBS Lett.* 120:163–70.

[36] PESCHLE, C. 1980. Erythropoiesis. *Ann. Rev. Med.* 31:303–14.

[37] PHILLIPS, L. S., and R. VASSILOPOULOU-SELLIN. 1980. Somatomedins. *New Engl. J. Med.* 302:371–80, 438–46.

[38] RINDERKNECHT, E., and R. E. HUMBEL. 1978. Primary structure of insulin-like growth factor II. *FEBS Lett.* 89:283–86.

[39] ROSS, R. 1979. The arterial wall and atherosclerosis. *Ann. Rev. Med.* 30:1–15.

[40] ROSS, R., and A. VOGEL. 1978. The platelet-derived growth factor. *Cell* 14:203–10.

[41] SARA, V. R., K. HALL, C. H. RODECK, and L. WETTERBERG. 1981. Human embryonic somatomedin. *Proc. Natl. Acad. Sci. USA* 78:3175–79.

[42] SHERWOOD, L. M., Y. BURSTEIN, and I. SCHECHTER. 1980. Similarities in the structure and function of both the mature forms and biosynthetic precursors of placental lactogen and growth hormone. *Ann. New York Acad. Sci.* 343:155–67.

[43] VAN WYK, J. J. 1980. Growth hormone, somatomedins, and growth failure. In *Neuroendocrinology*, eds. D. T. Krieger and J. C. Hughes, pp. 299–309. Sunderland, Mass.: Sinauer Assoc. Inc.

[44] VESELY, D. L. 1981. Human and rat growth hormones enhance guanylate cyclase activity. *Am. J. Physiol.* 240:E79–E81.

[45] ZAPF, J., H. WALTER, and E. R. FROESCH. 1981. Radioimmunological determination of insulinlike growth factors I and II in normal subjects and in patients with growth disorders and extrapancreatic tumor hypoglycemia. *J. Clin. Invest.* 68:1321–30.

13

Thyroid Hormones

INTRODUCTION

Anatomists of the fifteenth and sixteenth centuries described the thyroid gland in detail, and an enlargement of the thyroid as the anatomical basis for goiter was subsequently noted [23]. The etiological basis for goiter, however, was discerned centuries later after a number of important discoveries in chemistry. Courtois, a French pharmacist, discovered iodine in 1811 and Davy, an English chemist, discovered its elemental nature in 1813. Gay-Lussac named the element iodine in 1814. Iodine was discovered to be abundant in seaweed and other marine products; if eaten, these marine substances had a beneficial effect on goiter. Burnt sponge was recommended as a treatment for goiter in the mid-thirteenth century. It was subsequently surmised and proved correct that iodine might aid in the cure of goiter. Evidence for a connection between iodine deficiency and endemic goiter was obtained from studies of several European locales; the suggestion was put forward in 1849 that the disease was due to a deficiency of iodine in drinking water [20].

In 1895 Magnus-Levey demonstrated that the feeding of dried animal thyroids to normal men increased their metabolic rate. This suggested that the thyroid gland might contain a substance that affected the cellular activity of other organs. It was hypothesized that thyroid tissue might contain iodine which was known to be beneficial to hypothyroid individuals. In 1895 Kocher of Bern demonstrated the high concentration of iodine in a thyroid concentrate. He named this substance *iodothyrin*. Iodothyrin was active in hypothyroid patients, whereas an iodine-free fraction of the thyroid was not. In 1918 Kendall isolated the active component of the thyroid which he named *thyroxin* (thyroxine), and proposed its structural formula. Harrington in England revised the constitution of thyroxine and synthesized the definitive structure of L-thyroxine (Fig. 13.1). Thyroxine was later isolated from the thyroid gland in pure form.

It was soon discovered that the physiological activity of thyroid material could not be accounted for entirely by its thyroxine content. Kendall suggested that the "active" hormone might contain less iodine than thyroxine. Gross and Pitt-Rivers were then able to isolate a triiodinated thyronine from animal thyroid glands. In 1952 triiodothyronine (Fig. 13.1) was synthesized and found to be more active than thyroxine. It was then suggested that triiodothyronine was the peripheral physiological hormone and thyroxine its precursor [29, 30].

THE THYROID GLAND

The thyroid gland is derived from endoderm of the cephalic portion of the alimentary canal of the embryo. A saclike diverticulum first appears in the midline of the ventral surface of the pharynx. This glandular organ becomes bilobed but remains connected to the pharynx by a thyroglossal duct. The thyroglossal duct becomes a solid stalk which usually atrophies. The two lateral lobes of the human thyroid become solid masses of tissue and remain connected to each other by a narrow isthmus of tissue. The thyroid tissue in mammals lies over the trachea at a position just below the cricoid cartilage (Fig. 9.1). A pyramidal lobe near the isthmus of the thyroid may persist as a remnant of the thyroglossal stalk (Fig. 13.2). The thyroid gland of humans weighs about 15 to 20 g. In nonmammalian species the thyroid gland consists of a pair of glands separated from each other at varying distances lateral to the esophagus.

The functional components of the thyroid gland are the individual thyroid follicles, which consist of a cuboidal epithelium arranged as a single layer surrounding a lumen which contains a colloid material (Fig. 13.3). In humans an individual thyroid follicle may reach a diameter of almost 1 cm. In the mammal so-called clear (C) cells are present within the follicular wall and the extracellular space between the follicles. These cells are the source of calcitonin, an important hormone involved in calcium homeostasis in some animals (Chapter 9).

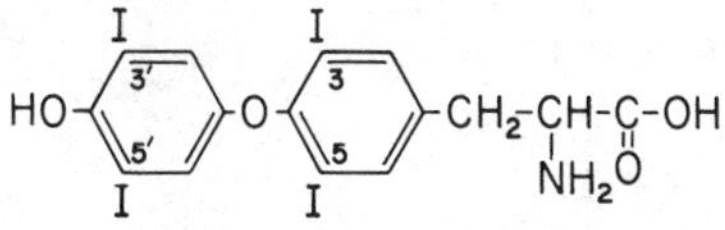

Thyroxine (3,5,3',5'-Tetraiodothyronine, T_4 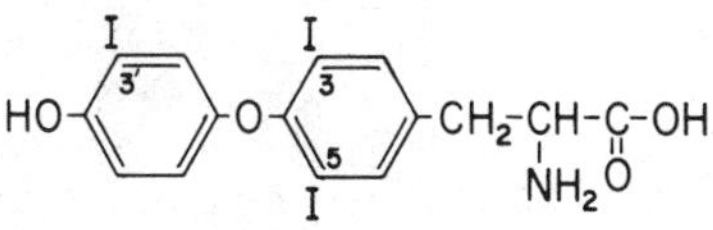)   Triiodothyronine (3,5,3'-Triiodothyronine, T_3)

Figure 13.1 Structures of thyroxine (T_4) and triiodothyronine (T_3).

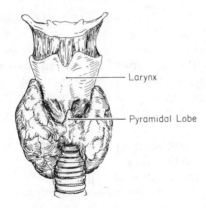

Larynx

Pyramidal Lobe

Figure 13.2 The human thyroid gland.

The follicular cells synthesize a protein, *thyroglobulin*, which is released into the colloid space by vesicular exocytosis. Thyroglobulin is important as substrate for tyrosine iodination and the subsequent synthesis of thyroid hormones. In response to endocrine stimulation follicular cells engulf the colloid by phagocytosis. The colloid within the endocytotic vesicles is enzymatically degraded to yield thyroid hormones, which are released from the follicular cells into the extracellular space where they enter the abundant capillaries.

The thyroid of some mammalian species, including humans, is richly supplied with sympathetic postganglionic neurons which not only serve a vasomotor function, but appear to innervate the individual follicular cells. In mice unilateral sympathetic stimulation induces secretion of thyroid hormones from those areas of the thyroid supplied by the stimulated nerve. Sympathetic innervation of the thyroid may provide a means for effecting prompt, short-term alterations in the rate of thyroid hormone secretion [25]. Amine-containing mast cells are present between the

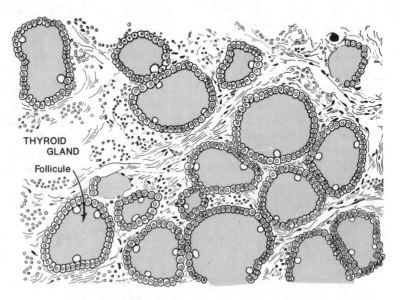

THYROID GLAND

Follicule

Figure 13.3 Diagrammatic histological representation of the human thyroid gland.

thyroid follicles of mammals; they respond to TSH by releasing histamine and serotonin (5-hydroxytryptamine, 5-HT) as well as other substances. The released biogenic amines may act directly on the follicle cells to initiate thyroid hormone secretion or to increase blood flow through the thyroid gland.

SYNTHESIS AND CHEMISTRY

Thyroid hormones are unique in that they are complexed through covalent bonds to iodine. The availability of iodine to the terrestrial vertebrate is limited and, therefore, some interesting cellular mechanisms have been adopted for the ultimate utilization and conservation of the element. The thyroid follicular cells are able to trap iodide at the base of the cell and transport it against an electrical gradient across the cell. Iodide is then converted by a *peroxidase*, most likely at the luminal surface of the cell, to an oxidized species of iodine which is incorporated into tyrosyl groups of thyroglobulin (TG) as monoiodotyrosine (MIT) and diiodotyrosine (DIT) residues. Within the TG, iodinated tyrosines apparently undergo an *oxidative coupling* which results mainly in the formation of T_4 and smaller amounts of T_3. This oxidative coupling may be catalyzed by the same peroxidase responsible for conversion of iodide to iodine. Iodination of TG tyrosyl residues and subsequent oxidative coupling to form *iodothyronines* may be facilitated by intraluminal ciliary action and the subsequent movement of TG to reactive sites of the apical surface of the follicular cells [42].

Through the processes of micropinocytosis and macropinocytosis, the colloid is engulfed by follicular cell pseudopods and transported into the cells as *colloid droplets*. These colloid-containing vesicles which then fuse with lysosomes are referred to as *secondary lysosomes*. Much of the TG within these vesicles is degraded by lysosomal proteolytic enzymes. The thyroid hormones are then released (presumably by diffusion) into the cytoplasm and enter the extracellular space by diffusion, apparently through the basal or lateral follicular membranes [13]. Exocytosis of vesicular products, including T_3 and T_4, is not excluded as TG is also secreted into the circulation. The iodinated tyrosines that are released into the cytosol through lysosomal proteolysis are then deiodinated by a *deiodinase* and recycled for use within the cell. The scheme of the events involved in thyroid hormone synthesis and secretion is depicted (Fig. 13.4).

Thyrotropin Stimulation of Thyroid Hormone Synthesis

Follicular thyroid hormone synthesis is regulated through the action of thyrotropin (TSH). Continued stimulation of the thyroid by TSH results in a great increase in the quantity and activity of the synthetic machinery (rough endoplasmic reticulum and Golgi) of the follicular cells. The cells become columnar in shape and the luminal content of the colloid is greatly decreased. In the absence of TSH, synthesis of thyroid hormones is minimal or nonexistent. Subsequently, there is a loss of most protein-synthesizing elements of the cell; the individual follicular cells become flattened (cuboidal) and the lumen remains enlarged and full of colloid.

In response to TSH there is an immediate activation of follicular cell thyroid

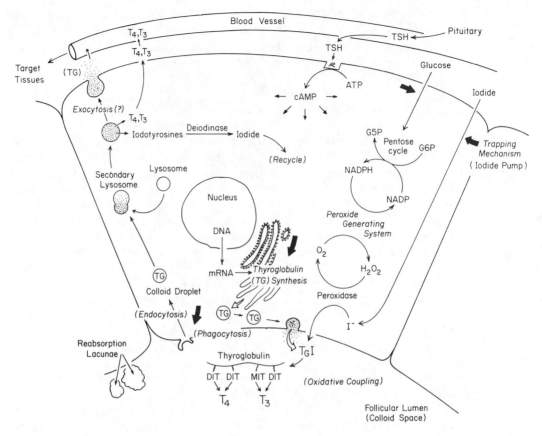

Figure 13.4 Summary scheme of thyroid hormone biosynthesis and secretion. The actual oxidative coupling of iodinated tyrosine residues probably takes place at the apical surface of the follicular cell, rather than in the lumen [42].

hormone synthesizing activity. TSH interacts with follicular cell membrane receptors with resulting activation of adenylate cyclase and cAMP production. All the subsequent follicular activities may be mediated through cAMP phosphorylation of substrate proteins, as theophylline and cAMP analogs added to thyroid tissue mimic most actions of TSH. TSH stimulates the in vitro incorporation of radiolabeled iodide into thyroglobulin, which suggests that the iodide pump and peroxidase activities are stimulated by the hormone. In response to TSH oxygen consumption is increased in incubated thyroid tissue and glucose is taken up from the medium and metabolized via the *pentose monophosphate shunt*. In this pathway NADPH is generated from NADP; this reduced adenine nucleotide is required for the reduction of molecular oxygen to hydrogen peroxide. The H_2O_2 is then utilized in the oxidation of iodide to an active form of iodide. The reaction is catalyzed by a thyroidal peroxidase which may be present within the Golgi-derived vesicles containing newly synthesized TG. Conversion of iodide to active iodide and organification of iodide into tyrosine residues of TG may occur as TG is secreted into the follicular lumen.

Immediately upon stimulation of the thyroid by TSH, there is enhanced pino-cytotic activity at the apical follicular membrane. Thus, colloid is actively engulfed and carried into the cell by this endocytotic process. The active removal of colloid from the lumen can be visualized as so-called *reabsorption lacunae* (Figs. 13.3 and 13.4).

Although thyrotropin stimulates TG biosynthesis, and a mRNA is obviously required for TG production, it is unclear if TSH-generated cAMP stimulates thyro-globulin mRNA production. Thyroglobulin may be composed of two polypeptide subunits, each with a molecular weight of about 300,000. Although tyrosyl residues are essential for iodine incorporation, the actual amount of tyrosine within TG is low (about 2%). The main intrathyroidal storage form of thyroid hormones is TG, and the individual iodinated thyronines are liberated from TG as T_4 and T_3 within the colloid droplets by the action of proteolytic enzymes.

Iodination of TG initially requires the conversion of inorganic iodide to some molecular species of "active iodide." This active iodide then reacts with tyrosine moieties of the TG. Incorporation of a single iodide into the phenolic ring of tyro-sine yields a 3-monoiodotyrosine (MIT). A second iodide may be incorporated into the 5 position to yield a 3,5-diiodotyrosine (DIT). Iodination specifically involves initial iodination of the 3 position, which is usually followed by iodination of the 5 position as 5-monoiodotyrosine is never formed.

Coupling of iodinated tyrosyl residues within TG is undoubtedly facilitated by the three-dimensional structure of TG, but the exact mechanism remains undeter-mined. For example, the extent to which intramolecular or intermolecular coupling by tyrosyl moieties predominates is unknown. Coupling is enzymatically controlled and apparently involves the cleavage of a phenolic ring from tyrosine, and its incor-poration through an ether (—O—) linkage, to another iodinated tyrosine. Coupling usually involves the joining of two DIT moieties to form 3,5,3',5'-tetraiodothyro-nine, T_4, while the addition of MIT to a DIT residue yields 3,5,3'-triiodothyronine, T_3. All iodinated tyrosines do not become coupled, and much extractable organic iodide remains in the form of MIT or DIT.

One suggested coupling scheme involves free radical formation. In this model free DIT radicals are generated within the TG matrix through the action of thyro-peroxidase. In this particular pathway a serine residue would remain in the position formerly occupied by the phenolic residue cleaved from the tyrosine (Fig. 13.5). The formation of T_3 may occur by a similar scheme except the coupling would be be-tween MIT (contributing a phenolic group) and DIT [41].

Antithyroid Drugs

Certain drugs inhibit thyroid function by antagonizing formation of thyroid hor-mones. These drugs are generally classified into those compounds which inhibit iodide transport (iodide trapping) into the thyroid gland and those that inhibit iodine incorporation into tyrosine. Univalent inhibitors of iodide transport include thio-cyanate and other monovalent cations (perchlorate, chlorate, periodate, etc.). Even iodide in large doses is transiently inhibitory to thyroid function (Wolff-Chaikoff ef-fect), but the mechanism of this inhibition remains unexplained. Iodide pump in-hibitors probably antagonize iodide transport through *competitive inhibition*. Other

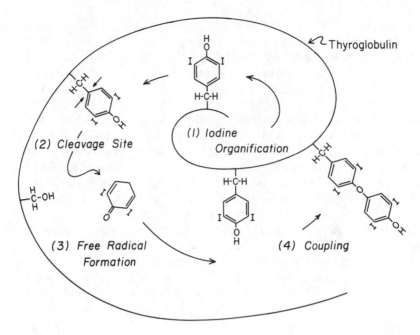

Figure 13.5 Hypothetical coupling scheme for iodothyronine formation.

antithyroid compounds include the thionamides, the sulfonamides (para-aminobenzoic acid), and the sulfonylureas (carbutamide, tolbutamide). Maintenance of an effective concentration of these antithyroid drugs for a sufficient time will usually cause thyroid hypertrophy and goiter [22]. These agents are therefore often referred to as *goitrogens*. A number of these drugs are of clinical importance in the treatment of excess thyroid hormone production (thyrotoxicosis) (Fig. 13.6).

Dietary goitrogens may be responsible for *endemic goiter* in parts of the world. Certain *cyanogenic glucosides* (found in cassava, sorghum, sweet potatoes, maize, apricots, cherries, almonds, etc.) are hydrolyzed by glucosidases and release free cyanide which is converted to thiocyanate. Thioglucosides found in certain plants (e.g., genus *Brassica:* cabbage, Brussels sprouts, cauliflower, turnips, and rutabagas) are metabolized within the body to thiocyanates and isothiocyanates (Fig. 13.7). These plant products are usually not consumed in large enough quantities to produce goiter, although they may augment endemic goiter in areas deficient in iodine. Involvement of dietary goitrogens in the pathogenesis of human goiter has been discovered in a population of natives in Zaire, Africa [14]. Cassava forms an important

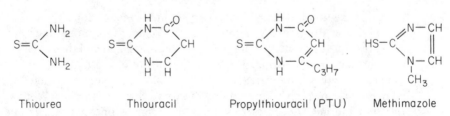

Figure 13.6 Structures of some thionamide type antithyroid drugs.

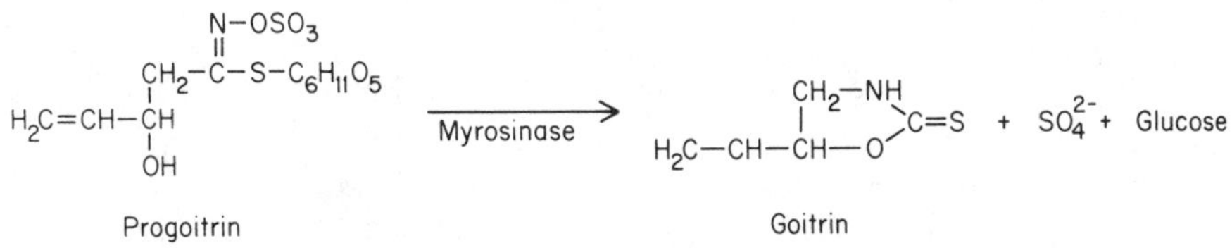

Figure 13.7 Synthesis and structure of goitrin.

part of the natives' diet, and it has been shown that ingestion of cassava from this area depresses the radioiodide uptake by the normal human thyroid. The nature of the putative goitrogen remains unclear. Congenital goiter in lambs of ewes fed various species of *Brassicae* has also been reported [22].

Thyroid Hormones or Thyroid Hormone?

Normally thyroxine (T_4) is produced in greater quantity than triiodothyronine (T_3). In human serum the concentration of T_4 is about 50 times greater than the T_3 level. Because T_4 is converted to T_3 in athyreotic human subjects [4], extrathyroidal mono-deiodination of T_4 appears, therefore, to be the major source of T_3 in the body. If T_3 is the physiologically relevant hormone, is T_4 therefore the prohormone of T_3? Is it possible that both T_4 and T_3 are hormones, each with their own specific target tissues? There is strong evidence that T_3 is the major physiologically active thyroid hormone regulating cellular activity in many species, but T_4 is thought to exert a negative feedback action on the hypothalamus. In newborn infants serum T_3 levels are very low in cord blood, whereas T_4 concentrations are high, suggesting that T_4 may serve a direct functional role during certain developmental stages of animals.

The pituitary gland of the rat binds T_3 more strongly than T_4. These binding sites are apparently specific for T_3 and exhibit a high affinity but low capacity for this iodothyronine. The inhibitory action of the thyroid hormones on pituitary TSH secretion in the rat would therefore appear to be regulated through T_3. There is convincing evidence that the effects of thyroid hormones are related to the concentration of iodothyronines bound to specific nuclear binding sites, that these sites are similar in various tissues, and that iodothyronines in plasma are in equilibrium with nuclear T_3–T_4 receptors [27]. It appears that T_3 contributes between 85% to 90% of the nuclear binding of T_3 and T_4 in the liver and kidney taken from the athyreotic rat. Thus, T_3 may contribute a like percentage of the thyroidal effects in the euthyroid (normal) rat. The remaining 10% to 15% thyroid hormone responsiveness may result from the intrinsic activity of T_4 [40]. In this text the term thyroid hormones will refer to the putative activities of both T_3 and T_4, but it is to be tentatively understood that T_3 is the most effective thyroid hormone under normal serum levels of iodothyronines, at least in mammals.

Other Iodothyronines in Biological Fluids

Although T_4 and T_3 are the major thyroid hormones in the human circulation, other iodothyronines are also present [6] (Fig. 13.8). The relative concentrations of these iodinated thyronines vary in healthy and disease states, but the significance of these

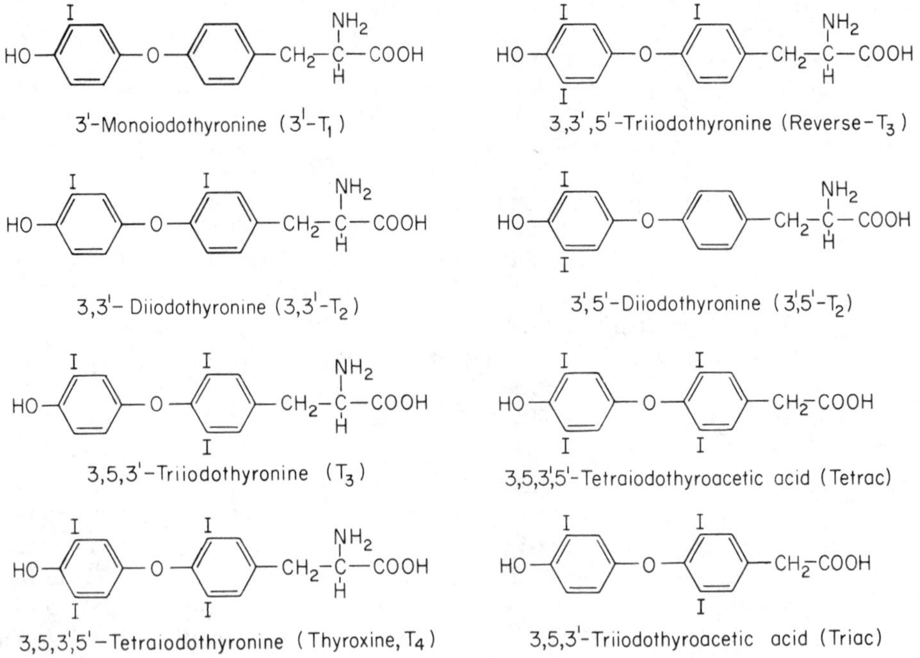

Figure 13.8 Structural formulas of iodothyronines found in human plasma.

differences is presently unknown. T_3, T_4, triac (3,5,3'-triiodothyroacetic acid), and tetrac (3,5,3',5'-tetraiodothyroacetic acid) have calorigenic activity; the relative potency of these compounds is approximately 300:100:21:11, respectively. Although reverse triiodothyronine (5,3',5'-triiodothyronine, rT_3) has little thermogenic activity, it is more potent than T_3 in a number of systems [8]. Nevertheless, it is argued that the concentrations of these iodothyronines required to cause physiological responses in vitro exceed by several orders of magnitude those concentrations present in vivo. Thus the physiological significance, if any, of the actions of these iodothyronines is questionable [6].

The T_3 and rT_3 present in body fluids are derived from monodeiodination of T_4 within peripheral tissues. Subsequent metabolism of these iodothyronines provides the major sources of the T_2's and $3'-T_1$. Ultimately, these iodinated thyronines are made soluble through sulfation or glucuronide formation within the liver and are excreted in the urine or with bile salts. Recent evidence suggests that high concentrations of T_0 (completely deiodinated thyronine) are present in the plasma and urine and may represent a major end product of thyronine deiodination in humans.

CONTROL OF THYROID HORMONE SECRETION

Thyroid hormone secretion is regulated by TSH from the pituitary gland which, in turn, is controlled by TRH of hypothalamic origin (Chapter 6). Thyroid hormones feed back at the pituitary and hypothalamic levels to inhibit TSH secretion (Fig. 13.9). TSH secretion is inhibited by stress in a number of species, including humans,

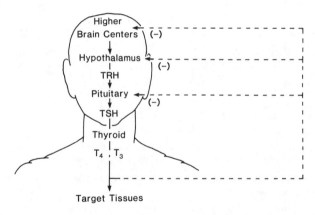

Figure 13.9 Central nervous system-pituitary-thyroid axis.

and it is likely that more than one mechanism is involved [24]. A primary neural event is clearly indicated, but corticosteroids and other hormones may have secondary modulatory effects at the hypothalamic level [38].

In many mammals activation of the pituitary-thyroid axis occurs during exposure to a lowered ambient temperature. Acute cold exposure of the rat, for example, leads to a rapid release of TSH, probably involving a neuroendocrine reflex mechanism. TSH release in response to a cold stimulus occurs in the infant but is minimal or absent in the adult human. Present evidence suggests that an acute neuroendocrine reflex exists for TSH release in some mammals and in human infants and is mediated initially by peripheral sensory receptors and then relayed to the hypothalamus where stimulation of TRH release occurs. This is substantiated by the observation that prior administration of T_4 inhibits pituitary TSH release in response to a cold stimulus. In addition peripheral plasma levels of TRH increase in hypophysectomized cold-exposed rats. Finally, TRH synthesis is increased in vitro in hypothalamic tissue taken from cold-exposed rats [16].

TSH mediates its action at the level of the follicular cell membrane. Radiolabeled TSH, for example, binds to follicle cell plasma membranes; this binding is partially inhibited by unlabeled TSH, but not by other polypeptide hormones. TSH activates adenylate cyclase in thyroid follicle membranes and theophylline and DcAMP mimic the action of TSH on thyroid tissue (Fig. 13.2).

CIRCULATION AND METABOLISM

The thyroid hormones are water-insoluble molecules that require specific binding proteins in the plasma and the cell cytosol to gain access to nuclear receptors. This protein-bound iodine (PBI) consists of two major thyroxine-binding proteins present in human plasma: *thyroxine-binding prealbumin* (TBPA) and *thyroxine-binding globulin* (TBG). Prealbumin has a molecular weight of 55,000 and is composed of four identical subunits, each consisting of 127 amino acid residues arranged in a tetrahedral symmetry and possessing a pair of T_4-binding sites [3]. These binding sites are located deep inside a cylindrical channel that runs completely through the molecule and are almost completely removed from the surrounding medium. TBG consists of a single polypeptide chain; although it is similar in molecular weight to TBPA, much less is known about its chemical constitution. About 70% to 75% of T_4 is bound to TBG, 15% to 20% to TBPA, and 5% to 10% may be bound to albumin. These binding proteins are synthesized within the liver.

During pregnancy in the human there is a doubling of TBG concentration which may result from estrogen stimulation of binding protein synthesis within the liver [34]. Increased TBG production is followed by increased thyroid T_4 synthesis and secretion, but the plasma concentrations of unbound iodothyronines remain unchanged. In normal individuals less than 0.5% of the total serum T_4 and about 0.3% of the serum T_3 are present in the free or unbound state. Teleosts lack high affinity T_4-binding plasma proteins. If one function of the binding proteins is to provide a large extrathyroidal pool of iodide, these proteins may not be required in a marine environment where iodide is always abundant.

PHYSIOLOGICAL ROLES

The first scientific experiment to determine the role of the thyroid gland was reported in 1858 and involved the removal of the gland from dogs. Although the animals died soon after, the symptoms preceding death resembled closely those following complete removal of goitrous glands in humans. Transplantation of thyroid tissue from a thyroidectomized animal into the body cavity resulted in survival of the animals for a long duration, thus demonstrating that death was due to an absence of the thyroid rather than to the operation itself. Many experiments led to the erroneous belief that the thyroid gland is essential to life. Only later was it realized that death from thyroidectomy was due to removal of the parathyroid glands present within the thyroid tissue. The essential role of the thyroid glands in the control of numerous physiological processes is now well documented.

Thyroid hormones influence most bodily functions. They directly affect a number of physiological processes and, although without observable actions, they are required for the (permissive) actions of other hormones on these processes. For example, they are obligatory with somatotropin for early growth and development. Thyroid hormone deficiencies in humans produce major abnormalities in growth, development, reproduction, behavior, and metabolism. Thyroid hormones are unique in that they exert effects within almost every tissue of the body throughout the life of an individual. Many actions of thyroid hormones are mediated through the hormones' effects on stimulation of cellular protein synthesis [27].

Growth and Development

The absence of thyroid hormones results in severe growth retardation, which is associated with arrest of bone elongation as well as retarded bone maturation. Somatotropin secretion is diminished in the absence of thyroid hormones and renewed when thyroid hormones are administered. Thus, one cause of growth retardation is the absence of circulating levels of STH. Nevertheless, administration of STH to hypothyroid individuals is without effect if thyroid hormones are not also given. Thus, the role of thyroid hormones in normal growth is twofold: They are required both for the production of STH and for its systemic actions.

Levels of hyaluronic acid are high in proliferating tissue and decrease as division ceases and the cells become more differentiated. The enzyme *hyaluronidase* (an endoglycosidase), which splits hyaluronic acid into smaller oligosaccharides, is apparently induced at a time when tissues mature and may, therefore, serve as a signal for differentiation [2]. Thyroid hormones stimulate tadpole tissue differentiation, which is paralleled by a decrease in hyaluronic acid levels and an increase in hyaluronidase concentrations. In myxedematous tissue from subjects with hypothyroidism there is an increase in hyaluronic acid. These observations suggest that thyroid hormones stimulate differentiation through stimulation of hyaluronidase production.

Thyroid hormones in concert with prolactin play an important role in the regulation of development of the mouse mammary gland. Decreased serum levels of thyroid hormones result in retarded growth of the ductal system and little or no alveolar development [43]. Thyroid hormones may also be required for the synthesis of normal levels of PRL by the pituitary gland. Thyroid hormones are required for the normal development of the brain; without them there is decreased protein synthesis, decreased myelinogenesis, and retarded axonal ramification. These developmental processes, unlike general body growth, are irreversibly compromised and lead to mental deficiency, as is evident in cretins. Nerve growth factor (NGF) induces dendritogenesis and regeneration of sympathetic neurons (Chapter 12). It may be significant, therefore, that thyroid hormone administration increases the concentration of NGF in the brain. Thyroid hormones also accelerate axonal regeneration in the cerebrum of lesioned adult rats, and the hormones appear to be selectively concentrated within adrenergic nerve terminals. These observations suggest that thyroid hormones may control CNS development through stimulation of NGF biosynthesis.

Thermogenesis

The evolution from poikilothermy to homeothermy required the acquisition of some mechanism for heat production. Active sodium transport uses a high proportion (possibly as much as 20% to 45%) of the total cellular energy supply. In the process of ATP hydrolysis by the sodium pump heat is liberated, which contributes greatly to the maintenance of an elevated body temperature in homeotherms. The activity of the sodium pump requires a source of ATP, which is produced mainly within the mitochondria. There is strong evidence that thyroid hormones stimulate mitochondrial oxygen consumption and production of ATP and also increase the number of active plasmalemmal sodium pumps [12]. Inhibition of Na^+-K^+ APTase activity by ouabain and other sodium pump antagonists markedly reduces the action of thyroid hormones on heat production and oxygen consumption. This *sodium pump theory* of thermogenesis differs from an earlier hypothesis. It was originally believed that thyroid hormones increased heat production by an uncoupling of oxidative phosphorylation within mitochondria.

Diet and Thyroid Hormone Function

The increase of caloric intake (mixed diet or carbohydrates) in individuals results in an increased diet-induced thermogenesis. The production of T_3 is increased during short-term overfeeding; the increased serum levels of T_3 apparently derive from altered (increased) peripheral conversion of T_4 to T_3 and a decreased conversion of T_3 to rT_3. Individuals fed isocaloric diets low in carbohydrates or containing no carbohydrates develop changes in T_3 and rT_3 opposite to those resulting from feeding excess carbohydrates. Here may be an adaptation in which the resting metabolic rate is increased, in the presence of an excess of poor-quality food (carbohydrates), to provide enough of a scarce nutrient, such as protein, or even minerals and not be burdened with a weight gain [36].

Plasma levels of T_3 decrease during prolonged fasting, which is correlated with a decrease (down regulation) in hepatic nuclear T_3 receptors. A decrease in serum T_3 concentration per se does not diminish hepatic nuclear T_3 receptor content as brain T_3 receptor number is not concomitantly changed. A particular cell type may be able to modify its nuclear T_3 receptor content in response to its own metabolic status, which "infers the possibility of individual target cell acceptance or rejection of the hormonal directive" [35]. This may represent a homeostatic protective mechanism to prolong survival of the organism under conditions of food deprivation [37].

Permissive Actions

Thyroid hormones are required for the actions of other hormones on target tissues. This permissive action of thyroid hormones is also a characteristic of gonadal and adrenal steroids on some of their target tissues. Because thyroid and steroid hormones mediate most of their actions at the level of the genome to induce protein synthesis, it is likely that these proteins function as substrates in the pathway of action of other hormones (Fig. 4.14).

Thyroid hormones induce STH production in cultured rat pituitary tumor (GH_1) cells. Glucocorticoids also stimulate STH synthesis but only in the presence of thyroid hormones. There is a dramatic synergistic activation of STH production when both hormones are present together in the medium, suggesting that the ability of glucocorticoids to stimulate STH synthesis is controlled by thyroid hormones [2]. This is another example of the permissive action of thyroid hormones; it is likely that many actions of these hormones are indirect and involve modulation of the activities of other hormones. Some of the more prominent actions of thyroid hormones are summarized in Table 13.1.

MECHANISMS OF ACTION

The action of T_3 is analogous to the model for steroid hormone action (Chapters 4 and 18) [37]. T_3 enters a target cell either by passive diffusion or by an unclarified *carrier-mediated process*. Within the cytoplasm T_3 interacts with a proteinaceous cytosol receptor. However, unlike the model for steroid hormone action where the cytosolic receptor translocates with bound steroid to the nucleus and combines with

TABLE 13.1 Some Physiological Roles and Actions of Thyroid Hormones in Mammals

---

Inhibits feedback inhibition of pituitary TSH secretion

Is permissive to the action of many other hormones:
  Enhances lipolytic response of adipose tissue to hormones
  Required for the growth-promoting activity of STH
Increases activity of the sympathoadrenal system

Regulates basal metabolic rate:
  Increases mitochondrial oxidative phosphorylation
Is required for hepatic conversion of carotenes to vitamin A
Is required for bone growth and maturation
Is required for nervous system differentiation in early development
Is required for pituitary prolactin and growth hormone synthesis
Increases the rate of intestinal glucose absorption
Increases human red blood cell Ca^{2+}-ATPase activity

Induces enzyme synthesis:
  Na^+-K^+ ATPase (or a protein component or activator of the sodium pump)
  Carbamoyl phosphate synthetase (a phosphotransferase)
  α-Lactalbumin (lactose synthetase system proteins)
  Hepatic pyruvate carboxylase (converts pyruvate to oxaloacetate)
  Chromatin protein kinase
  Mitochondrial α-glycerophosphate dehydrogenase
  Malic dehydrogenase (converts malic acid to oxaloacetate)
  Hyaluronidase (dissolves intercellular ground substance)
Causes induction of cellular proteins (other than enzymes):
  Prolactin, growth hormone, lung surfactants, brain nerve growth factor (NGF)

---

the chromatin, T_3 exists within cytoplasm of the cell in equilibrium with its receptors. T_3 is free to interact directly with chromatin; the cytosolic receptor may, however, provide a mechanism for concentrating the hormone within the thyroid hormone target cells (Fig. 13.10).

Thyroid hormones and their analogs bind to nuclear (nonhistone) chromatin protein, a binding which is correlated with the biological activity of the hormone analogs. The distribution of nuclear T_3 receptors is also correlated with those tissues which are physiologically responsive to the hormone. Interaction of T_3 with chromatin results in stimulation of protein synthesis. One effect of T_3, for example, is stimulation of protein kinase activity by liver chromatin nonhistone proteins. The nuclear effects of T_3 involve transcriptional as well as translational events as mRNA synthesis is increased.

The actions of T_3 may not be restricted to a genomic locus; rather, they may induce effects on the plasma membrane and mitochondria. Thyroid hormones stimulate the rapid uptake of amino acids into cells, an action not blocked by actinomycin D or puromycin. These results suggest a direct action of thyroid hormones at the level of the plasma membrane. In addition 2-deoxyglucose (a nonmetabolizable glucose substrate) uptake into cells is rapidly stimulated by T_3 at physiological concentrations. These effects are also not blocked by inhibitors of transcriptional and translational processes. Thyroid hormones also stimulate plasmalemmal Na^+-K^+-ATPase (the sodium pump). This enhanced activity may be an indirect action of the hormones and result from an increased number of pump units rather than

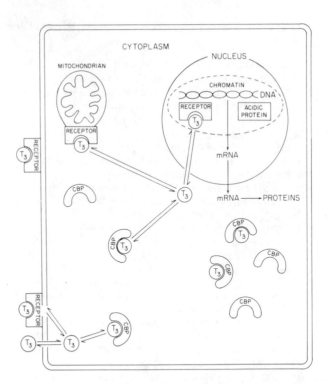

Figure 13.10 Model for the mechanism of action of thyroid hormone on target tissues. The sequence of events is believed to be similar for thyroxine (T_4) and triiodothyronine (T_3). T_3 (circled) indicates the unbound hormone, which diffuses or is transported into the cell and bound by CBP (cytosol-binding protein[s]). Instead of being translocated into the nucleus, the CBP-T_3 complex is in reversible equilibrium with a minute moiety of intracellular unbound T_3 that can interact with the binding proteins of the effector loci, the nucleus and the mitochondria. There are more than 20 million primary sites in the cytosol of rat-liver cells; hence, many CBP molecules would not have a bound T_3 molecule. The plasma membrane receptor is indicated. The relative importance of hormone entry by diffusion into the cell versus carrier-mediated transport is under study. (From Sterling, [37], reprinted, by permission of *The New England Journal of Medicine*, vol. 300, pp. 117–123, 1979.)

any direct increase in the activity of the ATPase. It is believed that newly synthesized ATPase derives from actions of the thyroid hormones at the level of the genome.

For many years there was argument if thyroid hormones mediated their effects through direct actions on mitochondria. The following data provide convincing evidence that, indeed, another site of thyroid hormone action is the mitochondria. In the hypothyroid state mitochondria are altered both morphologically and functionally, and the uptake of ADP by mitochondria is increased after administration of T_3 or T_4 to thyroidectomized rats. A specific receptor for T_3 and T_4 is a component of the inner mitochondrial membrane, which is known to be the site of oxidative phosphorylation. These receptors are present in mitochondria from thyroid hormone-responsive tissues but not in brain, spleen, and testes, tissues known to be refractory to thyroid hormones. Most interesting is the observation that mitochondria from neonatal rat brain but not from brain tissues of older animals possess thyroid hormone receptors. These data are compatible with the known temporal responsiveness of this tissue to thyroid hormones. Finally, mitochondrial oxygen consumption is increased in vitro by thyroid hormones. This effect is not inhibited by cycloheximide, an inhibitor of protein synthesis, suggesting an acute action of the hormones on the mitochondria. The marked changes in mitochondrial nucleic acid synthesis in vivo that are associated with altered thyroid states suggest that thyroid hormone action in mitochondria may involve both acute and long-term actions, the latter involving mRNA and protein synthesis.

The enzyme ornithine decarboxylase (ODC) is essential for polyamine biosynthesis and is intimately related to the regulation of nucleic acid and protein biosynthesis. Somatotropin stimulates ODC activity in brain tissue but only in the presence of thyroid hormones. Thyroid hormones do not, however, stimulate brain ODC activity. This demonstrates dramatically the permissive action of a hormone. In the liver, in contrast, STH and thyroid hormones stimulate ODC activity independently. These results demonstrate the tissue specificity to these hormones within an individual animal.

In summary thyroid hormones act on a number of cellular receptor sites. The actions of most hormones that mediate their effects at the plasmalemma involve changes in the intracellular levels of one or more cyclic nucleotides, whose activities appear restricted to substrate phosphorylation. The actions of steroid hormones appear to be restricted to the nucleus. There appears to be no single intracellular effector mechanism for thyroid hormone action; rather, several pathways contribute to an integrated cellular response of these hormones [38]. The nuclear actions of thyroid hormones may be related to slower anabolic effects such as are involved in growth and differentiation. The actions of thyroid hormones on the plasmalemma (sodium pump hypothesis) and mitochondria (mitochondrial receptor hypothesis) are rapidly initiated events which control increased heart rate, oxygen consumption, and ATP production. Thyroid hormones stimulate human red cell Ca^{2+}-ATPase activity, which clearly documents the extranuclear actions of these hormones.

PATHOPHYSIOLOGY

Because thyroid hormones affect many physiological processes and are necessary for the optimal activity of numerous hormones, it is not surprising that abnormalities of thyroid function lead to gross alterations in the normal physiology of an individual. Thyroid hormone underproduction or overproduction, referred to as primary hypothyroidism or hyperthyroidism, respectively, can occur at birth or later in life. A defect at the level of the pituitary or hypothalamus would result in decreased or increased production and secretion of TSH with resulting secondary or tertiary hypothyroidism or hyperthyroidism, respectively. Abnormalities of thyroid function may be familial (genetic) in nature and involve failure in growth or normal function of the thyroid gland. Other genetic defects may result in biosynthetic defects related to thyroid hormonogenesis, which may involve a defect in iodine trapping or organification, defective thyroglobulin synthesis and secretion, and other abnormalities [17].

At the level of the hypothalamus, abnormalities in TRH production could relate to anatomical or biochemical derangements in CNS function, possibly involving alterations in neurohormonal inputs to TRH-producing neurons. At the level of the pituitary, there may be a failure in total pituitary development, resulting in panhypopituitarism, or an isolated defect in thyrotroph development and function. Although only a few documented cases have been reported, pituitary neoplasm, either adenoma or carcinoma, may result in overproduction of TSH, which may lead to overstimulation of thyroid gland production of thyroid hormones.

Overstimulation of the thyroid may also result from an autoimmune response involving antibodies to the TSH receptor. *Long-acting thyroid stimulator* (LATS) is the name given the antibody believed responsible for TSH receptor stimulation. This type of hyperthyroidism has been referred to as Graves' disease, but a large number of affected patients have no measurable plasma levels of LATS. Present evidence is that LATS is probably not the etiologic factor in Graves' disease. Graves' thyrotoxicosis is uniquely associated with an exophthalmos (protruding of the eyes). In rare instances hyperthyroidism may result from the ectopic production of TSH or even from a trophoblastic (placental) tumor secreting either excessive amounts of choriogonadotropin (structurally somewhat related to TSH) or a TSH-like molecule. Primary hyperthyroidism may derive from development of a thyroidal adenoma or carcinoma and involve gross overproduction of thyroid hormones.

In the *low T_3 syndrome* hypothyroidism results from a failure in the peripheral conversion of T_4 to T_3 which is the physiologically relevant thyroid hormone [5]. A genetic failure in development of thyroid hormone receptors results in a familial peripheral (end organ, target tissue) resistance with resulting hypothyroidism. The clinical manifestations of tissue resistance to the action of thyroid hormones differ dramatically depending on tissues involved. Individuals with the general resistance syndrome are clinically euthyroid; they may have goiter and plasma levels of thyroid hormones may even be elevated. The variable biochemical defects responsible for end organ thyroid hormone resistance may be caused by the following: (1) decreased binding affinity; (2) decreased binding capacity (decrease in receptor number); and (3) an abnormal postreceptor mechanism [32]. For example, a genetic defect in development of thyroid hormone receptors results in a familial peripheral resistance with resulting clinical hypothyroidism that is not, however, characterized by goiter. On the other hand, individuals with a pituitary (thyrotroph) resistance to thyroid hormone feedback are hyperthyroid and, as might be expected, plasma TSH and thyroid hormone levels are elevated. This example of TSH-dependent hyperthyroidism represents one of the *syndromes of inappropriate TSH secretion*.

Cretins are individuals who suffer from a deficiency or total absence of thyroid hormones. *Athyreotic cretinism* may result from an in utero (congenital) thyroiditis or from a failure in thyroid development. Thyroid dysgenesis is responsible for decreased thyroid function in most infants with hypothyroidism and is most prevalent in females. Although sporadic, it may be familial in origin and may also occur in association with maternal autoimmune thyroiditis. Congenital goiter may also be associated with thyroid dyshormonogenesis due to hereditary defects in hormone synthesis or metabolism. The major symptoms of cretinism are failure of skeletal growth and maturation and a marked retardation in development of intellect. Hypothyroidism in the adult is referred to as *myxedema* (Greek: *myxa*, mucus + *oidema*,

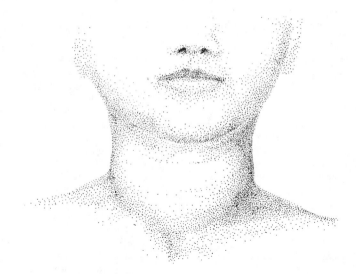

Figure 13.11 Simple goiter.

swelling) because of the characteristic mucinous protein deposit in the subcutaneous tissues.

Failure of the thyroid to produce T_4 and T_3 may lead to the development of a goiter (Fig. 13.11) as, in the absence of any negative feedback to the hypothalamus and pituitary gland, there is excessive secretion of TSH. In the absence of thyroid hormone production TSH stimulation continues to lead to hypertrophy of the thyroid follicular cells. Thyroid glands from such hypothyroid individuals are hyperplastic and exhibit grossly columnar follicular cells with a decreased amount of colloid (due to enhanced engulfment and degradation). Goiters may also develop under conditions of thyroiditis due to autoantibodies against thyroid TSH receptors. In the past a lack of iodine in the diet resulted in hypothyroidism; with the general availability of iodized salt this problem has been eradicated throughout much of the world. Clinically, *endemic* (*simple*) *goiter* is treated with iodized salt, but prolonged hypothyroidism may lead to irreversible stunting and cretinism.

Thyroxine has been used as replacement therapy in hypothyroidism. For the treatment of thyrotoxicosis, such antithyroid drugs as propylthiourea, methimazole, or carbimazole are used most commonly. These thionamide-type drugs inhibit the coupling of iodotyrosyl residues in thyroglobulin to form T_4 and T_3. Propylthiourea (PTU) is the preferred drug as, in addition to the effects in the thyroid common to all these drugs, it blocks the peripheral conversion of T_4 to T_3 in the liver. Radioactive iodine, administered one time only, is a preferred treatment of hyperthyroidism in patients who have difficulty adhering to the medical regimen of taking antithyroid drugs three times per day for a year or more.

The general symptoms of hypothyroxinemia and thyrotoxicosis are summarized in Table 13.2. Many general manifestations of underproduction or overproduction of thyroid hormones relate to decreased activity of the sympathoadrenal system (Chapter 14). A summary of the general etiology of hypothyroidism and hyperthyroidism is provided in Table 13.3.

TABLE 13.2 Major Physiological Manifestations of Hyperthyroidism and Hypothyroidism

Hyperthyroidism	Hypothyroidism
Elevated T_4-T_3 levels	Decreased (or absent) T_4-T_3 levels
Elevated basal metabolic rate (BMR) (hypermetabolism)	Low basal metabolic rate (BMR) (hypometabolism)
Increased perspiration	Decreased perspiration
Rapid pulse (increased cardiac output, hypertension)	Slow pulse (decreased cardiac output, hypotension)
Increased body temperature (sensation of warmness)	Lowered body temperature (sensation of coldness)
Heat intolerance	Cold intolerance
Warm, moist palms	Coarse, dry skin, subdermal thickening
Nervousness, anxiety, excitability, restlessness, insomnia	Lethargy, decreased mentation, depression, paranoia, sleepiness, tiredness
Weight loss	Weight gain
Muscle wasting	Loss of hair, dry and brittle texture
Increased appetite	Edema of face and eyelids
Menstrual irregularities	Menstrual irregularities
Exophthalmos (in some individuals)	Carotenemia (increased plasma levels of carotenes)
Goiter (primary or secondary origin)	Goiter (may or may not be present)

TABLE 13.3 Pathophysiology of the Human Thyroid Gland

HYPOTHYROIDISM (Hypothyroxinemia)
  Primary hypothyroidism
    Familial or constitutional thyroid dysgenesis
    Failure of thyroid hormonogenesis (usually of genetic origin)
  Secondary hypothyroidism
    Pituitary hypothyroidism (isolated TSH deficiency or pituitary dysgenesis)
    Hypothalamic hypothyroidism (tertiary hypothyroidism)
  Cretinism (childhood hypothyroidism)
    Goitrous cretinism (endemic)
    Athyreotic cretinism (congenital absence of thyroid; thyroid dysgenesis)
  Myxedema (adult hypothyroidism)
    Simple goiter (endemic)
    Primary myxedema
      Idiopathic (atrophic thyroiditis)
      Iatrogenic (surgical removal or chemical inactivation)
      Spontaneous (autoimmune destruction: Hashimoto's thyroiditis)
  Familial peripheral (end-organ) resistance to thyroid hormones (e.g., lack of T_3, T_4 receptors)
  Familial thyroid hormone binding globulin (TBG) deficiency syndrome
  Low T_3 syndrome (failure of peripheral conversion of T_4 to T_3)
  Thyroid gland resistance to TSH
HYPERTHYROIDISM (Thyrotoxicosis)
  Primary hyperthyroidism
    Neoplasia (adenoma, carcinoma)
  Secondary hyperthyroidism
    Hypothalamic hyperthyroidism (Tertiary hyperthyroidism)
    Pituitary hyperthyroidism (neoplasia producing excessive TSH)
    TSH-dependent hyperthyroidism (pituitary thyrotroph unresponsiveness to T_3 feedback inhibition)
    Ectopic TSH secretion (rare)
    Long-acting thyroid stimulator (LATS) (autoimmune agonistic antibodies of thyroid TSH receptors) (Graves' disease)

Tests for Thyroid Function

A variety of tests are utilized to determine the functional status of the thyroid gland. These tests are generally designed to identify the particular site of malfunction in the hypothalamic-hypophysial-thyroid axis [31].

Plasma T_4, T_3 levels.   Plasma concentrations of T_4 and T_3 are measured by radioimmunoassay. As noted, most serum content of thyroid hormones is bound to one or more serum proteins. It is the minute quantities of free T_4 and T_3 that best reflect the tissue metabolic activities of these hormones. The most commonly used tests of thyroid metabolic function measure the concentrations of total serum TBG-bound T_4 and T_3 and some measure the quantities of the free T_4 and T_3 moieties. An important consideration is the total amount of serum proteins available to bind T_4 and T_3 and the extent to which these protein-binding sites are saturated by thyroid hormones.

Serum thyrotropin.   In the normal individual there is usually an inverse correlation between the serum concentrations of thyroid hormones and TSH. Serum levels of TSH are elevated in patients with primary hypothyroidism and are usually undetectable in thyrotoxicosis of primary or autoimmune origin. A discrepancy in the reverse correlation between serum thyroid hormone levels and TSH concentrations might be suggestive of pituitary or hypothalamic dysfunction (secondary and tertiary hypothyroidism or hyperthyroidism).

Tests of pituitary TSH reserve.   In this test an increase in serum TSH in response to administration of synthetic TRH is measured. Thyroid hormones, also released in response to the TSH, are measured as an increase in plasma levels of T_4 and T_3. The TRH test clearly distinguishes between a hypothalamic or pituitary defect in TSH secretion as functional thyrotrophs will usually respond by releasing TSH.

TSH stimulation test.   This test measures the ability of the thyroid to respond to exogenous TSH. It was originally used to differentiate primary hypothyroidism due to thyroid gland failure from other defects in the pituitary thyroid axis.

Tests of thyroid gland activity and hormone synthesis.   Radioisotopes of iodine, ^{131}I and ^{125}I, are used to assess a number of facets in the pathway of thyroid gland hormonogenesis. Increased or decreased uptake of these radioisotopes is associated with excessive or diminished production of thyroid hormones, respectively. The isotope is given intravenously or orally, and the amount of radioactive iodine accumulated by the thyroid at various times following administration is measured by epithyroid radioisotope decay detection. Other tests are designed to determine the intrathyroidal organification of iodine.

Tissue sensitivity to thyroid hormones.   Numerous other tests are used in clinical medicine to determine other aspects of thyroid function. For example, to determine tissue responses to thyroid hormones an increase in basal metabolic rate is often measured in response to the administration of thyroid hormones.

COMPARATIVE ENDOCRINOLOGY

Some classical experiments in endocrinology were performed early in this century on amphibian larvae, most often the anuran (frog, toad) tadpole. These experiments established a role for the thyroid in the control of metamorphosis in the amphibian [18]. The following experimental observations were made:

1. Preparations (desiccated tissue) of the thyroid gland fed to frog tadpoles induced metamorphosis.
2. Removal of the thyroid glands prevented metamorphosis of tadpoles.
3. Implantation of thyroid glands into tadpoles caused accelerated development.
4. Hypophysectomy of tadpoles resulted in thyroid gland atrophy and prevented metamorphosis.
5. Injections of pars distalis extracts induced metamorphosis of hypophysectomized tadpoles.
6. Implantation of the pars distalis, but not the neurointermediate lobe, accelerated development in normal and hypophysectomized larvae, but not in thyroidless tadpoles.

The conclusion that emerged was that "metamorphosis is due to the combined action of both the anterior lobe of the hypophysis and the thyroid gland" [1]. Evidence has now shown that a thyroid stimulating hormone (TSH) is specifically produced by thyrotrophs of the pars distalis and that thyrotropin of any source will stimulate metamorphosis of larval amphibians. Both thyroxine and triiodothyronine induce metamorphosis of amphibian larvae, and they are the likely thyroid hormones controlling metamorphosis in these animals.

Metamorphosis involves radical changes in body structure and function to allow successful transition of the amphibian from an aquatic to a terrestrial habitat. The following metamorphic changes occur in amphibians:

1. Loss of the tail as a locomotory organ and acquisition of the characteristic tetrapod appendages.
2. Change in the integument from a smooth, moist skin (for respiration and increased locomotion) to a thicker, keratinized skin that is more resistant to water loss.
3. Loss of the major respiratory structure, the gills, and acquisition of lungs.
4. Radical changes in structural components of the gastrointestinal tract: loss of the horny, rasping beaklike mouth and development of a new mouth with distensible tongue; shortening of the long intestine (needed for an essentially vegetarian diet) to a much shorter one for a generally carnivorous diet.
5. Development of corneal reflex, eyelids, and ocular muscles to control eye movements (eye movements in larvae are essentially nonexistent).
6. Biochemical changes in numerous organs:
   (a) From predominantly amylase to protease production within the GI tract.
   (b) From larval hemoglobins to adult hemoglobins. Larval hemoglobins bind

more avidly to O_2 than do adult hemoglobins because O_2 is usually more limiting in the aquatic environment than in the terrestrial habitat [21].

(c) From larval visual pigments to those of the adult, a change from predominantly rhodopsin to mostly porphyropsin.

(d) From ammonia excretion (ammonotelism) to urea excretion (ureotelism) [9].

Amphibian larvae are voracious omnivores and spend most of their time eating and converting the ingested metabolic substrates into body structures, essentially proteins. After reaching a particular body size or in response to environmental cues, the larvae undergo irreversible metamorphic changes that lead ultimately to their adult forms. Clearly, thyroid hormones control metamorphic change, but what are the particular endocrine events involved? Are circulating levels of thyroid hormones increased? If so, what physiological events are responsible for such changes? What causes the destruction of one tissue (e.g., the tail) and the development of another (e.g., tongue)? The activity of the thyroid gland (amount of rough ER, follicular height) is clearly increased at metamorphic climax [33]. A popular hypothesis is that the low circulating levels of thyroid hormones in the premetamorphic tadpole cause a slow maturation of hypothalamic neurosecretory centers, resulting in time in greater thyroid hormone secretion. The increase in these hormones, in turn, provides a positive feedback to the hypothalamus, which causes an accelerated maturation of the hypothalamus and its neurosecretory neurons. The resulting activation of TRH secretion and subsequent stimulation of pituitary TSH secretion would provide the final stimulus to thyroid gland maturation and maximal T_4-T_3 secretion [15]. Injection of a minute amount of T_4 directly into the hypothalamus is capable of activating the hypothalamo-hypophysial-thyroid axis in larval salamanders [26].

A body of evidence suggests that prolactin is a larval growth hormone with antimetamorphic actions in amphibians. Normal metamorphic processes may depend on an interplay between PRL and thyroid hormones. For example, thyroxine-induced metamorphosis in the frog is accelerated by injections of antiserum to PRL [7]. Hypophysectomized larval amphibians administered PRL continue to grow with time, even beyond their normal size range; although they never metamorphose, they may be made to do so by injections of high concentrations of thyroid hormones. Both in vivo and in vitro experiments have provided data that PRL antagonizes the action of thyroid hormones on metamorphic processes. For example, thyroxine added to tadpole tails incubated in vitro causes their resorption, a process which normally takes place in the intact animal during metamorphosis. In contrast, PRL added to the incubation medium inhibits the actions of thyroid hormones on tail resorption. It was proposed that the actions of the PRL are also exerted at the level of the thyroid to inhibit thyroid hormone synthesis and secretion (a goitrogenic action). In the *hypothalamic maturation model of metamorphosis* the action of thyroid hormones at the level of the hypothalamus would also involve the establishment of an inhibitory influence on the release of pituitary PRL secretion. This might be effected by the developmental acquisition of functional prolactin-inhibiting factor neurons, resulting in establishment of a tonic inhibitory control over pituitary PRL secretion, as in mammals [15].

Acceleration of the metamorphic process may involve more than an increase in circulating levels of thyroid hormones. There appears to be an increased sensitivity of target tissues, such as the tail, during the progress of metamorphosis. Experimental evidence suggests that the number of binding sites for T_3 in nuclei from tail tissue increases during spontaneous metamorphosis; nuclear receptors for T_3 increase after exposure of intact cells to thyroid hormones. It has been proposed, therefore, that the elevated levels of endogenous thyroid hormones at the onset of metamorphic climax in the tadpole regulate the number of their own nuclear receptors, thus increasing tissue sensitivity to the hormones [45].

Further evidence for thyroid hormone-prolactin interactions during amphibian metamorphosis is available and provides interesting insights into the developmental roles of these two hormones. Certain urodeles, such as the red-spotted newt (*Notophthalmus viridescens*), undergo a second metamorphosis. After an initial metamorphosis from an aquatic larva to a terrestrial tetrapod, the young salamander migrates back to water (so-called water drive). Young newts can be induced to undergo precocious water drive by injections of prolactin. Thyroid hormones, on the other hand, antagonize the actions of PRL. All actions of PRL and thyroid hormones are not exerted in opposition to each other; their actions are indeed often synergistic [10]. For example, binding of PRL to the kidney of the bullfrog tadpole increases during metamorphic climax and in response to treatment with thyroxine [44]. It was suggested that, during metamorphosis, the role of PRL as a growth-promoting agent is lost with its action of ion regulation on the gill. The osmoregulatory function of PRL may nevertheless persist beyond the larval period and be directed through the actions of the thyroid hormones from the gills (which are lost) to the kidneys.

Role of the Thyroid in Other Vertebrates

Evidence is lacking for a clearly defined role of the thyroid gland in cyclostomes and elasmobranchs. In teleost fishes the thyroid gland is required for normal gonadal maturation. Thyroxine increases the sensitivity of the teleost olfactory epithelium to detection of salinity [28]. Thyroid hormones also increase O_2 consumption in fishes and amphibians, but the increase in metabolic activity is easily obscured by other factors. In reptiles a calorigenic action of thyroid hormones has been documented under certain environmental conditions. Thyroid hormones in birds appear to assume roles similar to those in mammals. In amphibians, reptiles, and birds thyroid hormones have prominent effects on the growth and differentiation of the integument and are required for moulting. Thyroxine is involved in the normal moulting of the pelage in mammals; in addition it stimulates the rate of hair growth in rodents and increases the rate of wool growth in sheep [11].

Because of the diverse physiological roles of thyroid hormones in mammals, it can be confidently conjectured that the thyroid gland probably subserves many other functions in nonmammalian vertebrates that have not hitherto been documented [19].

It has been hypothesized that in the evolution of endothermy, thermoregulatory responses to cold, thyroxine, and the sodium pump are related functionally and phylogenetically [39]. In this evolutionary scheme thyroxine was selected as the hormonal regulator because its major role in fishes is ion regulation. Thyroxine increases spontaneous motor activity in all classes of vertebrates; thus, thyroxine enhances behavioral thermoregulation through heat generation from muscular activity. Any increase in oxygen demand results in a concomitant stimulation of the Na^+ pump, and it is speculated that the evolution of nonshivering (metabolic) thermogenesis involved a bypassing of behavioral thermogenesis to a direct stimulation of the Na^+ pump by thyroid hormones to produce heat.

REFERENCES

[1] ALLEN, B. M. 1927. Influence of the hypophysis upon the thyroid gland in amphibian larvae. *Univ. Calif. Publ. Zool.* 31:53–78.

[2] BAXTER, J. D., N. L. EBERHARDT, J. D. APRILETTI, L. K. JOHNSON, R. D. IVARIE, B. S. SCHACHTER, J. A. MORRIS, P. H. SEEBURG, H. M. GOODMAN, K. R. LATHAM, J. R. POLANSKY, and J. A. MARTIAL. 1979. Thyroid hormone receptors and responses. *Rec. Prog. Horm. Res.* 35:97–153.

[3] BLAKE, C. C. F., and S. J. OATLEY. 1977. Protein-DNA and protein-hormone interactions in prealbumin: a model of the thyroid hormone nuclear receptor? *Nature* 268:115–20.

[4] BRAVERMAN, L. E., S. H. INGBAR, and K. STERLING. 1970. Conversion of thyroxine to triiodothyronine in athyreotic human subjects. *J. Clin. Invest.* 49:855–64.

[5] CAVALIERI, R. R., and B. RAPOPORT. 1977. Impaired peripheral conversion of thyroxine to triiodothyronine. *Ann. Rev. Med.* 28:57–65.

[6] CHOPRA, I. J., D. H. SOLOMON, U. CHOPRA, S. Y. WU, D. A. FISHER, and Y. NAKAMURA. 1978. Pathways of metabolism of thyroid hormones. *Rec. Prog. Horm. Res.* 34:521–67.

[7] CLEMONS, G. K., and C. S. NICOLL. 1977. Effects of antisera to bullfrog prolactin and growth hormone on metamorphosis of *Rana catesbeiana* tadpoles. *Gen. Comp. Endocrinol.* 31:495–97.

[8] CODY, V. 1978. Thyroid hormones: crystal structure, molecular configuration, binding, and structure-function relationships. *Rec. Prog. Horm. Res.* 34:437–75.

[9] COHEN, P. P., R. F. BRUCKER, and S. M. MORRIS. 1978. Cellular and molecular aspects of thyroid hormone action during amphibian metamorphosis. In *Hormonal proteins and peptides*, vol. 6, ed. C. H. Li, pp. 273–381. New York: Academic Press, Inc.

[10] DENT, J. N. 1975. Integumentary effects of prolactin in lower vertebrates. *Am. Zool.* 15:923–35.

[11] EBLING, F. J., and P. A. HALE. 1970. The control of the mammalian moult. In *Hormones and the environment*, eds. G. K. Benson and J. G. Phillips, pp. 215–37. London: Cambridge University Press.

[12] EDELMAN, I. S. 1974. Thyroid thermogenesis. *New Engl. J. Med.* 290:1303–1308.

[13] ERICSON, L. E. 1981. Exocytosis and endocytosis in the thyroid cell. *Molec. Cell. Endocrinol.* 22:1–24.

[14] ERMANS, A. M., F. DELENGE, M. VAN DER VELDEN, and J. KINTHAERT. 1972. Possible role of cyanide and thiocyanate in the etiology of endemic cretinism. In *Human development and the thyroid gland*, eds. J. B. Stanbury and R. L. Kroc. New York: Plenum Publishing Corporation.

[15] ETKIN, W. 1978. The thyroid: a gland in search of a function. *Perspectives Biol. Med.* 22:19–30.

[16] FISHER, D. A., J. H. DUSSAULT, J. SACK, and I. J. CHOPRA. 1977. Ontogenesis by hypothalamic-pituitary-thyroid function and metabolism in man, sheep, and rat. *Rec. Prog. Horm. Res.* 33:59–116.

[17] FISHER, D. A., and A. H. KLEIN. 1981. Thyroid development and disorders of thyroid function in the newborn. *New Engl. J. Med.* 304:702–12.

[18] GILBERT, L. I., and E. FRIEDEN. 1981. *Metamorphosis: a problem in developmental biology.* New York: Plenum Publishing Corporation.

[19] GORBMAN, A. 1978. Evolution of thyroid function. In *Hormonal proteins and peptides,* vol. 6. ed. C. H. Li, pp. 383–89. New York: Academic Press, Inc.

[20] HOSKINS, R. G. 1946. *The tides of life.* New York: W. W. Norton & Co., Inc.

[21] JUST, J. J., and B. G. ATKINSON. 1972. Hemoglobin transitions in the bullfrog *Rana catesbeiana* during spontaneous and induced metamorphosis. *J. Exp. Zool.* 182:271–80.

[22] LANGER, P., and M. A. GREER. 1977. *Antithyroid substances and naturally occurring goitrogens.* Basel: S. Karger.

[23] LASON, A. H. 1946. *The thyroid gland in medical history.* New York: Frogen Press.

[24] MARTIN, J. B. 1974. Regulation of pituitary-thyroid axis. In *MTP Intern. Rev. Science, Physiol.* Series 1, vol. 5, *Endocrine Physiology,* ed. S. M. McCann, pp. 67–107. Baltimore, Md.: University Park Press.

[25] MELANDER, A., L. E. ERICSON, F. SUNDLER, and S. H. INGBAR. 1974. Sympathetic innervation of the mouse thyroid and its significance in thyroid hormone secretion. *Endocrinology* 94:959–66.

[26] NORRIS, D. O., and W. A. GERN. 1976. Thyroxine-induced activation of hypothalamo-hypophysial axis in neotenic salamander larvae. *Science* 194:525–27.

[27] OPPENHEIMER, J. H. 1979. Thyroid hormone action at the cellular level. *Science* 203:971–79.

[28] OSHIMA, K., and A. GORBMAN. 1966. Olfactory responses in the forebrain of goldfish and their modification by thyroxine treatment. *Gen. Comp. Endocrinol.* 7:398–409.

[29] PITT-RIVERS, R. 1978. The thyroid hormones: historical aspects. In *Hormonal proteins and peptides,* vol. 6, ed. C. H. Li, pp. 391–422. New York: Academic Press, Inc.

[30] PITT-RIVERS, R., and J. R. TATA. 1959. *The thyroid hormones.* New York: Pergamon Press, Inc.

[31] REFETOFF, S. 1979. Thyroid disease: thyroid function tests. In *Endocrinology,* eds. L. J. DeGroot, G. F. Cahill, Jr., L. Martini, D. H. Nelson, W. D. Odell, J. T. Potts, Jr., E. Steinberger, and A. I. Winegrad, pp. 387–428. New York: Grune & Stratton, Inc.

[32] REFETOFF, S. 1982. Syndromes of thyroid hormone resistance. *Am. J. Physiol.* 243: E88–E98.

[33] REGARD, E. 1978. Cytophysiology of the amphibian thyroid through larval development and metamorphosis. *Int. Rev. Cytol.* 52:81–118.

[34] ROBBINS, J., S.-Y. CHENG, M. C. GERSHENGORN, D. GLENOER, H. J. CAHNMANN, and H. EDELNOCH. 1978. Thyroxine transport proteins of plasma. Molecular properties and biosynthesis. *Rec. Prog. Horm. Res.* 34:477–519.

[35] SCHUSSLER, G. C., and J. ORLANDO. 1978. Fasting decreases triiodothyronine receptor capacity. *Science* 199:686–87.

[36] SIMS, E. A. 1979. Syndromes of obesity. In *Endocrinology,* eds. L. J. DeGroot, G. F. Cahill, Jr., L. Martini, D. H. Nelson, W. D. Odell, J. T. Potts, Jr., E. Steinberger, and A. I. Winegrad, pp. 1941–62. New York: Grune & Stratton, Inc.

[37] STERLING, K. 1979. Thyroid hormone action at the cell level. *New Engl. J. Med.* 300: 117–23, 173–77.

[38] STERLING, K., and J. H. LAZARUS. 1977. The thyroid and its control. *Ann. Rev. Physiol.* 39:349–71.

[39] STEVENS, E. D. 1973. The evolution of endothermy. *J. Theor. Biol.* 38:597–611.

[40] SURKS, M. I., and J. H. OPPENHEIMER. 1977. Concentration of L-thyroxine and L-tri-iodothyronine specifically bound to nuclear receptors in rat liver and kidney. *J. Clin. Invest.* 60:555–62.

[41] TAUROG, A. 1977. Hormone synthesis. In *Endocrinology*, eds. L. J. DeGroot, G. F. Cahill, Jr., L. Martini, D. H. Nelson, W. D. Odell, J. T. Potts, Jr., E. Steinberger, and A. I. Winegrad, pp. 331–42. New York: Grune & Stratton, Inc.

[42] VAN HERLE, A. J., G. VASSART, and J. E. DUMONT. 1979. Control of thyroglobulin synthesis secretion. *New Engl. J. Med.* 301:239–49, 307–14.

[43] VONDERHAAR, B. K., and A. E. GRECO. 1979. Lobulo-alveolar development of mouse mammary glands is regulated by thyroid hormones. *Endocrinology* 104:409–18.

[44] WHITE, B. A., and C. S. NICOLL. 1979. Prolactin receptors in *Rana catesbeiana* during development and metamorphosis. *Science* 204:851–53.

[45] YOSHIZATO, K., and E. FRIEDEN. 1975. Increase in binding capacity for triiodothyronine in tadpole tail nuclei during metamorphosis. *Nature* 254:705–707.

14

Catecholamines and the Sympathoadrenal System

INTRODUCTION

The physiologically relevant catecholamines are epinephrine (E), norepinephrine (NE), and dopamine (DA). The chemical structure of epinephrine (also referred to as adrenaline) was the first determined; the structure of NE (also referred to as noradrenaline) was elucidated much later. Although E has generally been considered a classic example of a hormone (a humoral messenger) and NE a truly representative neurotransmitter, both catecholamines are now realized to function reciprocally as humoral effectors or neurotransmitters. Dopamine's major physiological roles are relegated to the CNS and certain autonomic nervous system ganglia. A chronological history of research related to the catecholamines provides a fascinating example of the growth and development of endocrine physiology [20].

Historical Perspective

1895 Oliver and Schafer discovered that extracts of the suprarenal (adrenal) glands (specifically the chromaffin component) of a number of mammalian species produced a pressor response when injected into animals [34].

1899 The pressor principle of the adrenal gland was isolated and named epinephrine by Abel.

1901 The true structural identity of epinephrine was determined by Aldrich (Fig. 14.1).

1904– Stolz (1904) and subsequently Dakin (1905) synthesized epi-
1905 nephrine.

1898– Lewandowsky and Langley noted that injections of adrenal ex-
1901 tracts produced effects similar to stimulation of sympathetic neurons.

1904 Elliot postulated that sympathetic nerve impulses release an epinephrine-like substance onto adjacent effector cells. This was the first suggestion of a neurohumor and the concept of neurotransmission.

1905 Administration of epinephrine was found to exhibit both excitatory (vasopressor) and inhibitory (vasodepressor) effects on the cardiovascular system. Langley therefore proposed that autonomic effector cells may possess excitatory and inhibitory receptive substances and that the particular response elicited depended on which substance was present.

1906 Dale discovered that a drug, an ergot alkaloid, specifically antagonized the pressor activities of sympathetic nervous stimulation or epinephrine administration [13]. Indeed, the drug actually reversed the actions of such stimuli, producing instead a vasodepressor response. These observations again revealed that epinephrine could elicit two opposing actions, even in the same tissue.

1910 Barger and Dale studied the action of a large number of synthetic amines related to epinephrine in structure and termed the actions of these drugs sympathomimetic.

1921 Loewi provided evidence that, indeed, an excitatory substance similar to epinephrine is released from the vagus nerve upon electrical stimulation. In this same year Cannon and Uradil noted that although stimulation of certain sympathetic neurons released an epinephrinelike substance which increased blood pressure and heart rate, other smooth muscle responses differed qualitatively from the effects produced by epinephrine. Cannon and Bacq referred to the substance released as sympathin. Barger and Dale had noted earlier (1910) that the effects of sympathetic nerve stimulation were more similar to those of a primary amine than epinephrine or other secondary amines.

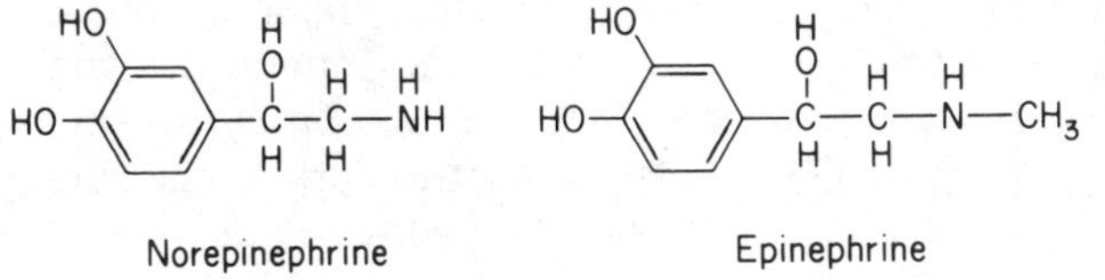

Norepinephrine   Epinephrine

Figure 14.1 Structures of norepinephrine and epinephrine.

1931   Bacq advanced the thesis that sympathin might be norepinephrine (noradrenaline).

1933   Cannon and Rosenblueth formulated the concept that two sympathins might exist, a sympathin E (excitatory) and a sympathin I (inhibitory) [10].

1935   Although Bacq realized that sympathin was not identical to epinephrine, he objected to the view that both a sympathin E and I existed. Rather, a catecholamine could have opposite effects on the same cell.

1946   Von Euler established that the neurotransmitter released from the postganglionic neurons of the sympathetic system was norepinephrine (Fig. 14.1). Although the chemical nature of sympathin was elucidated, this putative neurotransmitter, norepinephrine, could elicit either smooth muscle contraction or relaxation depending on the particular muscle preparation studied. The hypothesis of two sympathins was still in vogue.

1948   Ahlquist studied a large number of sympathomimetic amines and determined that for each tissue a certain potency ranking could be established for the biological actions of these agents. He formulated the concept of dual adrenoceptors where different receptors controlled smooth muscle contraction and relaxation. These receptive substances were referred to as α- and β-adrenoceptors, respectively. Although the *adrenoceptor hypothesis* was not accepted immediately, the discovery of drugs that specifically inhibit either α- or β-adrenoceptors firmly established the validity of the concept.

1962   Sutherland and his colleagues discovered cAMP and proposed that this cyclic nucleotide be considered an intracellular second messenger of hormone action [40]. It was subsequently revealed that β-adrenoceptor stimulation always leads to cAMP production, whereas in some tissues α-adrenoceptor stimulation lowers cellular cAMP levels.

1973   The ying-yang hypothesis of hormone action, involving the production of either cAMP or cGMP which then subserves opposing intracellular functions (e.g., muscle relaxation or contraction, respectively), was formulated [21]. The extent to which this potentially important concept applies to all cells is being explored.

In retrospect the confusion relating to the roles and actions of the catecholamines is understandable. Both E and NE are similar in structure and are released from the adrenal or from neurons in response to a variety of stimuli. Also, both catecholamines can produce similar or opposing physiological responses within the same tissue; their actions at a particular concentration may even be different. The formulation of the adrenoceptor hypothesis by Ahlquist [1] substantiated the early suggestion of Langley that cells might possess different "receptive substances" (in this context, adrenoceptors) and that the particular response of a cell depended on which substance (receptor) was activated. A more thorough historical discussion of catecholamines and adrenoceptors is available [20].

THE SYMPATHOADRENAL SYSTEM

Epinephrine and norepinephrine are hormones of the adrenal chromaffin tissue and sympathetic neurons, respectively. Because these two catecholamines have similar structures and biological actions, it is customary to discuss their endocrinologies together, as components of the *sympathoadrenal system*. It is first necessary to review the general anatomical components of the autonomic nervous system (ANS) because both sympathetic neurons and chromaffin tissue are integral structural and functional components of the ANS [3, 8].

The Autonomic Nervous System

The *peripheral nervous system* consists of those nerves which arise from the brainstem and spinal cord—the cranial and spinal nerves, respectively. Cranial and spinal nerves which innervate skeletal (voluntary) muscle make up the somatic component (*somatic nervous system*) of the peripheral nervous system. The cell bodies of the somatic neurons lie within the spinal column and the long axons of these nerves directly innervate skeletal muscle. The other nerves of the peripheral nervous system comprise the autonomic nervous system. These nerves supply the skin and all visceral organs (heart, blood vessels, GI tract, pancreas, adrenals, kidneys, etc.). These nerves are mainly *vasomotor* and *secretomotor* in function; that is, the neurons innervate smooth muscles of blood vessels, and they innervate exocrine (salivary, pancreas) and endocrine (adrenals, pancreas) glands. Other smooth muscles of the GI tract, gallbladder, urinary bladder, spleen capsule, hair follicles, as well as the cardiac muscle of the heart are also innervated by neurons of the ANS.

The ANS can be subdivided into nerves which comprise the *parasympathetic nervous system* and the *sympathetic nervous system*. The nerves of both systems are composed of *preganglionic* and *postganglionic* neurons. The cell bodies of the preganglionic fibers of both divisions, which reside within the spinal cord, synapse with a second neuron within various ganglia. The postganglionic neurons then directly innervate the various *autonomic effector organs*. Neurotransmission between preganglionic and postganglionic neurons is effected by *acetylcholine* release from the presynaptic neurons. The neurotransmitter of the postganglionic neurons of the parasympathetic system is also acetylcholine, but the neurotransmitter released by the postganglionic neuron of the sympathetic system is norepinephrine.

Parasympathetic nerves arise in the cranial-sacral segments of the spinal column, whereas sympathetic neurons arise in the thoraco-lumbar region of the spinal cord. The very long parasympathetic preganglionic fibers usually synapse with postganglionic neurons within ganglia located in the autonomic effector organs that they regulate. The sympathetic preganglionic fibers, on the other hand, usually synapse with postganglionic neurons within ganglia located some distance from the target tissues they innervate. The general anatomy of the autonomic system and its effector organs is shown (Fig. 14.2).

The parasympathetic system is concerned mainly with the so-called vegetative (resting) processes of the body. Most of its actions are related to those processes concerned with the movement and digestion of food within the GI tract, the movement of metabolic substrates into the body proper, and the conservation (storage) of these substrates within such storage depots as the liver, adipose tissue, and muscle. The sympathetic nervous system, in contrast, is concerned with those processes related to the more active states of the body and plays a particularly important role under conditions of stress. The sympathetic system generally prepares the body for "fight or flight" [9]. For example, the muscular and secretory activities of the GI tract are depressed, whereas the force and rate of the heartbeat are increased, and consequently blood flow is increased, particularly to those areas, such as muscle, that are most active. Blood flow to the brain and coronary arteries is enhanced, whereas circulation to the skin and digestive tract and kidneys is diminished.

Although the individual actions of acetylcholine and norepinephrine are often viewed as opposite they are actually complementary to each other. For example, norepinephrine contracts the heart and forces blood out into the circulatory system. Acetylcholine, on the other hand, relaxes the heart so that it can again fill up with blood. The movement of food through the GI tract results from peristalsis, a process which involves the alternate contraction and relaxation of individual segments of the gut in temporal unison. Contractions of the gut are regulated by acetylcholine, whereas norepinephrine relaxes smooth muscle of the gut. Although their actions are opposite in direction, both neurotransmitters participate in the rhythmic (peristaltic) movement of food through the gut.

Adrenal Chromaffin Tissue

The adrenal gland of many vertebrates is composed of two distinct cellular types of different embryological origin that secrete structurally very different hormones. Chromaffin cells (pheochromoblasts) are derived from the neural crest, whereas the steroidogenic component of the adrenal is of mesodermal origin (Chapter 15). In most mammals the chromaffin tissue is surrounded by an outer adrenal cortex composed of steroid-producing cells. Therefore, the chromaffin tissue is often referred to as the *adrenal medulla*. In most nonmammalian species, however, the chromaffin tissue is not associated with any surrounding mass of cortical tissue; hence the term adrenal medulla is without anatomical justification unless used in reference to a restricted number of mammalian species. The term chromaffin (Greek: *chroma*, color; Latin: *affinis*, affinity) tissue derives from the observation that the pheochromocytes become brown when placed in contact with oxidizing agents such as chromate.

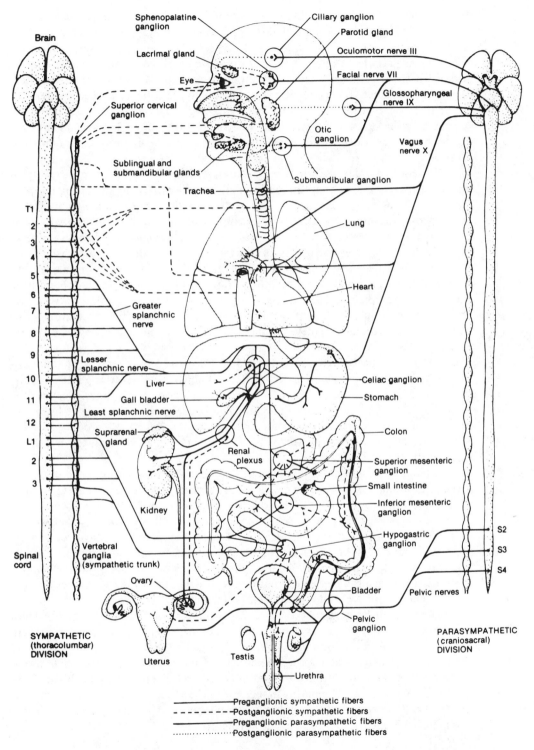

Figure 14.2 The autonomic nervous system. (From William F. Evans, ANATOMY AND PHYSIOLOGY 2nd ed. © 1976, p. 187. Reproduced by permission of Prentice-Hall, Inc., Englewood Cliffs, N.J.)

The human adrenal medulla consists of two cell types: adrenaline (A)- and noradrenaline (N)-storing cells. Chromaffin cells contain granules composed of catecholamines, adenine nucleotides (mainly ATP), proteins, and lipids. The protein of these granules is referred to as *chromogranin*. Histochemical studies demonstrate that the cells are not biochemically identical: The A cells apparently contain more glycoproteins. The ratio of these two cell types differs between species; the chromaffin tissue of the human and the guinea pig, for example, consists mainly of A cells. Less information is available relative to nonmammalian species, but the same two cell types have been recognized in species of elasmobranchs, amphibians, birds, and reptiles.

Extra-adrenal chromaffin tissue occurs as encapsulated and nonencapsulated masses scattered throughout the abdominal prevertebral sympathetic plexuses of the human fetus [11]. The encapsulated masses predominate and are richly vascularized from adjacent blood vessels. These numerous chromaffin masses are of varying size and are referred to as para-aortic bodies or *paraganglia*. The larger para-aortic bodies lie on the aorta near the origin of the inferior mesenteric artery and are known as the *organs of Zuckerkandl*. These groups of isolated chromaffin cells probably represent neural crest cells that "fail" to migrate into the adrenal during embryonic development. The extra-adrenal chromaffin tissue involutes after birth, but tumors may appear later from this tissue. The para-aortic chromaffin tissue may also proliferate and achieve a functional role if the adrenals are surgically removed or destroyed by disease.

Large amounts of extra-adrenal chromaffin tissue are present in the fetus. Although this tissue only contains NE, it is not known if it is secreted into the fetal circulation. The tissue, however, does have an endocrine appearance. Because the sympathetic nervous system is still incompletely developed at the time of birth, the vascular tone of the fetus may be under humoral control by NE produced by the para-aortic bodies; during postnatal life this function may be replaced by NE of sympathetic origin [11].

Comparative anatomical studies reveal that the distribution of chromaffin tissue and adrenal steroidogenic tissue differs considerably among the vertebrates. In elasmobranchs and teleost fishes the two tissues are well separated, whereas in mammals and birds they are always intermingled. The association of the two tissues in amphibians and reptiles is variable. The functional significance of what appears to have been an evolution of the two tissues to come together as a single anatomical entity—the adrenal gland—is nebulous. There is clearly a biochemical correlation between the degree of anatomical association of the two tissues and the relative amounts of NE and E produced by the chromaffin tissue.

In the dogfish shark where the chromaffin tissue is entirely separated from steroidogenic tissue NE is the only catecholamine produced. In the frog where chromaffin tissue is intermingled with steroidogenic tissue NE accounts for only about 55% to 70% of the catecholamines. In primates and other mammals where the two tissues are closely intermingled very little NE is produced and E is the exclusive product of the chromaffin tissue. From these observations it has been concluded that the presence of the adrenal steroidogenic tissue determines the degree to which NE is methylated to E in the chromaffin tissue.

Nature And Nurture In ANS Development

Elegant experimental techniques have provided fascinating observations related to the embryology of the ANS and continue to provide new insights into factors that may influence the autonomic neurons and chromaffin cells during development [5, 7]. There are preferential pathways located at precise levels of the embryo that direct neural crest cells to their definitive anatomical destinations. Nevertheless, differentiation of the autonomic neuroblasts is controlled by the environment in which the crest cells become localized at the end of their migration [30]. Neural crest cells destined to populate the ANS express an overt noradrenergic phenotype only upon reaching the primordium of the sympathetic chain. The initial metabolic commitment, however, appears to be mutable, and further differentiation may be influenced by the environment within which the cells reside. For example, those cells that populate sympathetic ganglia remain noradrenergic, whereas those that invade the adrenal gland begin to synthesize epinephrine [41].

The expression of the adrenergic phenotype of chromaffin precursor cells in the embryonic adrenal gland has been studied in some detail. In the 13.5-day-old mouse the medullary precursors lying in the sympathetic ganglia primordia—those migrating toward the adrenal as well as those within the adrenal—express noradrenergic characteristics (tyrosine hydroxylase and dopamine-β-hydroxylase activities). Phenylethanolamine-N-methyltransferase (PNMT), the enzyme required for conversion of NE to E, is not present but is detectable 3.5 days later at 17 days gestation. This initial expression of PNMT is not dependent on normal glucocorticoid levels and cannot be induced prematurely by glucocorticoids; it is also independent of the pituitary adrenal axis [6]. The normal ontogenetic increase in the activity of this enzyme after the initial expression has occurred does require the presence of an intact pituitary-adrenal axis. The synthesis of PNMT within the CNS indicates that development within the adrenal environment is not an absolute requirement for PNMT biosynthesis. Extra-adrenal chromaffin tissue is also capable of expressing PNMT activity in response to glucocorticoid stimulation.

Sympathetic neurons and adrenal chromaffin cells derive from a common neuroectodermal origin; the morphology and enzymatic profiles of the two cell types, however, differ considerably. Neural crest cell differentiation into sympathetic neurons is controlled by nerve growth factor (NGF). Prenatal and postnatal injections of NGF into rats can divert partially differentiated chromaffin cells into nerve cells that are morphologically and ultrastructurally indistinguishable from sympathetic neurons [2]. NGF can channel chromaffin cell precursors toward nerve cell differentiation, an action which apparently must override the effects of glucocorticoids which normally induce enzymes required for epinephrine synthesis. Sympathetic neurons disconnected from their autonomic effector organs die unless supplied with exogenous NGF. Apparently the effector organs normally provide a continuous supply of NGF to the sympathetic neurons which is a requirement for their structural and functional integrity. In the absence of NGF administration the transformed sympathetic cells also undergo massive destruction; injections of antisera to NGF into the rat fetus produce massive destruction of chromaffin cell precursors. Isolated adrenal medullary cells treated with NGF occasionally develop neurites, sometimes even in the absence of exogenous NGF. Addition of a gluco-corticoid to the incubation can inhibit neurite development. These results imply that normal growth and development of adrenal chromaffin tissue may depend on the temporal interactions of NGF and glucocorticoids.

SYNTHESIS, CHEMISTRY, AND METABOLISM

The pathways of catecholamine biosynthesis within the CNS, sympathetic post-ganglionic neurons, and adrenal chromaffin tissue appear to be identical. The number of steps in each pathway, however, depends on the definitive product—DA, NE, or E—to be secreted [4] (Fig. 14.3).

Synthesis. The conversion of tyrosine to E involves four steps: (1) hydroxylation at the three position of the phenolic ring; (2) side-chain decarboxylation; (3) side-chain hydroxylation; and (4) *N*-methylation [4]. Hydroxylation of phenylalanine, although essential for tyrosine production, may not make an important contribution to tyrosine availability within sympathetic neurons and chromaffin cells. Tyrosine is transported into the cell where it is converted to dihydroxyphenylalanine (DOPA) by the enzyme *tyrosine hydroxylase*. This is the rate-limiting enzyme in catecholamine biosynthesis. The activity of this enzyme is regulated by feedback (end-product) inhibition by cytoplasmic catecholamines. Chronic stimulation of catecholamine synthesis and secretion leads to elevation of cellular tyrosine hydroxy-

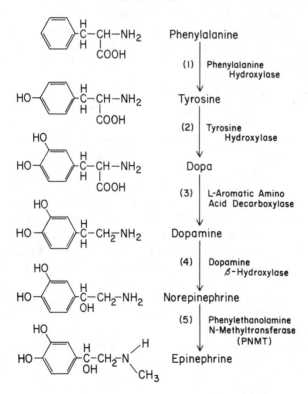

Figure 14.3 Pathway of catecholamine biosynthesis.

lase levels. In the subsequent step DOPA is decarboxylated to dopamine by *DOPA decarboxylase*, a nonspecific decarboxylase (L-aromatic amino acid decarboxylase) found in many tissues. Dopamine is then hydroxylated by *dopamine β-hydroxylase* (DBH) by addition of an —OH group to the side-chain carbon (β-carbon adjacent to the phenolic ring). The NE produced is converted to E by PNMT; this enzyme is only found in cells that synthesize E, adrenal chromaffin tissue of many vertebrates, and within specific neuronal tracts in the brain. It should be noted that NE is a primary amine, whereas E is an *N*-methylated secondary amine; these differences provide an important structural basis for the differing potency of these two catecholamines on adrenoceptors.

Storage and release. Catecholamines (NE and E, but not dopamine) are stored within granules where they are complexed with ATP and a specific protein, *chromogranin*, and DBH. The secretory vesicles are released through a stimulus-secretion coupling requiring calcium. All the contents of the storage granules are released during vesicular exocytosis [16].

Metabolism. Catecholamines are catabolized by two enzymes, catecholamine-O-methyltransferase (COMT) and monoamine oxidase (MAO). Norepinephrine and E are metabolized extracellularly by COMT to normetanephrine and metanephrine, respectively (Fig. 14.4). COMT is localized within the cytosol of sympathetic effector cells and is also found in close proximity to the NE receptor of autonomic effectors. MAO is found on the surface of the outer membrane of mitochondria where it limits the accumulation of catecholamines within the cytoplasm. Because of the sequential action of these two enzymes, the main metabolite of catecholamines excreted in the urine is 3-methoxy-4-hydroxymandelic acid (also known as vanillylmandelic acid, VMA) (Fig. 14.4).

Most NE released from sympathetic neurons is taken back up into the neuron where it is either transported back into the secretory vesicles or destroyed by MAO.

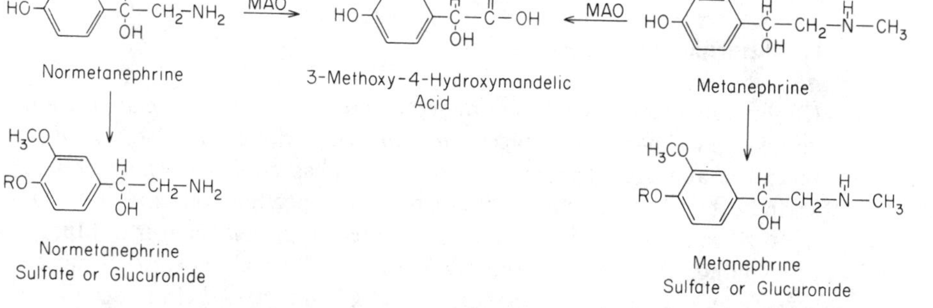

Figure 14.4 Pathways of catecholamine metabolism.

The NE accumulated within the synaptic cleft feeds back to α-adrenergic receptors within the presynaptic membrane, which stimulates uptake of the catecholamine and inhibits further synthesis of NE.

Hormonal control. In species where the chromaffin tissue is separated from the adrenal steroidogenic tissue NE is usually the main synthetic product. In those species (e.g., human, rat) where the chromaffin cells are contiguous with steroidogenic tissue, however, E is the predominant catecholamine synthesized. Levels of PNMT decline in hypophysectomized rats, and normal levels are restored by administration of ACTH or glucocorticoids. Actinomycin D and puromycin block hormonal restoration of PNMT levels, suggesting de novo synthesis of the enzyme. Levels of tyrosine hydroxylase and DBH are also lowered somewhat in the absence of adrenal glucocorticoids.

Catecholamine Regulation Of COMT Activity

COMT is one of the enzymes responsible for termination of the actions of catecholamines and occurs in cytoplasmic soluble and membrane-bound forms. The membrane-bound form appears to reside in close juxtaposition to postsynaptic β-adrenoceptors, and its activity is enhanced by β-adrenoceptor stimulation. However, although β-adrenoceptors are linked to adenylate cyclase activation and cAMP production, activation of COMT activity is not mediated through cAMP [45]. Increased activity of COMT in response to catecholamines provides a homeostatic mechanism for the rapid removal of catecholamines from the circulation and the synaptic cleft.

MECHANISMS OF ACTION

The terms *adrenergic* and *cholinergic* were introduced by Dale [14] to designate those nerves that release the sympathetic transmitter (unknown at that time) and acetylcholine, respectively. These terms are now used to designate the receptors through which these neurotransmitters of the postganglionic neurons of the sympathetic (norepinephrine) and parasympathetic (acetylcholine) nervous system mediate their effects. These receptors are localized to the postsynaptic membranes of the innervated effector cells (e.g., smooth muscle, salivary gland cells).

Cholinergic Receptors

Cholinergic receptors respond to acetylcholine and several related analogs of acetylcholine. Two plant substances, *nicotine* and *muscarine*, also stimulate cholinergic receptors and are appropriately referred to as *cholinomimetic* agents. The effects of these two cholinergic agonists are tissue specific. Nicotine, for example, stimulates skeletal muscle and autonomic postganglionic neurons. Muscarine, on the other hand, stimulates autonomic effector cells such as smooth muscle. These observations suggest that these nicotinic and muscarinic cholinoceptive sites are not identical. This is further substantiated by the observation that the drug curare (and also tubucurare) specifically blocks *nicotinic* cholinergic receptors, whereas the drug atropine is inhibitory to acetylcholine stimulation of *muscarinic* cholinergic receptors. For example, the muscles lining the gut of a teleost fish, the tench, are composed of both striated and smooth muscle. Electrical stimulation of the vagus nerve innervating these muscles results in contraction of both types of muscle producing a recorded response that contains both a quick and a slow component of contraction. After curarization, however, only the slow component can be elicited. After atropinization, on the other hand, only the fast component of contraction is evident. The slow and fast components of muscle contraction are abolished, however, after administration of both curare and atropine [20].

Adrenergic Receptors

After studying the actions of a number of sympathomimetic amines on smooth muscle contraction and relaxation, Ahlquist [1] concluded that two types of adrenergic receptors might exist: α- and β-adrenergic receptors or, as they are also designated, α- and β-adrenoceptors. These putative receptors differed in their relative responsiveness (sensitivity) to certain sympathetic amines. The response of α-adrenoceptors provided the following potency ranking: epinephrine (E) > norepinephrine (NE) > isoproterenol (ISO). The potency ranking for β-adrenoceptors was ISO > E > NE. The α-adrenoceptors subserve smooth muscle contraction, the β-adrenoceptors, relaxation. A number of drugs were then discovered that could stimulate specifically the putative adrenoceptors or antagonize the response of these receptors to catecholamines. It was noted, for example, that phenylephrine was a very specific agonist of α-adrenoceptors, whereas isoproterenol was a very specific β-adrenoceptor agonist. Used at high (unphysiological) concentrations sympathoamines can usually stimulate either adrenoceptor as these agents are structurally related.

After α-adrenoceptor blockage certain smooth muscle preparations relaxed rather than contracted as they normally did in response to epinephrine [33]. This epinephrine reversal was reminiscent of that noted by Dale [13] using an ergot alkaloid preparation. The subsequent discovery of a compound that specifically blocked β-adrenoceptor-stimulated smooth muscle relaxation provided an explanation for the phenomenon of epinephrine reversal. Epinephrine stimulates both α- and β-adrenoceptors simultaneously, but the actions of the hormone on α-adrenoceptors dominate (Fig. 14.5). However, in the presence of α-adrenoceptor blockage the response of the "silent" β-adrenoceptor is revealed. Simultaneous incubation of smooth muscle in the presence of both α- and β-adrenoceptor antagonists (blocking agents) totally inhibits smooth muscle responses to the agonists. The *dual receptor hypothesis* provided a rational explanation for the contrasting effects of catecholamines on autonomic effectors. It was no longer necessary to think of a sympathin E and a sympathin I to account for the excitatory and inhibitory activities of a catecholamine; rather, a single sympathetic neurotransmitter was conceived whose actions are determined by the nature of the particular adrenoceptor stimulated.

There is evidence that β-adrenoceptors represent at least two pharmacologically different subgroups [28]. The lipolytic response of adipose tissue and the contraction of cardiac muscle typify so-called β_1-adrenoceptors where the potency ranking for certain agonists is ISO >> E $\simeq$ NE. Bronchodilation and vasodepres-

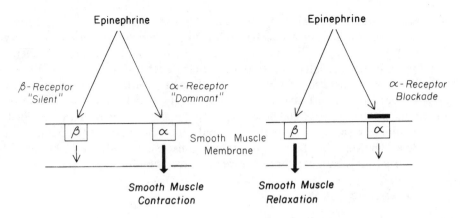

Figure 14.5 Experimental demonstration of epinephrine (catecholamine) reversal.

sion, on the other hand, are regulated by β_2-adrenoceptors where the agonist potency profile is ISO > E >> NE. The existence of two functionally distinct types of α-adrenoceptors has also been proposed. α_1-Adrenoceptors mediate responses typified by smooth muscle vasoconstriction where the agonists methoxamine and phenylephrine have high potency with respect to NE. The α_2-adrenoceptors mediate feedback inhibition of NE release at synapses where clonidine and α-methyl norepinephrine have high potency, relative to phenylephrine and methoxamine which are much less effective [39]. α_2-Adrenoceptors may also be found at some postsynaptic sites (liver, brain, some smooth muscles) [18, 26].

Autonomic effector cells may possess α- and β-adrenoceptors or only β-adrenoceptors. Smooth muscle contraction with one exception (intestinal smooth muscle) is regulated through α-adrenoceptors, whereas relaxation with one exception (cardiac muscle) is controlled through β-adrenoceptor stimulaton. Where α-adrenoceptors are present they dominate (mask) β-adrenoceptors. The β-adrenoceptors, noted earlier, can only be demonstrated in some tissues after α-adrenoceptor blockade. Some smooth muscles (e.g., bronchial smooth muscle) possess β-adrenoceptors but not α-adrenoceptors; these muscles always relax in response to catecholamines.

It is important to note that, depending on which adrenoceptors are present, a catecholamine can either contract or relax smooth muscle. Nevertheless, catecholamines normally only control one component of smooth muscle activity—contraction or relaxation—depending on the nature of the adrenoceptors present. Because smooth muscle must normally contract and relax, another neurotransmitter is required for the nonadrenergic component of muscle activity. Acetylcholine subserves that role. For example, acetylcholine controls the contractile components of bronchial smooth muscle as well as gastrointestinal smooth muscle.

β-adrenoceptors. The major difference between β_1- and β_2-adrenoceptors is their sensitivity to norepinephrine. The β_1-receptors respond readily to circulating E or to neurally released NE. On the other hand, the natural agonist of the β_2-adrenoceptors is probably E. From these observations it has been suggested that the β_2-receptor is a hormonal adrenoceptor, whereas the β_1-adrenoceptor is a neuronal adrenoceptor [37].

β-adrenoceptor blocking agents do not block responses associated with α-adrenoceptors and they do not inhibit the actions of other hormones or drugs. For example, E and glucagon both stimulate hepatic glycogenolysis, but only the actions of E are antagonized by the blocker (Fig. 11.10). On the adipocyte β-adrenoceptor antagonists block the lipolytic action of E but not ACTH. *N*-methylation of NE to yield E apparently enhances affinity for the β-adrenoceptor. The structures of β-adrenoceptor agonists and antagonists bear resemblance to isoproterenol (Fig. 14.6).

α-adrenoceptors. Presynaptic α_2-adrenoceptors occur at all noradrenergic synapses where they subserve an autoinhibition in which released NE inhibits its own further release (Fig. 14.7). An understanding of the pharmacology of α-adrenoceptors is relatively limited primarily because the structures of the α-adrenoceptor agonists and antagonists generally bear no structural resemblance to each other. The structures of phenylephrine and clonidine, α_1- and α_2-adrenoceptor agonists, respectively, are shown as is the structure of a mixed α-adrenoceptor antagonist, phentolamine (Fig. 14.8).

The silent β-adrenoceptor. The adrenoceptor hypothesis of Ahlquist explains adequately the vasopressor and vasodepressor responses of smooth muscle to catecholamines. The presence of dominant α-adrenoceptors also explains the vasodepressor response to E or NE after α-adrenoceptor blockade. Nevertheless, catecholamine reversal is a pharmacological phenomenon. The physiological significance of the β-adrenoceptor in the presence of the dominant α-adrenoceptor is

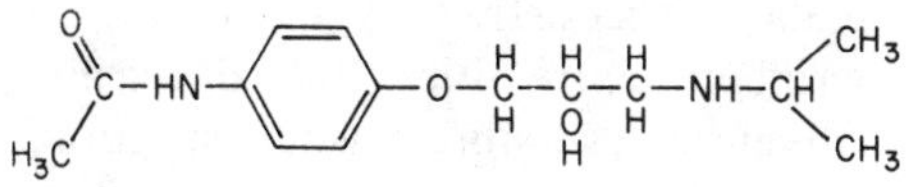

Practolol
(β_1-Antagonist)

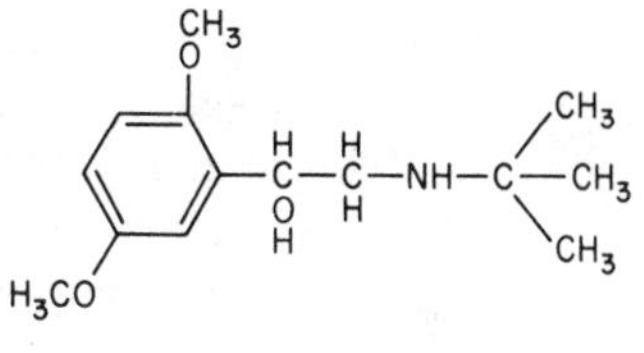

Butoxamine
(β_2-Antagonist)

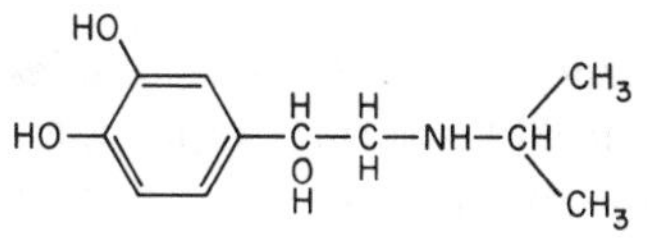

Isoproterenol

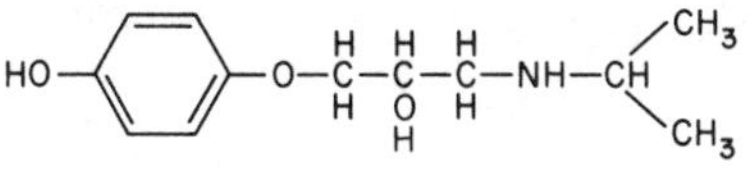

Prenalterol
(β_1-Agonist)

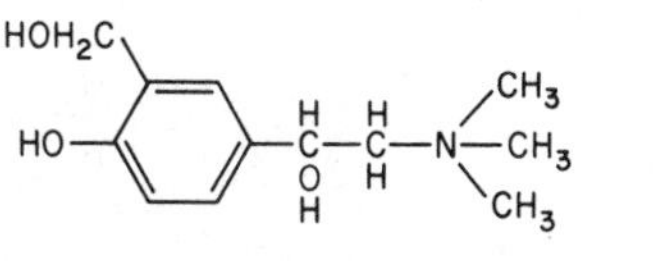

Salbutamol
(β_2-Agonist)

Figure 14.6 Examples of β-adrenoceptor agonist and antagonist structures.

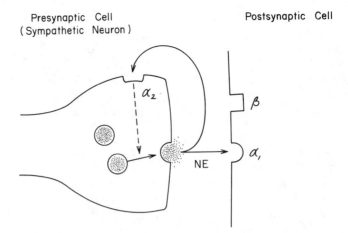

Figure 14.7 Sympathetic negative feedback mechanisms for inhibition of sympathetic neuron secretion.

unclear. Although there are examples of smooth muscles that lack α-adrenoceptors and only possess β-adrenoceptors, there apparently are no examples of smooth muscles that possess α-adrenoceptors in the absence of β-adrenoceptors. It is reasonable to hypothesize, therefore, that the β-adrenoceptor provides a mechanism for auto-inhibition. For example, although there is an initial contraction in response to dominant α-adrenoceptors, there follows a reversal of the vasopressor response due to a slowly developing β-adrenoceptor response. Autoinhibition can be prevented by β-adrenoceptor blockade. The silent β-adrenoceptor may provide a mechanism for protection against continuous vascular vasoconstriction that would lead to oxygen deprivation and gangrene in the peripheral extremities. Indeed, certain drugs, ergot alkaloids, which establish a relatively irreversible vasoconstriction, have been known to cause gangrene of the legs.

Cyclic Nucleotides

β-adrenoceptors. In the initial studies of Sutherland it was established that cAMP is the intracellular second messenger in the hepatic glycogenolytic response to β-adrenoceptor stimulation by epinephrine [40]. All subsequent studies have

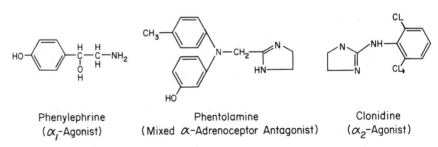

Phenylephrine
(α_1-Agonist)

Phentolamine
(Mixed α-Adrenoceptor Antagonist)

Clonidine
(α_2-Agonist)

Figure 14.8 Examples of α-adrenoceptor agonist and antagonist structures.

Catecholamines and the Sympathoadrenal System   Chap. 14

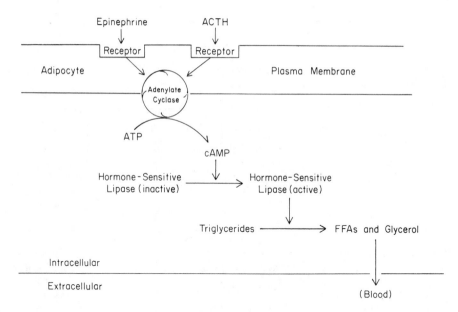

Figure 14.9 Lipolytic action of catecholamines on adipocytes.

established that cellular responses to β-adrenoceptor stimulation are, without exception, linked to adenylate cyclase activation and cAMP formation. Although both glucagon and E stimulate hepatic glycogenolysis, they do so through separate receptors which are, nevertheless, linked through a common adenylate cyclase (Fig. 11.10). Similarly E and ACTH stimulate fat cell lipolysis and do so through separate receptors, again linked to a common adenylate cyclase (Fig. 14.9). The transduction mechanism linking these separate receptors to adenylate cyclase are, however, not identical. For example, ACTH activation of adenylate cyclase requires Ca^{2+}, whereas activation of the enzyme through β-adrenoceptor stimulation is without such a divalent metal ion requirement. This lack of a Ca^{2+} requirement for β-adrenoceptor signal transduction appears to be a common feature of this receptor in many but not all tissues [25].

α-adrenoceptors. In those tissues where α-adrenoceptors are present they dominate over β-adrenoceptors, at least temporally. The mechanism of this domination may differ between α_1- and α_2-adrenoceptors, but the details of these differences are unclear. Stimulation of α-adrenoceptors may cause a rapid decrease in intracellular cAMP levels, apparently as a result of a direct inhibition of adenylate cyclase. In other tissues α-adrenoceptor stimulation may result in an activation of guanylate cyclase and the production of cGMP without concomitant reduction in cAMP levels. Calcium is required for α-adrenoceptor signal transduction in some tissues but not in others. Calcium may also be required for activation of guanylate cyclase in some tissues, and in others Ca^{2+} may be introduced into the cytosol either from the extracellular compartment or from an intracellular source, most likely the mitochondria [18]. Calcium may then bind with an intracellular Ca^{2+}-binding protein (calmodulin) and through this protein stimulate phosphodiesterase activity which would result in a lowering of intracellular cAMP levels.

TABLE 14.1 Tissue Adrenoceptor Responses To Catecholamines[a]

α-Adrenoceptor response	Tissue	β-Adrenoceptor response
↑ cGMP production	Many tissues	↑ cAMP production
↓ cAMP production	Many tissues	
Contraction	Vascular smooth muscle	Relaxation
Contraction	Urinary bladder smooth muscle	Relaxation
Contraction	Spleen smooth muscle capsule	Relaxation
Contraction	Uterine smooth muscle	Relaxation
	Bronchial smooth muscle	Relaxation
Relaxation	Intestinal smooth muscle	Relaxation
	Heart (cardiac muscle)	Contraction
	Skeletal muscle	↑ Glycogenolysis
	Hepatocyte	↑ Glycogenolysis
	Adipose tissue	↑ Lipolysis
↓ Insulin secretion	Pancreatic islet β cell	↑ Insulin secretion
	Bone marrow	↑ Erythropoiesis
↑ K$^+$ and H$_2$O secretion	Salivary gland	↑ Amylase secretion
	Pineal gland (pinealocyte)	↑ Melatonin synthesis-secretion
↓ MSH secretion	Pars intermedia	↑ MSH secretion
	Stomach	↑ Gastrin secretion
↓ Renin secretion	Kidney (JG cells)	↑ Renin secretion
↓ Parathormone secretion	Parathyroid gland	↑ Parathormone secretion

[a]Increased (↑) and decreased (↓) physiological responses are indicated.

Yin-yang hypothesis. It has been suggested that cGMP and cAMP serve as opposing regulatory effectors in many bidirectionally controlled cellular processes. This hypothesis has been termed the yin-yang hypothesis of hormone action [21]. For smooth muscle there is unequivocal evidence that acetylcholine stimulation of cholinergic receptors leads to guanylate cyclase activation and cGMP production followed by contraction. In contrast, catecholamines acting on smooth muscle β-adrenoceptors stimulate adenylate cyclase production, which leads to relaxation of the muscle. In cardiac muscle cAMP and cGMP mediate the positive and negative inotropic (force) and chronotropic (rate) effects of NE and acetylcholine, respectively. Increases in cGMP and cAMP in response to acetylcholine and NE, respectively, precede the changes in isometric tension, and these responses are blocked by atropine (cholinergic antagonist) and practolol (β-adrenoceptor antagonist). In many other tissues there is evidence that these two cyclic nucleotides similarly regulate bifunctional responses (Table 14.1).

Prostaglandins. Although intracellular cyclic nucleotides have generally been considered second messengers of hormone action, there is good evidence in smooth muscle at least that prostaglandins may also participate as intracellular messengers of hormone action. From studies on smooth muscle, β-adrenoceptor stimulation leads to PGE$_2$ synthesis which is followed by cAMP production and muscle relaxation. Stimulation of cholinergic receptors, on the other hand, often leads to PGF$_{2\alpha}$ synthesis which is immediately followed by cGMP production and muscle contraction. A general scheme depicting the role of prostaglandins in smooth muscle contraction in response to a variety of stimuli is shown (Fig. 14.9).

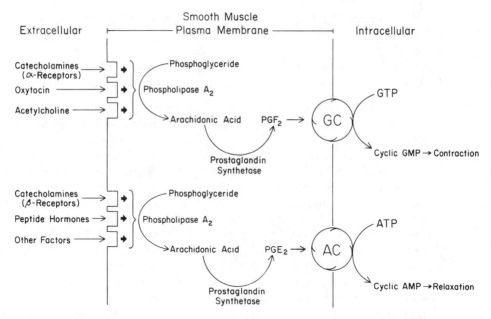

Figure 14.10   Role of adrenergic receptors and prostaglandins in smooth muscle contraction and relaxation.

Autoinhibition.   The role of the silent β-adrenoceptor in autoinhibition of smooth muscle contraction in response to α-adrenoceptor stimulation was discussed. The myometrium of the uterus provides a good model for understanding the role of cyclic nucleotides in autoinhibition of uterine muscle contractility in response to E [43]. In vitro, the isolated uterus always contracts in response to E, a response that can be blocked by α-adrenoceptor antagonists. However, the contractile response to subsequent doses of E is usually completely inhibited. This autoinhibition can be prevented by the β-adrenoceptor antagonist, propranolol; each subsequent addition of epinephrine to the rinsed uterus will produce a contraction as long as a β-antagonist is present. Epinephrine stimulates adenylate cyclase activity of uterine muscle, an action antagonized by β-adrenoceptor antagonists. Dibutyryl cAMP added to the incubation medium mimics the inhibitory action of E. Thus, the initial contractile response of the myometrium to E is mediated through α-adrenoceptors, but simultaneous stimulation of β-adrenoceptors also elevates the intracellular levels of cAMP which are inhibitory to myometrial contractility.

Hormonal Modulation of Adrenoceptors

The tissue density of adrenoceptors varies and depends on the presence or absence of stimulation; adrenoceptors increase (up regulation) in the absence of stimulation and decrease (down regulation) under continuous stimulation. The density of β_1- and β_2-adrenoceptors can be independently regulated, providing strong evidence that the receptors are separate [31]. An increase in the sensitivity of adrenergic effector organs to catecholamines has been noted after denervation. The denervated

Mechanisms of Action

heart of the dog and the denervated rat pineal, for example, respond to catecholamines by an enhanced production of cAMP over that of intact control tissues. This *denervation supersensitivity* is due to an increase in tissue β-adrenoceptors. On the other hand, the density of these receptors decreases in tissues subjected to continued elevated levels of the β-adrenoceptor agonist, isoproterenol [32].

Gonadal steroids. Adrenoceptor responses to catecholamines are affected by gonadal steroids. Steroid hormones affect sympathetic function by modulating adrenoceptor responses to catecholamines. Estrogens and progesterone may modulate sympathoadrenal activity by altering catecholamine metabolism and, in addition, produce qualitative changes in the contractile response of smooth muscle to stimulation by catecholamines. The response of the human oviduct and uteri from several species changes from contraction to relaxation depending on the concentrations of gonadal steroids present. Contraction is mediated through α-adrenoceptors in the estrogen-dominated uterus, whereas β-adrenoceptor-induced relaxation predominates during pregnancy or when incubated in vitro in the presence of progesterone.

It has been hypothesized that α- and β-adrenoceptors may be interconvertible; in other words, they may represent alternate configurations of the same active site. Experimental evidence, however, favors the view that these receptors are separate identities. Estrogen-treated uteri contain three times more α-adrenoceptors than the same uteri subsequently treated with progesterone; the β-adrenoceptor number remains constant in either steroidal milieu. Thus, gonadal steroids may affect smooth muscle responses by modulation of adrenoceptor number rather than conversion from one receptor type to the other [36].

Adrenal steroids. Glucocorticoids play a permissive role in regulating cAMP-mediated effects of hormones on the liver and other organs. In adrenalectomized rats the stimulation of liver gluconeogenesis and glycogenolysis in response to catecholamines is greatly reduced. The lipolytic response of adipose tissue to epinephrine in vitro is blunted in tissues removed from adrenalectomized animals. Glucocorticoid treatment restores the lipolytic response of fat tissue removed from adrenalectomized animals. Catecholamine-induced pressor effects on the cardiovascular system are dependent on permissive actions of glucocorticoids. One mechanism of glucocorticoid enhancement of cardiovascular responses to catecholamines may involve inactivation of COMT [15]. Glucocorticoids therefore play vital roles in the regulation of tissue responses to catecholamines during stress.

Thyroid hormones. Thyroid hormones profoundly affect the activity of the sympathoadrenal system. Sympathoadrenal activity is enhanced under conditions of hyperthyroidism and depressed under conditions of low levels of thyroid hormones, as in myxedema. As discussed, the actions of catecholamines are mediated through adrenergic receptors. In general the activity of these receptors is increased in response to thyroid hormones and, in states of hypothyroidism or hyperthyroidism, the activity of these receptors is greatly affected. Therefore, the major symptoms of patients with a thyroid dysfunction relate to functional alterations of those organs regulated by the sympathetic nervous system (Table 13.2).

SYMPATHOADRENAL FUNCTIONS

The unique role of the sympathoadrenal system is to maintain the constancy of the internal environment of the body. Any decrease in blood pressure, blood glucose level, or oxygen availability leads to an acute enhancement of sympathoadrenal activity with resulting elevation in plasma catecholamines. In addition the sympathoadrenal system is activated in anticipation of events that may affect adversely an individual. Stress is a term generally used to designate the state resulting from events (stressors) of external or internal origin, real or imagined, that tend to affect the homeostatic state. Although an acceptable definition of stress may not be available [44], in the present context stress refers to any condition tending to elevate plasma catecholamine levels in response to exogenous or endogenous stimuli. For example, the early experiments of Cannon [9] revealed that the barking of a dog was a stimulus to E secretion from the adrenal gland of the cat. In humans plasma levels of NE and E are immediately elevated upon standing, during exercise, during and after surgery, and whenever plasma glucose levels fall below normal [12].

Norepinephrine is released by sympathetic neurons to provide localized autonomic effector control, whereas E is released from the adrenal as a humoral messenger which may also provide an additional stimulus to autonomic effectors. Catecholamines communicate with their effector cells through adrenoceptors; the distribution and nature of these receptors will determine the response generated. These tissues must therefore possess the "correct" type of adrenoceptor to provide the response that will be most appropriate (adaptive) under conditions of stress. By inference, therefore, it should be possible to predict the nature of both the response and the type of adrenoceptor that must be possessed by any particular tissue. The following guidelines should assist in the formulation of such predictions. First, α-adrenoceptors (with one exception, those possessed by gastrointestinal smooth muscle) mediate smooth muscle contraction, whereas β-adrenoceptors mediate smooth muscle relaxation. Second, α-adrenoceptors when present dominate over β-adrenoceptors. Third, β-adrenoceptors are generally stimulatory to cellular secretion, whereas α-adrenoceptors (with few exceptions) are inhibitory to cellular secretion. Table 14.1 provides a list of effector organs and their responses to α- and β-adrenoceptor stimulation.

Intermediary Metabolism

One would expect that under conditions of stress blood glucose levels would need to be elevated to provide this metabolic substrate for energy production within critical tissues (brain, heart, skeletal muscle). Glycogen is available as a storage form of glucose within the liver. Epinephrine is stimulatory to hepatic glycogenolysis and glucose release through its action on β-adrenoceptors. Skeletal muscle may provide an even greater total source of glycogen and, in response to β-adrenoceptor stimulation, glycogen is converted through the glycolytic pathway to lactic acid. This lactic acid is cycled to the liver and through E-stimulated gluconeogenesis converted to glucose.

Adipose tissue cells possess β-adrenoceptors and, in response to catecholamines of either sympathetic or adrenal origin, lipolysis is stimulated. Epinephrine-induced cAMP production activates a hormone-sensitive lipase, a triglyceride lipase, which metabolizes fats into FFA's and glycerol (Fig. 14.10). The FFA's released into the blood are then utilized directly by certain tissues (brain, cardiac muscle) as sources of energy (a glucose-sparing action), or they may be utilized within the liver in the formation of glucose.

Most interesting is the demonstration that catecholamines are inhibitory (through α-adrenoceptors) to insulin secretion. (The actions of insulin are antagonistic to those of E.) On the other hand, catecholamines are stimulatory to glucagon secretion through an action on β-adrenoceptors of pancreatic A cells. It is interesting that glucagon is reciprocally stimulatory to adrenal E secretion.

Epinephrine acting through β-adrenoceptors and cAMP decreases the release of amino acids from skeletal muscle [19]. A reduced rate of muscle proteolysis appears to be the mechanism which causes adrenergic inhibition of amino acid release. This adrenergic modulation of protein degradation may be of physiological importance to the short-term fight or flight response associated with increased adrenal epinephrine secretion. Under these conditions, lactate, glycerol, and glucose levels are increased and additional gluconeogenic substrates might not be needed [19].

Both fasting and feeding induce changes in sympathoadrenal activity. In rats fasting suppresses and overfeeding stimulates the sympathetic nervous system. It was hypothesized that during fasting suppression of sympathetic activity would conserve calories by decreasing metabolism and heat production, whereas during feeding the increased sympathetic activity would expend the excess calories. Further, increased sympathetic activity might account for some of the increased incidence of cardiac arrhythmias, angina, and hypertension in populations known for overeating [29].

Cardiovascular System

Epinephrine increases both the force and rate of the heartbeat through stimulation of cardiac muscle β-receptors. This is the only example known where β-adrenoceptors induce muscle contraction. The particular distribution of vascular smooth muscle adrenoceptors provides a mechanism for the shunting of blood to various body compartments during stress. For example, blood is shunted from the skin, mucosa, connective tissue, and kidneys; as expected, vascular smooth muscle of these organs possesses α-adrenoceptors. In contrast, smooth muscle of coronary arteries as well as skeletal muscle and brain, as might be expected, possesses β-adrenoceptors. If dominant α-adrenoceptors were present, blood flow to these vital organs would be diminished when these organs are maximally active. The decreased blood flow to the kidneys reduces glucose clearance from the circulation, and this reduced clearance may be primarily responsible for the prolonged hyperglycemia induced by catecholamines.

Bronchial smooth muscle is relaxed in response to catecholamines and only β-adrenoceptors are present. Relaxation of these muscles would dilate the bronchial passageways so that increased amounts of air containing oxygen are made available to the blood under conditions of increased exertion. The spleen capsule is contracted through catecholamine stimulation of α-adrenoceptors, which increases the circulating levels of erythrocytes. These erythrocytes provide the blood with an increased capacity for oxygen uptake from the lungs. Epinephrine enhances blood platelet adhesiveness and reduces clotting time by its actions on platelet β-adrenoceptors.

In those smooth muscles where α-adrenoceptors subserve contraction the parasympathetic nervous system through the release of its neurotransmitter, acetylcholine, controls relaxation. This holds true for cardiac muscle as well. Where β-adrenergic receptors regulate relaxation of smooth muscle, however, acetylcholine regulates the contractile component of the muscle.

Norepinephrine: Humoral Hormone And Neurotransmitter In Humans

Epinephrine, in humans at least, is generally considered the only humoral catecholamine normally serving an endocrine function. Nevertheless, NE does escape into the circulation during sympathetic activity. Is this extrasynaptic NE destined only for metabolic degradation or might it not also subserve some role as a hormone? NE was infused into normal men and a variety of physiological parameters were monitored concomitantly. Only NE levels in excess of 1800 pg/ml caused hemodynamic and metabolic effects. Thus, under usual conditions, NE's biological actions may only relate to its sympathetic neurotransmitter function. Because NE levels can exceed 1800 pg/ml, during stress, for example, it is conceivable that NE might subserve some role in stress with epinephrine of adrenal origin [38]. Also, posturally stimulated NE concentrations occur in normal and even adrenalectomized individuals, suggesting that the adrenals are not the only source of plasma NE.

Comparative Endocrinology

The comparative physiology and pharmacology of adrenoceptors in vertebrates has not been studied systematically. Because NE, E, and possibly dopamine are the only catecholamines produced by the sympathoadrenal system, it might be expected that the adrenoceptors of all vertebrates are similar, although the particular response elicited might show some species specificity. (The turkey erythrocyte, for example, has been used for detailed studies on the β-adrenoceptor). Melanosome aggregation and dispersion within dermal melanophores of elasmobranchs, teleosts, amphibians, and reptiles are stimulated by catecholamines interacting through α- and β-adrenoceptors, respectively. These responses can be blocked by the classical α- and β-adrenoceptor antagonists [22].

CONTROL OF SYMPATHOADRENAL ACTIVITY

Both postganglionic sympathetic neurons and adrenal chromaffin cells are directly innervated by cholinergic neurons. Acetylcholine released from these neurons interacts with cholinergic receptors present on the effector cells, which leads to vesicular exocytosis of catecholamines into the synapse between sympathetic neurons and autonomic effector cells or, in the case of epinephrine, directly into the blood. Experimental studies show that under stress adrenal chromaffin cell enzymes are regulated by both neuronal and endocrine pathways. Tyrosine hydroxylase and DBH are regulated mainly by neuronal transynaptic stimulation, whereas PNMT is primarily under endocrine control [42]. For example, denervation of an adrenal gland by cutting the splanchnic nerve prevents elevations in tyrosine hydroxylase and DBH in response to stress, whereas PNMT is still enhanced. PNMT and DBH activities in the adrenal decrease following hypophysectomy and can be restored by administration of ACTH or glucocorticoids. Levels of tyrosine hydroxylase, on the other hand, are increased by ACTH but not by glucocorticoids. Thus, in addition to neuronal influences tyrosine hydroxylase activity appears to be directly affected by ACTH [27].

If the blood glucose concentration is reduced by fasting or administration of insulin, an immediate release of epinephrine follows. The denervated adrenal is, however, insensitive to a hypoglycemic stimulus. Adrenal catecholamine secretion in response to hypoglycemia can be blocked by local anesthetic application to the hypothalamus and adjacent brain areas [24]. In addition intracerebroventricular injection of a nonmetabolizable analog, 5-thioglucose, increases sympathoadrenal-mediated hyperglycemia. These observations suggest that some glucoreceptors that regulate sympathoadrenal discharge reside within the brain. The cellular receptors that mediate the hyperglycemic response to glucoprivation are apparently localized caudal to the forebrain [35].

SYMPATHOADRENAL PATHOPHYSIOLOGY

Tumors may arise within the sympathoadrenal system. Adrenal chromaffin tumors (pheochromocytomas) are generally benign. Neuroblastoma is a highly malignant neoplasm of early life which arises from primitive sympathogonia and neuroblasts. Although found wherever sympathetic nervous tissue is located, it most often arises from the adrenal medulla or along the sympathetic chain. Pheochromocytomas that contain only E are comprised entirely of A cells, whereas those containing only NE consist entirely of N cells. Both cells are present in mixed pheochromocytomas containing both NE and E. The excessive secretion of catecholamines, characteristic of pheochromocytoma and neuroblastoma, results in severe hypertension as well as increased basal metabolic rate, increased oxygen consumption, weight loss, psychosis, tremulousness, and increased respiratory rate. Competitive inhibitors of tyrosine hydroxylase, such as α-methyltyrosine, are often effective in the treatment of pheochromocytoma.

β-Adrenoceptor antagonists play an important role in the pharmacological therapy of such cardiovascular disorders as hypertension, ischemic heart disease, and arrhythmias. Rapid relief of symptoms is often achieved using β-adrenoceptor antagonists and with few side effects [23]. The demonstration that adrenoceptors could be classed into subgroups based on their selective response to pharmaceutical agonists and antagonists raises hopes that other drugs might be developed that would be selective for these adrenoceptor subtypes; such selectivity might decrease the severity of side effects. β_1- and β_2-Adrenoceptors are components of other tissues which may limit their effectiveness until further specificities of the receptors are discovered [32].

REFERENCES

[1] AHLQUIST, R. P. 1948. A study of the adrenotropin receptors. *Am. J. Physiol.* 153:586–600.

[2] ALOE, L., and R. LEVI-MONTALCINI. 1979. Nerve growth factor-induced transformation of immature chromaffin cells *in vivo* into sympathetic neurons: effect of antiserum to nerve growth factor. *Proc. Natl. Acad. Sci. USA* 76:1246–50.

[3] APPENZELLER, O. 1982. *Autonomic nervous system.* Amsterdam: Elsevier Biomedical Press.

[4] AXELROD, J. 1974. Neurotransmitters. *Sci. Amer.* 230:58–71.

[5] BLACK, I. B. 1982. Stages in development of autonomic neurons. *Science* 214:1198–1204.

[6] BOHN, M. C., M. GOLDSTEIN, and I. B. BLACK. 1981. Role of glucocorticoids in expression of the adrenergic phenotype in rat embryonic adrenal gland. *Develop. Biol.* 82:1–10.

[7] BUNGE, R., M. JOHNSON, and C. D. ROSS. 1978. Nature and nurture in development of the autonomic neuron. *Science* 199:1409–16.

[8] BURNSTOCK, G., and M. COSTA. 1975. *Adrenergic neurons.* New York: Chapman & Hall.

[9] CANNON, W. B. 1932. *The wisdom of the body.* New York: W. W. Norton & Co. Inc.

[10] CANNON, W. B., and A. ROSENBLUETH. 1937. *Autonomic neuroeffector systems.* New York: Macmillan, Inc.

[11] COUPLAND, R. E. 1953. On the morphology and adrenaline-noradrenaline content of chromaffin tissue. *J. Endocrinol.* 9:194–203.

[12] CRYER, P. E. 1980. Physiology and pathophysiology of the sympathoadrenal neuroendocrine system. *New Engl. J. Med.* 303:436–44.

[13] DALE, H. H. 1906. On some physiological actions of ergot. *J. Physiol.* 3:163–206.

[14] DALE, H. H. 1934. Chemical transmission of the effects of nerve impulses. *Br. Med. J.* 1:835–41.

[15] DEAVERS, D. R., and X. J. MUSACCHIA. 1979. The function of glucocorticoids in thermogenesis. *Fed. Proc.* 38:2177–81.

[16] DOUGLAS, W. W. 1968. Stimulus-secretion coupling: the concept and clues from chromaffin and other cells. *Br. J. Pharmacol.* 34:451–74.

[17] EVANS, W. F. 1976. *Anatomy and physiology.* Englewood Cliffs, N.J.: Prentice-Hall Publishing Co., Inc.

[18] EXTON, J. H. 1981. Molecular mechanisms involved in α-adrenergic responses. *Mol. Cell. Endocrinol.* 23:233–64.

[19] GARBER, A. J., I. E. KARL, and D. M. KIPNIS. 1976. Alanine and glutamine synthesis and release from skeletal muscle. *J. Biol. Chem.* 251:851–57.

[20] GILMAN, A. G., L. S. GOODMAN, and A. GILMAN. 1980. *Goodman and Gilman's, The pharmacological basis of therapeutics.* 6th ed. New York: Macmillan, Inc.

[21] GOLDBERG, N. D., and M. K. HADDOX. 1977. Cyclic GMP metabolism and involvement in biological regulation. *Ann. Rev. Physiol.* 46:823–96.

[22] HADLEY, M. E., and J. T. BAGNARA. 1975. Regulation of release and mechanism of ac-

tion of MSH. In *Trends in comparative endocrinology*, ed. E. J. W. Barrington, pp. 81–104. New York: Thomas J. Griffiths Sons.

[23] HEIKKILÄ, J., A. JOUNELA, M. KATILA, K. LUOMANMÄKI, and M. H. FRICK. 1979. Beta-blockade: selection and use. *Ann. Clin. Res.* 11:267–89.

[24] HIMSWORTH, R. L. 1970. Hypothalamic control of adrenaline secretion in response to insufficient glucose. *J. Physiol.* 206:411–17.

[25] HIRATA, F., and J. AXELROD. 1980. Phospholipid methylation and biological signal transduction. *Science* 209:1082–90.

[26] HOFFMAN, B. B., and R. J. LEFKOWITZ. 1980. Alpha-adrenergic receptor subtypes. *New Eng. J. Med.* 302:1390–96.

[27] KOPIN, I. J. 1976. Catecholamines, adrenal hormones, and stress. *Hosp. Prac.* 11(3): 49–55.

[28] LANDS, A. M., A. ARNOLD, J. P. MCAULIFF, F. P. LUDUENS, and T. G. BROWN, Jr. 1967. Differentiation of receptor systems activated by sympathomimetic amines. *Nature* 214: 597–98.

[29] LANDSBERG, L., and J. B. YOUNG. 1978. Fasting, feeding and regulation of the sympathetic nervous system. *New Engl. J. Med.* 278:1295–1301.

[30] LE DOUARIN, N. M., and M. A. M. TEILLET. 1974. Experimental analysis of the migration and differentiation of neuroblasts of the autonomic nervous system and of neuro-ectoderm of mesenchymal derivatives, using a biological cell marking technique. *Develop. Biol.* 41:162–84.

[31] MINNEMAN, K. P., M. D. DIBNER, B. B. WOLFE, and P. B. MOLINOFF. 1979. β_1- and β_2-Adrenergic receptors in rat cerebral cortex are independently regulated. *Science* 204: 866–68.

[32] MINNEMAN, K. P., R. N. PITTMAN, and P. B. MOLINOFF. 1981. β-Adrenergic receptor subtypes: properties, distribution, and regulation. *Ann. Rev. Neurosci.* 4:419–61.

[33] NICKERSON, M., and L. S. GOODMAN. 1947. Pharmacological properties of a new adrenergic blocking agent: N,N-dibenzyl-β-chloroethylamine (dibenamine). *J. Pharmac. Exp. Therap.* 89:167–85.

[34] OLIVER, G., and E. A. SCHAFER. 1895. The physiological effects of extracts from the suprarenal capsules. *J. Physiol. Lond.* 18:230–76.

[35] RITTER, R. C., P. G. SLUSSER, and S. STONE. 1981. Glucoreceptors controlling feeding and blood glucose: location in the hindbrain. *Science* 213:451–53.

[36] ROBERTS, J. M., P. A. INSEL, R. D. GOLDFIEN, and A. GOLDFIEN. 1977. α Adrenoceptors but not β adrenoceptors increase in rabbit uterus with oestrogen. *Nature* 270:624–25.

[37] ROSELL, S., and E. BELFRAGE. 1975. Adrenergic receptors in adipose tissue and their relation to adrenergic innervation. *Nature* 253:730–39.

[38] SILVERBERG, A. B., S. D. SHAH, M. W. HAYMOND, and P. E. CRYER. 1978. Norepinephrine: hormone and neurotransmitter in man. *Am. J. Physiol.* 234:E252–56.

[39] STARKE, K. 1977. Regulation of noradrenaline release by presynaptic receptor systems. *Rev. Physiol. Biochem. Pharmacol.* 77:1–124.

[40] SUTHERLAND, E. 1972. Studies on the mechanism of hormone action. *Science* 177:401–408.

[41] TEITELMAN, G., H. BAKER, T. H. JOH, and D. J. REIS. 1979. Appearance of catecholamine-synthesizing enzymes during development of rat sympathetic nervous system: possible role of tissue environment. *Proc. Natl. Acad. Sci. USA* 76:509–13.

[42] THOENEN, H., and U. OTTEN. 1978. Role of adrenocortical hormones in the modulation

of synthesis and degradation of enzymes involved in the formation of catecholamines. *Front. Neuroendocrinology* 5:163–84.

[43] TRINER, L., N. I. A. OVERWEG, and G. G. NAHAS. 1970. Cyclic 3′,5′-AMP and uterine contractility. *Nature* 225:282–83.

[44] USDIN, E., R. KVETNANSKY, and I. J. KOPIN, eds. 1979. *Catecholamines and stress: recent advances.* New York: Elsevier North-Holland, Inc.

[45] WRENN, S., C. HOMEY, and E. HABER. 1979. Evidence for the β-adrenergic receptor regulation of membrane-bound catechol-O-methyltransferase activity in myocardium. *J. Biol. Chem.* 254:4708–5712.

15

Adrenal Steroids

INTRODUCTION

The adrenal gland of most vertebrates is composed of two tissues of different origin which produce two classes of hormones which are unrelated in structure. Nevertheless, the hormones of both the adrenal steroidogenic tissue and the adrenal chromaffin tissue play important roles in response to stress. The discoveries that led to present knowledge of the hormones of adrenal steroidogenic tissue and their role in endocrine physiology are presented in the following chronological summary. A number of treatises on adrenal structure and function are available [7, 8, 25, 26, 28, 29, 30].

Historical Perspective

1815   Meckel described the gross comparative anatomy of the adrenals.

1846   Ecker provided a detailed description of the histology of the adrenal medulla and cortex.

1854   Kölliker recognized the cortex and medulla as functionally different structures in humans.

1855   Addison described a disease (Addison's disease) which involved a degeneration of the adrenals.

1856   Brown-Séquard studied the effects of adrenalectomy in animals and concluded that the glands are indispensable for life.

344

1866 Arnold described the cellular zonation of the cortex.

1927– Smith established that although the adrenals of the rat atrophied
1930 after hypophysectomy, they could be restored to normal size by administration of pituitary extracts.

1927 Baumann showed that longevity in animals after adrenalectomy was prolonged by injections of sodium salts. Other investigators noted that there was excessive excretion of sodium and chloride by the kidneys in the absence of normal adrenal function.

1928– Baumann and colleagues were among the first to employ adrenal
1929 cortical extracts as replacement therapy in adrenalectomized animals and in patients with Addison's disease. Swingle and Pfiffer (1931), as well as Hartman and Brownell (1930), described the beneficial actions of adrenal extracts on survival of adrenalectomized animals.

1936 Kendall and coworkers obtained crystalline extracts of the adrenal cortex and demonstrated the effectiveness of compound E (cortisone) in ameliorating the symptoms of adrenalectomy in rats.

1936 Selye described the *general adaptation syndrome* which provided a major impetus to stress research and the subsequent recognition of the essential role of the adrenal in the stress response.

1940 Long and associates established the importance of the adrenal cortex relative to carbohydrate metabolism.

1945 By 1945 six active and more than 20 inactive steroids were extracted from the adrenal cortex. The four compounds with greatest biological activity were 11-dehydrocorticosterone, corticosterone, cortisone, and hydrocortisone (cortisol).

1950 Hench and associates described the effectiveness of cortisone in relieving the symptoms of rheumatoid arthritis. It was noted, however, that patients treated with ACTH excreted cortisol rather than cortisone. Cortisol was found to be the principal glucogenic steroid secreted by patients with Cushing's disease.

1951 It was established that cortisol is the major steroid released from the adrenal gland following stimulation by ACTH.

1953 Tait and colleagues demonstrated the presence of an adrenal steroid that is extremely active in retaining sodium.

1954 The structure of the salt-retaining hormone, aldosterone, was determined.

1954 Conn described primary hyperaldosteronism (Conn's disease) [10].

1955 Li and coworkers isolated the pituitary factor, ACTH (corticotropin), which regulates adrenal cortisol secretion. As early as 1940 Swann proposed that there were separate controls for adrenal glucocorticoid and mineralocorticoid secretion.

1960 Laragh described the renin-angiotensin system that controls adrenal aldosterone secretion.

These studies established that cortisol, a *glucocorticoid*, and aldosterone, a *mineralocorticoid*, play important roles in carbohydrate and Na$^+$ balance, respectively, in humans and many other vertebrates. Abnormal secretion of either of these hormones has profound pathophysiological consequences in humans.

THE ADRENAL GLANDS

The adrenal gland is composed of steroidogenic as well as chromaffin tissue. In many mammals the steroidogenic tissue forms a cortical mass surrounding an inner medullary component of chromaffin tissue. In humans and many other mammals these tissue components may appropriately be referred to as the adrenal cortex and adrenal medulla. In many vertebrates including some mammals these two tissues are intermingled; therefore, the comparative endocrinologist prefers the functional designations adrenal steroidal and adrenal chromaffin. In some poikilotherms the two tissue components are totally separate masses of tissues.

Anatomy and Embryology

Steroidogenic and chromaffin tissues originate from separate primordia. Chromaffin cells are derived from the neural crest (Chapter 14), while the steroidogenic tissue arises from the coelomic mesoderm (corticogonadal analgen) in the genital ridge of the embryo. During migration to definite anatomical sites, some steroidogenic tissue becomes located in extra-adrenal sites. These aberrant adrenal *rests* may hypertrophy and become more active after adrenalectomy. In humans adrenal rests are usually distributed in the celiac plexus and the adjacent fatty tissue, or along the path of the spermatic cord.

In the primate the adrenals are located adjacent to the upper surface of each kidney (Fig. 15.1). Each human adrenal gland weighs approximately 3.5 to 4.5 g and is well vascularized by arterial branches from the aorta. Smaller arterial branches spread over the adrenal capsule, pierce it, and pass as sinusoids between adjacent

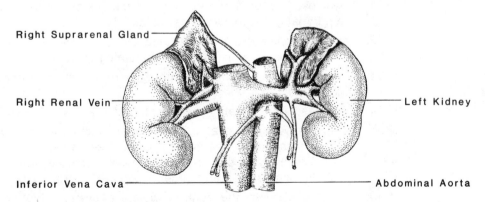

Right Suprarenal Gland

Right Renal Vein

Left Kidney

Inferior Vena Cava

Abdominal Aorta

Figure 15.1 Gross anatomy of the human adrenal glands.

rows of cortical cells to a subcapsular plexus at the corticomedullary junction. A few venules flow through the medullary chromaffin tissue to a central vein which connects directly or indirectly (via the renal vein) to the inferior vena cava.

The adrenal functional unit. In humans and many other mammals the chromaffin tissue is surrounded by steroidogenic tissue and the vascular relationships are such that the secretory products of the cortex perfuse the medulla through a portal network. In addition sphincter-like muscles in the central adrenal vein may alter the rate of flow of adrenal cortical effluent. As noted, adrenal chromaffin epinephrine synthesis is dependent on steroid hormonal support (Chapter 14) [2]. There is evidence that chromaffin tissue has the capacity to carry out many enzymatic reactions characteristic of the cortex and is therefore capable of converting incomplete steroid intermediates passing through the medulla into active glucocorticoids. The close anatomical coupling and the functional interrelationship between the cortex and medulla suggest that these two tissues, although of diverse origin, may constitute an integrated functional unit, at least in higher vertebrates. This relationship may be of particular adaptive importance under conditions of stress when both epinephrine and glucocorticoids are in particular demand [6].

Histology

In most mammals the adrenal cortical tissue can be divided into three morphologically and functionally different layers: a thin outer *zona glomerulosa;* a thicker middle *zona fasciculata;* and an innermost, moderately thick *zona reticularis* (Fig. 15.2).

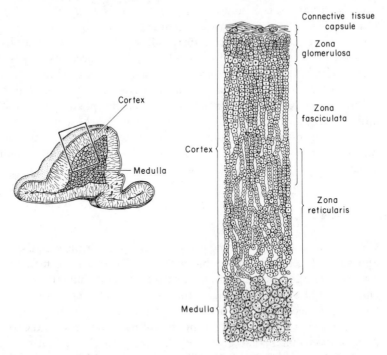

Figure 15.2 Diagrammatic representation of the microanatomy of the human adrenal cortex.

Steroidogenic cells are filled with lipid droplets (liposomes) containing cholesterol, the substrate for steroid biosynthesis. These droplets are stainable with lipid-soluble dyes such as sudan red or sudan black. In the typical alcohol dehydration preparation the cells appear full of vacuoles due to alcohol extraction of the lipids from their contained vesicles; these cells are often referred to as spongiocytes. Ultrastructurally, the steroidogenic cells (like those of the gonads) contain abundant mitochondria and an especially conspicuous smooth endoplasmic reticulum [40]. Although the cortical tissue may be grossly divided into three separate regions, the histological picture reveals that the three cell types are parts of the same cords of cells that extend from the capsule to the medulla. These cell cords are surrounded by a capillary network, thus providing steroids ready access into the blood.

The Fetal Adrenal Cortex and the X Zone

In the fetus a specialized region of the human adrenal cortex has been described between the maturing (permanent) cortex and the medulla. This primate *fetal adrenal cortex* may exceed the size of the kidney and is about one-third the size of the kidney at birth. The fetal cortex regresses during the last month of gestation and is then only one-tenth or less the size of an individual kidney. A transient adrenal cortex is also present in the monkey, armadillo, sloth, members of the cat family, elephant seal, and pig [22]. The permanency of the fetal cortex may depend on the pituitary, either ACTH or possibly α-MSH of pars intermedia origin (Chapter 8).

In the mouse the cortex possesses a juxtamedullary zone where morphological expression varies according to sex and age. This zone, generally referred to as the *X zone*, degenerates in the male at maturity and in the female early during the first pregnancy. Castration before puberty allows the X zone to survive, apparently in response to increased secretion of pituitary LH. Injections of LH into the postpubertal castrated mouse reestablish the X zone. The X zone does not disappear in the unmated female. Androgens of gonadal origin appear to be responsible for degeneration of the X zone in some strains of mice, but possibly not in other strains. The adrenal X zone degenerates in Tfm mutant mice whose cells are insensitive to androgens, suggesting that in this strain the X zone atrophy is not directly dependent on androgens [44]. The product(s) that the X zone might secrete is unknown as is the significance of this specialized area.

SYNTHESIS AND CHEMISTRY

Cholesterol, a sterol consisting of 27 carbon atoms, is the precursor for both gonadal and adrenal steroid hormone biosynthesis. The first step in the biosynthetic pathway of steroidogenesis involves cleavage of the terminal six carbons of the side chain of cholesterol, resulting in the formation of pregnenolone. A number of key enzymes, collectively known as the *desmolase system*, are requisite for side-chain cleavage. From pregnenolone a number of pathways lead to the formation of metabolic intermediates that give rise ultimately to the definitive steroid hormones characteristic of the species (Fig. 15.3). The steroid hormones of the adrenal glands may be categorized into three groups according to their principal effects: gluco-

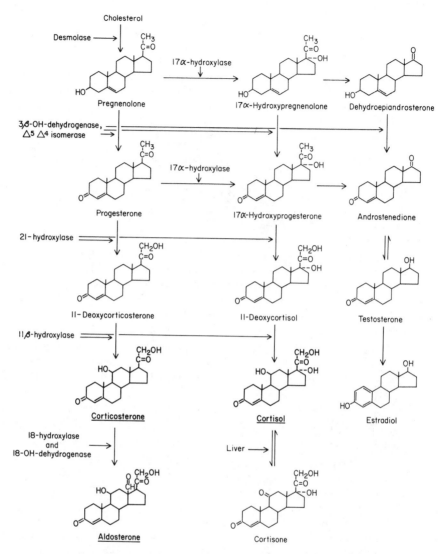

Figure 15.3 Pathways of adrenal steroid hormone biosynthesis.

corticoids, mineralocorticoids, and androgens. Cortisol and aldosterone are the major glucocorticoid and mineralocorticoid hormones, respectively, of humans. Note that all the steroids of the adrenal contain the *cyclopentanoperhydrophenanthrene* nucleus (Fig. 15.4).

Cortisol and aldosterone are examples of C-21 steroids, whereas androgens (androstenedione and testosterone) are C-19 steroids (Fig. 15.4). Estradiol, a C-18 steroid, is derived from testosterone, but estrogen production is of minor significance in the adrenal. Androgens that have a keto group at the C-17 position are appropriately referred to as *17-ketosteroids*. Those C-21 steroids that have a hydroxyl group at the 17-position are often referred to as *17-hydroxycorticoids*.

The double bond between positions 4 and 5 and the presence of the keto group

Synthesis and Chemistry

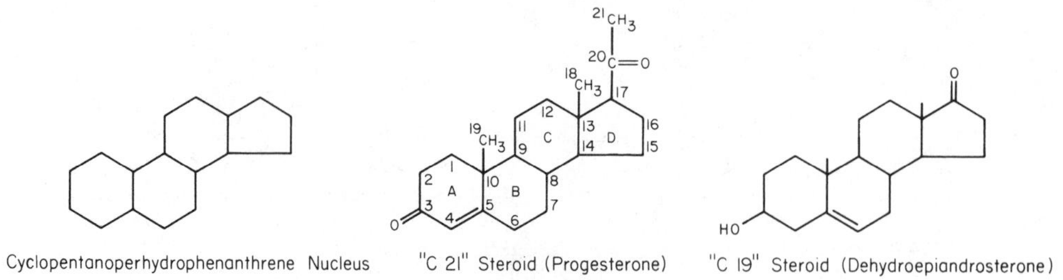

Figure 15.4 Steroid hormone structure and nomenclature.

at position 3 of the A ring are essential for the biological activities of adrenal steroids. Because of the dearth of comparative studies, it is difficult to assess the relative roles of hydroxyl groups at the 11 or 12 position of the steroid nucleus as determinants of either glucocorticoid or mineralocorticoid activity. Introduction of a 1,2 double bond in cortisone (prednisone, Δ^1-cortisone) or cortisol (prednisolone, A^1-cortisol) enhances the ratio of glucocorticoid to mineralocorticoid activity by increasing the former. Incorporation of fluoride into the 9α position enhances both the glucocorticoid and mineralocorticoid activity of cortisol (9α-fluoro-cortisol). Dexamethasone (9α-fluoro-16α-methylprednisolone) is a very potent glucocorticoid with minimal salt-retaining activity.

Conversion of cholesterol to pregnenolone occurs within the mitochondria. Pregnenolone is then released from the mitochondria and, in the smooth endoplasmic reticulum, the double bond is shifted from the 5 to the 4 position and the hydroxyl group at position C-3 is oxidized to a keto group by an enzyme, Δ^5,3-β-hydroxysteroid dehydrogenase-isomerase. All the remaining steps in corticosteroidogenesis consist of additional hydroxylations, at either positions 11, 17, or 21, by various NADPH-dependent hydroxylases [6, 25]. The pathway leading to aldosterone synthesis involves an initial hydroxylation at position 18 followed by dehydrogenase activity, resulting in formation of an aldehyde group at that position. A genetic defect in the function of any one of these enzymes can have a profound effect on the particular steroids produced by the adrenal.

Several different systems of nomenclature are used to refer to individual steroid structures (Tables 15.1 and 15.2). The Greek capital letter Δ (delta) is often used to indicate a double bond, and it is important to note that a Δ^4 bond is common to nearly all the adrenal steroids. The orientation of hydroxyl groups at either the 11 or 17 position of the steroid nucleus is indicated by a β sign and a solid line (—OH), or an α sign and a dashed line (- - -OH). The latter designation indicates that the group projects below the plane of the steroid nucleus, while the former indicates that it is above. Cortisol, for example, has a Δ^4-3-keto configuration in the A ring and β- and α-hydroxyl groups at positions 11 and 17, respectively, of the molecule. Aldosterone is unique in having an aldehyde group at the 18 position of the molecule. The systemic names of some steroids are provided (Table 15.2).

The bulk of adrenal cholesterol is derived by uptake from plasma cholesterol rather than by intracellular synthesis as previously believed [18]. Low density lipoproteins (LP) are the major cholesterol transport complexes in human plasma. Cholesterol esters, with triglycerides, are packaged into lipoprotein particles where

TABLE 15.1 Terms Used In Steroid Nomenclature

Term	Description
Hydroxy-	Indicates an —OH (hydroxyl) group
-ol	Indicates an —OH (hydroxyl) group
Oxo-	Indicates an $=O$ (keto) group
Keto-	Indicates an $=O$ group
-one	Indicates an $=O$ (keto) group
-al	Indicates an aldehyde (—CHO) group
Δ	Signifies location of a double bond in the steroid nucleus (e.g., Δ^4 =bond between C-4 and C-5 positions).
-ene[a]	Indicates one double bond in the steroid nucleus
-diene	Indicates two double bonds in the steroid nucleus
-triene	Indicates three double bonds in the steroid nucleus
α- and β-	Designates if a substituted group lies above (β) or below (α) the plane of the molecule
Estrane$_{(C_{18})}$[b]	Indicates basic steroid skeleton with a methyl group attached at C-13 in addition to the 17 carbon atoms of the ring structure
Androstane$_{(C_{19})}$[b]	Indicates steroid structure with methyl groups at both the C-13 and C-10 positions
Pregnane$_{(21)}$[b]	Indicates basic steroid skeleton with methyl groups at C-13 and C-10 and a two-carbon atom side chain attached at the C-17 position

[a]The suffix -ene is currently used more often than Δ.

[b]Hypothetical parent compound.

they form a hydrophobic core surrounded by a monolayer of polar phospholipids and small amounts of proteins called *apoproteins*. The apoproteins bind to LP receptors of adrenal target cells which may stimulate endocytosis and the transport of the lipoproteins into the cells, an event enhanced by ACTH. The number of LP binding sites is highest in membranes of the adrenal cortex and ovarian corpus luteum, two tissues that synthesize steroids and therefore have a high requirement for cholesterol. The sequence of reactions by which LP's are taken up by cells is known as the low density lipoprotein receptor pathway [3, 4].

A model for cholesterol homeostasis in the adrenal gland is presented in Figure 15.5 [3]. In the basal state the amount of cholesterol delivered to the cell by LP's is balanced by cholesterol conversion to steroid hormones that are then secreted.

TABLE 15.2 Systematic Names Of Vertebrate Steroids

Class name	Trivial name	Systematic name[a]
Glucocorticoids	Cortisol (hydrocortisone)	11β,17α,21-Trihydroxy-pregn-4-ene-3,20-dione
	Corticosterone	11β,21-Dihydroxy-pregn-4-ene-3,20-dione
Mineralocorticoids	Aldosterone	11β,21-Dihydroxy-pregn-4-ene-3,20-dione-18-al
	11-Deoxycorticosterone	21-Hydroxy-pregn-4-ene-3,20-dione
Androgenic steroids	Dehydroepiandrosterone	3β-Hydroxy-androst-5-ene-17-one
	Testosterone	17β-Hydroxy-androst-4-ene-3-one
Estrogenic steroids	Estradiol	1,3,5(10)-Estratriene-3,17β-diol
Progestens	Pregnenolone	3β-Hydroxy-pregn-5-ene-20-one
	Progesterone	Pregn-4-ene-3,20-dione

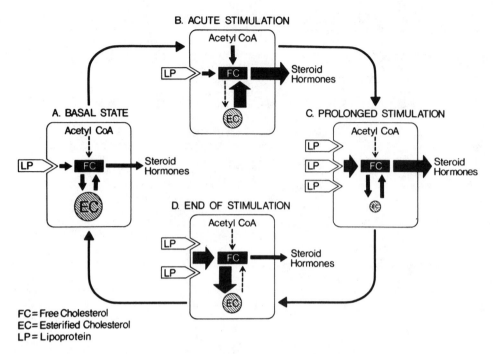

B. ACUTE STIMULATION

A. BASAL STATE

C. PROLONGED STIMULATION

D. END OF STIMULATION

FC = Free Cholesterol
EC = Esterified Cholesterol
LP = Lipoprotein

Figure 15.5 Model for cholesterol homeostasis in the adrenal. (From Brown, Kovanen, and Goldstein, [3], with permission.)

The metabolically active pool of free cholesterol is derived from LP internalization, limited endogenous synthesis (through acetyl-CoA), and hydrolysis of cholesterol esters. In response to ACTH there is an enhancement of intracellular cholesterol synthesis as well as hydrolysis of cholesterol esters. Esterified cholesterol reserves are limited, and endogenous cholesterol synthesis apparently soon returns to basal levels; consequently, extracellular lipoproteins must provide the cholesterol for continued steroid hormone biosynthesis. This is apparently accomplished by an increase in the number of LP receptors (Fig. 15.5).

Functional Zonation of the Adrenal Cortex

It is generally believed that in most mammals mineralocorticoids are produced in the zona glomerulosa, glucocorticoids in the zona fasciculata, and androgens in the zona reticularis [7]. Functional separation of the zones was suggested when Greep and Deane [17] noted that the zona fasciculata may atrophy or become grossly hyperactive without any conspicuous alteration in the zona glomerulosa. These investigators also noted that, on a gross morphological basis, the gland could be separated into two zones, and they were the first to comment on the dual nature of control of the adrenal cortex. The mammalian zona glomerulosa lacks a 17α-hydroxylase, and therefore synthesizes corticosterone, a glucocorticoid which does not contain a 17α-hydroxyl group. Sequential actions by the enzymes 18-hydroxylase and 18-hydroxysteroid dehydrogenase convert corticosterone to aldosterone.

The latter enzyme is found only in the glomerulosa. In humans and cattle 17-hydroxysteroids are produced by the zona fasciculata and zona reticularis. Because corticosterone is the principal steroid of the rat, the zones of the adrenal, except for the zona glomerulosa which also produces aldosterone, are alike in their synthesized products [49].

CONTROL OF SYNTHESIS AND SECRETION

The biological roles of adrenal glucocorticoids and mineralocorticoids differ considerably. It is not unexpected, therefore, that the control of synthesis and secretion of these two classes of steroid hormones is also different. Adrenal glucocorticoid synthesis and secretion are controlled by pituitary adrenocorticotropin (ACTH), whereas aldosterone secretion is controlled primarily by the *renin-angiotensin system*.

Glucocorticoids

Glucocorticoid production by the cells of the zona fasciculata is regulated by pituitary ACTH. The release of ACTH is in turn regulated by a hypothalamic corticotropin releasing hormone (CRH) as discussed in Chapters 5 and 6. Unilateral adrenalectomy is followed by contralateral adrenal hypertrophy and hyperplasia. After bilateral adrenalectomy or in primary adrenal insufficiency (Addison's disease), there is a striking increase in plasma ACTH levels. These elevated levels of ACTH can be returned to normal by administration of glucocorticoids, suggesting a negative feedback regulation of ACTH secretion by the steroids. Glucocortocoid negative feedback may be mediated at the level of the pituitary, hypothalamus, or even higher brain centers (Fig. 15.6).

ACTH interacts with the plasmalemma of zona fasciculata cells to increase intracellular cAMP levels; activation of one or more protein kinases follows. During ACTH stimulation increased cAMP production precedes the steroidogenic event. Calcium is required for ACTH activation of adenylate cyclase but not for binding of the peptide to adrenal cells [41]. The effects of ACTH on adrenal fasciculata cell steroidogenesis are mimicked by methylxanthines and cAMP analogs, suggesting that cAMP is the second messenger regulating ACTH action. There is strong experimental evidence that cGMP plays no role in adrenal steroidogenesis [20].

Acute stimulation by ACTH involves transformation of an inactive precursor protein to an active labile one by phosphorylation [38]. Concomitant activation of an inactive phosphatase may provide a mechanism for the rapid termination of the steroidogenic response (Fig. 15.7). The function of the active phosphorylated protein may be to activate a cholesterol ester hydrolase to convert sequestered cholesterol into a free form available for steroidogenesis. In addition to its acute stimulatory effects on steroidogenesis ACTH also has a prolonged trophic action on the adrenal cell. This is manifested in part by increases in the levels of key mitochondrial steroidogenic enzymes.

In humans there is a diurnal rhythm of ACTH and cortisol secretion and 17-hydroxycorticoid excretion [30, 45]. The regularity of this rhythm appears to be a func-

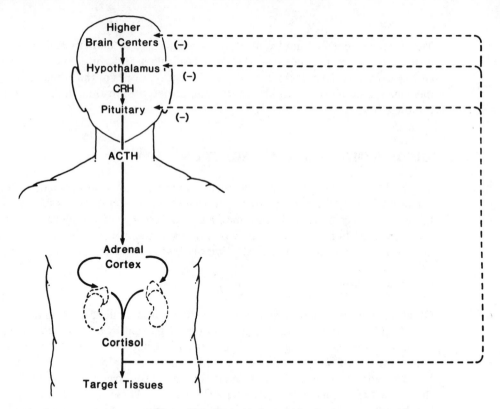

Figure 15.6 Brain-pituitary-adrenal axis.

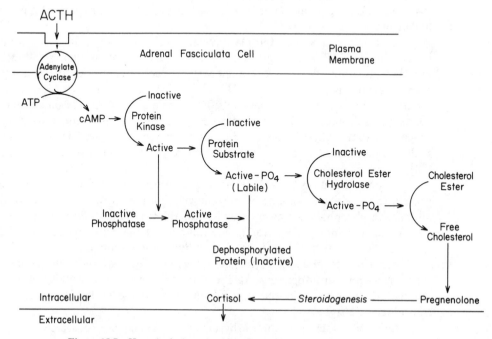

Figure 15.7 Hypothetical mechanism of ACTH action on adrenal steroidogenesis.

tion of the sleep-wake habits of the individual. In those individuals who sleep regularly at the same hours each day a sharp increase in ACTH-cortisol secretion occurs during the third to fifth hours of sleep and becomes maximal about an hour after awakening. Minimal levels of these hormones are reached a few hours before and after resumption of sleep. In humans this rhythm of activity is first established at about 3 months of postnatal life. The circadian rhythm has a cycle length of about 24 hours and cannot be synchronized with environmental lighting regimes. In a free-running environment with an absence of clues to the true local time the rhythm persists but is slightly and consistently longer or shorter than 24 hours [45].

Aldosterone

Aldosterone secretion from the zona glomerulosa is mainly controlled by *angiotensin II*, an octapeptide which is derived from a decapeptide, angiotensin I, through the action of a *converting enzyme* [36, 37]. Angiotensin I is derived from a precursor protein, appropriately designated as *angiotensinogen* (or renin substrate), which originates in the liver. The conversion of angiotensinogen to angiotensin I results from the enzymatic action of an enzyme, *renin*, which is released from specialized granular cells, *juxtaglomerular (JG) cells*, in the afferent arteriole of the vascular pole of the renal glomerulus. The action of angiotensin II on adrenal glomerulosa cells is terminated by *angiotensinases* which split the octapeptide into smaller inactive fragments (Fig. 15.8). Extrarenal sources of renin, *isorenins*, have been described (brain, uterus, adrenal glands) but their significance is undefined. Angiotensin I converting enzyme has been localized to a variety of vascular beds. The presence of this enzyme in these vessels may be indicative of a functional role of angiotensins in the local control of blood flow. These extrarenal sites of angiotensin production comprise so-called tissue angiotensinogenase systems.

Renin is secreted in response to hypovolemia or to an increase in the osmolarity of the blood. According to the *baroreceptor hypothesis*, the afferent arteriole responds to a change in mean renal perfusion pressure. These changes result in either a stretching or a decreased transmural (vessel-wall) pressure in the afferent arteriole, which results in an observable altered juxtaglomerular cell granularity (the granules being the cellular source of renin). In this theory the JG cells are modified smooth muscle cells and function as baroreceptors.

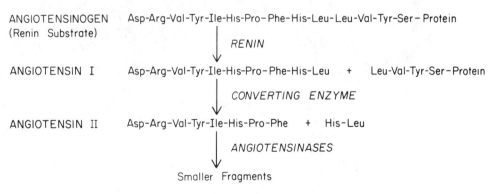

Figure 15.8 Angiotensin biosynthesis.

Another theory suggests that specialized cells of the distal tubular epithelium play a pivotal role in the control of renin release. These cells are in close apposition to the JG cells and may function as chemoreceptors and monitor the urinary sodium load within the distal tubule. According to the *macula densa theory*, this information is in some manner relayed to the JG cells where appropriate modifications of renin release take place. The renal functional unit of renin secretion, which consists of the macula densa cells and the JG cells, is referred to as the *juxtaglomerular apparatus* (Fig. 15.9) [11].

Renin secretion may also be regulated by the ANS [39]. Renin release is increased in response to sympathetic nerve stimulation; the normal reduction in resting plasma renin levels in response to volume depletion is reduced by renal sympathectomy, and catecholamines stimulate renin release from kidney slices incubated in vitro. Norepinephrine released from sympathetic neurons apparently acts on β-adrenoceptors of the JG cells and the resulting increase in cAMP is the stimulus to vesicular exocytosis of the renin secretory granules.

The angiotensin II produced in response to renin release acts on adrenal glomerulosa cell membranes. The cAMP produced stimulates aldosterone synthesis and secretion. Aldosterone mediates its action at the level of the distal convoluted tubules and possibly, to a lesser degree, the cortical collecting tubules of the kidney. Sodium resorption increases the osmolarity of the blood which is monitored by the JG cells and they respond by decreased renin secretion (Fig. 15.10). Increasing the plasma Na^+ concentration may be a direct inhibitory stimulus to further aldosterone secretion. In the absence of aldosterone the ratio of K^+ to Na^+ increases; high K^+ is a direct stimulus to aldosterone secretion. Besides its action on the cells of the zona glomerulosa, angiotensin II stimulates vasoconstriction. This adaptive vasopressor

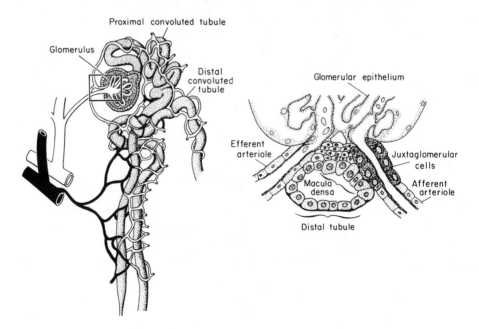

Figure 15.9 Renal juxtaglomerular apparatus.

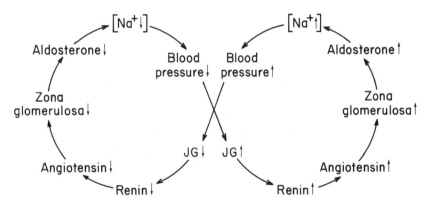

Figure 15.10 Renin-angiotensin system and Na⁺ homeostasis. Arrows indicate increases (↑) or decreases (↓) in the factors indicated. (From Goss, [16], with permission.)

response results in elevation of the blood pressure. Afferent sensory neurons respond to the vasoconstriction and, by a reflex mechanism, inhibit sympathetic stimulation of renin secretion.

Removal of the N-terminal aspartic acid residue from angiotensin II gives rise to a heptapeptide referred to as angiotensin III. Although originally considered only a degradative product of angiotensin II metabolism, this peptide produces levels of aldosterone secretion in the rat similar to that of angiotensin II but possesses very little pressor activity. It has been suggested, therefore, that angiotensin III may serve as a specific hormone for aldosterone secretion.

Renal Kallikrein-Kinin System

Kinins are polypeptide hormones released from plasma protein precursors by plasma and tissue enzymes termed *kallikreins* [35]. The protein precursors are referred to as *kininogens*, and they serve as substrates for the enzymatic actions of the kallikreins which may themselves become activated after they are enzymatically released from proenzymes referred to as *prekallikreins*. The kinins are subsequently inactivated by enzymes referred to as *kininases* (Fig. 4.10). Glandular kallikreins are a group of kinin-forming enzymes found in many glands such as the kidney. Glandular kallikreins from different tissue may not be identical in primary structure. Activation of these enzymes and their subsequent activation of kininogens may provide a mechanism for the local production of kinins. Within the kidney kallikrein activation leads to the production of a nonapeptide, *lysylbradykin*, which is then converted (apparently by an angiotensinase) to the octapeptide *bradykinin* (Fig. 15.11).

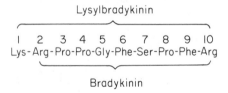

Figure 15.11 Structures of lysylbradykinin and bradykinin.

In the kidney renin is derived from an inactive zymogen precursor, a prorenin. There is evidence that renal kallikrein is responsible for the enzymatic activation of renin from prorenin in addition to its role in the activation of a kininogen to bradykinin [42]. Most interesting is the discovery that the angiotensin I converting enzyme is apparently identical to kininase II. Thus, this enzyme is responsible for the conversion of angiotensin I to its active form, angiotensin II, as well as the conversion of bradykinin to inactive fragments (Fig. 15.12) [23].

It is of interest that renal kallikrein participates in the activation of two polypeptides that have vasoactive actions. Angiotensin II can be considered a systemic vasoconstrictor whose direct actions on the arterial tree elevate blood pressure. Within the kidney, on the other hand, bradykinin may function as a localized vascular smooth muscle relaxant. It has been suggested that the concurrent release of two enzymes which produce peptides with diametrically opposing actions would seem counterproductive. However, it would be important that maintenance of blood pressure via constriction does not occur at the expense of renal blood flow. The role of bradykinin would be confined to the renal vascular bed so that kidney perfusion is protected. Thus, this dual system would function to maintain a normal renal blood flow and at the same time increase systemic pressure [42].

Within the kidney kallikrein is localized to the basal membrane of the epithelial cells of the distal tubules. There is evidence that aldosterone increases kallikrein excretion in humans and other animals and also enhances renin activity [33]. A stimulus may be required to release prorenin so that prorenin can be acted on by kallikrein. There is strong evidence that bradykinin mediates its renal vasodepressor action through activation of one or more E-series prostaglandins. Bradykinin also increases the concentration of prostaglandinlike substances in the renal venous blood. Prostaglandins released from renal tissues may therefore participate in the regulation of renin release. Prostacyclin I_2 (PGI_2) appears to be the arachidonic acid product that is responsible for renin release. It is possible that the roles of PGE_2 and PGI_2 differ in different compartments of the kidney. A summary scheme of the possible relationships of aldosterone and the renal kallikrein-bradykinin system to renin production is shown (Fig. 15.13).

CIRCULATION AND METABOLISM

Steroid hormones are only sparingly soluble in water and most are transported to their target tissues by plasma proteins. Within the plasma, cortisol is reversibly bound to two proteins, *transcortin* or *corticosteroid-binding globulin* (CBG) and,

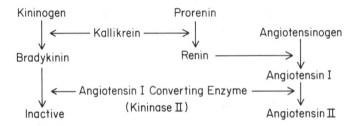

Figure 15.12 Kallikrein role in renin activation and bradykinin production. (From Inagami and Murakami, [23], with permission.)

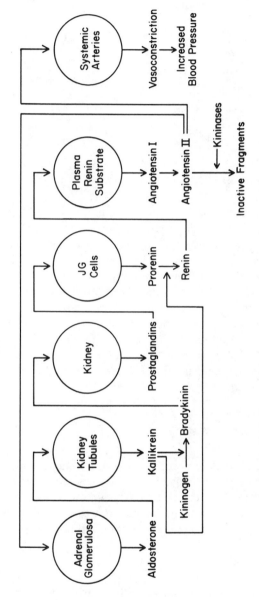

Figure 15.13 Summary scheme of the role of aldosterone in renal renin production.

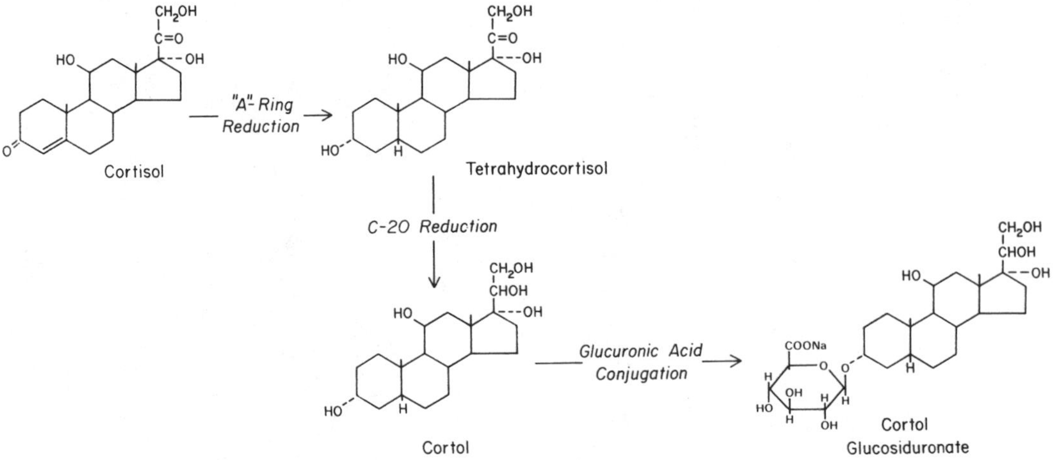

Figure 15.14 One pathway of cortisol metabolism and glucuronide formation.

to a lesser extent, an α-2 globulin. About 6% of cortisol is unbound, and it is this pool that apparently represents the hormone available for uptake by target tissues. The bound cortisol provides a large buffer pool of the corticosteroid that can be made immediately available as the free cortisol.

Greater than 50% of circulating aldosterone is unbound. The biological half-life of cortisol in the human is about 80 minutes, whereas that for aldosterone is about 30 minutes. The short half-life of aldosterone may be because most aldosterone circulates in an unbound form and is therefore readily available for metabolism and excretion. Metabolism of adrenal steroids occurs primarily in the liver where side-chain and A-ring reductions take place. Structurally altered steroids are then conjugated to glucuronic acid to form water-soluble derivatives. One pathway of cortisol metabolism is shown in Figure 15.14.

PHYSIOLOGICAL ROLES

The biological roles of cortisol and aldosterone, the major glucocorticoid and min-eralocorticoid, respectively, in humans are quite different. In pathophysiological states of cortisol hypersecretion (Cushing's disease) or aldosterone hypersecretion (Conn's disease) each hormone may, however, exhibit both glucocorticoid and min-eralocorticoid activity because they share structural similarities.

Glucocorticoids

Intermediary metabolism. Glucocorticoids affect carbohydrate, lipid, and protein metabolism. They increase synthesis of a number of key enzymes in the gluconeogenic pathway within hepatocytes. Although the actions of glucocorticoids on the liver are anabolic, the actions on skeletal muscle and adipose tissue are catabolic. Catabolic actions may result because glucose uptake by these tissues is inhibited by glucocorticoids. In the absence of a metabolic substrate for ATP production proteolysis of muscle proteins and lipolysis of fat occur. The FFA's and amino acids that are released from these tissues become available as substrates for gluconeo-genesis within the liver (Fig. 15.15). The glucose produced is either stored as glyco-gen or released into the blood. Excessive secretion of glucocorticoids is antagonistic to the actions of insulin and predisposes the individual to diabetes mellitus as the actions of glucocorticoids elevate blood glucose levels. Glucocorticoids also reduce the affinity of certain cells for insulin, which further encourages diabetes.

Permissive actions. Most, if not all, effects of glucocorticoids may be con-sidered permissive to the actions of other hormones [24]. In particular, glucocorti-coids are required for functioning of the sympathoadrenal system. Under conditions of stress and in the absence of glucocorticoids there is vascular collapse which leads usually to death. Glucocorticoids are necessary for catecholamine synthesis within sympathetic nerve terminals and for the process of catecholamine reuptake from the synaptic cleft; they may also decrease the rate of catecholamine degradation by COMT. Evidence for these statements includes a diminished sympathoadrenal ac-tivity in the absence of glucocorticoids. Fat mobilization in response to catechol-amines is impaired after hypophysectomy but is corrected by treatment with ACTH or glucocorticoids. Glucocorticoids themselves have little if any fat-mobilizing activity, but they apparently maintain levels of lipolytic enzymes that are activated through the actions of catecholamines. Hypothermia usually follows adrenalec-tomy, and adrenalectomized animals soon die under conditions of cold stress. Glu-cocorticoids maintain body temperature in homeotherms through their permissive actions on liver gluconeogenesis and adipose tissue metabolism.

Role in reproduction. In sheep and other domestic animals the pituitary-adrenal axis is clearly involved in the process of parturition. Plasma levels of corti-costerone increase in fetal sheep several days before birth and infusions of ACTH or dexamethasone induce premature parturition. The fetal adrenal is relatively un-responsive to ACTH until 7 to 9 days before term, but no adequate explanation is

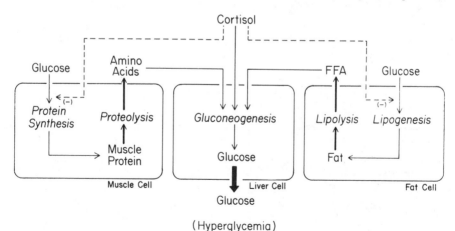

Figure 15.15 Major effects of excess cortisol in intermediary metabolism.

available why adrenal sensitivity to ACTH changes just prior to parturition. One hypothesis is that large molecular weight forms of ACTH-like peptides are present in the plasma and may inhibit the steroidogenic response of the adrenal to ACTH. A fall in levels of these large peptides late in gestation is suggested to be one of the factors initiating parturition [27].

Cortisol and prolactin are the principal hormones required for lactogenesis in the mouse mammary gland. In mammary tissue cortisol is expressed through a specific glucocorticoid receptor. There is about an 85% decrease in the level of casein mRNA after adrenalectomy. A single injection of cortisol will then cause an increase in casein mRNA to a level above that of the adrenalectomized animal.

Nervous system effects. Neonatal administration of corticosterone can reduce both the basal level and amplitude of the diurnal rhythm of plasma corticosterone in the adult rat, depending on the age at which exposure to the steroid occurs. This suggests that, as for gonadal steroids, adrenal steroids of fetal or maternal origin may play an important role in early "imprinting" of the CNS (Chapter 16). It is also possible that the presence of maternal steroids in excessive concentrations adversely affect the normal development of the fetal nervous system and thus contribute to birth defects.

Antiinflammatory and immunosuppressive actions of glucocorticoids. At higher than physiological concentrations, as in Cushing's disease, glucocorticoids inhibit inflammatory and allergic reactions. It is suggested that these actions may result from stabilization of lysosomal membranes which prevents the secretion of enzymes that normally occurs during inflammation. Glucocorticoids inhibit the infiltration of leukocytes into the affected tissue and also exert an immunosuppressive action through their lympholytic actions.

In addition to the catabolic actions of glucocorticoids on muscle tissue and the protein matrix of bone, glucocorticoids cause atrophy of the lymphatic system (lymph nodes, thymus gland, spleen) which results in decreased levels of circulating lymphocytes. Ultimately, this lymphocytopenia results in failure of the body to provide antibodies during an infection. Although glucocorticoids may be useful in combating the undesirable effects of local infections, excessive use of these agents may render the individual susceptible to severe systematic bacterial infection as many protective mechanisms are suppressed but the underlying cause of the disease remains.

Glucocorticoids and the general adaptation syndrome. In 1936 Selye published the paper, "A Syndrome Produced By Diverse Nocuous Agents." This syndrome was later referred to as the *general adaptation syndrome* or GAS. In response to stress a body responds in a stereotypic manner, which, if the stress is prolonged, may proceed through a number of stages: (1) an initial *alarm reaction;* (2) *resistance;* and eventually (3) *exhaustion* [43]. These stages may be characterized more precisely if one understands the underlying physiological processes involved in the adaptation syndrome.

In response to stress the sympathoadrenal system is activated (Chapter 14). Through the actions of epinephrine released from the adrenal chromaffin tissue and norepinephrine released from sympathetic nerve endings the general body metabolic and motor activity is increased (alarm reaction). The basal metabolic rate is elevated and blood flow is increased, particularly to those organs that are more physiologically active. A major effect of circulating catecholamines is the utilization of liver glycogen stores for the production of glucose. This depot source of readily available carbohydrate, though limited, may be sufficient for an immediate stress (alarm) response.

The release of adrenal glucocorticoids is also activated in response to stress. Through the permissive actions of these hormones there is an enhancement of sympathoadrenal activity. In fact, in the absence of adrenal steroids sympathoadrenal actions are greatly depressed, which may lead to the individual's demise. Glucocorticoids enhance the lipolytic actions of catecholamines on adipose tissue. The FFA's released from fat cells provides metabolic substrates necessary for survival in the absence of hepatic glycogen stores. However, hepatic glycogen depots are restored through gluconeogenesis. The actions of glucocorticoids are slower than the initial rapid actions of catecholamines on metabolic processes, but they provide the secondary response (resistance) necessary for continued sympathoadrenal activity and hepatic gluconeogenesis.

Under prolonged conditions of stress the individual enters the third stage of the adaptation syndrome, exhaustion. In effect the prolonged hypercortisolism eventually leads to muscle wasting, hyperglycemia (diabetes mellitus), atrophy of the immune system, vascular derangements, gastrointestinal ulceration, and other symptoms of excessive sympathoadrenal activity.

It is clear that adrenal steroid hormones are essential for survival under stress. Continued stress eventually leads to gross pathophysiological alterations of bodily processes due to prolonged excessive actions of adrenal hormones. A little stress may be of adaptive necessity; too much, however, may be disastrous.

Aldosterone

Aldosterone accelerates the reabsorption of Na^+ by the kidney tubules, salivary and sweat glands, and gastrointestinal mucosa. Through its major action on renal tubular Na^+ retention aldosterone also profoundly affects the plasma concentration of potassium and hydrogen ions. In the nephron the uptake of Na^+ in response to aldosterone is usually balanced by a concomitant loss of K^+ (Fig. 15.16). Under condi-

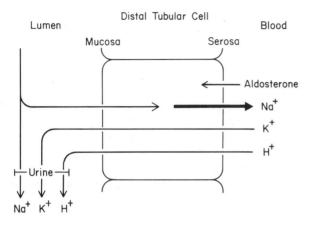

Figure 15.16 Physiological effects of aldosterone on renal distal tubular Na^+ resorption and K^+ and H^+ excretion. In response to aldosterone sodium is actively transported across the tubular serosal membrane into the peritubular space. Potassium and hydrogen ions are passively shunted across the mucosal membrane in exchange for sodium.

Physiological Roles

tions of plasma K^+ deficiency (hypokalemia) there is an increase in distal tubular H^+ secretion, whereas during states of K^+ excess distal tubular secretion of K^+ is enhanced. One of the important elements in acclimatization to heat is the ability to reduce the amount of Na^+ in sweat. Injections of a mineralocorticoid into an individual not exposed to heat produce a drop in the Na^+ content of sweat within 2 to 3 days. These observations suggest the Na^+ concentration of sweat is regulated in the human by aldosterone. High affinity sites for aldosterone have been identified in the rat brain. These receptors may represent extrarenal sites of aldosterone action and one of these may affect salt intake (Chapter 20).

Adrenal Androgens

The production of androgens by the adrenal is minimal compared to the production of these hormones by the gonads. In the female adrenal androgens may contribute to pubertal changes, and postmenopausally these androgens may serve as substrates for extragonadal estrogen production. Abnormal adrenal steroid production due to a defect in the normal steroidogenic pathway or to a tumorous condition has profound morphogenetic consequences, particularly in the pregnant female. There is evidence that adrenal steroids may help support growth of mammary and prostatic carcinomas. Regression of steroid-dependent tumors although accelerated after gonadectomy is further enhanced by adrenalectomy.

MECHANISMS OF ACTION

Adrenal steroid hormones, like other steroid hormones, mediate their actions by an initial interaction with cytoplasmic receptors. Three separate renal receptors for aldosterone have been identified and arbitrarily defined based on their specificity for corticoids: type I (mineralocorticoid, binds aldosterone), type II (glucocorticoid, binds dexamethasone), and type III (glucocorticoid, binds corticosterone). The cytoplasmic receptor-hormone complex then translocates to the nucleus where it is believed that the hormone attaches to a chromatin nonhistone protein. This results in a derepression of specific sequences of DNA (genes) and the synthesis (transcription) of messenger RNA's which then travel out of the nucleus to the cytoplasm where they attach to ribosomes and initiate protein synthesis. The particular proteins synthesized (translated) vary with each target tissue and relate specifically to those functions characteristic of the tissue.

Glucocorticoids

Glucocorticoids regulate the activity of a variety of tissues. Most actions involve de novo synthesis of cellular proteins, most often enzymes. In addition glucocorticoids as well as other steroid hormones enhance guanylate cyclase activity, at physiological concentrations, in a variety of tissues [48]. Glucocorticoids also inhibit prostaglandin synthesis by an inhibition of phospholipase activity. One mechanism of glucocorticoid action may be to modulate the number of cell membrane receptors for hormones.

Enzyme induction. Glucocorticoids increase the activity of a number of enzymes. This action could come about either by controlling the number of mRNA templates for enzyme synthesis or by changing the translational efficiency of a fixed level of mRNA. There is evidence that glucocorticoids stimulate the de novo synthesis of mRNA; thus, glucocorticoids stimulate both transcriptional and translational processes related to protein synthesis. Many of these enzymes, such as hepatic tyrosine amino transferase, play important roles in the anabolic actions of steroid hormones. A majority of the actions of cortisol are, however, catabolic in nature. There is evidence that the catabolic actions of glucocorticoids may, in part, result from the synthesis of one or more inhibitory proteins.

Aldosterone

Both kidney and (toad) urinary bladder have been utilized extensively for studies on the mechanism of action of aldosterone. Aldosterone increases the rate of Na^+ transport across epithelial cells of these organs. This movement of Na^+ is generally viewed as a two-step process: (1) there is entry of Na^+ from the fluid bathing the mucosal surface of the cell; (2) there is subsequent extrusion of Na^+ through the serosal membrane into the interstitial space. Numerous experiments have been directed toward determining which step in the transport process is stimulated by aldosterone.

Aldosterone mediates its action through the induction of the synthesis of proteins within target tissues. Three different mechanisms have been postulated by which these hormone-inducible proteins augment transepithelial Na^+ transport (Fig. 15.17). The sodium pump theory postulates that these proteins directly stimu-

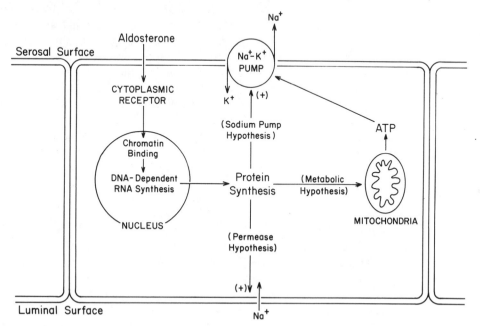

Figure 15.17 Hypothetical mechanisms of aldosterone action on the kidney.

Mechanisms of Action

late the activity of a sodium pump which is localized in the serosal side of the cell. The metabolic theory suggests that the aldosterone-inducible proteins increase the supply of ATP to the pump. In the permease theory these proteins enhance the permeability of the luminal mucosal membrane to Na^+. Experimental evidence strongly supports the view that both the passive apical entry of Na^+ and the active extrusion of Na^+ across the basal-lateral serosal membranes depend on the induction of enzymes that modulate energy metabolism [13]. Aldosterone also stimulates fatty acid synthesis and the turnover of membrane phospholipid fatty acids in the toad bladder. Aldosterone alteration of the lipid composition of membranes may be an important component of the mechanism of action.

Vasopressin (AVP) also increases the rate of Na^+ transport and the permeability to water of the urinary bladder of the toad, two responses mediated through cAMP. Although aldosterone stimulates Na^+ transport in these tissues, it does so without affecting permeability to water. Aldosterone stimulation of Na^+ transport does not involve cAMP production, but it enhances cAMP-induced Na^+ transport and water permeability. The action of the steroid may involve the inhibition of the degradation of cAMP as suggested by the following observations. In response to AVP or theophylline cAMP levels are higher in aldosterone-treated tissue, and the activity of cyclic nucleotide phosphodiesterase, the enzyme that catalyzes the degradation of cAMP, is depressed [13].

PATHOPHYSIOLOGY

The clinical manifestations of abnormal levels of adrenal glucocorticoids or mineralocorticoids in humans are predictable from a knowledge of the biological actions of these corticosteroids (Table 15.3). A total loss of adrenal function may derive from a congenital developmental defect or destruction during a particular disease state (e.g., tuberculosis). The adrenal abnormality may be of primary origin and involve a failure of corticosteroid biosynthesis due to a genetic defect related to an absence or faulty structure of a particular enzyme. Overproduction of a particular corticoid may be due to an adrenocortical adenoma or carcinoma, resulting in excess cortisol (Cushing's syndrome) or, as in primary aldosteronism, in excess aldosterone secretion (Conn's disease). Hyposecretion or hypersecretion of adrenal steroids may be of secondary origin and involve a defect in mechanisms involved in the control of cortisol or aldosterone secretion.

Disorders Of Cortisol Secretion

Addison's disease. In a manuscript published in 1855, "On the Constitutional and Local Effects of Disease of the Supra-Renal Capsules," Addison provided the classical description of the disease that bears his name. The disease may be of primary origin and involve total destruction of the glands. Most often the etiology is due to bilateral tubercular destruction of the glands. Atrophy due to tuberculosis involves the medulla as well as the cortex, whereas in idiopathic (unknown cause) atrophy only the cortex is usually affected. The most frequent symptoms of Addison's disease include weakness, increased melanin pigmentation of the skin,

TABLE 15.3   Endocrine Pathophysiology Of The Adrenal Cortex

Adrenocortical Hypofunction
  Addison's disease
    Primary adrenocortical insufficiency
    Secondary adrenocortical insufficiency
      Pituitary origin (no ACTH secretion)
      Hypothalamic origin (no CRH secretion?)
  Hypoaldosteronism
    Primary (adrenocortical insufficiency)
    Secondary
      Hyporeninemic hypoaldosteronism
Adrenocortical Hyperfunction
  Syndromes of excess cortisol secretion (Cushing's disease)
    Cushing's syndrome (primary origin)
      Adrenal adenoma or adenocarcinoma
    Cushing's syndrome (secondary origin)
      Bilateral adrenal hyperplasia
        Pituitary origin (microadenoma secreting ACTH)
        Hypothalamic origin
        Ectopic ACTH syndrome
  Syndromes of excess aldosterone secretion
    Primary hyperaldosteronism, Conn's syndrome (adrenal adenoma, aldosteronoma)
    Secondary hyperaldosteronism
      Bartter's syndrome (hyperreninism)
      Malignant hypertension
      Renin-secreting tumor
  Syndromes of excess adrenal androgen secretion (virilizing adrenal tumors)
    Male (precocious pseudopuberty in the preadolescent boy)
    Female (masculinization)
  Syndromes of excess estrogen production (feminizing adrenal tumor)
    Male (gynecomastia)
    Female (precocious puberty in the preadolescent girl)
Adrenal Enzyme Deficiency Syndromes
  Congenital (lipoid) adrenal hyperplasia (fatal)
  Congenital virilizing adrenal hyperplasia
    3 β-Dehydrogenase deficiency
    11 β-Hydroxylase deficiency (hypertensive form)
    21 β-Hydroxylase deficiency (salt-losing form)
  Congenital 17 α-hydroxylase deficiency
  Corticosterone methyl oxidase (type II) deficiency (hypoaldosteronism)

weight loss, hypotension, salt craving, and hypoglycemia. These symptoms result from a combination of both glucocorticoid and mineralocorticoid deficiencies. The increased integumental pigmentation, a cardinal symptom, is because in the absence of cortisol feedback to the hypothalamus, excessive amounts of ACTH are secreted. Because the nearly complete structure of α-MSH is contained within the ACTH molecule (Fig. 8.1), it is probable that ACTH acts on integumental melanocytes to increase melanin production of the skin. In Addison's disease of secondary or tertiary origin the defect may reside at the level of the pituitary or hypothalamus, respectively. A failure of the hypothalamus to secrete CRH or the absence of functional pituitary corticotrophs could explain the etiology of some forms of adrenal insufficiency.

Cushing's syndrome. This disease, first described by Cushing in 1932, refers to any clinical entity due to excessive and prolonged secretion and action of glucocorticoids, although the cause of the disease may relate to any one of a number of origins. Primary hypercortisolism may be due to an adrenal cortical tumor (adenoma or carcinoma). Cushing's disease of secondary origin may derive from a pituitary tumor secreting an excess of ACTH or to ectopic ACTH production, or to pituitary corticotroph hyperplasia. The simultaneous measurement of plasma ACTH and cortisol is useful in differentiating between adrenal hyperplasia (due to excess pituitary ACTH stimulation) and adrenal tumors as the cause of Cushing's syndrome. In patients with adrenal tumors plasma cortisol levels are high but the concentration of ACTH is low or undetectable. In contrast, both cortisol and ACTH plasma levels are elevated in bilateral adrenal hyperplasia.

Some symptoms of cortisol excess are central (trunkal) obesity, hypertension, glucose intolerance, hirsutism, osteoporosis, polyuria, and polydipsia. The hyperglycemia resulting from excess glucocorticoids leads to a so-called steroid diabetes, where prolonged elevated levels of glucose may in time lead to pancreatic β-cell exhaustion (diabetes mellitus). The change in fat distribution is due to the lipolytic action of ACTH and glucocorticoids on the normal fat depots. The redistribution of fat may not be due to the direct actions of glucocorticoids but rather to the insulin that is secreted in response to increased hepatic glucose formation. Although the actions of insulin on the normal fat depots are apparently antagonized by cortisol, insulin appears able to exert a lipogenic effect in other areas of the body such as the face, upper back, and supraclavicular fat pads. The catabolic actions of glucocorticoids on skeletal muscle cause thinning of the extremities. Loss of the protein matrix of bones causes severe osteoporosis which may severely affect the spinal column. The excess androgens produced are the cause of hirsutism in the female. Again, the hyperpigmentation that may be present in Cushing's disease of secondary origin may be due to the presence of increased circulating levels of ACTH. Polyuria and polydipsia are due to the loss of large volumes of water as a result of solvent drag during the process of excessive glucose excretion by the kidneys.

Disorders Of Aldosterone Secretion

Conn's syndrome. In 1955 Conn published a classical report, "Primary Aldosteronism, A New Clinical Syndrome" [10]. The cause of aldosterone hypersecretion is almost always an adrenal adenoma but in some instances may be due to adrenal carcinoma, hyperplasia, or other unknown causes. The oversecretion of aldosterone increases renal distal tubular secretion of K^+ (K^+ diuresis) and H^+ in exchange for reabsorbed sodium. This leads to the cardinal findings of plasma *hypernatremia* and *hypokalemia;* because hydrogen ions are also lost, this leads to serum *alkalosis* and nephropathy. The hypernatremia is usually associated with water retention, leading to severe hypertension. Therefore, plasma renin levels are low in primary aldosteronism.

Renin-secreting tumors. The rare occurrence of a renin-secreting tumor is associated with hypertension due to excessive renin secretion. The larger precursor molecule, prorenin, may be present in the plasma and may prove useful as a potential peptide marker for this disorder.

Malignant hypertension. This disease state develops whenever renal damage decreases the flow of blood to the afferent arteriole of the glomerulus. The localized decrease in blood pressure is the stimulus to renin secretion which becomes excessive due to the constancy of the restricted blood flow to the glomerulus. The resulting overproduction of angiotensin II, due to increased renin secretion, causes a chronic hypertension.

Hyporeninemic hypoaldosteronism. As the clinical name implies, this disease state is associated with reduced plasma renin levels. It is not known, however, whether the etiology involves a defect in stimulatory cues to renin secretion or resides at the level of the JG cell itself. Clinical evidence suggests that in some cases the defect involves destructive lesions of the JG cells, most often associated with diabetes mellitus.

Bartter's syndrome. Hyperaldosteronism due to hyperreninism has been associated with hyperplasia of the JG cells in some individuals. This disease is usually associated with increased urinary excretion of E-series prostaglandins. The increased production of these prostaglandins may contribute to several functional abnormalities usually associated with this syndrome. Prostacyclins are directly stimulatory to JG cell renin secretion and may be implicated in JG cell hyperplasia [15, 33, 35].

Disorders Due to Adrenal Enzyme Deficiencies

Genetic defects can lead to inherited inborn errors of metabolism that lead to specific enzymatic deficiencies in the biosynthesis of adrenal steroids. The severity of such a defect depends on whether the block occurs early or late in the steroidogenic biosynthetic pathway.

Congenital adrenal hyperplasia. This rare condition results from a defect in the conversion of cholesterol to pregnenolone. In the absence of cortisol production and negative feedback to the hypothalamus or pituitary there is enhanced secretion of ACTH. Corticotropin stimulates adrenal cortical cells; although cholesterol is taken up, it is not used as substrate for steroid hormone production. This leads to a condition referred to as adrenal lipoidal hyperplasia. This defect in enzyme activity in the initial stage of steroid biosynthesis would also involve a concomitant failure in synthesis of gonadal steroids.

Congenital virilizing adrenal hyperplasia. A defect in 3 β-hydroxysteroid dehydrogenase, 11 β-hydroxylase, or 21 β-hydroxylase leads to virilizing syndromes of differing severity depending on whether the defect is partial or complete. In the absence of 3 β-hydroxysteroid dehydrogenase activity there is impaired formation of both cortisol and aldosterone, thus this defect in steroidogenesis is usually fatal. Because ACTH secretion is elevated and the desmolase system is intact, as is 17 α-hydroxylase activity, the major product formed is dehydroepiandrosterone. Although a weak androgen with minimal masculinizing activity, excessive levels of this androgen are indeed masculinizing.

In the absence of 11 β-hydroxylase activity diminished cortisol secretion leads to excessive ACTH secretion, resulting in adrenal cortical hyperplasia. The subsequent excessive production of cortisol precursors leads to an increased availability of substrates for androgen production (mainly androstenedione), causing excessive virilization in both male and female. There is enhanced deoxycorticosterone production (at the expense of cortisol synthesis), and the excessive secretion of this mineralocorticoid leads to hypertension. Glucocorticoid replacement therapy will correct the abnormal steroid synthesis and secretion by suppressing the excessive pituitary ACTH production.

A defect in 21 β-hydroxylase may be partial or complete. In the female the excessive secretion of androgens may lead to complete masculinization of the external genitalia (Chapter 16). In the salt-losing form of the syndrome there is an almost total lack of 21 β-hydroxylase activity which is essential for mineralocorticoid production. Both mineralocorticoid and glucocorticoid replacement therapies are essential for survival.

Corticosterone methyl oxidase (type II) deficiency. Hypoaldosteronism due to an inborn error in the terminal step of aldosterone biosynthesis has been discovered within related members of a family. These individuals exhibit hyperreninemia and elevated plasma and urinary levels of specific 18-hydroxysteroids. The genetic basis for this disease involves a defect in the function of corticosterone methyl oxidase (type II), the enzyme involved in the oxidation of the hydroxyl group at the C-18 position to the aldehyde [47].

17-hydroxylase deficiency. Deficient activity of 17-hydroxylase results in deficient biosynthesis of cortisol and androgens. The enzymic defect is also in ovarian tissue and, as testosterone is the precursor to estradiol synthesis, estrogen deficiency is also present, resulting in primary amenorrhea and defeminization (breast and genital atrophy), depending on whether the defect is congenital or occurs later in life. With diminished 17-hydroxylase activity adrenal metabolism is shunted toward increased production of aldosterone as well as the production of the precursor mineralocorticoids, 11-deoxycorticosterone, and corticosterone. Absence of glucocorticoid feedback to the brain results in an aggravated production of precursors to mineralocorticoid synthesis (Fig. 15.18). The resulting hypertension can be alleviated by the administration of dexamethasone which feeds back to the hypothalamus, resulting in decreased ACTH secretion.

Adrenal Steroid Hormone Pharmacology

A number of drugs have been produced which are useful in the treatment of overproduction or underproduction of adrenal steroids or their actions. One approach to secondary hyperaldosteronism is to prevent the production of angiotensin II from its precursors by inhibition of converting enzyme activity. Other enzyme inhibitors have been developed to prevent specific enzyme-regulated hydroxylations in the aldosterone biosynthetic pathway. Renin secretion may normally be regulated by a renal prostaglandin; indomethacin, an inhibitor of PG synthesis, has been used successfully in some cases to lower renin secretion and aldosterone production in Bartter's syndrome.

Spironolactone, an aldosterone antagonist, is a competitive inhibitor of aldosterone binding to receptors, primarily those of the distal renal tubule. Spironolac-

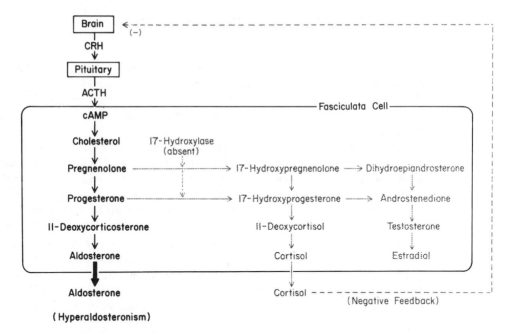

Figure 15.18 Genetic defect in 17 α-hydroxylase activity leading to hyperaldosteronism.

tone is used clinically to suppress the action of excess aldosterone on renal Na⁺ retention.

Metyrapone, an inhibitor of cortisol production, is used to test the capacity of the pituitary to respond to decreased circulating levels of plasma cortisol. Metyrapone is particularly useful in the differential diagnosis of Cushing's syndrome as it will usually enhance ACTH secretion if the disease is of pituitary origin but not if the excess cortisol is due to ectopic production of ACTH.

COMPARATIVE ENDOCRINOLOGY

An adrenal gland is present in all vertebrate species. In most vertebrates a steroidogenic component is intermingled with chromaffin tissue. In some poikilothermic vertebrates the two tissues may be completely separated from each other. In most vertebrates the adrenal tissues are closely adherent to the kidneys and the eponym ad-renal is clearly appropriate. In elasmobranchs the adrenal steroidogenic tissue is confined to a single mass of cells localized between the kidneys and is usually referred to as the *interrenal gland*. In cyclostomes a putative site of adrenal steroidogenic tissue remains undetermined.

Adrenal function in the vertebrates studied is controlled by a hypothalamopituitary-adrenocortical axis. The primary structures of ACTH are known for a number of mammals (Fig. 5.8) but are unavailable for most nonmammalian species. There is evidence from a wide variety of vertebrates (reptiles, amphibians, teleosts) that, as in mammals, ACTH regulates corticosteroid production in adrenal steroidogenic tissue through a mechanism involving cyclic nucleotide formation.

Phylogenetic Relationships Of Vertebrate Steroid Hormones

More than 50 different steroids have been isolated from the adrenal, but only a small number are secreted into the blood and even fewer are known to have significant biological activity. Although steroids are generally classified as glucocorticoids or mineralocorticoids, these functional designations essentially have been derived from studies on mammals.

The distribution of the major steroids produced by the adrenal steroidogenic tissues of vertebrates is known (Table 15.4). From available phylogenetic evidence, aldosterone may be the most recently evolved steroid hormone. In the amphibian aldosterone clearly influences Na^+ metabolism by its actions on the skin and the urinary bladder. A role for aldosterone in fishes is yet to be determined. Cortisol may, however, function in the control of Na^+ exchange across the gills. Thus cortisol or other glucocorticoids may function as a mineralocorticoid in teleosts and possibly other lower vertebrates. The reason a distinct adrenocortical hormone evolved to regulate electrolyte metabolism in tetrapods is unknown. It is likely that the role of aldosterone arose, or was perpetuated, because a dual function for a single hormone would be restrictive, whereas a more distinct separation of roles would be advantageous for the control of specific target tissues [1].

Physiological Roles Of Adrenal Steroids

It would appear that glucocorticoids and mineralocorticoids generally regulate similar physiological processes in most vertebrates. In some species the glucocorticoids may function as mineralocorticoids. Within nonmammalian vertebrates adrenal steroid hormones act on a number of structures unique to each vertebrate group: urinary bladder and skin of toads, gills of fishes, nasal salt glands of birds, and so on. A few examples of the roles of steroids in nonmammalian animals will be discussed.

TABLE 15.4 Major Adrenal Steroids Of Vertebrates

Vertebrate group	Aldosterone	Corticosterone	Cortisol
Mammals[a]	x		x
Aves	x	x	
Reptiles	x	x	
Amphibians	x	x	
Teleosts[b]		x	x
Lung fish[c]	x	x	x
Elasmobranchs[d]		x	
Cyclostomes		x	x

[a]The mouse and the rat produce corticosterone rather than cortisol.

[b]Aldosterone is absent in teleosts, except in very few species.

[c]Large amounts of aldosterone are present in lungfish plasma; these fish are often regarded as "transitional" forms between bony fishes and amphibians.

[d]No 17-hydroxylating enzyme systems are present.

Teleosts. In euryhaline fishes, the temporal interaction of cortisol and PRL may play an important role in migratory behavior. It has been demonstrated that seasonal changes in salinity preference apparently relate to a shift in the phase relationships of the rhythms of cortisol and PRL secretion. Increases in gonadal weights and body fat stores are also affected by the temporal synergistic actions of these two hormones. Thus, it is likely that seasonal changes in reproduction, fat metabolism, and salinity preference may be regulated and coordinated by a common endocrine mechanism [14]. These coordinated responses are necessary for reproductive success.

Birds. Circadian rhythms and temporal interactions of corticosterone and prolactin may regulate seasonal migrations in some birds (e.g., white-throated sparrow) [34]. The phases of corticosterone and PRL rhythms of secretion change seasonally, and this apparently determines the sequential seasonal changes in metabolism and migratory behavior in some birds. Migratory restlessness can be stimulated in these birds by timed daily injections of corticosterone and PRL [32]. Depending on the time PRL is injected, after corticosterone administration, the hormone can induce locomotor restlessness oriented southward or northward. Thus, orientation of migratory behavior is apparently controlled by a temporal synergism of corticosterone and PRL. It has been debated whether seasonal changes in migratory orientation result from seasonal changes in environmental cues or from physiological differences in the birds during the spring and fall migratory periods. Nocturnal cues existent during the vernal and autumnal migratory seasons are apparently used interchangeably by some birds to orient northward or southward. How these cues are employed, however, appears to depend, at least in part, on the temporal relation of the daily rhythms of corticosterone and PRL secretion [32].

A pair of extrarenal secretory nasal glands are situated above the ocular orbit of birds. These glands are usually small and nonfunctional in most terrestrial and freshwater species. In coastal and pelagic species, however, they secrete a highly concentrated solution of electrolytes onto the external surface of the bill [21]. In those species living in both environments the adrenal glands increase in size in response to seawater or hypertonic saline drinking water. The normal secretory response of the nasal glands is dependent on an intact pituitary-adrenal axis. Nasal gland salt secretion is abolished almost completely by adrenalectomy, but administration of glucocorticoids restores nasal gland salt secretion to normal. Normal salt gland secretion in these birds is most likely regulated by corticosterone of adrenal origin. The parasympathetic nervous system probably provides the direct stimulus to nasal salt gland secretion, but corticosterone is necessary for the integrity of the secretory capacity of the glands.

Reptiles. The comparative anatomy and ultrastructure of the reptilian adrenal have been characterized [31] as has the general physiology of the glands [5]. As in birds, salt glands are present in many reptiles. In marine and desert species faced with a limited supply of fresh water and high salt intake the salt glands provide an important means for reducing the total salt load. Adrenal steroids regulate electrolyte balance in reptiles by actions at both renal and extrarenal sites. Aldosterone is clearly salt retaining through its action on the kidneys, whereas corticosterone is hyponatremic by its sodium-excreting action on salt glands. As in birds [34] and fishes

[14] cortisol and prolactin may play important integrated roles in seasonal storage and utilization of fat in some reptiles.

Amphibians.   The structure and function of the adrenal steroidogenic tissue and its hormones in amphibians have been described [19]. Much work on the mechanism of action of aldosterone and related adrenal steroids has been done on the amphibian bladder and skin. It is clear from a number of studies [8, 19] that amphibian adrenal steroids, as in other vertebrates, affect water and electrolyte exchanges [1] and the metabolism of carbohydrates, proteins, and fats.

Adrenal hormones and self-regulation of mammalian populations.   Within natural populations of animals adrenal hormones may play an important role in the control of population density. Within some animal populations mammals establish social hierarchies where there is a dominant animal, a second-ranking animal, and so on to the lowest ranking animal that is subordinate to all others [9]. Adrenocortical morphology and function (corticosterone output) are negatively related to social rank or dominance in these populations. In subordinate animals adrenal hypertrophy is followed by thymic involution, diminished resistance to disease, and many symptoms related to excessive glucocorticoid and sympathoadrenal activity. Increases in population density also enhance the number of encounters between members of a group which can lead to further subordination of the less dominant individuals. Increased mortality follows as well as diminished reproductive capacity. Therefore, the ultimate effect of increased population density is, through the actions of adrenal hormones, to inhibit recruitment of new individuals into the population and thus to maintain the population at a level below that which might exhaust environmental resources [9].

Renin-Angiotensin System

Morphological and biochemical studies indicate that the renin-angiotensin system may have first appeared during the early evolution of the bony fishes [46]. Renin and angiotensins are in the plasma of all vertebrates except cyclostomes and cartilaginous fishes. There are species differences in the primary sequences of the angiotensins, even among some mammals. A number of kinins have even been isolated from wasp venom; within their primary sequences is contained the nonapeptide sequence of bradykinin.

Kallikrein-Kinin Systems

Little information is available regarding the kallikrein-kinin systems in nonmammalian vertebrates. There is no evidence for a plasma kallikrein-kinin system in elasmobranchs, holocephalians, and teleosts [12]. Only traces of the system have been found in amphibians, and among reptiles the system may (turtles) or may not (snakes) be present. Birds and all mammals appear to possess all elements of the system.

REFERENCES

[1] BENTLEY, P. J., and W. N. SCOTT. 1978. The actions of aldosterone. In *General, comparative and clinical endocrinology of the adrenal cortex*, vol. 2, eds. I. Chester Jones and I. W. Henderson, pp. 497–564. New York: Academic Press, Inc.

[2] BLACK, I. B. 1982. Stages of neurotransmitter development in autonomic neurons. *Science* 215:1198–1204.

[3] BROWN, M. S., P. T. KOVANEN, and J. L. GOLDSTEIN. 1979. Receptor-mediated uptake of lipoprotein-cholesterol and its utilization for steroid synthesis in the adrenal cortex. *Rec. Prog. Horm. Res.* 35:215–57. New York: Academic Press, Inc.

[4] ———. 1981. Regulation of plasma cholesterol by lipoprotein receptors. *Science* 212:628–35.

[5] CALLARD, I. P., and G. V. CALLARD. 1978. The adrenal gland in reptilia. In *General, comparative and clinical endocrinology of the adrenal cortex*, vol. 2, eds. I. Chester Jones and I. W. Henderson, pp. 419–94. New York: Academic Press, Inc.

[6] CARBALLEIRA, A., and L. M. FISHMAN. 1980. The adrenal functional unit: a hypothesis. *Perspect. Biol. Med.* 23:573–97.

[7] CHESTER JONES, I. 1957. *The adrenal cortex*. Cambridge, England: Cambridge Univ. Press.

[8] CHESTER JONES, I. 1977. Evolutionary aspects of the adrenal cortex and its homologues. *J. Endocrinol.* 71:3P–32P.

[9] CHRISTIAN, J. J. 1971. Population density and reproductive efficiency. *Biol. Reprod.* 4:248–94.

[10] CONN, J. W. 1955. Primary aldosteronism: a new clinical entity. *J. Lab. Clin. Med.* 45:3–17.

[11] DAVIS, J. O., and R. H. FREEMAN. 1976. Mechanisms regulating renin release. *Physiol. Rev.* 56:1–56.

[12] DUNN, R. S., and A. M. PERKS. 1975. Comparative studies of plasma kinins: the kallikrein-kinin system of poikilotherm and other vertebrates. *Gen. Comp. Endocrinol.* 26:165–78.

[13] EDELMAN, I. S., and D. MARVAR. 1980. Mediating events in the actions of aldosterone. *J. Steroid Biochem.* 12:219–24.

[14] FIVIZZANI, A. J., and A. H. MEIER. 1978. Temporal synergism of cortisol and prolactin influences on salinity preference of Gulf killifish, *Fundulus grandis. Can. J. Zool.* 56:2597–2602.

[15] GILL, J. R. 1980. Bartter's syndrome. *Ann. Rev. Med.* 31:405–19.

[16] GOSS, R. J. 1978. *The physiology of growth*. New York: Academic Press, Inc.

[17] GREEP, R. O., and H. W. DEANE. 1947. Cytochemical evidence for the cessation of hormone production in the zona glomerulosa of the rat's adrenal cortex after prolonged treatment with desoxycorticosterone acetate. *Endocrinology* 40:417–25.

[18] GWYNNE, J. T., and J. F. STRAUSS III. 1982. The role of lipoproteins in steroidogenesis and cholesterol metabolism in steroidogenic glands. *Endocrine Rev.* 3:299–329.

[19] HANKE, W. 1978. The adrenal cortex of amphibia. In *General, comparative and clinical endocrinology of the adrenal cortex*, vol. 2, eds. I. Chester Jones and I. W. Henderson, pp. 419–95. New York: Academic Press, Inc.

[20] HAYASHI, K., G. SALA, K. CATT, and M. L. DUFAU. 1979. Regulation of steroidogenesis by adrenocorticotropic hormone in isolated adrenal cells. *J. Biol. Chem.* 254:6678–83.

[21] HOLMES, W. N., and J. G. PHILLIPS. 1976. The adrenal cortex of birds. In *General, comparative and clinical endocrinology of the adrenal cortex*, vol. 1, eds. I. Chester Jones and I. W. Henderson, pp. 293–420. New York: Academic Press, Inc.

[22] IDELMAN, S. 1978. The structure of the mammalian adrenal cortex. In *General, comparative and clinical endocrinology of the adrenal cortex*, vol. 2, eds. I. Chester Jones and I. W. Henderson, pp. 1–199. New York: Academic Press, Inc.

[23] INAGAMI, T., and K. MURAKAMI. 1980. Prorenin. *Biomed. Mater. Res.* 1:456–75. New York: John Wiley and Sons.

[24] INGLE, D. J. 1954. Permissivity of hormone action, a review. *Acta. Endocrinol.* 17:172–86.

[25] JAMES, V. H. T., ed. 1979. *Adrenal gland.* New York: Raven Press.

[26] JAMES, V. H. T., G. GIUSTI, and L. MARTINI, eds. 1978. *The endocrine function of the human adrenal cortex.* New York: Academic Press, Inc.

[27] JONES, C. T., and M. M. ROEBUCK. 1980. ACTH peptides and the development of the fetal adrenal. *J. Steroid Biochem.* 12:77–82.

[28] JONES, I. C., and I. W. HENDERSON, eds. 1976. *General, comparative and clinical endocrinology of the adrenal cortex*, vol. 1. New York: Academic Press, Inc.

[29] JONES, I. C., and I. W. HENDERSON, eds. 1978. *General, comparative and clinical endocrinology of the adrenal cortex*, vol. 2. New York: Academic Press, Inc.

[30] JONES, M. T. 1979. Control of adrenocortical hormone secretion. In *The adrenal gland*, ed. V. H. T. James, pp. 93–130. New York: Raven Press.

[31] LOFTS, B. 1978. The adrenal gland of reptiles. In *General, comparative and clinical endocrinology of the adrenal cortex*, vol. 2, eds. I. Chester Jones and I. W. Henderson, pp. 419–95. New York: Academic Press, Inc.

[32] MARTIN, D. D., and A. H. MEIER. 1973. Temporal synergism of corticosterone and prolactin in regulating orientation in the migratory white-throated sparrow (*Zonotrichia albicollis*). *Condor* 75:369–74.

[33] McGIFF, J. C. 1981. Prostaglandins, prostacyclin, and thromboxanes. *Ann. Rev. Pharmacol. Toxicol.* 21:479–509.

[34] MEIER, A. H. 1973. Daily hormone rhythms in the white-throated sparrow. *Amer. Scientist* 61:184–87.

[35] NASJLETTI, A., and K. U. MALIK. 1981. The renal kallikrein-kinin and prostaglandin systems interaction. *Ann. Rev. Physiol.* 43:597–609.

[36] PEACH, M. J. 1977. Renin-angiotensin system, biochemistry and mechanisms of action. *Physiol. Rev.* 57:313–70.

[37] PEART, W. S. 1982. Renin-angiotensin system. *Quart. J. Exp. Physiol.* 67:401–406.

[38] PODESTA, E. J., A. MILANI, H. STEFFEN, and R. NEHER. 1979. Adrenocorticotropin (ACTH) induces phosphorylation of a cytoplasmic protein in intact isolated adrenocortical cells. *Proc. Natl. Acad. Sci. USA* 76:5187–91.

[39] REID, I. A., B. J. MORRIS, and W. F. GANONG. 1978. The renin-angiotensin system. *Ann. Rev. Physiol.* 40:377–410.

[40] RHODIN, J. A. G. 1971. The ultrastructure of the adrenal cortex of the rat under normal and experimental conditions. *J. Ultrastruc. Res.* 34:23–71.

[41] SAYERS, G., R. J. BEAL, and S. SEELIG. 1972. Isolated adrenal cells: adrenocorticotropic hormone, calcium, steroidogenesis, and cyclic adenosine monophosphate. *Science* 175:1131–32.

[42] SEALEY, J. E., S. A. ATLAS, and J. H. LARAGH. 1978. Linking the kallikrein and renin systems via activation of inactive renin. *Am. J. Med.* 65:994–1000.

[43] SELYE, H. 1976. *The stress of life.* New York: McGraw-Hill Book Company.

[44] SHIRE, J. G. M. 1976. Degeneration of the adrenal X-zone in Tfm mice with inherited insensitivity to androgens. *J. Endocrinol.* 71:445–46.

[45] SIMPSON, H. W. 1976. A new perspective: chronobiochemistry. *Essays Med. Biochem.* 7:115–87.

[46] SOKABE, H., T. NAKAJIMA, M. OGAWA, and T. Y. WATANABE. 1980. Evolution of the renin-angiotensin mechanism. In *Endocrinology, 1980,* eds. I. A. Cumming, J. W. Funder, and F. A. O. Mendelsohn, pp. 166–69. New York: Elsevier North-Holland, Inc.

[47] VELDHUIS, J. D., H. E. KULIN, R. J. SANTEN, T. E. WILSON, and J. C. MELBY. 1980. Inborn error in the terminal step of aldosterone biosynthesis. *New Engl. J. Med.* 303:117–21.

[48] VESELY, D. L. 1980. On the mechanism of action of adrenocortical steroids: cortisol and aldosterone enhance guanylate cyclase activity. *J. Pharmacol. Exp. Therap.* 214:561–66.

[49] VINSON, G. P., and C. J. KENYON. 1978. Steroidogenesis in the zones of the mammalian adrenal cortex. In *General, comparative and clinical endocrinology of the adrenal cortex,* vol. 2, eds. I. Chester Jones and I. W. Henderson, pp. 201-64. New York: Academic Press, Inc.

16

Endocrinology of Sex Differentiation and Development

INTRODUCTION

No other component of the vertebrate endocrine system is as complex as the reproductive system. Although the *genetic sex* of an individual is determined by the chromosomal complement of the fertilized egg, the direction in which the gonads differentiate to produce either ovaries or testes depends on hormones secreted by the gonads. The *gonadal sex* then regulates the *phenotypic sex*. Even the development of the brain into a male or female type is dependent on early exposure to gonadal steroid hormones. The brain, in turn, affects the temporal characteristics of pituitary gonadotropin secretions which regulate further development of the gonads into functional organs capable of producing mature gametes. In addition adult behavior is dependent on both early and late effects of gonadal steroids on the brain (Fig. 16.1).

Compared to the human female, the human adult male might be considered to possess a rather uncomplicated reproductive system. After puberty the male reproductive system is rather invariant in its structural and functional characteristics. The female, on the other hand, is cyclic in her hormonal output and gonadal function. The female may also become pregnant, which entails radical changes in the reproductive organs to provide an environment for fetal growth and development. Unique female hormones are involved in the maintenance of pregnancy and parturition, and additional special hormones are required for milk synthesis

378

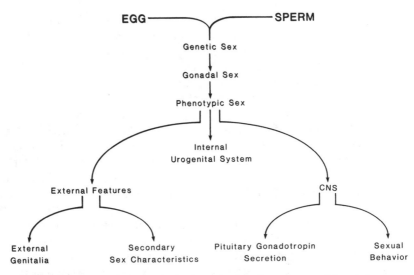

EGG ——————— SPERM

Genetic Sex

Gonadal Sex

Phenotypic Sex

Internal
Urogenital System

External Features   CNS

External   Secondary   Pituitary Gonadotropin   Sexual
Genitalia   Sex Characteristics   Secretion   Behavior

Figure 16.1 Sequential events in the determination of genetic, gonadal, and pheno-typic sex.

and secretion. These sexually dimorphic female functions are regulated by a variety of hormones acting in concert or sequentially.

SEX DETERMINATION, DIFFERENTIATION, AND DEVELOPMENT

Genetic sex, established at the time of conception, governs the development of the gonadal sex of the individual [8]. Gonadal sex, in turn, regulates the development of phenotypic sex, that is, the differentiation of internal and external sex organs as well as attainment of adult secondary sexual characteristics [17, 33].

Chromosomal (Genetic) Basis of Sex Determination

The genetic sex of an individual is realized at the moment of fertilization of the egg by a sperm. The genes specifically related to the determination of sex are grouped together on particular chromosomes. Initially, all cells of the human body contain 22 pairs of somatic chromosomes (*autosomes*) plus a pair of *sex chromosomes*. The female possesses a pair of X chromosomes (homogametic sex), whereas the cells of the male contain an X and a Y chromosome (heterogametic sex). During gameto-genesis the diploid number (46) of chromosomes is reduced through meiotic division to the haploid number (23). The female can normally only contribute an X chromosome, whereas the male may contribute either an X or a Y chromosome. The fertilized egg, the zygote, will normally develop in a female or male direction depending on whether a pair of XX or XY chromosomes are present, respectively.

The Y chromosome in the mammal appears to be mainly responsible for sex differentiation as any embryo without a Y chromosome develops as a female. Even humans with as many as four X chromosomes and a single Y chromosome develop into males. Random union of the male gamete with the egg ensures that approximately half the progeny will be females and half will be males. The possible differential survival or other attributes of the X- and Y-bearing sperms may thwart the theoretical sex ratio.

The majority of vertebrates have a sex-determining scheme (XX/XY) of male heterogamety or a ZW/ZZ scheme of female heterogamety. In birds and reptiles the W chromosome of the heterogametic female (ZW) induces differentiation of the ovary. In fishes and amphibians the male or female of certain species may be heterogametic. Some species of fishes are even *synchronous* or *asynchronous hermaphrodites*, that is, they are able to shed both eggs and sperm at the same time or, alternately, one or the other of the gametes during a particular developmental state. In reptiles all-female parthenogenic (egg development in the absence of activation by a sperm) or gynogenic (activation of the egg by a sperm without any genetic material being contributed) species have been discovered. Although the genetic sex of the species determines the direction in which the gonads initially differentiate, the exogenous administration of sex steroids at a critical time (which differs between species) can induce permanent gonadal sex reversal. Although interesting, the possible relevance, if any, of these experimentally induced observations to normal sex differentiation is unclear.

Gonadal Sex

The undifferentiated gonad has generally been considered to be composed of cortical and medullary regions. In the male sex differentiation of the gonads involves differentiation of the medullary primordium and suppression of the cortex. In the female, on the other hand, the cortical region develops, whereas medullary differentiation is suppressed. The directions of these two anatomical components were for years theorized to be controlled by hypothetical corticomedullary inductive substances the production of which was related to whether an XX or XY chromosomal complement was present. It is now proposed that the undifferentiated primordium normally tends to develop toward the female in the mammal unless influenced by genes located on the Y chromosome [26]. Mammalian testicular organogenesis is dependent on an *H-Y antigen*, a protein produced by cells containing XY chromosomes [26, 35, 36]. This inducer substance is released early in embryonic development and causes differentiation of the somatic elements of the primordial gonads. In the absence of this H-Y antigen the mammalian gonads will differentiate to form ovaries. The H-Y antigen can be considered as a protein hormone which is ubiquitous in its production by cells of the early embryo. The H-Y receptor sites, on the other hand, are confined to the gonadal cells of both sexes. Although the expression of the H-Y receptor is common to both the testes and the ovary, this is of no consequence as production of the H-Y antigen is male specific. Thus, although the H-Y receptor is present in the prospective female gonad, the H-Y antigen is not available for receptor occupancy. That such receptors are present in the female gonad is demonstrated by the observation that addition of H-Y antigen to an organ culture of the bovine embryonic (indifferent) gonad causes precocious testicular conversion of these gonads. If, on the other hand, the H-Y antigen is removed (lysostripped) from the membranes of dispersed cells of the neonatal testis, the cells organize into ovarianlike cells in culture [27].

Normal testicular differentiation is invariably associated with the presence of the H-Y antigen. The testes differentiate under the influence of the Y chromosome during the seventh week of gestation in the human, whereas ovarian development usually does not proceed before 13 to 16 weeks [38]. Two X chromosomes appear to be essential for the development of normal ovaries as individuals with a single X chromosome develop gonads which are only partially differentiated. It is not yet clear where the chromosomal locus of the H-Y gene is located. It has been argued that certain X-linked genes are regulatory and control the expression of H-Y antigen production by a structural gene located on the Y chromosome. It has also been suggested that H-Y structural genes may be X-linked or even autosomal [13]. Thus, the primary sex of mammals is believed determined not so much by the presence or the absence of the Y chromosome, but by the expression or nonexpression of H-Y antigen [27] (Fig. 16.2). There are, for example, H-Y antigen positive XX males (human, mouse, dog, goat). In contrast, in some rodent species failure to express H-Y antigen results in fertile XY females.

In 1916 Lillie, who had long reflected on the problem of sex differentiation, provided the theory of the *freemartin* [19]. A freemartin is a term used by cattle breeders to characterize a barren (sterile) female born cotwin to a normal bull calf. Lillie noted that in cattle a twin pregnancy is almost always the result of fertilization of an ovum from each ovary. Although development begins separately in each horn of the uterus, the elongating fetal membranes fuse and blood vessels from each side may anastomose so that a constant interchange of blood takes place between the two fetuses. No harm results if both animals are females or males. But if one is a male and one a female, then, as Lillie noted, the reproductive system of the female is largely suppressed and certain male organs may actually develop in the female. According to Lillie's hormonal theory, the transformation of the freemartin gonad was mediated by circulating hormones of the bull twin. However, androgens do not

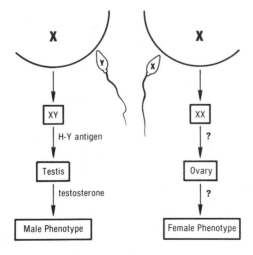

Figure 16.2 Role of the H-Y antigen in the determination of gonadal sex. (Reprinted with permission from The American College of Obstetricians and Gynecologists. *Obstetrics and Gynecology*, 54:671–685, 1979; from Wachtel [36].)

alter the development of the fetal ovary when injected into a pregnant cow; hormone-mediated sex reversal has not been demonstrated in any eutherian (placental) mammals. Thus, an endocrine basis for the theory of the freemartin remained unresolved for many years. Experimental evidence now suggests that ovarian masculinization is due to H-Y antigen produced and disseminated in the blood by the male during early fetal development.

A basic dogma is that the homogametic sex is the neutral state in which maleness (in mammals) and femaleness (in birds) is superimposed by the hormonal secretions of the heterogametic gonad [33]. The H-Y antigen has been detected in a number of species of vertebrates including, besides mammals, amphibians and birds. Because the H-Y antigen is a marker for the sex-determining gene [35, 36], the gene would code for a testis where the male is the heterogametic sex as in mammals. In birds and some amphibians where the female is the heterogametic sex the H-Y antigen directs the differentiation of the gonad into an ovary.

Whether the male or the female is the heterogametic sex has an important bearing on the role of hormones in gonadal and phenotypic development. In those species which bear young outside their body (e.g., egg layers) the heterogametic sex may be either male or female. Most mammals, on the other hand, grow and develop in a maternal environment characterized by elevated levels of estrogens. It is likely, therefore, that to protect the genetic male from the influence of estrogens, evolution favored development of the female as the neutral sex. Rather than devising a mechanism of protecting the male from the feminine influence, differentiation toward the male gonadal and body phenotype requires the inductive actions of gonadal androgens. All aspects of female development, ovarian as well as internal genital ducts and external genitalia, are essentially an automatic process apparently requiring no hormonally active inductive substances. It has been said that the male mammal is "merely a female which has been subjected to induction by testosterone" [29].

The presumptive gonadal primordia are composed of coelomic epithelia, underlying mesenchyme, and primordial germ cells. The gonadal anlagen are visible in the 4-week-old human embryo as a pair of genital ridges. The primordial germ cells, the gonocytes, arise in the yolk sac endoderm, move to the mesoderm of the gut, and seed the undifferentiated gonads by migration from the hindgut. The course of migration of the gonocytes may be oriented by some chemotactic substance elaborated by the gonadal anlagen. During the migration of the primordial germ cells, the coelomic epithelium invades to varying degrees the underlying mesenchyme of the presumptive gonads to form the primary sex cords. At this stage the gonads are *indifferent*, or *bipotential*, in that, depending on the genetic sex of the individual, the gonads will develop into either testes or ovaries. An early sign of sexual differentiation is seen in the distribution pattern of the primordial germ cells. The germ cells of XX embryos remain in the periphery away from the central somatic blastema of the gonad, whereas the germ cells of the XY embryo invade the center of the blastema. Thus, not only are germ cells attracted to the primordial gonads but also to the cortical or medullary regions depending on whether they are of XX or XY genotype, respectively. Whether these primordial germ cells subsequently undergo spermatogenesis or oogenesis depends on early organizational influences of the H-Y antigen on gonadal differentiation into either a testis or an ovary. In some nonmammalian vertebrates, although the germ cells normally become spermatocytes or oocytes, *sex reversal* is easily accomplished by early administration of steroids. For example, in the goldfish presumptive male (XY) embryos can be transformed into phenotypic females by estrogens; they can be subsequently mated to normal males (XY) to produce viable male (YY) offspring [39]. In the medaka (*Oryzias latipes*) in which the presumptive female fish (XX) was converted to a phenotypic male by an androgen, subsequent mating with a normal female (XX) resulted in all-female (XX) progeny.

The primitive gonads of the male and female embryos, which appear morphologically identical, are composed of three components: the primordial germ cells, the mesenchyme of the genital ridge, and a covering layer of epithelium. In the male the primitive sex cords, which are initially solid, develop into the seminiferous tubules (Fig. 16.3). These ducts subsequently branch and their terminal endings anastomose to form the rete testis, which transports sperm to the epididymus. The seminiferous tubules are lined with epithelial cells which differentiate into *Sertoli cells;* the gonocytes become embedded within these sustentacular cells of Sertoli. The *interstitial cells of Leydig* arise from intertubular elements of the seminiferous tubules; these cells are the source of androgen necessary for development of the accessory sexual organs (e.g., prostate gland), but they disappear shortly after birth and do not become abundant until the onset of adolescence. The developing seminiferous tubules become separated by a connective tissue layer, the tunica

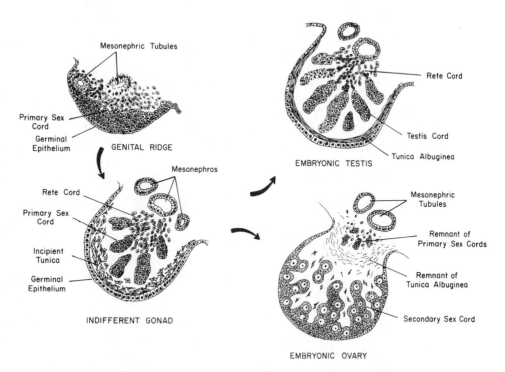

Figure 16.3 Diagrammatic representation of the development of the mammalian ovary and testis from a bipotential primordial gonad. (Prepared by Dr. R. B. Chiasson, University of Arizona.)

Sex Determination, Differentiation, and Development

albuginea, from the remnant of the coelomic epithelium which atrophies into the so-called tunica vaginalis.

In the primitive ovary the coelomic epithelium undergoes proliferation, and strands of epithelial cells, the primary sex cords, move into the interior of the gonad to form a rete ovarii which subsequently degenerates and disappears. Later in fetal development secondary sex cords extend into the underlying mesenchyme (Fig. 16.3). The primordial germ cells are carried along within the proliferating inward migration of the secondary sex (cortical) cords. Some germ cells within the sex cords become isolated and form primordial follicles at about 16 weeks of gestation in the human female.

Differentiation of the Genital Ducts

The definitive internal reproductive organs consist of tubular passageways for the exit of gametes produced by the gonads. Glands associated with these structures may contribute various secretions that aid in the dissemination and function of the gametes. During the undifferentiated stage, both Müllerian and Wolffian ducts are present. Development of the female or male accessory sex organs involves differentiation of the Müllerian or Wolffian ducts, respectively, with the concomitant loss of the other. Differentiation of the Müllerian ducts results in formation of the Fallopian tubes with associated uterus and vagina. Differentiation of the Wolffian ducts, on the other hand, results in the development of the epididymus, ductus deferens, and seminal vesicles.

In the absence of the ovaries or testes, the Müllerian duct system develops and Wolffian ducts atrophy, suggesting that these events are not dependent on any gonadal directive. Atrophy of the Wolffian ducts in the female may represent *programmed cell death*, a common phenomenon of developmental processes. In the male fetus, on the other hand, the testes apparently produce a *Müllerian regression factor* (MRF), which is a glycoprotein (about 70,000 MW). MRF acts to induce Müllerian duct atrophy [16]. Maintenance and further development of the Wolffian ducts, however, is dependent on the presence of testicular androgen (and possibly, to some minor extent, MRF). MRF is believed to be secreted by the Sertoli cells of the fetal testes. It exerts a local effect rather than a systemic one, as unilateral castration in the fetal male rat and rabbit results in female duct development on the side where the testis was removed, and the contralateral duct develops along male lines.

Occasionally male infants are born with morphologically normal testes but an apparent inability to synthesize androgenic steroids. In these individuals the Müllerian ducts still atrophy, suggesting that MRF is nevertheless still present and not an androgen. In the *persistent Müllerian duct syndrome* genetic and phenotypic males have Fallopian tubes and a uterus together with male Wolffian duct structures. The underlying defect may be a failure to produce MRF or an inability of the tissue to respond to the hormone. The effects of the presence or absence of testosterone and MRF on development of the male and female urogenital tracts are shown schematically (Fig. 16.4A).

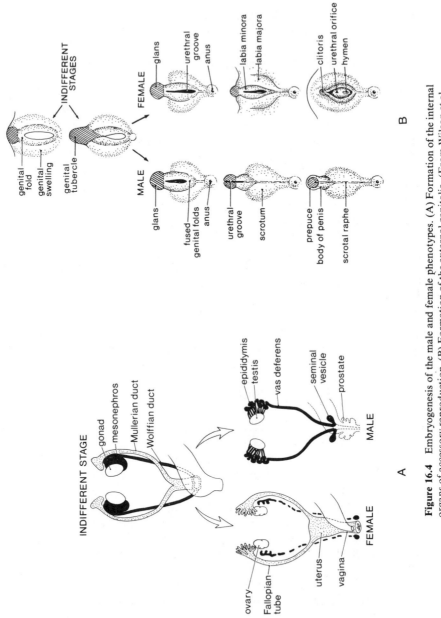

Figure 16.4 Embryogenesis of the male and female phenotypes. (A) Formation of the internal organs of accessory reproduction. (B) Formation of the external genitalia. (From Wilson et al., [32], "The Hormonal Control of Sexual Development", *Science*, vol. 211, pp. 1278–1284, Fig. 2, March 20, 1981. © 1981 by The American Association for the Advancement of Science.)

Sex Determination, Differentiation, and Development

385

Differentiation of the External Genitalia

As with the ovary and internal urogenital ducts, the external genitalia develop a female phenotype in the absence of the Y chromosome. Differentiation of the male external genitalia is dependent solely on androgen production by the testes. Development of the penis and scrotum commences shortly after onset of Wolffian duct development. The genital folds elongate and fuse to form the penis and male urethra. The urogenital swellings on each side of the urethral orifice form a bilobed scrotum into which the testes descend (Fig. 16.4B). In the female embryo the genital tubercle becomes the clitoris and the adjacent genital swellings give rise to the labia majora; the genital folds become the labia minora (Fig. 16.4B). Removal of the gonads from indifferent embryos of either sex results in development of a female genotype, demonstrating that the male is the induced phenotype [1, 27].

Of critical importance in development of the external genitalia is the timing of androgen action. In the female fetus, for example, the external genitalia may become masculinized if androgen levels are elevated as in *congenital adrenal hyperplasia*. Androgens originating from the maternal circulation can also cause genital masculinization in the female fetus; except for clitoral hypertrophy, androgen excess at a later time (eleventh to twelfth week) is without effect.

GONADAL STEROID HORMONE SYNTHESIS AND CHEMISTRY

Gonadal steroids are produced by mesodermally derived tissues of the testes and ovaries. The same demolase system as found in the adrenal is responsible for this first biosynthetic step in steroidogenesis. The nature of the stimulus that activates testosterone biosynthesis in the fetal testis is unknown. There is experimental evidence that testes or ovaries of rabbit embryos synthesize testosterone or estradiol, respectively, in media devoid of hormones. It appears, therefore, that differentiation of gonads as endocrine organs is controlled by factors intrinsic to the gonads themselves [38]. It is also possible that during early development the need for gonadotropins, which in the adult normally control conversion of cholesterol to pregnenolone, is circumvented by the presence of C-21 steroids of placental origin.

Unlike the adrenal, 17 α-hydroxylase activity is dominant and, through conversion of pregnenolone to 17-hydroxypregnenolone and 17 α-hydroxyprogesterone, provides substrates for androgen biosynthesis. In the testes testosterone is the major androgen secreted (Fig. 16.5). In the ovary androstenedione and testosterone serve as precursors for estrogen formation. Estradiol is the major estrogen produced by the ovaries. The key reaction in the ovary is *aromatization* of the A ring of the steroid nucleus. The first step in this reaction involves the hydroxylation of the C-19 carbon followed by removal of the newly formed hydroxymethyl group from the steroid nucleus. The A ring is then aromatized to yield a phenolic hydroxyl group at the C-3 position (Fig. 16.5).

In some tissues testosterone is converted by 5 α-reductase activity to dihydrotestosterone (DHT) (Fig. 16.6). The rudiments of the external genitalia and pros-

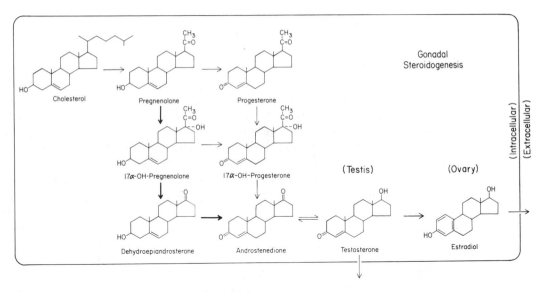

Figure 16.5 Biosynthesis of gonadal steroid hormones in the vertebrate testes and ovaries.

tate (the urogenital tubercle and sinus) convert testosterone to DHT which is then responsible for the development of these organs. The importance of DHT formation in certain tissues for normal virilization is revealed in rare anomalies of male development which are due to the absence of 5 α-reductase activity [14, 15].

Although the ovary differentiates much later than the testes, the enzymatic machinery for estrogen synthesis is developed at the same time as the processes for androgen biosynthesis in the testes. It is unclear whether ovarian estrogen synthesis is important in the development of the female fetus. Possibly estrogens synthesized by the ovary play a role, as testosterone in the testes, in the maturation of the ovaries.

Androgens, like other steroid hormones, are known to act by stimulating protein synthesis within their target tissues. After an initial uptake by a cell, the steroid interacts with a cytosolic protein receptor. The hormone protein complex then migrates to the nucleus where it interacts with specific binding sites on the chromosomes. Derepression of a segment of the genome results and leads to messenger RNA synthesis and the subsequent translation of the mRNA message into de novo protein synthesis. In the DHT-dependent cell testosterone is first converted to the DHT metabolite in the cytosol, which then combines with a specific receptor apparently not identical to the testosterone receptor.

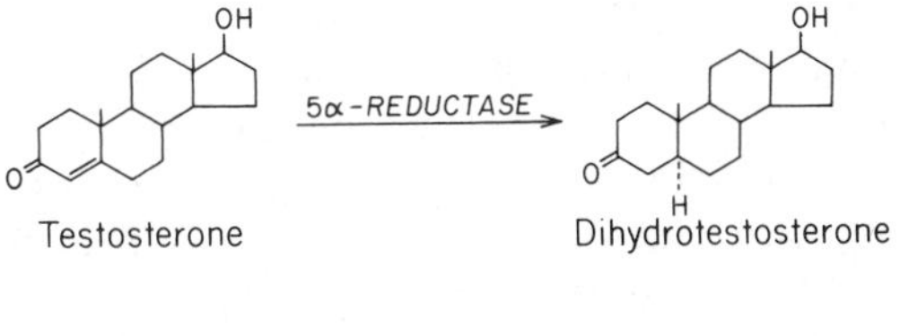

Figure 16.6 Cellular conversion of testosterone to dihydrotestosterone.

GONADAL STEROIDS AND BRAIN DIFFERENTIATION

In adult male mammals there is a tonic (generally uniform) secretion of pituitary gonadotropins, whereas in adult female mammals secretion of these pituitary hormones is cyclic in nature; that is, the amount of gonadotropins released usually follows a recurrent pattern characteristic of the species. Cyclic *estrous* behavior, the ovarian cycle of ovum maturation and ovulation, as well as the cyclic growth of the uterus, are phenomena dependent on the cyclicity of pituitary gonadotropin secretion (Chapter 18). Questions arise as to the mechanisms controlling such cyclic or noncyclic reproductive events in mammals. Experiments have established that transplantation of the pituitary from a male or female rat to the opposite sex did not alter the normal reproductive processes in either sex. These observations revealed that the pituitaries were equivalent and could not be responsible for the cyclicity or noncyclicity of pituitary gonadotropin secretion. In contrast to the tonic uniform secretion of pituitary gonadotropins in the intact adult male rat, these hormones are released cyclically (as in the female) in adult neonatally-castrated male rats. Transplantation of an ovary into adult rats of either sex that had been neonatally castrated did not alter the function of the ovary whether or not it was transplanted into the inappropriate sex. In other words in the adult (neonatally-castrated) male rat the ovaries cycled (ovulated) normally as in the female. Transplantation of ovaries into male rats castrated as adults produced different results. Ovaries transplanted into these rats failed to cycle. These results suggested that the control of pituitary hormone secretion and subsequent gonadal function depended upon a system that was programmed early in development and was not localized to the pituitary or gonads.

It was subsequently discovered that a single injection of testosterone into a female rat during a *critical period* (a few days postnatally) resulted in adults that were acyclic. In addition these females exhibited male sexual behavior (mounting of other females). These results were consistent with earlier observations that transplanted ovaries only became functional if the transplant were into a neonatally castrated male rat rather than an intact adult male rat. Apparently testosterone secreted by the neonatal testes of the male conditioned the animals so that pituitary gonadotropin secretion in the adult animal was tonic rather than cyclic. Similar results were obtained by implantations of testosterone into the hypothalamus (but not other sites), suggesting that the locus of testosterone action was at the level of the hypothalamus, a postulate compatible with the emerging evidence that pituitary hormone secretion is regulated by the brain, particularly the hypothalamus.

Organizational Roles

The studies just discussed suggest that deprivation of testosterone in the male animal during his species-specific critical time of brain differentiation will result in a female pattern of sex-dimorphic behavior. Such male animals will asume the female mating posture when administered estrogen but will not mount females even when injected with testosterone. From these studies of androgen effects on the neonatal rodent emerged the hypothesis that testosterone was not only responsible for differentiation of the internal and external genitalia but was of critical importance for normal differentiation of the brain into the male type (Fig. 16.7). Maximal sensitivity of the hypothalamus to testosterone may be associated with a particular stage of neuronal maturation [20]. Thyroid hormones are known to affect maturation of the CNS and an altered thyroid hormone status such as hyperthyroidism or hypothyroidism shortens or prolongs, respectively, the postnatal period during which the rat brain centers controlling gonadotropin secretion can be differentiated by testosterone. In species that are relatively less mature at birth (many rodents, pigeons) the critical period extends into postnatal life, whereas in animals more fully developed at birth the critical period may be predominantly prenatal.

One observation was particularly difficult to reconcile with this hypothesis: Estradiol also masculinized the brain of either the male or female rodent. This dilemma was solved when it was discovered that testosterone is aromatized to estradiol within the brain. Several experimental lines of evidence support the hypothesis of androgen-to-estrogen conversion: (1) The effects of testosterone treatment in neonatal female rats is blocked by prior administration of specific estrogen (but not androgen) receptor antagonists; (2) the brain possesses the aromatase enzymes required for conversion of testosterone to estradiol; (3) dihydrotestosterone does not mimic the effect of testosterone on neonatal brain differentiation, thus revealing that the actions of testosterone are not mediated through its conversion to DHT; in addition, DHT cannot be converted to estradiol; (4) [^{3}H]-labeled testosterone is recovered from the brain mainly as [^{3}H]-labeled estradiol; (5) aromatase inhibitors impair brain differentiation in response to perinatal testosterone administration; (6) in the Tfm (testicular feminization mutation) mouse, which has greatly reduced levels of androgen receptors, testosterone causes brain differentiation as it does in normal mice. Thus, it appears that in addition to its hormonal role on a number of target tissues testosterone serves as a prohormone for dihydrotestosterone biosynthesis in some tissues and for estradiol production within the brain (Fig. 16.8) [1]. If estradiol is indeed responsible for brain differentiation in the male, why is not the brain of the female also masculinized as estradiol is the major gonadal steroid of the fe-

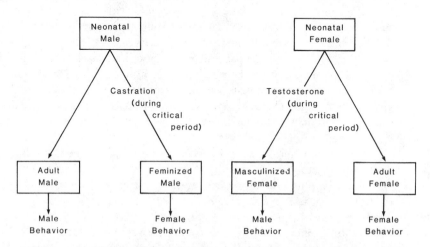

Figure 16.7 Effects of castration and testosterone administration in the neonatal rat on subsequent adult male and female behavior [21].

Gonadal Steroids and Brain Differentiation

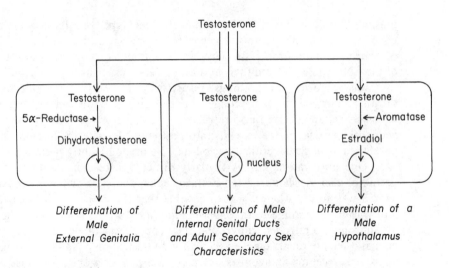

Figure 16.8 Testosterone: prohormone for dihydrotestosterone and estradiol in certain target tissues.

male? First, estradiol production by the fetal ovaries may be minimal. Second, a circulating α-fetoprotein (fetoneonatal estrogen-binding protein, FEBP) is present in high levels within the blood of the fetus and apparently has a specific binding affinity for estradiol. Theoretically, therefore, no estradiol is available to reach the brain of the female fetus. The *FEBP protection hypothesis* is supported by the observation that administration of antibodies to the protein produces effects similar to estradiol injections [20]. Synthetic estrogens that exhibit little binding affinity for FEBP also effectively masculinize the fetal brain.

Although estradiol is available in the male at a critical time in development to regulate the differentiation of the brain, the mechanisms by which estradiol is able to alter irreversibly the brain and subsequent sexual behavior are unclear. Although the brains of males and females differ physiologically, do they also differ anatomically? It has been discovered that in the rodent there are sex-related differences in the distribution of synaptic connections of nerve cells of the preoptic area (POA) of the brain [9]. The female pattern of synaptic contacts is established if males are castrated before the critical period of fetal development. On the other hand, the male pattern of synaptic distribution is established if newborn female animals are given testosterone. The *sexually dimorphic nucleus* of the preoptic area of the rat is actually visible with the naked eye, being at least five times larger in the male than in the female.

The cellular mechanisms by which estradiol affects neonatal brain maturation appear similar to those controlling steroid hormone effects on other tissues. Nuclear chromatin binding and subsequent transcriptional and translational events leading to protein synthesis are involved (Fig. 18.6). The ultimate effects of estradiol may involve neuronal growth and neurotransmitter synthesis. Using an in vitro system it was shown that estradiol and testosterone (but not dihydrotestosterone) enhanced neurite outgrowth from explants of newborn mouse preoptic tissue [34]. These steroid hormone effects are anatomically specific as other brain regions do not respond similarly.

Activational Roles

The permanent actions of gonadal steroid hormones on differentiation and development of the brain led to the proposal that gonadal steroids can have two types of action, depending on the developmental state of the CNS, either organizational or activational. The *organizational effects* of steroids refer to the actual maturation processes leading to development of the dimorphic nuclear center of the POA and possibly other nuclear centers of the brain. The *activational effects* of steroid hormones refer to the actions on acute release of pituitary gonadotropins and to sexual behaviors associated with reproductive processes. In contrast to the organizational effects of gonadal steroids on brain differentiation and function, the activational effects of hormones are reversible, repeatable, and not limited to a critical phase of development. In adult animals steroid hormones released by the gonads play important roles in regulating behavioral events that relate to reproductive success. Gonadal steroid hormones in the fetus, as discussed, affect the organization of the brain into a sexually dimorphic adult organ; the mechanisms by which the activational effects of steroid hormones are expressed shall now be considered.

Control of pituitary gonadotropin secretion. There is evidence, particularly from studies in the female rat, that the preoptic area (POA) of the brain may be an important site of gonadal steroid hormone action related to the cyclic release of pituitary gonadotropins. Estradiol receptors are abundant in this specific area of the brain [20, 21]. It is believed that during the estrous cycle of the female rat, for example, estradiol and progesterone (in a critical ratio) activate the POA which in turn stimulates the arcuate-ventromedial nuclear area of the hypothalamus. This stimulation results (possibly in combination with exteroceptive stimuli in some species) in a surge of gonadotropin releasing hormone (GnRH) secretion which is responsible for the midcycle surge of pituitary gonadotropin (LH) secretion which is then responsible for ovulation. In this model steroid hormones would interact with neuron bodies in the POA, which in turn would result in activation of neural pathways leading to the ventromedial hypothalamus where GnRH neurons would be stimulated to secrete GnRH into the hypophysial portal system to activate pituitary gonadotropin secretion. In the male rat the development of the sexually dimorphic nuclei of the POA results in a tonic stimulation of hypothalamic GnRH secretion.

Testosterone and behavior in the human male. Although aggressive behavior is a characteristic of violent individuals, it is not consistently related to increased plasma testosterone levels [32]. Individuals with chronic low levels of testosterone, due to genetic abnormalities in steroid biosynthesis especially if occurring before puberty, exhibit reduced aggression and diminished sexual drive. Exogenously administered testosterone is often effective in restoring sexual interest and overt sexual behavior.

Some synthetic progestins have androgenic activity. In recent decades millions of pregnant women have been treated for threatened abortion with progestins and estrogens. It has been discovered that individuals exposed during gestation to synthetic progestins show a significantly higher potential for physical aggression than their sex-matched unexposed siblings [31]. It would appear that the mechanisms controlling hormone-organized behaviors as reported in laboratory animals may also apply to human behavior.

Mood and the menstrual cycle. Changes in feelings and behavior can be characteristics of the menstrual cycle and are undoubtedly related to changing hormonal levels. Nevertheless, no clear correlation has been documented between gonadal steroid levels and the so-called premenstrual tension syndrome or other menstrual cycle-related behaviors [31].

Gonadal steroids and gender identification. Psychologists in general have argued that although sexual behavior is influenced by hormones, sexual identity is socially determined. In other words a child will identify with whatever sex he or she is brought up to be as a child. However, pubertal shifts from female to male gender identity in an interrelated group of male pseudohermaphrodites from two rural communities in the Dominican Republic have been described [15]. Feminization of the external genitalia in these males results from a defect or absence of 5 α-reductase activity. Although these individuals were brought up initially as girls, they took on male sexual identities at puberty. It was postulated on the basis of these observations that their prenatal exposure to testosterone irreversibly shaped their sexual behavior. According to these investigators, this "experiment of nature" emphasizes the importance of androgens in an organizational as well as activational role (at puberty) in the evolution of male-gender identity [15]. This interpretation has raised the argument of "nature versus nurture" relative to the basis of gender identification in humans. From other studies there is evidence that in male pseudohermaphrodites reared unambiguously as females their postpubertal gender remained consistent with their sex upbringing [5, 32].

Activational roles of gonadal steroids in nonmammalian vertebrates. Castration eliminates sex behavior in the frog, *Xenopus laevis*; clasping behavior is restored by administration of exogenous testosterone, but not by estradiol. Three distinct populations of gonadal hormone concentrating cells are present in the brain of *Xenopus*: "testosterone only" cells, "estradiol only" cells, and cells labeled after administration of either hormone. These latter cells may represent cells where testosterone is converted to estradiol [18]. The regions of hormone uptake are also known to be involved in the neural control of frog sex behavior. Sex behavior in some frogs may therefore depend on testosterone production by the testes and subsequent interaction with one or more nuclear centers within the brain where the hormone may act directly or be converted to estradiol. Seasonal initiation of sex behavior would necessitate pituitary gonadotropin secretion to initiate androgen production by the testes.

In birds the homogametic sex is male, and differentiation of the female CNS phenotype occurs as a result of exposure to ovarian hormones. Estradiol appears to be the ovarian product responsible for feminine differentiation. For example, embryonic exposure to an antiestrogen masculinizes behavior in female quail; these birds exhibit the male mating pattern as adults in response to testosterone. Androgens play an important role in the control of song in male birds. Castration abolishes song in some birds; singing can be restored by exogenous testosterone administration. There are specialized brain areas concerned with the production of sound in some birds. In the zebra finch all the brain nuclei of the song system are much larger in males than females. Early exposure of the chick to estradiol or dihydrotestosterone influences the establishment of the differences in functional capacity and brain architecture in the zebra finch [12]. When a neonatal female zebra finch is exposed to estradiol, her system is subsequently masculinized. Testosterone or dihydrotestosterone can then induce such a female to sing when an adult. These observations suggest that the female zebra finch is the neutral sex with respect to sexual differentiation of the song system [12].

Singing is also a typical behavioral characteristic of the male canary. Ovariectomized adult canaries can be induced to sing by administration of testosterone. Some brain nuclei which comprise the efferent pathway for control of song in the canary have been shown to concentrate tritiated androgen. The nucleus robustus archistriatalis (RA) of the forebrain is highly dimorphic in the adult canary, the overall volume being much greater in the male bird. Microscopically, injections of testosterone into ovariectomized female canaries increase the volume of the RA as well as the length of the dendrites of this nucleus to a state resembling that of the male canary. Although steroid hormones are normally responsible for an organizational effect on the neonatal brain, results reveal that steroid hormones can induce plasticity in the adult brain [4].

In the male canary two telencephalic nuclei that control song are much larger in the spring when the birds sing than in the fall after several songless months [24]. Such fluctuations may reflect an increase and then a reduction in the numbers of synapses within the brain and may be related to the yearly ability to acquire new motor coordination. According to this hypothesis, "The plastic substrate for vocal learning is renewed once yearly, a growing, then a shedding of synapses, much the way trees grow leaves in the spring and shed them in the fall" [24]. This species of bird truly has "a brain for all seasons" [24].

The distribution of gonadal steroid hormone receptors in the brains of members of all vertebrate classes has been determined [22]. Basically, estrophilic neurons are localized predominantly to the medial preoptic area, the tuberal hypothalamus, and in specific limbic areas of the brain. The distribution of androgen receptors is similar, but not identical between species. Generally, the neural distribution of gonadal steroid receptors, although characteristic of the species, is independent of genetic or phenotypic sex [22]. In the zebra finch (*Poephila guttata*) androphilic cells are exclusively found in brain regions that are the sites of the control of androgen-dependent song. In the spinal cord of the male rat a group of androgen-concentrating neurons are present in the lumbar region; these neurons, absent in the female, innervate striated muscles of the penis. The existence of gonadal steroid binding sites in the members of diverse vertebrate groups suggests that binding of these hormones by nerve cells is a general vertebrate phenomenon. It is likely that such binding is evidence for evolutionary divergence from vertebrate ancestors that also possessed such sites [23].

PUBERTY

Although androgens produced by the fetal testes play a prominent role in the early development of the internal urogenital system and the external genital organs, as well as in brain differentiation, the Leydig cells subsequently become quiescent and remain so until activated much later by gonadotropins from the pituitary. The ovaries of the female also remain relatively inactive during preadolescence. In response to gonadotropin-induced gonadal steroidogenesis, there is a growth spurt and maturation of the gonads. The state at which the gonads come to maturity relative to their endocrine and gametogenic potential for reproductive function is referred to as *puberty*. The average age of puberty is variable between ethnic groups and individuals within any one group, but is about 12.5 to 13 years for the female and 14 years for the male.

Precocious and Delayed Puberty

Sexual maturity may occur earlier or later than normal; a number of possible factors determine the etiology of such divergent development. *True precocious puberty* is defined as the attainment of sexual maturity at an earlier than normal age. This sexual precociousness may be of a constitutional (genetic) nature, or it may result from disorders of the hypothalamus which result in enhanced GnRH secretion. *Precocious pseudopuberty*, on the other hand, characterizes the situation where there is a development of secondary sexual characteristics without gametogenesis. The problem is that there are excessive levels of circulating steroids either of gonadal or adrenal origin. In *congenital adrenal hyperplasia* excessive amounts of adrenal androgens are produced and may cause early virilization and pseudohermaphroditism in the female. Interstitial cell tumors of the gonads or sex steroid-secreting tumors of the adrenal glands are also sources of excessive levels of estrogens or androgens (Table 16.1). The high levels of circulating steroids exert a negative feedback inhibition of hypothalamic release of GnRH. In the absence of pituitary gonadotropin secretion there is a failure of gametogenesis, but the secondary sexual characteristics that normally develop at puberty are well developed. The pubertal process can also be delayed due possibly to panhypopituitarism where all pituitary hormones including the gonadotropins are absent. A defect at the level of the hypothalamus or an isolated deficiency in FSH or LH secretion could also be responsible for a delayed onset of puberty.

Hormonal Control of Puberty

Large fluctuations in blood and urine levels of gonadotropins, androgens, and estrogens occur during development, but lowest levels are present in the preadolescent years. During the prepubertal period, the output of gonadotropins is rather constant except for minor fluctuations during the day and night. Surges in gonadotropin secretion occur during sleep in the early stages of puberty, which may indicate that pubertal maturation has begun. By late puberty there are rather large fluctuations in gonadotropin secretion that extend throughout the day and night. Gonadotropin secretion in the postpubertal period becomes more uniform again, but at a level about double that of prepubertal individuals [2, 11].

A number of theories have been promulgated to account for the onset of puberty. No one theory provides all the necessary information, but it is likely that there are elements of truth in all the models. The *missing link hypothesis* suggests that some component of the brain-pituitary-gonadal axis is missing or nonfunc-

TABLE 16.1 Endocrine Pathophysiology of Sexual Differentiation and Development

Chromosomal disorders (a few examples)
    Gonadal dysgenesis (Turner's syndrome), XO karyotype
      Female phenotype but lack of secondary sexual characteristics (sexual infantilism)
    Seminiferous tubule dysgenesis (Kleinfelter's syndrome) XXY karyotype
      Normal male genitalia and male characteristics but seminiferous tubules are abnormal
Hermaphroditism
    True hermaphroditism (mosaicism)
      Both ovarian and testicular components present; equivocal external genitalia
    Male pseudohermaphroditism (testes present but partial or nearly complete female internal and
      external phenotypes)
      Deficient 17-ketosteroid reductase activity
      Congenital adrenal hyperplasia (due to block in pregnenolone formation)
      Leydig cell ageneses (or hypoplasia)
      Syndromes of androgen resistance
        Testicular feminizing syndrome (absence of target tissue androgen receptors)
        Syndrome of 5 α-reductase deficiency (failure to convert testosterone to DHT)
    Female pseudohermaphroditism
      Congenital virilizing adrenal hyperplasia (due to enzyme defect in cortisol biosynthesis)
      Androgen administration to the mother during fetal development
Sexual precocity (precocious puberty)
    Complete (increased gonadotropin secretion of pituitary or ectopic origin)
    Incomplete (precocious pseudopuberty; development of secondary sex characteristics but lack of
      gametogenesis)
      Adrenal steroid-secreting tumors (androgens or estrogens)
      Adrenal hyperplasia (e.g., 11 β-hydroxylase or 21 α-hydroxylase deficiencies; increased adrenal
      androgen production)
        Early masculinization in the male, masculinization of the female

tional [30]. The pituitary of immature animals is competent as it secretes normal amounts of gonadotropins when transplanted under the hypothalamus of an adult animal. The ovaries and testes of immature animals are also potentially functional, as they too become active when transplanted into adult animals or when stimulated by gonadotropins. These observations reveal that the brain rather than the pituitary or gonads is the site that is functionally incompetent prior to puberty.

Another hypothesis suggests that there is a decrease in hypothalamic sensitivity to feedback inhibition by gonadal steroids. Such a change would account for the higher circulating titers of gonadotropins present after puberty. This *gonadostat hypothesis* is supported by the observation that lesions of the hypothalamus often result in enhanced gonadotropin secretion. Also, castration of immature animals leads to an increase in pituitary gonadotropin secretion. Individuals lacking functional ovaries (as in Turner's syndrome) have high circulating levels of FSH and LH long before puberty, which could be evidence that the gonads depress gonadotropic hormone secretion in infancy. The administration of an estrogen elicits the discharge of FSH and LH during puberty, but not in infancy, which suggests that the mechanisms involved in such positive feedback have matured. It is even possible that an increased rate of androgen aromatization in the brain may be responsible for an alteration in hypothalamic sensitivity that results in initiation of the pubertal process.

A change in gonadal sensitivity to LH is purported by yet another hypothesis. It is suggested that there is a change in sensitivity of the interstitial cells to LH and that this increased sensitivity from an FSH induction of LH receptors on the cells. There is evidence that FSH enhances the steroidogenic response of testicular Leydig cells to LH [25].

In the primate, however, there is convincing evidence that neither adenohypophysial nor ovarian competence is limiting in the initiation of puberty; rather, the process depends on the maturation of the neuroendocrine control system that directs the pulsatile secretion of GnRH from the hypothalamus. For example, normal ovulatory menstrual cycles have been initiated in the prepubertal female rhesus monkey by hourly infusions of GnRH. These animals revert to the immature stage when administration of GnRH is discontinued [37].

The events that result in maturation of the neuroendocrine control system regulating GnRH secretion are still unclear. It has been proposed that puberty occurs in the human female at a critical weight or with a particular body composition [6]. In the rat, for example, puberty is reached at a set body size rather than at a specific age. Compelling support derives from the clinical observation that patients with anorexia nervosa and amenorrhea have a prepubertal or early pubertal pattern of gonadotropin secretion, which is reversed to the adult pattern in response to a weight gain. Also, leanness associated with strenuous physical activity is linked with delayed puberty, whereas the menarche (time of first menstruation) is usually early in obese individuals. For example, among young ballet dancers, there is a high incidence of primary amenorrhea (failure to initiate the first menstrual cycle), secondary amenorrhea (loss of previously established menstrual cycle), and irregular cycles, which are clearly correlated with excessive thinness [7]. High school and college athletes also have a statistically significant later age of menarche than do nonathletes. A change in the fat/lean ratio may affect metabolism and hormone levels, which may delay menarche and menstrual cycles. For example, obesity in humans is associated with increased peripheral aromatization of androgens to estrogens and also with a decrease in the transformation of estrogens to certain inactive metabolites. The resulting hyperestrogenicity from an extragonadal source of estrogens could be instrumental in the induction of neuroendocrine events related to the pubertal increase in pituitary gonadotropin secretion.

PATHOPHYSIOLOGY OF SEX DIFFERENTIATION AND DEVELOPMENT

Because of the complexity of the reproductive system, it is no surprise that there are many events that can account for abnormalities in sexual development (Table 16.1). Most defects have a genetic basis, and they may result from a failure of steroid hormone biosynthesis or a failure of steroid hormone action on target tissues [3, 10, 25].

Hermaphroditism

In the male or female gonadal steroid imbalance in the fetus results in *hermaphroditism*. A *true hermaphrodite*, a rare condition, is one who possesses both ovarian as well as testicular tissue. A *male pseudohermaphrodite* is one whose gonads are exclusively testes but whose genital ducts or external genitalia or both exhibit a female phenotype or that of an incompletely differentiated male. Individuals possessing exclusively ovarian gonadal structures but whose external genitalia exhibit some masculine characteristics are considered *female pseudohermaphrodites.*

In those individuals in which female pseudohermaphroditism has an endocrine basis the ambiguity of the external genitalia is due to excess levels of circulating androgens. The degree of virilization depends on the amount and period of exposure to androgens. Female pseudohermaphroditism in most patients is due to *congenital adrenal hyperplasia.* There are a number of types of congenital adrenal hyperplasia, and the etiology of each relates to a specific defect in steroid biosynthesis, usually a failure in cortisol production. In the absence of cortisol biosynthesis there is a lack of negative feedback inhibition to the hypothalamus which results in increased ACTH release and subsequently enhanced stimulation of adrenocortical steroid biosynthesis. However, the metabolites that accumulate due to enzymatic failure to convert them to cortisol and aldosterone are shunted to pathways of androgen production. The androgens that are now secreted in excess are responsible for virilization of the external genitalia as well as development of masculine secondary sexual characteristics.

Male pseudohermaphroditism may result from sex chromosomal anomalies, mutant genes, or teratologic factors that lead to defective gonadogenesis. Only those factors whose etiology relates to endocrine dysfunction will be discussed. Testosterone is synthesized by the Leydig cells of the testes in response to LH of pituitary origin. There is evidence that male pseudohermaphroditism in some individuals may result from a defect in the LH receptors of fetal Leydig cells. A number of inborn errors of testosterone production can also account for development of hermaphroditism in the male. Three enzymes, which include the cholesterol desmolase complex, 3 β-hydroxysteroid dehydrogenase, and 17 α-hydroxylase, are present in both the adrenals and testes. Failure of their enzymatic function results in an abnormality of glucocorticoid and mineralocorticoid synthesis as well as androgen production. These enzyme defects may be partial or complete and are caused by autosomal or X-linked recessive mutations (Table 15.1 and Table 16.1).

Syndrome of 5 α-reductase deficiency. Evidence from a familial-related group of individuals in the Dominican Republic, has provided important insights into genetically based male pseudohermaphroditism. Failure to virilize certain androgen-dependent structures results from a lack of 5 α-reductase activity in these target tissues. The affected individuals had bilateral inguinal or labial testes and a labial-like scrotum at birth; there were no Müllerian structures, but Wolffian structures were well developed. These developmental characteristics clearly reveal the anatomically specific target tissue responses to testosterone and the near absence of DHT-dependent structures. At puberty there was striking virilization of testosterone-dependent secondary sex characteristics: axillary and pubic hair growth, deepening of the voice, increased muscle mass, and an enlargement of the phallus to a near functional size. The enhancement of the phallus mass, which is a DHT-dependent structure, may have been due to the very high circulating levels of testosterone in these individuals. Affected men had less facial and body hair and less temporal hairline recession than unaffected men from the same families. Acne was absent, and the prostate glands failed to develop. Thus, it appears that the sexual characteristics absent in these individuals are those mainly regulated by DHT. Because of the extreme defect in the development of the external genitalia, male pseudohermaphrodites are usually raised as females [10].

Syndrome of testicular feminization. A number of single gene mutations involve defects in production of androgen-binding proteins. Much is known about the syndrome of testicular feminization. Males with this syndrome have testes and normal (or higher) rates of testosterone secretion, but they are almost completely insensitive to exogenous or endogenous androgen action. These individuals are therefore phenotypic females, often with a truly feminine appearance. Although the external genitalia are ambiguously female and the clitoris normal, the vagina is short and blind ended and the internal genitalia are absent except for a testes which may be in the abdomen, inguinal canal, or labia majora. Androgen resistance is due to abnormalities of the androgen receptor; the receptor protein is either absent or defective in structure. That the Wolffian ducts fail to differentiate and external genitalia do not develop indicates that both testosterone and DHT receptors are involved. The absence of Müllerian ducts and their derivatives in these otherwise phenotypic females indicates that the action of MRF has not been comprised.

Androgen-insensitive male rats are capable of responding to ovarian hormones with a display of feminine sexual behavior if they are castrated at birth but not about 10 days after birth. Although genital differentiation in these animals is insensitive to testicular androgens, it appears that the neural substrate of sexual behavior is differentiated by the presence of the testes during the critical period of a few days after birth [28].

Receptor-positive resistance. Another type of androgen resistance does not appear to involve either a defect in 5 α-reductase activity or cytosolic androgen receptors. The site of the molecular abnormality is unclear, but could reside at one or more sites distal to the receptor [10].

Primary and Secondary Hypogonadism and Hypergonadism

As noted previously, hermaphroditism may result from a failure in steroid hormone biosynthesis or in end organ resistance. Defects in the normal development of secondary sex characteristics at puberty may result from defects that reside at the level of the gonads (primary) or at the level of the pituitary (secondary) or even the hypothalamus (tertiary) (Fig. 16.9A). Primary hypogonadism might relate to a failure in production of gonadal steroids due to any one of a number of causes. Failure in a negative feedback inhibition at the pituitary (or hypothalamus) by steroid hormones would lead to enhanced gonadotropin secretion in the face of hypogonadism (hypergonadotropic hypogonadism, Fig. 16.9B). Secondary hypogonadism, on the other hand, could result from a defect in pituitary gonadotropin secretion (hypogonadotropic hypogonadism, Fig. 16.9C). Hypergonadism involving overproduction of gonadal steroids could relate to a primary defect (hypogonadotropic hypergonadism) at the gonads involving a tumorous condition of the steroid-secreting cells (Leydig cells in the male or follicular thecal cells in the female, Fig. 16.9D) or to a secondary defect (hypergonadotropic hypergonadism) involving overproduction of pituitary gonadotropins (Fig. 16.9E).

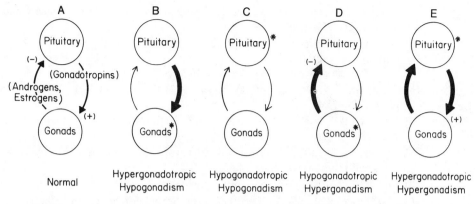

Figure 16.9 Primary (gonadal) or secondary (pituitary) defects causing underproduction or overproduction of gonadal steroids with concomitant effects on pituitary gonadotropin secretion are depicted. The site of the lesion, at either the gonads or the pituitary, is indicated (*).

REFERENCES

[1] BARDIN, C. W., and J. F. CATTERALL. 1981. Testosterone: a major determinant of extragenital sexual dimorphism. *Science* 211:1285–94.

[2] BOYER, R. M. 1978. Control of the onset of puberty. *Ann. Rev. Med.* 29:509–20.

[3] CONTE, F. A., and M. M. GRUMBACH. 1979. Pathogenesis, classification, diagnosis, and treatment of anomalies of sex. In *Endocrinology*, vol. 3, eds., L. J. DeGroot, G. F. Cahill, Jr., L. Martini, D. H. Nelson, W. D. Odell, J. T. Potts, Jr., E. Steinberger, and A. I. Winegrad, pp. 1363–79. New York: Grune & Stratton, Inc.

[4] DeVOOGD, T., and F. NOTTEBOHM. 1981. Gonadal hormones induced dendrite growth in the adult avian brain. *Science* 214:202–204.

[5] EHRHARDT, A. A., and H. F. L. MEYER-BAHLBURG. 1981. Effects of prenatal sex hormones on gender-related behavior. *Science* 211:1312–18.

[6] FRISCH, R. E. 1980. Pubertal adipose tissue: is it necessary for normal sexual maturation? Evidence from the rat and the human female. *Fed. Proc.* 39:2395–2400.

[7] FRISCH, R. E., G. WYSHAK, and L. VINCENT. 1980. Delayed menarche and amenorrhea in ballet dancers. *New Engl. J. Med.* 303:17–19.

[8] GORDON, J. W., and F. H. RUDDLE. 1981. Mammalian gonadal determination and gametogenesis. *Science* 211:1265–71.

[9] GORSKI, R. A. 1979. The neuroendocrinology of reproduction: an overview. *Biol. of Reprod.* 20:111–27.

[10] GRIFFIN, J. E., and J. D. WILSON. 1980. The syndromes of androgen resistance. *New Engl. J. Med.* 302:198–208.

[11] GRUMBACH, M. M. 1980. The neuroendocrinology of puberty. *Hosp. Prac.* 15(3):51–60.

[12] GURNEY, M. E., and M. KONISHI. 1980. Hormone-induced sexual differentiation of brain and behavior in zebra finches. *Science* 208:1380–83.

[13] HASELTINE, F. P., and S. OHNO. 1981. Mechanisms of gonadal differentiation. *Science* 211:1272–78.

[14] IMPERATO-McGINLEY, J., L. GUERRECO, T. GAUTIER, and R. E. PETERSON. 1974. Steroid

5 α-reductase deficiency in man: an inherited form of male pseudohermaphroditism. *Science* 186:1213–15.

[15] IMPERATO-MCGINLEY, J., R. E. PETERSON, T. GAUTIER, and E. STURLA. 1979. Androgens and the evolution of male-gender identity among male pseudohermaphrodites with 5 α-reductase deficiency. *New Engl. J. Med.* 300:1233–37.

[16] JOSSO, N., J. Y. PICARD, and D. TRAN. 1977. The antimüllerian hormone. *Rec. Prog. Horm. Res.* 33:117–67.

[17] JOST, A., B. VIGIER, and J. PREPIN. 1973. Studies on sex differentiation in mammals. *Rec. Prog. Horm. Res.* 29:1–41.

[18] KELLEY, D. B. 1978. Neuroanatomical correlates of hormone sensitive behaviors in frogs and birds. *Amer. Zool.* 18:477–88.

[19] LILLIE, F. R. 1916. The theory of the free-martin. *Science* 43:611–13.

[20] MACLUSKY, N. J., and F. NAFTOLIN. 1981. Sexual differentiation of the central nervous system. *Science* 211:1294–1302.

[21] MCEWEN, B. S. 1976. Interactions between hormones and nerve tissue. *Sci. Amer.* 235:48–58.

[22] _____. 1981. Neural gonadal steroid actions. *Science* 211:1303–12.

[23] MORRELL, J. I., D. B. KELLEY, and D. W. PFAFF. 1975. Sex steroid binding in the brains of vertebrates. In *Brain-endocrine interaction* II, eds. K. M. Knigge, D. E. Scott, H. Kobayashi, and S. Ishii, pp. 230–56. Basel: S. Karger.

[24] NOTTEBOHM, F. 1981. A brain for all seasons: cyclical anatomical changes in song control nuclei of the canary brain. *Science* 214:1368–70.

[25] ODELL, W. D. 1979. The physiology of puberty: disorders of the pubertal process. In *Endocrinology*, vol. 3, eds. L. J. DeGroot, G. F. Cahill, Jr., L. Martini, D. H. Nelson, W. D. Odell, J. T. Potts, Jr., E. Steinberger, and A. I. Winegrad, pp. 1363–79. New York: Grune & Stratton, Inc.

[26] OHNO, S. 1979. *Major sex-determining genes.* Berlin: Springer-Verlag.

[27] OHNO, S., Y. NAGAI, S. CICCARESE, and H. IWATA. 1979. Testis-organizing H-Y antigen and the primary sex-determining mechanism of mammals. *Rec. Prog. Horm. Res.* 35:449–76.

[28] OLSEN, K. L. 1979. Androgen-insensitive rats are defeminized by their testes. *Nature* 279:238–39.

[29] PRICE, D., J. J. P. ZAAIJER, E. ORTIZ, and A. O. BRINKMANN. 1975. Current views on embryonic sex differentiation in reptiles, birds, and mammals. *Amer. Zool.* 15(Suppl. 1):173–95.

[30] RAMALEY, J. A. 1979. Development of gonadotropin regulation in the prepubertal mammal. *Biol. Reprod.* 20:1–31.

[31] REINISCH, J. M. 1981. Prenatal exposure to synthetic progestins increases potential for aggression in humans. *Science* 211:1171–73.

[32] RUBIN, R. T., J. M. REINISCH, and R. F. HASKETT. 1981. Postnatal gonadal steroid effects on human behavior. *Science* 211:1318–24.

[33] SHORT, R. V. 1979. Sex determination and differentiation. *Brit. Med. Bull.* 35:121–27.

[34] TORAN-ALLERAND, C. D. 1978. Gonadal hormones and brain development: cellular aspects of sexual differentiation. *Amer. Zool.* 18:553–65.

[35] WACHTEL, S. S. 1979a. Immunogenetic aspects of abnormal sexual differentiation. *Cell* 16:691–95.

[36] _____. 1979b. The genetics of intersexuality: clinical and theoretical perspectives. *Obstetrics & Gynocology* 54:671–85. New York: Harper and Row Publishers, Inc.

[37] WILDT, L., G. MARSHALL, and E. KNOBIL. 1980. Experimental induction of puberty in the infantile female rhesus monkey. *Science* 207:1373–75.

[38] WILSON, J. D., F. W. GEORGE, and J. E. GRIFFIN. 1981. The hormonal control of sexual development. *Science* 211:1278–84.

[39] YAMAMOTO, T. 1975. A YY male goldfish from mating estrone-induced XY female and normal male. *J. Hered.* 66:2–4.

17

Hormones and Male Reproductive Physiology

INTRODUCTION

Castration of young males to provide eunuchs was a custom of some earlier societies. Eunuchs fail to develop the secondary sex characteristics that typify postadolescent development of the normal male. The physiological basis for this atypical male development was not understood, but it was undoubtedly obvious that the testes must have provided some stimulus to normal male development. As early as 1771 Hunter was able to induce male characteristics in the hen by transplantation of testes from a rooster; spontaneous sex reversal in the hen had been noted to be associated with conversion of the ovary to a testis. In 1849 Berthold showed that transplantation of the gonads into castrated roosters prevented loss of male secondary sex characteristics and sexual behavior (Chapter 1). Brown-Séquard (1889) popularized the role of the testes in the maintenance of virility by his claim that testicular extracts administered to himself restored vigor.

An active androgenic substance (androsterone) was first isolated from the urine of man by Butenandt in 1931. Testicular extracts were prepared in 1927 and the major androgenic principle was soon isolated in crystalline form. The chemical structure of this testicular androgenic principle was elucidated and synthesized by Ruzicka and Wettstein in 1935 and appropriately named *testosterone*. The role of testosterone and other hormones in the control of normal and abnormal development in humans and other vertebrates is the topic of this chapter.

ANATOMY OF THE MALE REPRODUCTIVE SYSTEM

In the human fetus the indifferent gonads of the genetic male are induced to differentiate into testes. The fetal testes, in turn, produce testosterone which is responsible for differentiation and development of the urogenital system characteristic of the male. The testes become quiescent until puberty when they are activated by pituitary gonadotropins (Chapter 16).

The Testis

The two major functions of the adult testes are to provide an environment for spermatogenesis and to secrete testosterone to regulate a variety of bodily functions related to male reproductive function. In the human adult male the testes are located within the scrotum; each testis is ovoid in shape and is about 4 to 6 cm in length and 2 to 3 cm in diameter. A connective tissue sheath, the tunica albuginea, encapsulates each testis. The testis consists of convoluted *seminiferous tubules* within which sperms are produced. These tubules converge into the rete testis which opens to efferential ductules to the *epididymus*. The epididymus is composed of a head (caput), body (corpus), and the tail which connects directly with the vas deferens (Fig. 17.1) The outer sheet of the seminiferous tubules is made up of connective tissue and smooth muscle; the inner lining is composed of Sertoli cells within which are embedded the spermatogonia and various differentiated stages of immature and mature sperms. The suggestion that the Sertoli cells provide nutrients and other factors necessary for sperm maturation is compatible with the observation that the germ cells are, indeed, embedded deeply within and between the Sertoli cells. The fully matured spermatozoa, sperms, are released into the lumen of the seminiferous tubules and subsequently

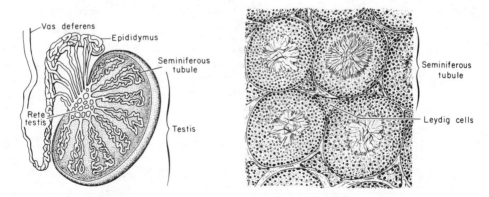

Figure 17.1   Gross and microscopic anatomy of the human testis.

advance slowly to the rete testis and epididymus where they are stored within the tail. Between the seminiferous tubules are found the interstitial cells of Leydig, the cellular source of androgen production within the testes (Fig. 17.1).

SOURCE, SYNTHESIS, CHEMISTRY, AND METABOLISM OF ANDROGENS

As in adrenal steroidogenic tissue, cholesterol serves as the substrate for pregnenolone biosynthesis in the Leydig cells. Extracellular low density lipoproteins are the major substrate for androgen production by Leydig cells of most mammalian species studied. Unlike in the adrenal, however, conversion of pregnenolone to 17-hydroxylated steroids provides the predominant steroidogenic pathway in testicular interstitial tissue. The conversion of pregnenolone to progesterone with subsequent 17-hydroxyla-tion appears not to provide an important pathway in humans. The 17-hydroxysteroids are converted by side-chain cleavage to 17-ketosteroids, and these, in turn, are converted to testosterone. *Testosterone* is the principal steroid produced by Leydig cells of the testis (Fig. 17.2). Androstenedione and dehydroepiandrosterone are also produced, but the physiological potencies of these androgens are so low that they will not substitute for normal Leydig cell function. Although some androgens are 17-

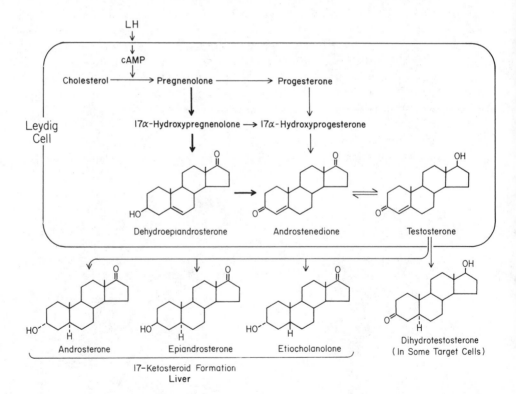

Figure 17.2 Testicular biosynthesis and hepatic metabolism of testosterone.

ketosteroids, not all 17-ketosteroids are androgens and not all androgens are 17-ketosteroids. For example, etiocholanolone has no androgenic action and testosterone is not a 17-ketosteroid. An oxygen atom at the C-3 position and a 17-hydroxyl or keto group are required for androgenic activity. In some tissues testosterone is converted to either dihydroxytestosterone (DHT) or estradiol, which are the biologically active steroids affecting these tissues (Fig. 16.8).

Almost 100% of the testosterone in the blood is bound to protein: About 40% is bound to a β-globulin called gonadal steroid-binding globulin, about 40% is bound to albumin, and 17% to other proteins. Inactivation of testosterone, which occurs primarily in the liver, involves the following metabolism: oxidation of the 17-OH group, reduction of the A ring, and reduction of the 3-keto group (Fig. 17.2). The primary urinary products of androgens in humans are androsterone and etiocholanolone which are excreted in the form of glucuronide and sulfate conjugates.

ENDOCRINE CONTROL OF TESTICULAR FUNCTION

The testis has two major functions: androgen production and spermatogenesis. The control of these diverse functions requires the coordinated activity of a number of pituitary hormones which are in turn regulated by a complex of neurohumoral inputs from the hypothalamus.

GnRH and Pituitary Gonadotropins

Early experiments established that hypophysectomy led to testicular atrophy (Chapter 5). Restoration of testicular function could be affected by administration of pituitary extracts or, after further purification, of pituitary gonadotropins. Pituitary gonadotropin secretion is enhanced after orchidectomy, whereas gonadotropin secretion is diminished after administration of exogenous androgens. These observations established that testicular androgens exert a negative feedback on pituitary gonadotropin secretion. Part of this feedback is apparently directed at the level of the hypothalamus. For example, testosterone implantations into the hypothalamus are inhibitory to pituitary gonadotropin secretion. Subsequent discovery of a hypothalamic gonadotropin releasing hormone provided evidence that the inhibitory feedback actions of testosterone involved inhibition of GnRH secretion. A number of neuronal inputs may be important to GnRH synthesis and secretion; the exact cellular site(s) of androgen feedback in the hypothalamus remains undefined. Hypothalamic lesions that are specifically inhibitory to pituitary gonadotropin secretion have provided insights into the neuronal pathways concerned with distribution of GnRH. By the use of a large armamentarium of drugs, the diverse neuronal circuits involved in the control of GnRH secretion are also being delineated. It is still unresolved whether there is one GnRH that regulates both FSH and LH secretion or two gonadotropin releasing factors (an FSH/RH and an LH/RH) that control the release of each individual gonadotropin from the pituitary.

Pituitary gonadotropin secretion in the male has generally been considered to be under a tonic regulatory control. There is evidence, however, that these hormones undergo wide fluctuations in their circulating concentrations over relatively short periods of time [11]. Apparently the release of GnRH from the hypothalamus is frequency coded and may be necessary to prevent pituitary gonadotrophs from becoming refractory (down regulated) to GnRH. In the adult human male there is a pulsatile release of LH about every 90 minutes. The precise pattern of this episodic release varies from day to day, suggesting that the mechanisms controlling gonadotropin secretion are not coupled to an endogenous oscillator.

In a number of mammals LH is released upon exposure of a male to a female. Successive presentation of the same female to a male mouse may lead to habituation where LH secretion is diminished upon subsequent presentations of the female. Introduction of a novel female, on the other hand, will initiate a burst of LH secretion [6]. This adaptive neuroendocrine response may be important in providing a stimulus to courtship and copulatory behavior in some species.

The following evidence clearly establishes the individual roles of pituitary gonadotropins in regulating testicular function [13]. Radiolabeled LH specifically binds to Leydig cells, whereas radiolabeled FSH binds only to Sertoli cells. LH increases cAMP levels in the interstitial cells of the testes but not the seminiferous tubules. FSH, on the other hand, does not increase cAMP levels in the Leydig cells but does stimulate production of the cyclic nucleotide in seminiferous tubules devoid of germ cells or in enriched fractions of Sertoli cells [29]. FSH also stimulates the conversion of testosterone to estrogens and $5\,\alpha$-reduced androgens within Sertoli cells [12]. Although the Sertoli cell is the major site of FSH action, there is evidence that FSH enhances the number of Leydig cell LH receptors (Chapter 16). Although FSH does not by itself stimulate steroid biosynthesis within purified testis interstitial tissue, in combination with LH it causes a dramatic increase (synergism) in the action of LH on Leydig cell 3 β-hydroxysteroid dehydrogenase-isomerase activity (Fig. 17.3).

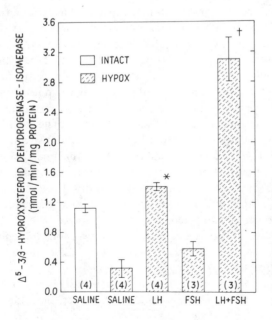

Figure 17.3 Effect of in vivo treatment with gonadotropins on isolated interstitial tissue 3 β-HSD activity in hypophysectomized mature male rats. Rats were injected twice daily for 14 days. Each value represents the mean, ± S.E., enzyme activity from the number of interstitial preparations indicated. *, significantly different from saline-injected hypox rats; [+], significantly different from LH- or FSH-treated hypox rats. (From Shaw, [35], with permission.)

Hormones and Male Reproductive Physiology   Chap. 17

Inhibin

It has been postulated that the testes produce a hormone whose putative role is to control the secretion of pituitary FSH. This factor, referred to as *inhibin*, which may be peptidergic in nature, is believed to be produced within the seminiferous tubules, most likely the Sertoli cells [37]. High levels of FSH and normal levels of LH are present in the plasma of oligospermic males [9] and in males after testicular irradiation and cytotoxic chemotherapy. Sertoli cells alone are not capable of reducing FSH levels in the absence of spermatogenesis. It is postulated that inhibin production by Sertoli cells may be regulated by influences deriving from maturing sperms. FSH secretion from cultured anterior pituitary cells is inhibited when pituitary cells are cocultured with Sertoli cells (but not spleen or kidney cells). Thus, pituitary FSH secretion may normally be regulated via negative feedback by an inhibitory factor of Sertoli cell origin. This is further substantiated by the observation that prior exposure of the pituitary to inhibin suppresses the elevation of FSH release following GnRH administration. Other evidence suggests that inhibin also suppresses FSH by a hypothalamic site of action. Because FSH release but not LH release is altered, it was postulated that inhibin might exert a selective inhibitory effect on the release of a hypothalamic FSH releasing factor [27].

   Granulosa cells from the ovarian follicle also secrete a substance during culture, presumably inhibin, that acts directly on pituitary cell cultures derived from the male or female to suppress preferentially FSH secretion. Administration of antiinhibin antisera to rats of either sex causes a rise in serum FSH levels; LH levels, in contrast, remain unchanged [14]. A summary scheme of the roles of FSH and inhibin in the control of testicular (and ovarian) function is provided (Fig. 17.4).

Prolactin

Hypophysectomy of the male rat results in a loss of testicular LH receptors; administration of FSH or LH does not, however, reestablish testicular LH receptor

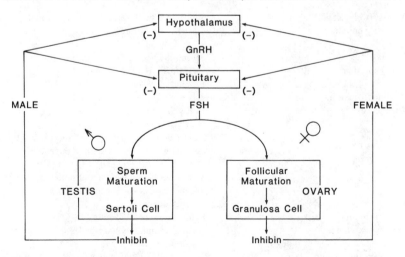

Figure 17.4   A summary scheme of the roles of FSH and inhibin in the control of testicular (and ovarian) function.

concentration. Inhibition of pituitary FSH and LH secretion from the rat pituitary by administration of anti-GnRH or by estradiol or testosterone treatment does not result in a loss of testicular LH receptors. These results suggest that one or more pituitary hormones other than the gonadotropins might be responsible for maintenance of testicular receptors. Inhibition of prolactin secretion by ergot alkaloids results in a decrease in testicular LH receptors, whereas PRL treatment prevents loss of LH receptors in hypophysectomized animals. These observations suggest that PRL may play a role in the control of testicular Leydig cell LH receptor number [40].

PHYSIOLOGICAL ROLES OF ANDROGENS

Testicular androgens are responsible for the growth and development of those tissues and organs which characterize the male (Table 17.1). The role of gonadal androgens in the differentiation and development of the male urogenital system, the accessory sex organs, and the external genitalia has already been described (Chapter 16). Although many target tissues respond directly to testosterone, this androgen must first be converted either to DHT or estradiol in some other tissues to mediate its actions. After the initial actions of testosterone in early fetal development, the gonads remain quiescent until puberty when gonadal activity is increased in response to secretion of pituitary gonadotropins. The elevated circulating levels of androgens that ensue are responsible for initiating spermatogenesis (gametogenesis) and for growth and development of the secondary sex characteristics that first become evident during the pubertal process. Some of the established roles of androgens in the male are discussed below.

TABLE 17.1 Biological Effects and Roles of Testicular Androgens in the Human Male

Primary locus of action	Physiological response
Prepubertal	
Accessory sex glands	Wolffian duct differentiation and growth
External genitalia	Growth and differentiation (scrotum and penis)
Pubertal	
Skeletal Muscle	Masculine body growth and physique
(enhanced protein synthesis)	(Na^+, K^+, H_2O retention)
Bone	Epiphysial closure
(bone formation)	(Ca^{2+}, SO_4^{-2}, PO_4^{-3} retention)
Vocal cords	Voice change
Skin	Hair growth
	(beard, axilla, chest, pubic, and general body surface)
	Sebaceous gland growth and lipogenesis
	Hair loss (e.g., forehead)
	Sebaceous gland growth and sebum production
Testis	Sertoli cell maturation and androgen-binding protein synthesis
	Spermatogenesis
External genitalia	Penile and scrotal growth
Accessory sex glands	Prostate gland, seminal vesicles, bulbourethral gland growth, and secretion
Central nervous system	Sexual activity (libido increased)
Hypothalamo-pituitary axis	Inhibition of LH secretion

Spermatogenesis

FSH and testosterone are required for the initiation of spermatogenesis during sexual maturation. Administration of FSH to immature or mature hypophysectomized rats markedly increases the size of the testes but does not accelerate the appearance of mature sperm or increase the secretory activity of the Leydig cells. For completion of spermatogenesis, an androgenic influence is needed which can be provided by the administration of testosterone. Spermatogenesis can be maintained in hypophysectomized adult animals by testosterone in the absence of gonadotropins, but its initiation at puberty requires FSH. Resumption of spermatogenesis in regressed testes following hypophysectomy also requires administration of FSH. In immature animals FSH increases the number of Sertoli cells, which accounts for the testicular hypertrophy that follows hemicastration [8]. FSH is required for the normal reinitiation of sperm production during the breeding season of monkeys. Although LH alone stimulates sperm production in some patients with deficiencies in LH and FSH production, others have required a combination of FSH and LH to initiate spermatogenesis. Interestingly, FSH alone has never been reported to initiate or maintain spermatogenesis in males [38].

Although the details of the individual roles of FSH and testosterone in spermatogenesis remain unresolved, the following model has been proposed [37]. FSH interaction with Sertoli cell plasmalemmal receptors results in cyclic AMP production and the synthesis of an androgen binding protein (ABP). Presumably, cyclic AMP activates a protein kinase which leads to the genomic production of an mRNA coding for ABP. The ABP is then secreted into the lumen of the seminiferous tubules.

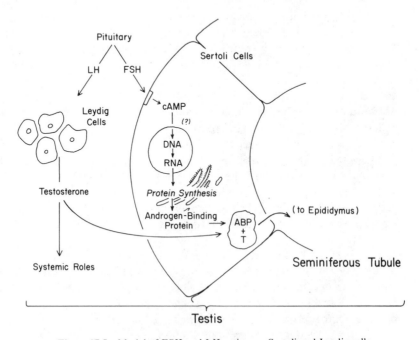

Figure 17.5 Model of FSH and LH action on Sertoli and Leydig cells.

Physiological Roles of Androgens

Testicular receptors for LH are specifically localized to the Leydig cells. In response to LH cyclic AMP is produced which causes Leydig cell testosterone production (Fig. 17.5). Testosterone is released from the Leydig cells and finds its way into the systemic circulation and the adjacent seminiferous tubules. Because the Sertoli cells are connected by tight junctions, they apparently provide a barrier (blood-testis) to most large molecules. Testosterone may be taken up by the Sertoli cells by an active transport mechanism or by facilitated diffusion [34]. The blood-testis barrier first appears at puberty and may function to create some special environment for spermatogenesis. The barrier may also protect the germ cells from the immunological system. Within the Sertoli cells testosterone is bound to ABP. This binding protein may provide a mechanism for testosterone sequestration close to the spermatocytes whose maturation may be androgen dependent. Because germ cells lacking androgen receptors develop into fertile spermatozoa in the presence of normal Sertoli cells, it is presumed that the hormonal effects of testosterone on spermatogenesis are mediated via the Sertoli cells.

Androgen binding protein may also provide a mechanism for the accumulation of androgen within Sertoli cells which can then be released (via vesicular exocytosis) into the lumen of the seminiferous tubules. Within the lumen ABP may function to transport testosterone to the epididymus. The spermatozoa mature in the caput and corpus regions of the epididymus where they develop the potential for fertilization and motility. These characteristics of mature sperm are soon lost in castrated animals, but can be maintained by testosterone administration [5].

Nervous System

Unlike in the female, gonadal steroids do not feed back to the pituitary or hypothalamus of the male to regulate the cyclic release of pituitary hormones. Nevertheless, pituitary gonadotropin secretion is increased after gonadectomy, and exogenous androgens depress the elevation of gonadotropin secretion in the castrated animal. Therefore, testicular androgens exert a tonic inhibitory feedback action on pituitary gonadotropin secretion. Nuclear androgen binding sites are present in the brain of vertebrates, and they represent loci of androgen activation of sexually related behavior (Chapter 16). For example, implantation of androgen within specific areas of the brain can induce copulatory behavior in fowl [2].

In the dove, *Streptopelia risoria*, male courtship depends on the action of androgen on the preoptic-anterior hypothalamus (AHPOA) of the brain. The aggressive components of courtship, as well as perch calling, are specifically testosterone dependent, whereas nest-oriented courtship activity and nest soliciting appear to be mediated by estrogens (derived from testosterone) acting on the AHPOA [20].

A sexually dimorphic nucleus is present in the fifth and sixth lumbar segments of the male rat spinal cord [4]. This nucleus contains motoneurons that innervate the perineal striated muscle of the penis. This nucleus is diminished or absent in the normal female and in males who are genetically insensitive to androgens. The cell bodies of these motoneurons accumulate androgens but not estradiol. These motoneurons probably represent a site of androgen action modifying penile reflexes during copulatory behavior. In the male frog, *Xenopus laevis*, spinal neurons projecting to muscles primarily involved in the clasp reflex during amplexus accumulate [^{3}H]-dihydrotestosterone. DHT added to an isolated spinal cord preparation containing these neurons changes the firing patterns of the neurons. Androgens or their metabolites may therefore regulate mating behavior in these animals by an initial action within specific spinal neurons that control muscle activity during mating.

Gonadal hormones alter the level of spontaneous electrical activity of anatomically defined populations of neurons within the brain and change the responses of peripheral and central neuronal pathways to sensory stimulation in some vertebrate species. For example, testosterone alters preoptic neuron responses to electrical stimulation of the olfactory bulb and to natural sexual odors. Therefore, in the adult animal, androgens may be significant in the interception and interpretation of olfactory cues important to reproductive success.

Gonadal androgens are essential for establishment and maintenance of male dominance and aggressive behavior in most birds (e.g., domestic fowl, mallards). Sexual aggressiveness is diminished after castration but can be reestablished by administration of androgens. In phalaropes (*Steganopes tricolor*), however, the female is more active than the male in courtship behavior. During the breeding cycle, female phalaropes produce more gonadal androgens than males [18]. In females the nuptial plumage is also more brilliant than that of males. Administration of testosterone (but not estradiol or PRL) to phalaropes of either sex in the dull juvenile or adult nonbreeding plumage results in formation of the full plumage pattern which normally only develops in the female [21]. These results clearly establish that androgens in the female phalarope are responsible for inducing nuptial plumage and dominant mating behavior during the breeding season.

Anabolic Actions

The major extragenital site of androgen action is skeletal muscle, which may account for part of the body weight difference between males and females of many species. Growth of the musculature and cartilage of the larynx of the human causes a permanent deepening of the voice. Because skeletal muscle cannot convert testosterone to DHT, it is likely that testosterone has a direct anabolic action on muscle. The myotropic actions of androgens result from their ability to increase retention of dietary nitrogen through protein synthesis. A great many derivatives of testosterone have been prepared with the hope that they might be of practical use in promoting general body growth without concomitantly producing masculinizing effects. These compounds are referred to as *anabolic steroids*. There is no clear consensus that the androgenic and anabolic actions of these steroids can be separated.

Erythropoiesis

Androgens stimulate erythropoiesis directly on the erythron (bone marrow red blood cell progenitor) and indirectly by stimulating renal erythropoietin production. The effects of androgens on the kidney are mediated through interaction with androgen receptors common to other target tissues. In bone marrow, on the other hand, the pluripotential stem cells respond to 5 β-androgen and 5 β-progestin metabolites which have no measurable effect on the reproductive tract [1]. Steroids with the 5 β-structure are more potent than their 5 α-epimers in stimulating hemoglobin synthesis within erythroblasts. The receptors for these 5 β-androgen metabolites differ from the classical androgen receptors. Animals that have a genetically determined deficiency for androgen receptors respond normally to these β-steroids but not to testosterone or 5 α-metabolites.

Secondary Sex Characteristics

The dramatic developmental and behavioral changes at puberty in the male result from enhanced testosterone secretion by the testes and the actions of testosterone or one of its metabolites on specific target tissues. Dimorphic secondary sex characteristics are typical of all vertebrates. These differences are most often modifications of the integument or underlying tissues: skin coloration; hair color, distribution, and coarseness; development of specialized integumental structures such as horns, antlers, beaks, claws, and spines [10]. In the male androgens profoundly affect such courtship behaviors as aggression, bodily movements and display, and even vocalization. Only a few representative examples of the role of androgens among the major groups of vertebrates shall be discussed.

Sex organs. The accessory reproductive glands are dependent on testosterone to enable them to contribute secretory products to the semen. Androgens increase the content of endoplasmic reticulum within the cells of the prostate, seminal vesicles, and bulbourethral glands. The spermatozoa contain only a relatively small amount of cytoplasm and apparently must be nourished by constituents of the seminal fluid. Fructose, a source of metabolic energy for the spermatozoa, is secreted by the seminal vesicles. The effects of testosterone on the prostate gland are greatly augmented by prolactin which is without effect on this gland in the castrated animal. The penis and scrotum also enlarge in response to testosterone or dihydrotestosterone.

Skin and hair. Sebaceous gland activity is stimulated by androgens most likely derived from testosterone. The acne often present in the male during the pubertal process is due to the increased activity of these glands in response to elevated plasma levels of androgens. The coarseness of hair in some animals is increased by androgens, and the pattern of hair growth is also affected. Androgens are stimulatory to hair growth in the axilla, the pubic area, and on the chin. In contrast, androgens cause recession of the male hairline. Androgens may even cause baldness (alopecia) in individuals with such a genetic predisposition. Castration of males who are becoming alopeic prevents further extension of the bald areas but does not promote general regrowth of hair. In females with adrenal virilism the excessive levels of androgens may induce baldness; loss of hair ceases when the abnormal masculinization ends [17].

The sexually dimorphic kidney. In Chapter 16, it was noted that gonadal steroids affect sexual dimorphic differentiation and development of nuclear centers within the vertebrate central nervous system. Other organs and tissues are also differentially affected by gonadal steroids. The proximal tubules of the kidneys of male mice, for example, contain mitochondria and lysosomes that are ultrastructurally different from those of females. Males also have higher kidney activities of mitochondrial cytochrome C oxidase and lysosomal hydroxylases. The female pattern of organellar structure develops after orchidectomy. Testosterone administration induces the male pattern of cellular structure and function in castrated male mice or in female mice [23]. Sex differences in kidney function and metabolism as well as pathophysiology have been documented and may relate to differences in the hormonal milieu between the two sexes.

Submaxillary glands of mice. As noted in Chapter 12, submaxillary gland production of nerve growth factor (NGF) and epidermal growth factor (EGF) in the mouse is acutely controlled by androgens. Several enzymes are more abundant in the male submaxillary gland than in the female. The cellular synthesis of these enzymes is androgen dependent and can be induced in the female by administration of an androgen. In boars, salivary glands utilize nonandrogenic steroids of testicular origin and secrete them into the saliva where they may function as sex attractants (e.g., musk).

Skin coloration. In most vertebrates skin coloration differs between the sexes and can be striking in some teleosts and birds. Often the color of the skin changes during the breeding season. These pigmentary changes are usually androgen dependent and involve increases or decreases in the number of pigment cells and the amount and kind of pigment within integumental chromatophores. In some birds, such as the weaver finch, the bill becomes melanized in response to androgens during the breeding season.

Brood patches. Some birds develop a brood patch on the abdomen during the breeding season. Feathers are lost from this area and the skin becomes thick and hypervascularized so that warmth can be imparted to the incubating eggs. In female passerine birds where the female develops a patch estrogen and PRL synergize to cause brood patch development [22]. In those species in which both sexes develop a patch (e.g., quail), estrogens or androgens synergize with PRL to initiate patch development. In the phalarope, in which only the male develops a patch, patch development is regulated by the synergistic actions of PRL and androgens.

Epidermal cornifications. In many amphibians black, cornified structures may occur on the forelimbs or hindlimbs. These nuptial pads, as they are designated, assist the male in grasping the female during amplexus. These are androgen-dependent structures that regress after castration and can be reinstated following androgen replacement therapy. In the newt, nuptial pads develop in response to androgens but only if prolactin and thyroid hormone are also present.

Antlers. A vast array of morphological outgrowths of the integument characterize the male of the species and are often enlarged or otherwise exaggerated during the breeding season. The growth of antlers in some species of deer might be considered the most conspicuous of integumental growths. The antlers are solid bony outgrowths that arise from the frontal bones and are borne usually by the male. The growth and shedding of antlers is under the control of androgens, except in caribou where both the male and female possess antlers. In the red deer stag (*Cervus elaphus*) the cycle of testosterone secretion is responsible for the redevelopment of the secondary sexual characteristics each year; the animal undergoes a type of "annual puberty and senescence" [24]. Testosterone stimulates development of the neck mane and rutting odor and is responsible for loss of velvet from the antlers. Changes in photoperiod affect testicular androgenesis. Increasing day length is inhibitory to testicular androgenic activity in the Sitka deer (*Cervus nippon*) [16]. Testicular activity resumes at the summer solstice when day length stops increasing.

Breeding tubercles. Androgens increase the thickness of the skin of the salmon and also increase integumental mucous production. In some fishes breeding tubercles develop on the head of the male. These structures apparently evolved to enable breeding individuals to maintain close contact during spawning and may be particularly important in fishes that spawn in fast-moving water [36, 39].

MECHANISMS OF ANDROGEN ACTION

Androgens mediate their actions through the classical scheme of steroid hormone action (Fig. 4.13): They interact with cytoplasmic and nuclear receptors, a two-step mechanism, to stimulate transcriptional and translational processes related to protein synthesis. For example, $\alpha_{2\mu}$-globulin is a protein synthesized by the liver of the male but not the female rat. Androgen treatment of spayed female rats or castrated male rats induces the appearance of both $\alpha_{2\mu}$-globulin and its corresponding messenger RNA. Glucocorticoids, thyroid hormones, and STH are required for the action of androgens on $\alpha_{2\mu}$-globulin production. The physiological role of this protein is presently undetermined.

Most unusual, however, is the observation that skeletal muscle does not contain specific receptors for androgens; nevertheless, androgens have anabolic actions in a variety of skeletal muscles. It has been proposed that the anabolic actions of androgens (at least in pharmacological doses) in skeletal muscle may derive from androgen competition for cytosolic glucocorticoid receptors [28].

Antiandrogens

Some of the most potent antiandrogens are derivatives of progesterone. Although they may possess weak androgenic activity, they are inhibitory to the actions of testosterone because of their receptor occupancy. Cyproterone acetate is one of the most potent antiandrogens (Fig. 17.6). For example, treatment of the pregnant rat with cyproterone acetate results in male fetuses that are morphologically feminized, and the male rat adult behavior is that of the female. Administration of the antiandrogen in the mature male causes atrophy of the seminal vesicles, prostate, and other androgen-responsive target organs. Pituitary gonadotropin secretion is enhanced after antiandrogen treatment, as after castration, and in the human male cyproterone acetate causes a loss of libido. In the female, on the other hand, this antiandrogen has been used successfully to treat hirsutism and virilization. In the male acne and the development of baldness are reversed by antiandrogen treatment. Although cyproterone acetate has been used with some success to treat precocious puberty, its inhibition of the anabolic actions of androgens may preclude its use in the treatment of sexual precocity.

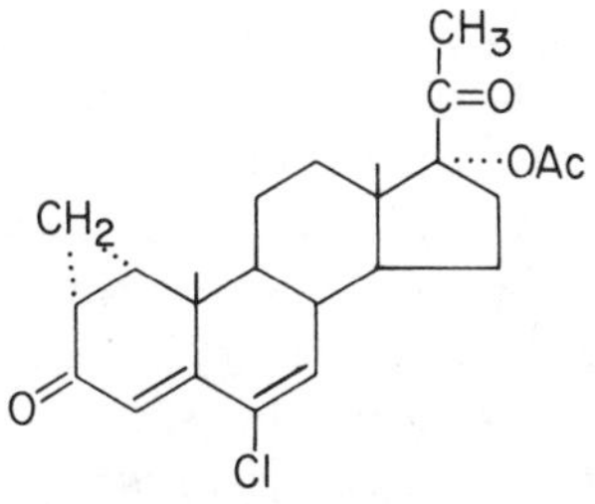

Cyproterone Acetate

Figure 17.6 Structure of cyproterone acetate, an active antiandrogen.

CONTROL OF MALE FERTILITY

Ideally, contraception in the male by endocrine manipulation should be limited to inhibition of spermatogenesis without undue side effects. Unfortunately, this goal has not been realized. Because testosterone is most directly responsible for maintenance of spermatogenesis, most strategies would be expected to be directed toward inhibition of either testosterone biosynthesis or its action on the testis. Theoretically, the following methods might be employed:

1. Production of androgen receptor antagonists (e.g., cyproterone acetate). Ideally such an antagonist would be specific for the gonadal androgen receptor.
2. Inhibition of testosterone biosynthesis by one or more enzymes in the biosynthetic pathway. Such an inhibitor would have to antagonize one of the terminal steps in androgen biosynthesis or adrenal steroid hormone production would also be compromised.
3. Production of antibodies against testosterone. The effects of this accomplished "immunological castration" are similar to those following surgical castration: loss of sexual activity, atrophy of accessory reproductive glands, and an increase in pituitary gonadotropin secretion. However, these phenomena are accompanied by hyperplasia of the Leydig cells and increased testosterone production [30].
4. Production of antibodies against pituitary gonadotropins.
5. Production of antibodies to GnRH. This small peptide has little immunogenicity, but antigenicity has been enhanced by coupling the peptide to larger molecules [33].
6. Production of GnRH receptor antagonists. Inhibitory analogs of GnRH have been demonstrated to be active in males [33]. Research is in progress.

The problem with all these approaches is that when testosterone levels are lowered or the actions of the androgens blocked all other target tissues are also affected. There would be, for example, loss of libido as well as decreased muscle mass and development of a negative nitrogen balance and osteoporosis. Most interesting is the observation that superactive analogs of GnRH, originally developed with the expectation that they might be stimulatory to reproductive function, cause antifertility effects. One mechanism of action of these superagonists may be to cause desensitization of pituitary gonadotrophs and a subsequent decrease in serum gonadotropin and testosterone levels [25]. There is evidence that these agents also cause marked loss of testicular LH receptors [19]. A substance related to GnRH has been localized by immunohistochemical methods in the cytoplasm of the interstitial cells of Leydig and the nuclei of spermatogonia within the seminiferous epithelium of the rat testis [31]. This material is not identical to GnRH. It was suggested that this GnRH-like substance might be synthesized within the Leydig cells and subsequently transported to the germ cells where it is translocated to the nucleus to mediate its inhibitory action.

If the putative inhibin can be isolated, its structure determined, and subsequently synthesized, it is possible that it might prove to be the most ideal male (and female) contraceptive. Because inhibin's actions might be expected to be directed mainly at inhibition of FSH secretion, it might preferentially inhibit spermatogenesis without any effects on testosterone action and metabolism.

Gossypol, a phenolic compound (Fig. 17.7) isolated from the seed, stem, and roots of the cotton plant, may offer a new approach to male contraception. This drug inhibits the enzyme, lactate dehydrogenase, most specifically the LDH isozyme found in sperm cells. Gossypol does not appear to affect sex hormone levels or libido and its contraceptive effects may be fully reversible.

PATHOPHYSIOLOGY

Hypogonadism may result from a failure in pituitary gonadotropin secretion because of an isolated defect in one or the other of the gonadotrophs or to some defect in the hypothalamus resulting in a failure to secrete GnRH. Leydig cell agenesis due to a congenital defect would lead to male pseudohermaphroditism, whereas adult Leydig cell dysfunction may be responsible for the male climacteric experienced by some men [26].

Primary hypergonadism may derive from tumors that secrete excess androgens. Feminizing tumors that secrete estrogens have even been documented in the male. Secondary hypergonadism may result from any factors leading to excessive pituitary gonadotropin secretion. Some few endocrine disorders are outlined in Table 17.2 and discussed below.

Endocrine Disorders

Male pseudohermaphroditism. As noted in Chapter 16, male pseudohermaphroditism may be classified into three broad categories related to defects in the following: (1) testosterone synthesis; (2) androgen receptor synthesis or function; and (3) absent or defective activity of Müllerian regression factor. In addition an isolated

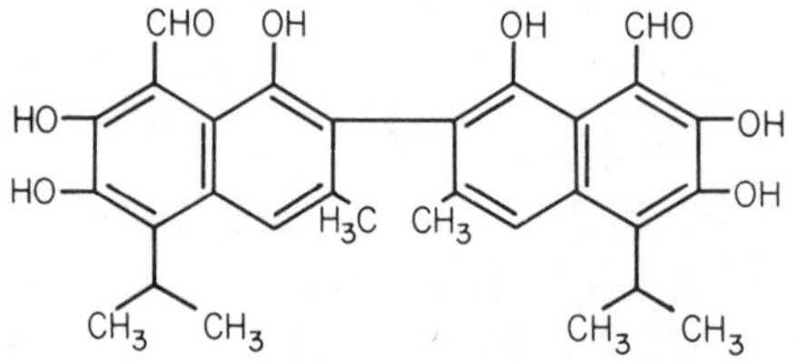

Figure 17.7 The structure of gossypol, a potential male contraceptive drug.

TABLE 17.2 Endocrine Pathophysiology of the Human Male Reproductive System

Hypogonadism
  Primary
    Leydig cell deficiency (Leydig cell agenesis)
    Adult Leydig cell failure (male climacteric phase)
    Germinal cell aplasia (Sertoli-cell-only syndrome)
  Secondary
    Gonadotropin deficiency (hypogonadotropic hypogonadism)
    Hypothalamic hypogonadism (defect in GnRH secretion)
Hypergonadism
  Primary (steroid-secreting testicular tumors)
    Virilizing (androgen-secreting) Leydig (interstitial) cell tumors (macrogenitosomia in the prepubertal
      male)
    Feminizing (estrogen-secreting) Leydig (interstitial) cell tumors
  Secondary
    Hypothalamic origin (enhanced GnRH secretion)
    Pituitary origin (hypergonadotropic hypergonadism)
Syndromes of androgen resistance
  Testicular feminizing syndrome (absence of target tissue androgen receptors)
  Syndrome of 5 α-reductase deficiency (failure to convert testosterone to DHT)
Gynecomastia (breast enlargement)

deficiency of Leydig cells and a defect in any one of the five enzymes required for testosterone biosynthesis will individually lead to male pseudohermaphroditism [15].

Gynecomastia. Growth of the mammary tissue of the male, gynecomastia, may be common during the neonatal period. This enlargement of the breasts is generally attributed to maternal hormones reaching the fetus during gestation. Prepubertal gynecomastia may result from a peripheral conversion of androgens produced by the testes and adrenals to estrogens. Adolescent gynecomastia may be associated with a decreased testosterone/estradiol ratio of unknown etiology. The slow increase in the prevalence of gynecomastia in adult males, which is accentuated over the age of 45, may also be accounted for by the increase with age in estrogen to testosterone levels. Although uncommon, gynecomastia may occur unilaterally rather than bilaterally. If gynecomastia is accompanied by galactorrhea, the possibility of a PRL-secreting tumor should be considered [32].

Premature adrenarche (pubarche). Premature adrenarche refers to the isolated development of sexual hair at an early age due to adrenal androgens. In the female it is known that adrenal androgens are responsible for growth of sexual hair. In the male the penis is of normal size, therefore it is believed that adrenal androgens are also responsible for early sexual hair growth rather than testosterone.

Adult Leydig cell failure (male climacteric phase). In some men Leydig cell function may decline with age; the fall in serum testosterone levels may produce symptoms similar to those of the postmenopausal woman. The age of onset is variable and may be caused by a variety of factors (e.g., secondary to mumps). Although androgen therapy may not improve sexual function, muscle function may be restored thus counteracting the negative nitrogen balance that is a sequel of androgen deficiency.

Feminizing adrenocortical carcinoma. Increased estrogen production by an adrenal tumor may inhibit pituitary-hypothalamic function, resulting in decreased pituitary gonadotropin secretion which, as expected, leads to testicular atrophy.

Sertoli-cell-only syndrome (germinal cell aplasia). This syndrome may arise from a congenital absence of germ cells. The seminiferous tubules are therefore populated only by Sertoli cells. As noted, FSH levels may preferentially be elevated in this syndrome.

Pharmacological Considerations

Cannabinoids (substances present in marihuana, e.g., Δ^9-tetrahydrocannabinol, Δ^9-THC) inhibit testicular function in all vertebrate species studied [3]. Testicular testosterone synthesis is decreased, which is correlated with lowered plasma levels of testosterone and involution of the prostate, seminal vesicles, and epididymus. Prolonged cannabinoid intake also leads to diminished spermatogenesis. The immediate effects of cannabinoids on the male reproductive system appear to be reversible. In humans marihuana smoking decreases plasma testosterone levels and the sperm count. In mice cannabinoids reduce fertility and increase the incidence of chromosomal abnormalities, not only in the treated mice but also in their untreated male offspring. The occurrence of congenital birth defects indicates that cannabinoids are capable of inducing genetic mutations which are transmissible to offspring [7]. Alcoholism may also lead to gonadal dysfunction, possibly by diminishing the number of gonadotropin receptors possessed by Leydig cells.

REFERENCES

[1] BARDIN, C. W., and J. F. CATTERALL. 1981. Testosterone: a major determinant in extragonadal sexual dimorphism. *Science* 211:1285–94.

[2] BARFIELD, R. J. 1969. Activation of copulatory behavior by androgen implanted into the preoptic area of the male fowl. *Horm. Behav.* 1:37–52.

[3] BLOCH, E., B. THYSEN, G. A. MORRELL, E. GARDNER, and G. FUJIMOTO. 1978. Effects of cannabinoids on reproduction and development. *Vit. Horm.* 36:203–58.

[4] BREEDLOVE, S. M., and A. P. ARNOLD. 1980. Hormone accumulation in a sexually dimorphic motor nucleus of the rat spinal cord. *Science* 210:564–66.

[5] BROOKS, D. E. 1981. Metabolic activity in the epididymus and its regulation by androgens. *Physiol. Rev.* 61:515–55.

[6] COQUELIN, A., and F. H. BRONSON. 1979. Release of luteinizing hormone in male mice during exposure to females: habituation of the response. *Science* 206:1099–1100.

[7] DALTERIO, S., F. BADR, A. BARTKE, and D. MAYFIELD. 1982. Cannabinoids in male mice: effects on fertility and spermatogenesis. *Science* 216:315–16.

[8] DAVIES, A. G. 1981. Role of FSH in the control of testicular function. *Arch. Androl.* 7:97–108.

[9] DE KRETSER, D. M., H. G. BURGER, and B. HUDSON. 1974. The relationship between germinal cells and serum FSH levels in males with infertility. *J. Clin. Endocrinol. Metab.* 38:787–93.

[10] DENT, J. N. 1975. Integumentary effects of prolactin in the lower vertebrates. *Amer. Zool.* 15:923-35.

[11] DESJARDINS, C. 1981. Endocrine signaling and male reproduction. *Biol. Reprod.* 24:1-21.

[12] DORRINGTON, J. H., and D. T. ARMSTRONG. 1979. Effects of FSH on gonadal function. *Rec. Prog. Horm. Res.* 35:301-42.

[13] DUFAU, M. L., and K. J. CATT. 1978. Gonadotropin receptors and regulation of steroidogenesis in the testis and ovary. *Vit. Horm.* 36:461-592.

[14] FRANCHIMONT, P., J. VERSTRAELEN-PROYARD, M. T. HAZEE-HAGELSTEIN, CH. RENARD, A. DEMOULIN, J. P. BOURGUIGNON, and J. HUSTIN. 1979. Inhibin: from concept to reality. *Vit. Horm.* 37:243-302.

[15] GIVENS, J. R., W. L. WISER, R. L. SUMMITT, I. J. KERBER, R. N. ANDERSON, D. E. PITTAWAY, and S. A. FISH. 1974. Familial male pseudohermaphroditism without gynecomastia due to deficient testicular 17-ketosteroid reductase activity. *New Engl. J. Med.* 29:938-44.

[16] GOSS, R. J. 1968. Inhibition of growth and shedding of antlers by sex hormones. *Nature* 220:83-85.

[17] HAMILTON, J. B. 1942. Male hormone stimulation is prerequisite and incident in common baldness. *Am. J. Anat.* 71:451-80.

[18] HÖHN, E. O., and S. C. CHENG. 1967. Gonadal hormones on Wilson's phalarope (*Steganopus tricolor*) and other birds in relation to plumage and sex behavior. *Gen. Comp. Endocrinol.* 8:1-11.

[19] HSUEH, A. J. W., and G. F. ERICKSON. 1979. Extra-pituitary inhibition of testicular function by luteinizing hormone releasing hormone. *Nature* 281:66-67.

[20] HUTCHISON, J. B., and T. STEIMER. 1981. Brain 5 β-reductase: a correlate of behavioral sensitivity to androgen. *Science* 213:244-46.

[21] JOHNS, J. E. 1964. Testosterone induced nuptial feathers in phalaropes. *Condor* 66:449-54.

[22] JONES, R. E. 1971. The incubation patch of birds. *Biol. Rev.* 46:315-39.

[23] KOENIG, H., A. GOLDSTONE, G. BLUME, and C. Y. LEE. 1980. Testosterone-mediated sexual dimorphism of mitochondria and lysosomes in mouse kidney promimal tubules. *Science* 209:1023-26.

[24] LINCOLN, G. A. 1971. The seasonal reproductive changes in the Red Deer stag (*Cervus elaphus*). *J. Zool. Lond.* 163:105-23.

[25] LINDE, R., G. C. DOELLE, N. ALEXANDER, F. KIRCHNER, W. VALE, J. RIVIER, and D. RABIN. 1981. Reversible inhibition of testicular steroidogenesis and spermatogenesis by a potent gonadotropin-releasing hormone agonist in normal men. *New Engl. J. Med.* 305:663-67.

[26] LIPSETT, M. B. 1980. Physiology and pathology of the Leydig cell. *New Engl. J. Med.* 303:602-88.

[27] LUMPKIN, M., A. NEGRO-VILAR, P. FRANCHIMONT, and S. MCCANN. 1981. Evidence for a hypothalamic site of action of inhibin to suppress FSH releae. *Endocrinology* 108:1101-104.

[28] MAYER, M., and F. ROSEN. 1975. Interaction of anabolic steroids with glucocorticoid receptor sites in rat muscle cytosol. *Am. J. Physiol.* 229:1381-86.

[29] MEANS, A. R., J. R. DEDMAN, J. S. TASH, D. J. TINDALL, M. VAN SICKLE, and M. S. WELSH. 1980. Regulation at the testis Sertoli cell by follicle stimulating hormone. *Ann. Rev. Physiol.* 42:59-70.

[30] NIESCHLAG, E., and E. J. WICKINGS. 1978. Biological effects of antibodies to gonadal steroids. *Vit. Horm.* 36:165-202.

[31] PAULL, W. K., C. M. TURKELSON, C. R. THOMAS, and A. ARIMURA. 1981. Immunohisto-

chemical demonstration of a testicular substance related to luteinizing hormone-releasing hormone. *Science* 213:1263–64.

[32] PENNY, R. 1979. The testis. *Pediat. Clin. North America* 26:107–21.

[33] SCHALLY, A. V., A. ARIMURA, and D. H. COY. 1980. Recent approaches to fertility control based on derivatives of LH-RH. *Vit. Horm.* 38:257–323.

[34] SETCHELL, B. P. 1980. The functional significance of the blood-testis barrier. *J. Androl.* 1:3–10.

[35] SHAW, M. J., L. E. GEORGOPOULOS, and A. H. PAYNE. 1979. Synergistic effect of follicle-stimulating hormone and luteinizing hormone on testicular Δ^5-3 β-hydroxysteroid dehydrogenase-isomerase: application of a new method for the separation of testicular compartments. *Endocrinology* 104:912–18. © 1979 The Endocrine Society.

[36] SMITH, R. J. F. 1974. Effects of 17 β-methyltestosterone on the dorsal pad and tubercles of flathead minnows (*Pimephales promelas*). *Can. J. Zool.* 52:1031–38.

[37] STEINBERGER, A., and E. STEINBERGER. 1976. Secretion of an FSH-inhibiting factor by cultured Sertoli cells. *Endocrinology* 99:918–21.

[38] STEINBERGER, E. 1971. Hormonal control of spermatogenesis. *Physiol. Rev.* 51:1–22.

[39] WILEY, M. L., and B. B. COLLETTE. 1970. Breeding tubercles and contact organs in fishes, their occurrence, structure and significance. *Amer. Mus. Natur. Hist. Bull.* 143:147–53.

[40] ZIPF, W. B., A. H. PAYNE, and R. P. KELCH. 1978. Prolactin, growth hormone, and luteinizing hormone receptors. *Endocrinology* 103:595–600.

18

Hormones and Female Reproductive Physiology

INTRODUCTION

It was noted earlier that in the mammal the female phenotype develops spontaneously, apparently in the absence of any gonadal hormone directive. At puberty, however, ovarian steroid hormone secretion is essential for development of female secondary sex characteristics. In addition gonadal hormone production regulates the cyclic pattern of pituitary gonadotropin secretion characteristic of the female which is responsible for other cyclic phenomena as egg maturation, ovulation, and the menstrual cycle.

It has long been known that ovariectomy results in uterine atrophy and the loss of sexual activity and reproductive function. The role of the ovaries in the control of reproductive function was established in 1900 by Knauer who found that ovarian transplants prevented the atrophic symptoms of gonadectomy. Ovarian extracts were then found to maintain the integrity of reproductive structures following ovariectomy. Allen and Doisy identified the Graffian follicle as a major source of estrogenic activity [2]. A putative female sex hormone was then discovered in the blood of a number of animals, and it was further observed that the concentration of the substance varied with the phase of the menstrual cycle in the human female. An important discovery was the finding that this substance, a steroid, was present in the urine in large amounts during pregnancy. Chemists were able to isolate the active substance from urine in crystalline form and to determine its chemical structure. This steroid hormone, *estradiol*, plays an essential role in the control of secondary sex characteristics in the female of most vertebrate species. It was also established that the corpus luteum of the ovary secreted a steroid hormone which is necessary for normal reproductive function during pregnancy. This hormone, *progesterone*, was isolated and subsequently synthesized in 1934.

Although ovarian estrogens and progestins play pivotal roles in the regulation of female reproductive function, it is now realized that many other hormones of neural, placental-uterine, and adrenal origin are also essential in the female [16].

ANATOMY OF THE FEMALE REPRODUCTIVE SYSTEM

The female reproductive system consists of a pair of ovaries which serve gametogenic and endocrine functions (Fig. 18.1). The female gametes, ova, are released (ovulated) from the ovary into the abdominal cavity where they find their way into the closely adherent uterine tubes (Fallopian tubes, oviducts). The eggs may become fertilized en route down the oviducts by spermatozoa previously introduced into the vagina by the male ejaculate. If fertilization occurs, the fertilized egg, the *zygote*, may then become embedded within the lining of the uterus and through embryogenesis develop into a fetus. The general morphological and functional features of the human female reproductive system will be described.

Ovary

The gonad in the homogametic species develops in the absence of any apparent endocrine influence (Chapter 16). In the human female the gametogenic potential of the ovary is established early in fetal development, but the endocrine role of the ovary is not realized until puberty. Each of the embryonic ovaries is initially populated by about 1000 to 2000 *primordial germ cells* which through rapid proliferation give rise in each ovary to about 3 million oocytes. At birth this number is reduced through cell death to about 1 million oocytes in each ovary and by puberty each ovary may only be populated by about 250,000 oocytes. Only an exceedingly small fraction of these viable oocytes will develop fully into mature egg cells. Indeed, because a single ovum is usually ovulated during each reproductive cycle, only about 400 to 500 oocytes are released from the ovary; the remaining 99.9% are destined for atresia during the years of ovarian activity (puberty to menopause).

As discussed, the ovary consists of both epithelial and mesenchymal components. The mesenchymal tissue differentiates into interstitial tissue which will be the primary source of estrogen production by the ovary. The epithelial tissue will become closely associated with the germinal elements of the ovary and, in addition to providing a nutritive environment for the oocytes, will also provide an important source of hormones during particular phases of the female cycle.

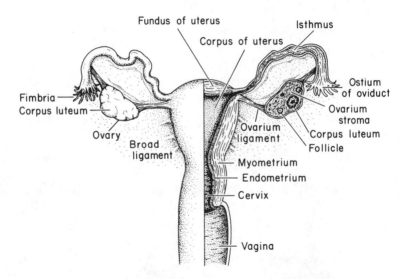

Figure 18.1   Reproductive organs of the human female.

At birth each oocyte is surrounded by a single layer of flattened epithelial-derived *granulosa cells;* the combined structure is termed a *primordial follicle* (Fig. 18.2). These primordial follicles lie mostly near the periphery (cortex) of the ovary but are separated from each other by stromal (connective) and interstitial tissue. Most primary follicles remain in an arrested state, which may last until puberty or even menopause, if they are not selected for further differentiation and development. Within the embryonic ovary the primordial follicles begin the reduction division of meiosis, but when meiotic division is delayed in the late prophase, the follicles and contained primary oocytes may continue to increase greatly in size. Further development of a primordial follicle involves development of the follicular epithelial cells into a single layer of cuboidal cells surrounding the oocyte; the composite structure is referred to as a *primary follicle* (Fig. 18.2).

Under endocrine stimulation once during each ovarian cycle after puberty, six to 12 primary follicles develop into *secondary follicles*. This process involves an increase in the size of the oocyte and in the number of layers of granulosa cells that surround each oocyte (Fig. 18.2). During the development of these secondary follicles, the granulosa cells secrete a mucoid material that forms the *zona pellucida* around the oocyte (Fig. 18.2). The granulosa cells develop protoplasmic processes that penetrate the zona pellucida and make contact with the plasmalemma of the oocyte. Although a number of primary follicles may be selected for further development into secondary follicles during each menstrual cycle, only one is usually destined to develop into a mature follicle. The others by some unknown process become atretic and disappear with time.

During each ovarian cycle selected primary oocytes complete the first meiotic division with resulting extrusion of the first polar body and formation of a *secondary oocyte* which contains most of the cytoplasm. The first meiotic division is completed shortly before ovulation. The secondary oocyte then immediately enters the second reduction division of meiosis, a process which is arrested in metaphase unless fer-

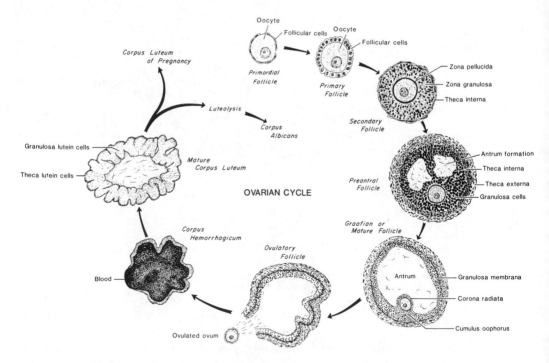

Figure 18.2 The primate ovarian follicular cycle.

tilization occurs subsequent to ovulation. The second polar body is extruded if the oocyte is penetrated by a sperm. The diploid state of the transiently haploid oocyte is therefore reconstituted by the haploid chromosomal contribution of the sperm to the zygote.

The granulosa cells of follicles destined for further maturation continue to increase in number. At the same time interstitial tissue adjacent to the follicle becomes arranged concentrically around the follicle to form the *theca* (theca folliculi). Those thecal cells adjacent to the follicle, the *theca interna*, are surrounded by an additional outer layer of interstitial cells, the *theca externa*, which merges somewhat imperceptively with the ovarian stroma. The theca interna remains separated from the granulosa cells by a basement lamella. Although the theca is penetrated by vascular elements, no capillaries penetrate into the granulosa.

Continued proliferation of granulosa cells and the incorporation of surrounding interstitial cells into the theca are accompanied by the accumulation of fluid in spaces or clefts within the granulosa cells. As the follicle enlarges, a single large vesicle or antrum is formed. Those granulosa cells that remain adherent to the ovum comprise the coronal granulosa cells; those granulosa cells that remain in contact with the surrounding theca constitute the *granulosa membrana*. A bridge of granulosa cells connects those cells adherent to the ovum with the granulosa membrana and constitutes the *cumulus oophorus*. During ovulation this connection is severed and the ovum is ejected with its surrounding layer of granulosa cells, the *corona radiata*. The fully developed mature follicle, shown in Fig. 18.3, is known as a *Graafian follicle*.

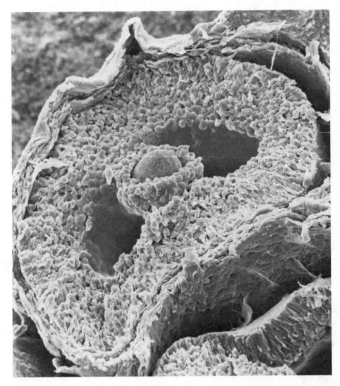

Figure 18.3 Scanning electron micrograph of the human Graafian follicle. (From
P. Bagavadoss. The Reproductive Endocrinology Program, Department of Anatomy,
The University of Michigan.)

The mechanisms controlling rupture of the mature ovarian follicle during ovulation have been debated and many hypotheses provided. In the hamster, for example, smooth muscle cells (SMC) are present within the theca externa at the base of the follicle. Contraction of these muscle cells is believed to squeeze the cumulus mass toward the apex of the cell. Tension within the follicle wall then results in a thinning of the apical layers leading to rupture of the follicle. Although it might be assumed that high levels of LH are responsible for follicular SMC contraction, it is not known whether the hormone directly or indirectly stimulates the cells. Local changes in the environment of the SMC could lead to their contraction. Whatever the stimulus may be, it appears to be mediated through the production of $PGF_{2\alpha}$ probably generated in response to an inward Ca^{2+} ion flux [14]. It might also be expected that cGMP would be an intracellular second messenger involved in myofilament activation within SMC (Fig. 14.10). Other models have suggested that production or activation of follicular proteases (collageneses) may be essential to the mechanism of ovulation.

After rupture of the mature follicle and liberation of the ovum during ovulation, the follicle promptly fills up with blood, forming what is called a *corpus hemorrhagicum*. The granulosa and thecal cells rapidly increase in number and the clotted blood is absorbed. Vascular elements from the theca now penetrate the granulosa cells. The granulosa cells begin to accumulate large quantities of cholesterol; this luteinization process leads to formation of the *corpus luteum*. The mature corpus luteum of some species appears to contain a number of distinct cell types. Cells derived from the theca interna migrate into granulosa-derived areas of the luteal tissue soon after ovulation to give rise to small luteal cells, theca lutein cells, and fibroblasts. The large luteal cells apparently differentiate from the membrana granulosa. Although luteal cell heterogeneity is commonly accepted, the definitive origin of each cell type and their individual functions within the corpus luteum of pregnancy remain unclear.

Fallopian Tubes

In the human female these paired oviducts are about 10 cm long and are closely adherent to the superolateral aspects of the uterus (Fig. 18.1). The ostium tubae, the fimbriated ovarian extremity of the oviduct, spread over most of the medial surface of the ovary, and the undulatory movements of the fimbriae assist ova transport into the lumen of the Fallopian tubes. The oviducts proper are composed of longitudinal and circular muscular layers covered by a simple columnar epithelium which comprises the mucosa. The ciliated mucosal cells beat toward the uterus and thus rapidly convey the ova toward the uterus. Fertilization of the egg takes place within the oviducts.

Uterus

The uterus, connected to the oviducts at superolateral angles, is a thick-walled, muscular organ that serves as a site for fetal development and as an endocrine organ during pregnancy. The bulk of the uterus is composed of smooth muscle, the *myometrium* (Fig. 18.1). An *endometrium* covers the mucosal aspect of the myometrium and is composed of connective tissue and an extensive vascular network. The endometrium, in turn, is covered by a simple epithelium. The thickness of the endometrium varies dramatically throughout the menstrual cycle in response to ovarian hormones. The myometrium is also similarly variable in thickness, most profoundly during pregnancy.

OVARIAN STEROID HORMONES

The ovarian follicle is the source of three types of steroid hormones: progestogens (progestins), androgens, and estrogens. The relative amounts of each class of steroid vary throughout the menstrual cycle and drastically change in the pregnant state. During the follicular phase of the menstrual cycle estradiol is the major steroid hormone secreted by the ovary, whereas during the luteal phase and during pregnancy progesterone is the major steroid hormone secreted. Controversy surrounds the source of estrogen production by the ovary.

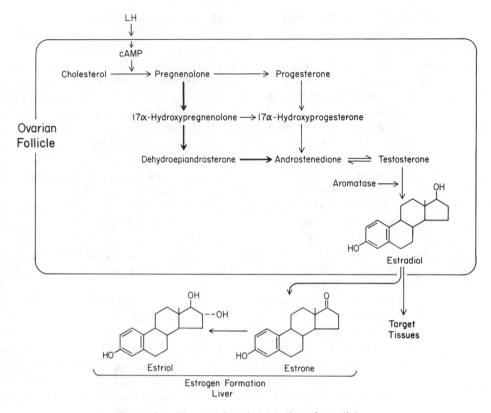

Figure 18.4 Biosynthesis and metabolism of estradiol.

Estrogen Biosynthesis

It has been believed that the thecal cells are the source of estrogen production which predominates during the follicular phase of the cycle (Fig. 18.4). The *two-cell theory* of estrogen production states, however, that the thecal cells produce C-19 androgens that are delivered to the granulosa cells where they are aromatized to estrogens (Fig. 18.5). This theory is supported by the observation that granulosa cells from several species secrete estrogens if given an androgen substrate. In addition thecal cells pro-

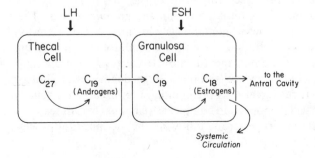

Figure 18.5 Two-cell, two-gonadotropin hypothesis of estrogen synthesis [11].

Ovarian Steroid Hormones

duce large amounts of androgens. Granulosa cells, on the other hand, have little or no capacity for producing C-19 androgens from C-21 steroids but do have an active aromatase system. There is evidence that as follicular maturation progresses the ability of granulosa cells to aromatize androgens increases. Estrogen production increases within the follicle during the preovulatory phase and is highest at the time of the LH/FSH surge. Before exposure to a high level of LH, androgen and estrogen levels predominate; after the LH surge and during the luteal phase of the cycle, however, progesterone is the major steroid produced. A complex number of interactions involving LH, FSH, androgens, progesterone, and estrogens are undoubtedly involved in the shift from estrogen to progesterone synthesis [8, 13].

A modified version [5] of the two-cell theory suggests that LH stimulates androgen production within the thecal cells. The androgens are then aromatized within the thecal cells but are also made available to the granulosa cells for aromatization to estrogens. The estrogens produced by the thecal cells would be the major source of circulating levels of the steroid, whereas estrogens synthesized by the granulosa cells would serve a local role, possibly related to ovum maturation. The granulosa cells are regulated through FSH stimulation of cAMP production and subsequent induction and activation of aromatase activity.

Estradiol is readily oxidized to *estrone* within the liver; estrone may be further hydrated to *estriol*. These three estrogens are excreted in the urine as glucuronides and sulfates. During pregnancy the placenta is an additional source of estrogens. Indeed, the formation of estrogens is not limited to the ovaries, placenta, or adrenals as some peripheral tissues (e.g., adipose tissue) can produce significant quantities of estrogens from steroid precursors. Aromatization of androstenedione and testosterone within these tissues is a major source of estrogens in the male and postmenopausal female. Incredibly, the stallion produces more estrogens than any other animal for which data are available.

Progesterone Biosynthesis

Progesterone synthesis is an early step in the biosynthesis of androgen and estrogen production with the thecal cell. Thecal cell progesterone production is not, however, considered an important source of vascular levels of progesterone. The corpus luteum is the major source of circulating progesterone. During the follicular phase of the cycle these cells, which are essentially devoid of a smooth endoplasmic reticulum characteristic of steroid-secreting cells, may utilize an androgen substrate for aromatization to estrogens as discussed. Just prior to the LH/FSH surge in some species, progesterone biosynthesis is initiated within the granulosa cells. The fact that granulosa cells from large follicles spontaneously luteinize in culture but fail to do so in the presence of follicular fluid obtained from small follicles suggests that a luteinization inhibitor may be present and function to keep granulosa cells from secreting prematurely [5]. Luteinized cells contain large quantities of cholesterol, and it has been shown that rat luteal cells preferentially utilize and are acutely dependent on plasma low density lipoprotein complexes (Chapter 15). Luteal cells are the major source of circulating progesterone following the luteinization process.

Androgens

With the commencement of ovarian estrogen synthesis at puberty, androstenedione and testosterone, precursors of estrogens, are secreted by the ovaries. The development of secondary sex characteristics during the pubertal process appears to be almost totally accountable by the actions of estrogens. Nevertheless, it is possible that the growth spurt that occurs at puberty may, in part, be influenced by androgens of ovarian origin. In addition acne, common to many females at puberty, results from sebaceous gland activation by ovarian androgens. Pubic and axillary hair growth are also attributed to androgens of ovarian or adrenal origin.

PHYSIOLOGICAL ROLES OF OVARIAN STEROID HORMONES

There is no evidence that the fetal or preadolescent human ovary produces significant quantities of estrogens or other gonadal steroids. At puberty, however, ovarian steroidogenesis is activated by pituitary gonadotropins. During the follicular phase of the ensuing menstrual cycles estrogens are the main steroidal products of the ovary, whereas during the luteal phase of each cycle progesterone is the hormonally important steroidal product of the postovulatory follicle.

Estrogens

Estrogens produced during pubertal maturation in the human female are responsible for growth and development of the vagina, uterus, and oviducts, organs essential to ovum transport and zygote maturation and implantation of the conceptus. Estrogens affect the distribution of fat deposition, a process that occurs in the postadolescent female. Mammary growth and development is also initiated by the actions of estrogens in concert with other hormones. Estrogens acting on specific nuclear sites within the brain affect the libido which is usually first evident in the adolescent female. Other physiological actions of estrogens are summarized in Table 18.1.

Progesterone

Progesterone is the ovarian hormone of pregnancy and is responsible for preparation of the reproductive tract for implantation by the zygote and the subsequent maintenance of the pregnant state. It has been speculated that preovulatory plasma levels of progesterone may trigger sexual behavior in some species. In some rodents, for example, progesterone appears necessary for induction of sexual receptivity. Progesterone may also play a role in the initiation of nest-building activity and brooding behavior in some avian species. It must be emphasized that many actions of progesterone are usually, if not exclusively, on estrogen-primed tissues. Table 18.1 summarizes the known physiological roles of progesterone in the human female.

TABLE 18.1 Some Physiological Effects and Roles of Ovarian Steroid Hormones in Mammals

Primary site of action	Physiological action
Estradiol	
CNS	Maintains libido and sexual behavior
Pituitary	Has negative and positive feedback effects on gonadotropin secretion
	Increases pituitary TRH receptor number
	Increases pituitary GnRH receptor number
	Increases oxytocin production
Ovary	Is required for ovum maturation (is luteolytic in some mammalian species)
Vagina	Causes proliferation and cornification of the mucosa
Oviducts	Causes growth and development in preparation for gamete transport
Uterus	
Cervix	Increases mucus secretion
Endometrium	Increases blood flow
	Increases prostaglandin biosynthesis at term
	Increases number of oxytocin receptors at term
	Causes decidualization response (increases the number of estrogen receptors in the decidua)
Myometrium	Synthesizes contractile proteins of smooth muscle cells
	Increases membrane excitability (increases sensitivity to oxytocin)
Mammary glands	Causes ductule and stromal growth and development, fat accretion
Skin	Induces sebaceous gland secretion (thinner fluid)
	Stimulates axillary and pubic hair growth (possibly in concert with gonadal and adrenal androgens)
General body effects	Causes H_2O and Na^+ retention, weight gain (anabolic action), and female type of fat distribution
	Maintains bone mineral deposition
Liver	Causes hepatic angiotensinogen production
	Causes hepatic production of thyroid binding globulin
Blood	Decreases plasma cholesterol formation
Progesterone	
CNS	Increases sexual receptivity (at least in some mammalian species)
	Inhibits pituitary gonadotropin secretion by an action on the hypothalamus during the ovarian luteal phase
Oviducts	Causes growth and development for gamete transport
Uterus	
Endometrium	Stimulates growth and development in preparation for blastocyst implantation
	Decreases estrogen receptor number (at least, in the rat)
Cervix	Increases mucus consistency
Myometrium	Causes antiestrogen effects (myometrial hyperpolarization, decreased sensitivity to oxytocin, decreased estrogen receptor number; "maintenance of pregnancy")
Vagina	Inhibits estrogen-induced vaginal cornification
Mammary glands	Is necessary for lobular-alveolar development (in some species)
	Inhibits prepartum prolactin-induced lactogenesis by decreasing PRL receptor number
General body effects	Causes thermogenic action (rise in basal metabolic rate)

MECHANISMS OF ACTION OF OVARIAN STEROID HORMONES

Ovarian steroid hormones stimulate their target tissues through an initial interaction with cytosolic receptors as described for steroid receptors in general (Fig. 4.13). The actions of steroid hormones on egg protein synthesis in nonmammalian vertebrates have provided particularly important insights into the detailed mechanisms of steroid hormone action, particularly those processes related to selective gene expression. The actions of estrogens in the amphibian liver and of progesterone in the oviduct of the chick will be described [19, 21].

Estrogens and Vitellogenesis

The maturation of the amphibian oocyte in some species provides a good model for understanding steroid hormone action. In response to environmental cues pituitary gonadotropins stimulate estrogen production by follicular cells of the ovary. Circulating estrogens then stimulate hepatic production of *vitellogenin*, a protein precursor of egg proteins. Vitellogenin is normally only produced by egg-producing females, not by males [23]. Nevertheless, the liver of the male frog, *Xenopus laevis*, can be induced by estrogens to produce large amounts of the protein which are then released into the blood; the response is specific to estrogens as other gonadal and adrenal steroids are similarly ineffective. The isolated liver of the male *Xenopus* has provided a model system for the study of estrogen action [23]. The immediate action of estrogen appears to involve an increase in the number of nuclear estrogen receptors, and the subsequent continued stimulation is responsible for the induction of vitellogen mRNA. Vitellogenin is then selectively taken up by the pinocytotic activity of the oocytes. After uptake the vitellogenin is converted mainly into two smaller proteins, lipovitellin and phosvitin, by proteolytic enzymes within the oocytes. The products of vitellogenin cleavage are incorporated into the crystalline lattice of the yolk platelets which may account for up to 90% of the protein content of mature oocytes.

Progesterone and Egg Protein Synthesis

The chick oviduct has provided an exquisite model system for understanding the mechanism of gonadal steroids, particularly progesterone [19]. Steroid hormones initially bind to cytoplasmic proteinaceous receptors which undergo activation and are translocated to the nucleus. Within the nucleus the hormone-receptor complex binds to chromatin receptor sites, which results in the activation of specific genes and the transcription of new species of mRNA which often code for proteins specific to the target tissue. The immature oviduct of the chick is a tubular structure consisting of relatively undifferentiated cells. In response to estrogen stimulation the cells differentiate and grow to produce tubular glands which comprise most cells of the oviduct of the mature egg-laying hen. These cells respond to estrogens by synthesizing proteins that comprise the egg white (e.g., ovalbumin). Although the undifferentiated oviduct does not respond to progesterone, the oviduct of the es-

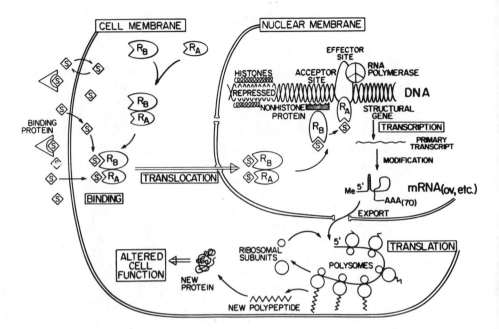

Figure 18.6 General scheme of steroid hormone action. (From O'Malley, B. W. and R. E. Buller, "Mechanisms of Steroid Hormone Action", The Journal of Investigative Dermatology, 68:1–4, 1977. © 1977 by The Williams & Wilkins Company.)

trogenized chick does by synthesis and secretion of the protein avidin. In addition to the production of egg proteins estrogen-stimulated differentiation of the chick oviduct also induces the production of progesterone receptors. If estrogen administration is discontinued, the oviductal cells atrophy to some extent and there is cessation of synthesis of mRNA's and protein synthesis. In response to a secondary stimulation, however, progesterone is able to stimulate the synthesis of ovalbumin as well as avidin [19].

Each of two nonidentical subunits of the progesterone receptor can bind the hormone. The polypeptide subunit is probably a product of a separate gene. Upon activation by progesterone, the inact cytosolic complex translocates to the nucleus where it binds with chick oviduct chromatin. The larger B subunit is responsible for

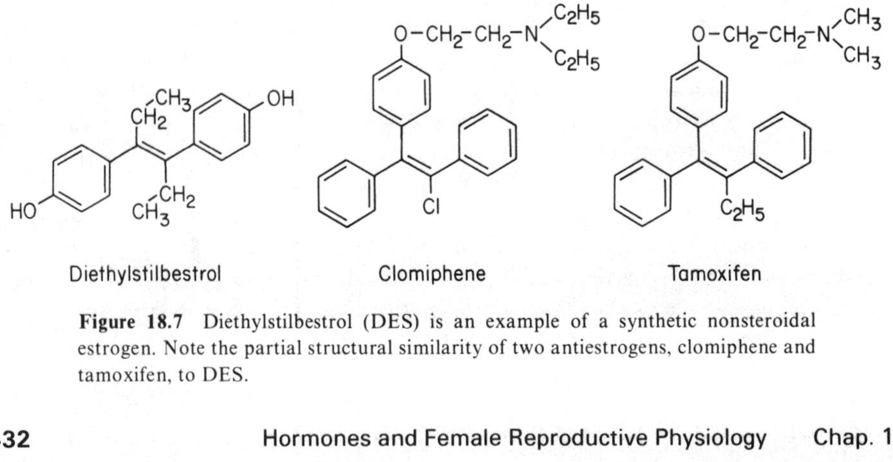

Diethylstilbestrol   Clomiphene   Tamoxifen

Figure 18.7 Diethylstilbestrol (DES) is an example of a synthetic nonsteroidal estrogen. Note the partial structural similarity of two antiestrogens, clomiphene and tamoxifen, to DES.

recognizing and interacting with a specific nonhistone chromatin protein (acceptor site). Following this initial interaction, the A subunit of the A-B complex is liberated and interacts with DNA to activate RNA synthesis. There appears to be no nucleotide sequence specificity (the A subunit binds to any DNA), but rather, it is likely that the interaction of the A subunit is with DNA near the chromatin binding site. The B subunit binding site has a helix-destabilizing effect which may result in an unwinding of the DNA, thus exposing nucleotide sites for the initiation of RNA synthesis. A model for the general mechanism of action of steroid hormones is depicted (Fig. 18.6).

Nonsteroidal Estrogens and Antiestrogens

A number of nonsteroidal compounds possess estrogenic activity, the most potent of which is diethylstilbestrol (DES). The similarity in structure of DES to the natural steroids is illustrated (Fig. 18.7). DES is highly active when given orally, apparently because it is degraded more slowly in the GI tract. Antiestrogens, such as clomiphene and tamoxifen (Fig. 18.7), are typically nonsteroidal compounds that, through competition of estrogen receptors, prevent actions of endogenous estrogens from expressing their full effects on their target tissues. By this action they antagonize a variety of estrogen-dependent processes such as uterine growth and negative feedback to the hypothalamus. Interest in these drugs derives from the hope that they might prove useful in preventing the growth of estrogen-dependent mammary tumors (Chapter 19).

NEUROENDOCRINE CONTROL OF OVARIAN FUNCTION

Activation and maintenance of normal follicular function is dependent on gonadotropins secreted by the adenohypophysis (Chapter 5). Both follicle stimulating hormone (FSH) and luteinizing hormone (LH) are required to stimulate ovarian changes leading to ovulation. Treatment of hypophysectomized immature female animals with purified LH causes thecal and interstitial cell stimulation but no follicular growth and, depending on the species, no significant estrogen production. When injections of purified FSH are given, follicular development proceeds only to antrum formation and only minimal amounts of estrogens are produced. Normal follicular development only occurs when both FSH and LH are administered to an animal. These observations support the two-cell, two-gonadotropin scheme of follicular development and steroid hormone production [18].

Pituitary gonadotropin secretion is initiated during pubertal development and, indeed, secretion of gonadotropins at this time is responsible for the development of secondary sex characteristics typical of the adult female [24]. The CNS organizational basis for cyclic release of pituitary gonadotropins in the adult female is established early in fetal development (Chapter 16). The detailed mechanisms controlling pituitary gonadotropin secretion are best understood in the primate and rodent; this text will discuss only the former.

Elegant studies on the rhesus monkey have established the role of the brain and pituitary in the control of ovarian function in the primate [12]. Pituitary gonadotropin secretion is critically dependent on hypothalamic GnRH release. Administration of antisera to GnRH causes an abrupt reduction in plasma gonadotropin concentrations. Discrete lesions within the medial basal hypothalamus of the female monkey result in a sudden decrease in plasma gonadotropin levels. There is a pulsatile pattern of gonadotropin secretion with a frequency of approximately one pulse per hour ("circhoral") [12]. The concentration of GnRH in pituitary stalk blood of ovariectomized monkeys fluctuates with a frequency similar to that of pituitary gonadotropin secretion. The circhoral rhythm of gonadotropin secretion is abolished by α-adrenoceptor antagonists, suggesting that pulsatile GnRH release is regulated by neural elements, most specifically, neurons of the arcuate nuclei. The neuroendocrine elements responsible for the regulation of gonadotropin secretion appear to be restricted to the medial basal hypothalamus. Unlike that of the rat, the preoptic-anterior hypothalamic area appears *not* to be required for the initiation of preovulatory surges of gonadotropin.

Although GnRH of hypothalamic origin is an obligatory requirement for gonadotropin secretion, its stimulatory action on the pituitary appears to be dependent on the permissive actions of estradiol. There is compelling evidence that the duration of the primate menstrual cycle is determined not by the brain but rather by the ovary itself, through estrogens acting directly on the pituitary. If the hypothalamic source of GnRH is removed by discrete lesions and GnRH is administered by chronic, intermittent intravenous infusion, the pituitary responds by pulsatile release of gonadotropins. These animals go through "normal" menstrual cycles including a preovulatory surge of LH/FSH and typical follicular and luteal phase levels of plasma estradiol and progesterone. The preovulatory gonadotropin surge does not require an increase of GnRH by the hypothalamus. The initial levels of estrogens during the early follicular phase of the menstrual cycle exert a negative feedback action directly on pituitary gonadotropin secretion. After estrogen levels rise and remain above a critical level for at least 36 hours, the negative feedback action is reversed and a positive feedback ensues which results in the preovulatory gonadotropin surge. The positive effect of estrogens on LH and FSH secretion may be due to an increase in pituitary GnRH receptors [1].

Apparently the duration of the ovarian cycle, at least in the rhesus monkey, is determined by the characteristic (genetically programmed) duration of follicular development as well as the functional life span of the corpus luteum. The sum of both processes is approximately 28 days [12]. Evidently there is activation of a hypothalamic arcuate (nucleus) oscillator from almost total inactivity before puberty to an adult frequency of about one pulse of GnRH secretion per hour. During the luteal phase of the cycle and during pregnancy ovarian progesterone inhibits estrogen-induced gonadotropin surges by an action on the central nervous system. This neuronal mechanism is inhibited again during pregnancy as a result of suckling-induced PRL secretion. This action may involve a reduction of the frequency of the arcuate oscillator [12].

Catecholestrogens

The first step in the metabolism of estradiol is oxidation to estrone which may be further metabolized through hydroxylation of the A and D rings. The principal product of A-ring hydroxylation is 2-hydroxyestrone, referred to as a *catecholes-*

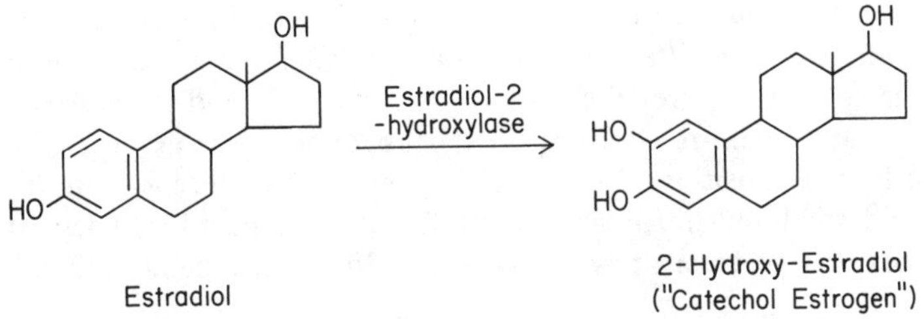

Figure 18.8 Biosynthesis of a catecholestrogen.

trogen because of the structural similarity of the hydroxylated A ring to the catechol nucleus (Fig. 18.8; Fig. 14.1). There is accumulating evidence that 2-hydroxyestrone may play a role in the control of pituitary gonadotropin secretion [9]. This catecholestrogen is reported to affect both LH and PRL secretion in humans, but the precise actions of the putative hormone are presently unclear. 2-Hydroxyestrone could act as a competitive inhibitor of estradiol on hypothalamic and pituitary estrogen receptors. Because catecholestrogens are competitive inhibitors of catechol-O-methyltransferase, they could also cause a decrease in the turnover of CNS catecholamine neurotransmitters. Catecholestrogens also inhibit tyrosine hydroxylase, the rate-limiting enzyme in catecholamine biosynthesis, and therefore decrease the catecholamine content of the CNS. Evidence that estradiol metabolism in the rat brain changes during the estrous cycle indicates that 2-hydroxylation of estradiol in the brain may be involved in the negative feedback control of estrogens on pituitary gonadotropin secretion [9].

Intrafollicular Polypeptide Regulatory Factors

Several peptides have been isolated from ovarian follicles and claimed to function as putative hormones in the regulation of oocyte maturation [10].

Oocyte maturation factor. Oocytes obtained from middle and late antral follicles of mice resume meiosis when removed from the follicle and cultured in vitro. In contrast, oocytes cultured with granulosa cells do not mature, and antral follicular fluid from a number of species is also inhibitory to oocyte maturation in culture [4]. The putative oocyte maturation inhibitor (OMI) appears to be a low molecular weight peptide whose concentration in antral fluid decreases as the follicle matures. The inhibitory action of granulosa cells on oocyte maturation is reversed by addition of LH to the medium. LH is not effective, however, in overcoming the inhibitory activity of granulosa cell-conditioned medium on oocyte maturation. These results suggest that LH may mediate its effect through an action on the granulosa cells. Gap junctions, present between cells of the corona radiata and the oocyte, may provide a structural pathway for cell-to-cell communication between these two cell types. In addition cumulus cell extensions project through the zona pellucida to the oocyte. Because follicular fluid extracts inhibit maturation of oocytes cultured with their intact cumuli but not maturation of denuded oocytes, the OMI may exert its action indirectly through an action on cumulus cells [5]. It might be postulated that LH-induced oocyte maturation results from an uncoupling between the cumulus cells and the oocyte.

Neuroendocrine Control of Ovarian Function

Ovarian growth factors. Induction of LH receptors is a critical aspect of granulosa cell differentiation and ovarian follicular development. By this process the follicle acquires the responsiveness to LH and the subsequent capacity to ovulate and luteinize. Pituitary FSH functions as the inducer of granulosa cell LH receptor acquisition. This FSH-dependent LH receptor induction is inhibited by epidermal and fibroblast growth factors (Chapter 12). These and other growth factors may represent physiological effectors that regulate follicle development [15].

Ovarian follicular inhibin. Evidence supporting the existence of a gonadal peptide inhibitory to pituitary FSH secretion in the male was reviewed (Chapter 17). Equally compelling evidence for a granulosa-derived peptide in the female has been marshalled [5]. A follicular inhibin has been shown in follicular fluid, ovarian and granulosa cell extracts, granulosa cell conditioned media, and ovarian venous plasma. This proteinaceous substance exerts a suppressive action on both basal and GnRH-stimulated pituitary FSH secretion. The precise cellular localization and factors that may regulate the synthesis and secretion of this putative peptide remain to be clarified. A model for the role of inhibin in the control of pituitary FSH secretion was shown (Fig. 17.4).

MAMMALIAN REPRODUCTIVE CYCLES

Females of most vertebrate species are subject to cyclic changes in reproductive activity [3]. Most often these changes are integrated with seasonal environmental changes so that the young are born under more favorable conditions of climate and food availability. In many mammals other than primates females experience recurring periods of sexual excitement referred to as *estrus* (Greek: *oistros*, mad desire; heat), during which time they are psychologically as well as physically receptive to the male. The female primate does not go through an *estrous cycle*, but eggs are nevertheless matured within the ovaries during a precise follicular cycle of events, and the genital tract is also cyclically prepared for passage and implantation of the zygote. The monthly cycle of uterine maturation and sloughing is therefore a characteristic feature of the primate *menstrual cycle*.

Primate Menstrual Cycle

Ovarian cycle. The production and secretion of pituitary gonadotropins in the primate are controlled by cyclic ovarian follicular events; the duration of the cycle appears to be dependent on the genetic program that is read out to completion once follicular maturation is initiated. FSH levels are elevated at the beginning of the cycle, but they become diminished through most of the early and middle follicular phases. Follicular selection and early maturation may be dependent on the initially elevated plasma levels of FSH. Increased estrogen (and inhibin) secretion by the maturing follicles exerts a negative feedback inhibition of pituitary gonadotroph FSH secretion. Luteinizing hormone levels also remain low during most of this follicular phase due to the negative feedback action of estrogens on the pituitary. With continued follicular maturation, estrogen levels become increasingly elevated to a peak at midcycle. The prolonged action of the higher concentrations of estrogens is the stimulus to the midcycle FSH/LH surge (through enhancement of pituitary gonadotroph GnRH receptor number). The subsequently elevated plasma levels of LH provide the stimulus to ovum release from the mature Graafian follicle. The granulosa cells, which have now become responsive to LH, initiate progesterone biosynthesis and secretion. At this stage, the postovulatory follicle has become an endocrine gland in the classical sense. During the follicular phase plasma progesterone levels are low, but with commencement of the luteal phase they become elevated. Progesterone levels are elevated just prior to the LH/FSH surge, apparently in response to increasing levels of LH which are also secreted at that time. The action of progesterone on the hypothalamus results in postovulatory decreases in both LH and FSH secretion. Under conditions of low circulating levels of these gonadotropins, there is no stimulus to folliculogenesis and estrogen levels therefore remain only minimally elevated during the luteal phase. As the corpus luteum matures during the subsequent week following ovulation, progesterone levels become increasingly elevated to a midluteal peak. Afterward they level off and decline unless the ovulated ovum is fertilized and takes up residence within the uterine lining. With the demise of the corpus luteum in the nonpregnant female and the sharp decline in plasma progesterone levels, pituitary gonadotropins are again secreted which leads to the initiation of the next round of ovarian folliculogenesis and steroid hormone production. The cyclic pattern of pituitary gonadotropin and gonadal steroid hormone secretion in the rhesus monkey is illustrated in Figure 18.9 [7].

Uterine cycle. The menstrual cycle of the human female is approximately 28 days in length and is numbered from the first day of the menses [24]. Menstruation is the process where the lining of the uterus is shed once during each cycle, a process that in most women takes 4 to 5 days. Under the influence of increasing titers of plasma estrogens, the endometrium of the uterus increases in thickness, reaching a maximal width of 3 to 5 mm just prior to ovulation (Fig. 18.10). Stromal connective tissue cells proliferate and extracellular collagen deposits are increased. In response to luteal phase progesterone levels, uterine glands increase in complexity from simple tubular elements during the follicular phase of the cycle to thick-coiled structures with a glandular lumen containing abundant secretory material. Spiral arteries within the endometrium become thickened and engorged with blood, particularly in response to luteal levels of progesterone. If implantation of a zygote fails to occur, by about 11 days following ovulation lymphocytes begin to invade the endometrium and by day 14 (day 1 of the cycle) sloughing of the endometrium occurs due to loss of ovarian steroid hormone support. In the absence of a hormonal directive the spiral arteries become constricted and the blood lost from these arteries with stromal debris is responsible for the bulk of the menstrual flow.

The nature of the cervical mucus is also characteristically altered during the menstrual cycle. During the follicular phase the mucus is rather thin and watery. In response to periovulatory levels of progesterone the mucus becomes thickened and is composed of innumerable tiny channels that apparently provide access of the sperm through the cervical os.

Vaginal cycle. In prepubertal and postmenopausal females the vaginal epithelium is thin, being composed of a few layers of epithelial cells. In response to

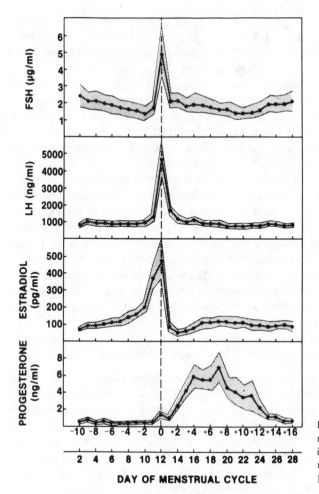

Figure 18.9 Serum concentrations of mFSH, mLH, estradiol, and progesterone in 20 rhesus monkeys during ovulatory menstrual cycles. (From DiZerega and Hodgen, [7], with permission.)

estrogens this epithelium proliferates and subsequently consists of many more layers of epithelial cells. The histological features of the vaginal epithelium change in a characteristic manner during the menstrual cycle. Early in the cycle the epithelium consists mainly of rounded basal cells that stain intensely with certain dyes. Maximal growth of the epithelium occurs during the periovulatory period. At this time the basal cells are overlain with layers of more flattened cells: The outermost cells are very flat and keratinized (cornified) and fail to stain, thus indicating that they are dead. Toward the end of the luteal phase the vaginal epithelium becomes invaded with leukocytes, and by the initiation of the next cycle cells of the outer layers of the epithelium are lost.

Induced and Spontaneous Ovulators

Most mammals (e.g., primates, hamsters, mice, rats) ovulate at the end of a follicular phase and then initiate development of corpora lutea. In contrast to these *spontaneous ovulators*, certain animals (domestic cats, rabbits, minks) go through a fol-

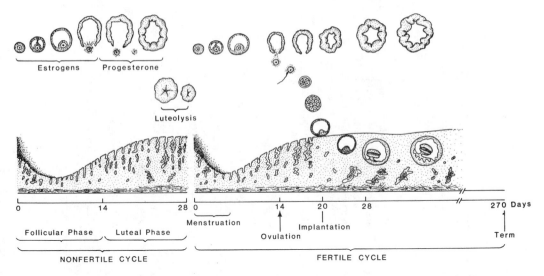

Figure 18.10 Cycle of uterine endometrial growth and development during nonfertile and fertile cycles in the human female.

licular phase but then remain in a state of sexual receptivity where the follicles mature and are usually released after copulation. These *induced* or *reflex ovulators* generally mate during estrus. Some animals may exhibit a *constant estrus* (e.g., rabbits), whereas estrus in other species may be a seasonal phenomenon with a long anestrous period between cycles where ovaries and follicles remain small.

During mating there is a reflex release of LH from the pituitary which leads to ovulation usually 12 to 48 hours later (Table 18.2). Although spontaneous ovulators are characterized by ovarian cycles that do not normally exhibit an estrous component, coitus can affect the time of ovulation in some of these species. These spontaneous ovulators can be divided into two major groups: (1) animals with nonfunctional corpora lutea and short (4- to 5-day) ovarian cycles (e.g., rats, mice, hamsters); and (2) animals with functional corpora lutea and long estrous cycles (e.g., pigs, cows, horses). The spontaneous ovulators with long cycles can be further subdivided into two groups: (1) animals with but one estrous cycle (monestrous) in a mating season; and (2) animals which have two or more estrous cycles (polyestrous) in the mating season.

Delayed Implantation

In some species the fertilized egg, the zygote, may reside within the uterine cavity for a considerable time. This *delayed implantation* allows flexibility between mating and birth. Most often, all reproductive events must be crowded into a short time interval. Of fundamental importance is that the young be born at the optimum season of the year for survival and growth [6]. In colonial animals, such as certain seals, the sexes are usually together only for a short time each year and must breed, give birth, and rear their young during this critical interval. In certain marsupials the suckling young may be lost due to harsh environmental conditions. The loss of the

TABLE 18.2 The Estrous Cycle of Various Mammalian Species[a]

Species	Length of cycle (days)	Duration of estrus	Ovulation Type	Ovulation Time
Cow (*Bos taurus*)	21	13–14 hours	Spontaneous	12–16 hours after end of estrus
Goat (*Capra hircus*)	20–21	1–3 days	Spontaneous	30–36 hours after onset of estrus
Sheep (*Ovis aries*)	16	20–48 hours	Spontaneous	12–24 hours before end of estrus
Pig (*Sus scrofa*)	21	2–3 days	Spontaneous	36 hours after onset of estrus
Horse (*Equus caballus*)	19–23	4–7 days	Spontaneous	1–2 days before end of estrus
Dog (*Canis familiaris*)	60	7–9 days	Spontaneous	1–3 days after start of estrus
Cat (*Felis catus*)	—	4 days with male 9–10 days without male	Induced	20–30 hours after mating
Ferret (*Mustela furo*)	8–9	Continuous	Induced	30 hours after mating
Mink (*Mustela vison*)		2 days	Induced	40–50 hours after mating
Fox (*Vulpes vulpes*)	90	1–5 days	Spontaneous	1–2 days after onset of estrus
Ground squirrel (*Citellus tridecemlineatus*)	16	6–11 hours	Induced	8–12 hours after mating
Guinea pig (*Cavia porcellus*)	16	6–11 hours	Spontaneous	10 hours after start of estrus
Golden hamster (*Mesocricetus auratus*)	4	20 hours	Spontaneous	8–12 hours after start of estrus
Mouse (*Mus musculus*)	4	10 hours	Spontaneous	2–3 hours after start of estrus
Rat (*Rattus norvegicus*)	4–5	13–15 hours	Spontaneous	8–10 hours after start of estrus
Rabbit (*Oryctolagus cuniculus*)	No cycle	Continuous	Induced	10 hours after mating
Rhesus monkey (*Macaca mulatta*)	28[b]	None	Spontaneous	14 days prior to onset of menstrual bleeding
Human (*Homo sapiens*)	28[b]	None	Spontaneous	14 days prior to onset of menstrual bleeding

[a] From van Tienhoven [22], with permission.
[b] Menstrual cycle.

suckling stimulus (absence of prolactin) causes an unimplanted blastocyst to break diapause (Greek: *dia*, through, completely; *paula*, pause; arrested embryonic development). Within each species the length of the implanted gestation period is rigidly fixed, but in some species of bats the young may experience a delayed development. The hormonal requirements for implantation of a delayed blastocyst are poorly understood. In the European badger there is a fertile postpartum coitus in February, but the fertilized eggs remain in the blastocyst stage until December when implantation occurs [22].

Environment and Reproduction

Reproductive success depends on successful mating, fetal growth and development, and the birth and rearing of young under appropriate environmental conditions. Success in these sequential events requires that eggs be ovulated at the right time, eggs become fertilized, and the nutritional state of the mother be adequate to provide for the needs of the growing offspring, whether in utero or postpartum. Environmental cues play important roles in synchronizing mating behavior in animals and provide signals indicative of when food sources may become available. For example, some desert species are opportunistic breeders and mate following rainfall [6]. In many small rodents reproductive activity is restricted to the spring and the fall; within the confines of the laboratory, however, these animals become continuous breeders.

A variety of exogenous factors—auditory, visual, tactile, and odoriferous— serve as signals to initiate reproductive behavior in some species. Lighting conditions as well as species-specific odors play particularly important roles.

Light. The most universal environmental synchronizing cue is light. Seasonal and daily changes in light duration and intensity are cyclic phenomena that usually directly or indirectly relate to other environmental factors such as the abundance of water and food. Light information must be received (sensed), transcribed (a neural processing mechanism), and translated into a physiological response. In vertebrates a neural sensory system ("eye") must monitor the presence or absence of light and transmit this information by neural afferents to the central nervous system, which then directly or indirectly affects pituitary gonadotropin secretion. In either case neurohormones released from the hypothalamus provide the initial input to pituitary hormone secretion. The important role of the pineal gland in the control of reproductive processes in the vertebrate is discussed in Chapter 20.

Olfaction. Smell is particularly crucial in eliciting mating behavior in many animals. Chemical messengers released by one member of a species may be received by a second member of the same species and produce a physiological response. These *pheromones* are volatile hydrocarbons (Fig. 2.5) which, in mammals at least, interact with receptors of olfactory epithelial cells of the recipient animal. Nervous afferents to the CNS then cause either a rapid behavioral response or slower physiological response involving the release of pituitary gonadotropins. Again, as for light stimuli, hypothalamic neurosecretory neurons provide the final common pathway linking sensory perception to pituitary-gonadal activation.

In the mouse a number of effects ascribed to pheromones have been noted

[20]. In the *Lee-Boot effect* female mice housed with four or more other female mice become *pseudopregnant;* that is, the corpora lutea are maintained in the absence of mating. If female mice are housed in very large groups, the incidence of anestrus increases. These observations suggest that female mice secrete one or more pheromones that affect the estrous cycle. In the *Whitten effect* the presence of a male mouse causes shortening and synchronization of the estrous cycle of grouped female mice. Bedding or urine from a male mouse is equally effective, suggesting that odor is the stimulus to synchronization and shortening of the estrous cycle. The *Vandenbergh effect* is demonstrated when prepubertal female mice, reared in the presence of a male (or his urine), attain first estrus several weeks earlier than if reared in the absence of the male. An additional observation made by Vandenbergh was that the odor of an adult female caused precocious testicular development of young males. In contrast, testes development is markedly retarded when young males are reared with adult males. The *Bruce effect* [17] results if a recently impregnated female mouse is exposed to a strange male; pregnancy is blocked and she returns to estrus within 1 week. The bedding or urine of the strange male is equally effective in terminating pregnancy. Females made anosmic by destruction of the olfactory bulbs are unaffected by the presence of the strange male. The source of the male odor is unknown but may be derived from the preputial glands.

Pheromones and other stimuli that activate reproductive behavior fall into two broad categories: *releaser effects* and *primer effects.* Releaser effects resulting from a visual or odoriferous signal involve an immediate behavioral response on the part of the recipient. This often involves activation of a stereotyped mating behavior in the female such as assuming a posture (lordosis) conducive to copulatory activity by the male. Primer effects also involve activation of central nervous system afferents, but in addition pituitary gonadotropin secretion is enhanced or inhibited most likely due to increases or decreases in hypothalamic secretion of GnRH. The Bruce effect appears to involve an inhibition of pituitary prolactin secretion as the hormone is required for maintenance of the corpus luteum and can repair the block to pregnancy induced by the strange male if administered to the female. It has been speculated that the block to pregnancy involves the reestablishment of prolactin inhibiting factor (dopamine) secretion by the hypothalamus.

REFERENCES

[1] ADAMS, T. E., R. L. NORMAN, and H. G. SPIES. 1981. Gonadotropin-releasing hormone receptor binding and pituitary responsiveness in estradiol-primed monkeys. *Science* 213:1388–90.

[2] ALLEN, E., and E. A. DOISY. 1923. An ovarian hormone: preliminary report on its localization, extraction, and partial purification and action in test animals. *JAMA* 81:819–21.

[3] AUSTIN, C. R., and R. V. SHORT, eds. 1972. *Reproduction in mammals. Book 4. Reproductive patterns.* Cambridge, England: Cambridge University Press.

[4] CENTOLA, G. M., L. D. ANDERSON, and C. P. CHANNING. 1981. Oocyte maturation inhibitor (OMI) in porcine granulosa cells. *Gamete Res.* 4:451–61.

[5] CHANNING, C. P., F. W. SCHAERF, L. D. ANDERSON, and A. TSAFRIRI. 1980. Ovarian and luteal physiology. *Int. Rev. Physiol.* 33:117–201.

[6] CONAWAY, C. H. 1971. Ecological adaptation and mammalian reproduction. *Biol. Reprod.* 4:239–47.

[7] DIZEREGA, G. S., and G. D. HODGEN. 1980. Changing functional status of the monkey corpus luteum. *Biol. Reprod.* 23:253–63.

[8] DORRINGTON, J. H., and D. T. ARMSTRONG. 1979. Effects of FSH on gonadal functions. *Rec. Prog. Horm. Res.* 35:301–42.

[9] FISHMAN, J. 1981. Biological action of catechol oestrogens. *J. Endocrinol.* 89:59P–65P.

[10] FRANCHIMONT, P., and C. P. CHANNING. 1981. *Intragonadal regulation of reproduction.* New York: Academic Press, Inc.

[11] HILLIER, S. G. 1981. Regulation of follicular oestrogen biosynthesis: a survey of current concepts. *J. Endocrinol.* 89:3P–18P.

[12] KNOBIL, E. 1980. Neuroendocrine control of the menstrual cycle. *Rec. Prog. Horm. Res.* 36:53–88.

[13] LEUNG, P. C. K., and D. T. ARMSTRONG. 1980. Interactions of steroids and gonadotropins in the control of steroidogenesis in the ovarian follicle. *Ann. Rev. Physiol.* 42:71–82.

[14] MARTIN, G. G., and P. TALBOT. 1981. Drugs that block smooth muscle contraction inhibit in vivo ovulation in hamsters. *J. Exp. Zool.* 216:483–91.

[15] MONDSCHEIN, J. S., and D. W. SCHOMBERG. 1980. Growth factors modulate gonadotropin receptor induction in granulosa cell cultures. *Science* 211:1179–81.

[16] NALBANDOV, A. V., and B. COOK. 1968. Reproduction. *Ann. Rev. Physiol.* 30:245–78.

[17] PARKES, A. S., and H. M. BRUCE. 1961. Olfactory stimuli in mammalian reproduction. *Science* 134:1049–54.

[18] RICHARDS, J. S. 1979. Hormonal control of ovarian follicular development: a 1978 perspective. *Rec. Prog. Horm. Res.* 35:43–73.

[19] SCHRADER, W. T., M. E. BIRNBAUMER, M. R. HUGHES, N. L. WEIGEL, W. W. GRODY, and B. W. O'MALLEY. 1981. Studies on the structure and function of the chicken progesterone receptor. *Rec. Prog. Horm. Res.* 37:583–633.

[20] STODDART, D. M. 1976. *Mammalian odours and pheromones.* London: Edward Arnold Publishers Ltd.

[21] TATA, J. R., and D. F. SMITH. 1979. Vitellogenesis: a versatile model for hormonal regulation of gene expression. *Rec. Prog. Horm. Res.* 35:47–95.

[22] VAN TIENHOVEN, A. 1968. *Reproductive physiology.* Philadelphia: W. B. Saunders Company.

[23] WAHLI, W., I. B. DAWID, G. U. RYFFEL, and R. WEBER. 1981. Vitellogenesis and the vitellogenin gene family. *Science* 212:298–304.

[24] YEN, S. S. C. 1979. Neuroendocrine regulation of the menstrual cycle. *Hosp. Prac.* 14(3):83–97.

19

Endocrinology of Pregnancy, Parturition, and Lactation

INTRODUCTION

The ovulated egg has two possible fates: (1) if it fails to become fertilized, it undergoes lysis; (2) if, on the other hand, the ovum becomes fertilized, it (the zygote) may develop into an offspring of the species. If such an event is to be successful, then in many animals a complex number of integrated neuroendocrine events between both conceptus and mother must transpire.

Oviparity, Ovoviviparity, and Viviparity

After fertilization embryonic development in *oviparous* species (all birds) takes place outside the body in eggs that are covered with one or more protective membranes (shell, jelly). In *ovoviparous* species the mother gives birth to live young which are nevertheless developed within a protective egg retained within the oviduct which receives no nutrition from the mother. In *viviparous* animals the young develop within the mother and receive nourishment through connections between embryo and mother. Except for the duckbilled platypus and spiny anteater, all mammals are viviparous.

Endocrines play essential roles in the processes of fetal growth and development, parturition at term, and, in most mammals, the control of lactation [41]. Unfortunately, only a few details of this complex topic can be discussed and these are limited mostly to the primate.

PREGNANCY

Fertilization and Implantation

In the primate usually a single egg is ovulated approximately midway through the menstrual cycle. During coitus spermatozoa released by the male into the vagina travel via the uterus to the oviducts where the ovum may become fertilized. Many spermatozoa may penetrate through the corona radiata surrounding the ovum and, although more than one sperm can penetrate through the zona pellucida, usually only one enters the ovum. In response to the sperm the oocyte completes the second meiotic division and expels the second polar body. The resulting female pronucleus comes in contact with the male pronucleus that has been formed after loss of the sperm tail. Fusion of the male and female pronuclei, to form the zygote, reestablishes the diploid chromosomal number of the egg. During passage down the uterine tube, which takes about 2 days, the zygote undergoes rapid mitotic divisions, and the resulting cells are referred to as *blastomeres*. By about 3 days a compact mass of cells, the *morula*, enters the uterus. Continued cell division produces a hollow sphere, the early *blastocyst*, which is composed of a single layer of cells, the *trophoblast*, and an inner cell mass, *embryoblast*, which is attached to the trophoblastic wall at the embryonic pole of the blastocyst. The inner cell mass through differentiation and growth will form the embryo, whereas the trophoblast will establish contact with the maternal circulation to provide the initial mechanism for the exchange of nutrients, oxygen, and waste products between fetus and mother. After residing within the uterus for about 2 days, the embryonic pole of the blastocyst becomes implanted in the endometrial epithelium on about day 6 (Fig. 19.1). In response to the blastocyst the underlying epithelium and endometrium undergo cellular changes, a so-called *decidualization* process. As a result, the endometrial tissue enlarges to form an implantation chamber, the *decidua*, to accommodate the growing embryo. The trophoblastic cells in contact with the uterine epithelium proliferate into an invasive *syncytiotrophoblast* which consists of a multinucleated protoplasmic mass (Fig. 19.1). By 10 days the conceptus is completely embedded within the endometrium. The syncytiotrophoblast forms lacunar networks which establish contact with the endometrial capillaries to form the primitive uteroplacental circulation.

Gonadal steroids may be required for implantation. There is evidence that the blastocyst synthesizes estrogens, and it has been proposed that steroids synthesized

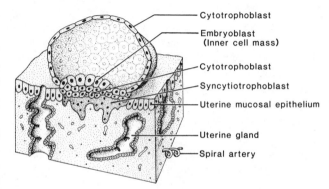

- Cytotrophoblast
- Embryoblast (Inner cell mass)
- Cytotrophoblast
- Syncytiotrophoblast
- Uterine mucosal epithelium
- Uterine gland
- Spiral artery

Figure 19.1 Implantation of the blastocyst within the uterus.

or accumulated by the blastocyst may play a role in implantation through a local action on the adjacent endometrium. Indeed, in the rat uterus the concentrations of nuclear receptors for both estradiol and progesterone are higher in implantation sites than in nonimplantation regions of the endometrium.

The Corpus Luteum

The corpus luteum normally regresses about 12 days after ovulation during an infertile cycle in the primate. If, however, the ovum is fertilized and subsequently implants within the uterus, by 10 days after ovulation a glycoprotein molecule unique to pregnancy is now present within the blood. This protein is secreted by the syncytiotrophoblast and, in humans, is referred to as *human chorionic gonadotropin* (hCG) or choriogonadotropin. Detection of this protein in the urine provides the basis for the most common determination of pregnancy.

The role of hCG is to stimulate progesterone biosynthesis by the luteal cells of the corpus luteum. Initially, LH of pituitary origin is stimulatory to progesterone production by the corpus luteum. But LH levels drop precipitously after the midcycle LH/FSH surge. During the menstrual cycle progesterone secretion by the corpus luteum reaches a peak about 8 days after its formation. If the egg is not fertilized, progesterone levels decline rapidly and menstruation follows. The role of hCG is to rescue the corpus luteum, thereby prolonging its life span by converting it into a corpus luteum of pregnancy. There is good evidence that luteal cell hCG receptors are identical to LH receptors; they are therefore often referred to as LH/hCG receptors, and either hormone may be utilized to study activation of progesterone synthesis by luteal cells. Plasma levels of hCG rise to their highest between about the ninth and fourteenth weeks of pregnancy and then begin to decline gradually, reaching a nadir at approximately 20 weeks of gestation [8]. Luteal function begins to decline while circulating levels of hCG are at their peak, suggesting that failure of luteal activity is not related to declining levels of hCG.

In many mammals (e.g., rats, rabbits, but not primates) the pituitary gland is essential for the initial development as well as the survival of the corpora lutea in the pregnant female [31]. Hypophysectomy in these animals results in atrophy of the corpus luteum which can, however, be maintained by administration of pituitary extracts. The pituitary hormone responsible for luteotropic action in these species is prolactin. In the rat transplantation of the adenohypophysis to an ectopic site, such as the kidney, shortly after ovulation will allow development of the corpora lutea to an active state and at the same time keep the female in a state of pseudopregnancy [26]. In the absence of an inhibitory hypothalamic control the ectopically transplanted adenohypophysis autonomously secretes PRL. Implantation of fertilized ova within the uterus is apparently perceived by sensory neural elements which through spinal afferents convey this information to the hypothalamus. This is believed to result in an inhibition of hypothalamic dopaminergic neurons and, in the absence of dopamine secretion into the hypophysial portal system, PRL is secreted autonomously.

Steroid hormone biosynthesis and secretion by the corpus luteum differ from that of the follicle in that there is a striking increase in progesterone production. In some species this increase is accompanied by a decrease in estrogen and androgen biosynthesis. A physiologic relationship between mammalian viviparity and the corpus luteum appears to be established in mammals as progesterone is necessary for growth and maintenance of pregnancy. However, such a relationship in other vertebrates is not as clear, although oviparous birds do not form a corpus luteum. Although a corpus luteum occurs in all reptilian species, only certain species of squamates (lizards and snakes) are viviparous. Some fishes and amphibians form a corpus luteum during pregnancy, but the relationship of the corpus luteum to viviparity is unclear [31].

The Fetal-Placental Unit

With the demise of the corpus luteum in the primate, estradiol and progesterone production is taken over by the placenta. However, the placenta is not capable of producing these steroid hormones without a supply of precursors from both the fetus and the maternal compartment [8].

Progesterone. The placenta, incapable of de novo progesterone biosynthesis, is dependent on cholesterol derived from the maternal blood supply (Fig. 19.2). The progesterone produced by the placenta is released into the maternal circulation to serve a multitude of functions related to pregnancy: maintenance of uterine structure and function, mammary growth and development, and inhibition of pituitary gonadotropin secretion. In addition placental progesterone is utilized as a substrate

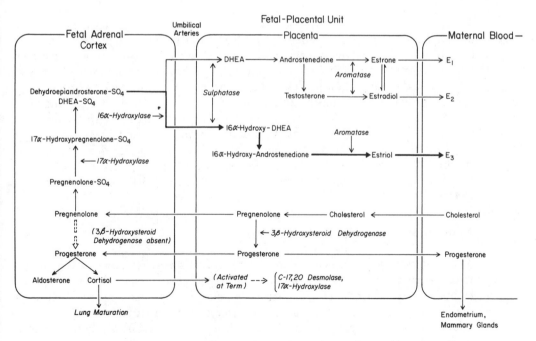

Figure 19.2 The fetal-placental unit.

for corticoid production by the fetal adrenals which lack an active 3 β-hydroxy-steroid-dehydrogenase.

Estrogens.   Pregnenolone of placental origin is also utilized by the fetal adrenals in the production of precursors for estrogen production within the placenta. The placenta itself has only a limited capability for estrogen synthesis due to minimal 17 α-hydroxylase activity. Within the fetal adrenal cortex, however, this enzyme is responsible for production of dehydroepiandrosterone sulfate (DHEA-SO$_4$). This steroid metabolite serves as a precursor substrate for estrone (E$_1$) and estradiol (E$_2$) synthesis by the placenta. Much of the substrate is, however, converted by a fetal adrenal 16 α-hydroxylase to precursors that lead to copious estriol (E$_3$) production. Measurements of E$_3$ levels in the maternal plasma or urine as a means of evaluating fetal well-being have been undertaken, but their usefulness is questionable [8]. It is obvious from the preceding discussion that the fetal adrenals and the placenta, with respect to steroid hormone production, are incomplete endocrine organs. There is a circular flow of steroid metabolites that passes from the maternal compartment to the placenta, to the fetal adrenals, and then back through the placental compartment to the maternal bloodstream. The evolution of this complex system and the intricate signals between these compartments, which must exist to ensure maintenance of pregnancy and yet provide the means for the eventual process of parturition, are still ambiguous.

PARTURITION

A functional corpus luteum is required for maintenance of pregnancy in many mammalian species (e.g., goat); its demise in these species initiates the process of parturition. In other placenta-dependent species (e.g., sheep, primates) in which the corpus luteum regresses well before term a decrease in particular placental steroids may be the key to the parturition process. The factors regulating placental hormone production probably vary considerably among these latter species. Prostaglandins of uterine origin participate in the initiation of delivery of the fetus at term by actions at a number of target sites. One or more pituitary hormones of maternal and fetal origin may also be instrumental in activating processes leading to parturition. The particular roles of neural and endocrine factors in parturition vary considerably among species and, therefore, no single model adequately describes the process in any one species [19, 22, 40].

Neuroendocrine Control of Parturition

Progesterone.   In most mammalian species a drop in circulating levels of progesterone occurs prior to labor. In corpus luteum-dependent species this may be accomplished by uterine luteolytic factors (prostaglandins in some species). In other placenta-dependent species changes in enzyme activities that increase estrogen production may lower progesterone levels. Progesterone is directly antagonistic to uterine smooth muscle contraction induced either by oxytocin or prostaglandins. The *progesterone block hypothesis* was formulated to provide a theoretically relevant mechanism by which the uterus might be protected from premature contraction and expulsion of the fetus [4]. In this model a lowering of progesterone levels at term would be the stimulus to parturition.

Estrogens. Estrogens increase myometrial excitability, possibly by lowering the membrane potential of uterine smooth muscle. The actions of estrogens on the myometrium are, however, antagonized by the action of progesterone. In the rat the number of uterine estrogen receptors increases as progesterone levels decline. Estrogens enhance uterine excitability by a number of mechanisms: increasing endometrial prostaglandin synthetase activity, increasing myometrial and endometrial oxytocin receptors, and increasing oxytocin production and secretion by the neurohypophysis (Chapter 7).

Prostaglandins. There is evidence that in most species studied prostaglandins play an important role in parturition. In many species increased synthesis and release of prostaglandins precede labor. In some large animals (e.g., goat, sow) that depend on the corpus luteum as a source of progesterone, prostaglandin $F_{2\alpha}$ ($PGF_{2\alpha}$) released from the endometrium may be the luteolytic factor responsible for luteal regression. The resulting drop in luteal progesterone production is followed by uterine contractions and parturition. As noted, uterine prostaglandin synthesis may be dependent on stimulation by placental estrogens.

Placental prolactin. Levels of PRL increase in the human fetus during late gestation, PRL levels are very high in amniotic fluid, and synthesis of PRL by chorion-decidual tissue has been demonstrated. This placental PRL is immunologically similar to pituitary PRL and should not be confused with placental lactogen (PL) which differs considerably in primary structure. Increased levels of PRL coincide with a stage in development during which major changes in organ growth occur in the fetus and may be responsible for increased growth and function of the fetal adrenal cortex (Chapter 12).

Autonomic motor innervation. The female reproductive tract is richly innervated by adrenergic neurons. The role, if any, of such innervation in parturition is unresolved. Both estrogens and progestins affect the norepinephrine content of these nerves as well as the turnover of NE, the activity of enzymes related to catecholamine biosynthesis, and the release of NE from nerve terminals. In the progesterone-dominated uterus catecholamine stimulation of myometrial smooth muscle β-adrenoceptors causes relaxation of the uterus. During the latter stages of pregnancy in some species stretch-induced hypertrophy of the uterus causes degeneration of the nerves in the uterine corpus. Withdrawal of this neural inhibitory influence to the corpus may allow spontaneous myogenic contractions to intensify [23].

It has been noted that gap junctions (nexuses, low resistance electrical pathways) are present between the uterine muscle cells of a number of species (including the human) immediately before, during, and immediately after delivery [13]. These junctions are absent at all other times during pregnancy and are also lacking in immature or nonpregnant animals. Ovariectomy of pregnant animals at midterm causes the rapid appearance of gap junctions, and the appearance of gap junctions at term is prevented by progesterone administration. The absence of gap junctions throughout the gestation period may be important in preventing electrical communication between uterine muscle cells. The acquisition of gap junctions at term may be an essential element in synchronizing uterine contractility for effective expulsion of the fetus [13]. Because gap junction formation may be initiated by progesterone withdrawal, this could provide the morphological and functional bases for the progesterone block hypothesis formulated much earlier by Csapo [4].

Oxytocin. Oxytocin, a neurohypophysial hormone, has a direct uterine contracting (oxytocic) action (Chapter 7). Fetal movements monitored by the uterine cervix and relayed by spinal afferents are stimulatory to oxytocin release during labor in the human. The sensitivity of the myometrium to oxytocin is enhanced by estrogens and depressed by progesterone. In the human female maternal plasma oxytocin levels increase with advancing gestation. It is not clear, however, whether oxytocin is an initiating factor or only facilitory to human labor. Plasma estrogen concentrations increase during gestation and in the rat are known to increase the affinity and number of uterine oxytocin receptors. The actions of oxytocin on the uterus could be mediated indirectly through stimulation of endometrial and myometrial prostaglandin $F_{2\alpha}$ production. $PGF_{2\alpha}$ might then stimulate cGMP production by uterine smooth muscle cells. This intracellular cyclic nucleotide would then be responsible for activating the contractile machinery of the cell leading to contraction of the uterus and expulsion of the fetus.

The fetal adrenal cortex. There is compelling evidence, particularly in sheep but also in other large mammals, that the onset of parturition is initiated by the activation of the fetal pituitary-adrenal axis [25]. The fetal adrenal gland increases in weight rapidly during the last 2 weeks of gestation. This growth is primarily due to hypertrophy and hyperplasia of adrenal cortical cells. Premature delivery can be induced in the pregnant ewe by infusion of ACTH or glucocorticoids (but not mineralocorticoids) and can be prevented by fetal adrenalectomy or hypophysectomy.

Increased fetal glucocorticoid production in sheep is stimulatory to placental production of estrogen from progesterone; this, therefore, leads to a subsequent fall in maternal plasma and tissue progesterone concentrations and a consequent rise in estrogen concentrations. The action of fetal adrenal glucocorticoids may be to induce synthesis of 17,20 desmolase and 17 α-hydroxylase activities within the placenta (Fig. 19.2). The resulting change in estrogen-progesterone levels may provide the stimulus to uterine production of prostaglandins or related hormones (prostacyclins) and to an increase in uterine oxytocin receptor number.

Relaxin. In 1926 Hisaw reported that an aqueous extract of the corpora lutea of the pregnant sow "relaxes" the pubic symphysis of the guinea pig. This biologically active substance was purified and named *relaxin* [10]. Because of difficulties in isolating this factor, the chemical structure was not determined until much later [32]. The development of a reliable radioimmunoassay made possible the determination of the blood levels of the peptide throughout pregnancy, the sites of production of the hormone, and the factors that may regulate relaxin secretion.

Most interesting was the discovery that the primary structures of relaxin and insulin are similar (Fig. 19.3). Although there is only about 40% homology between

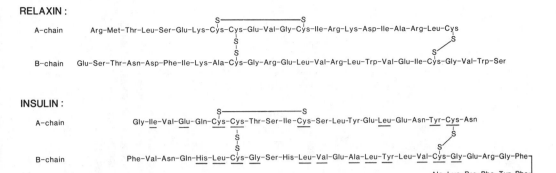

Figure 19.3 Comparative structures of porcine relaxin and insulin. The underlined residues within the insulin molecule indicate those that are either homologous or conservatively replaced relative to those at similar positions within the relaxin chains. (Modified from Schwabe and McDonald, [32].)

the residues, the conformations of the two peptides are comparable [32, 33]. The cross-linking pattern of the two hormones strongly suggests that they have come into existence by gene duplication. It has been concluded, a posteriori, that relaxin, like insulin, is synthesized as a prohormone in a single chain to facilitate the correct folding of the protein. At present there is only meager evidence for a prorelaxin.

A relaxinlike peptide is present in shark ovaries and bears structural similarity to porcine relaxin. However, the amino acid composition of shark relaxin resembles porcine insulin to a greater extent than it does porcine relaxin. It has been suggested that shark relaxin may represent a phylogenetically more primitive relaxin that has undergone fewer mutations than porcine relaxin since a putative duplication of the gene early in evolution. It is possible, therefore, that evolution of the relaxin molecule antedates the point at which sharks branched from the mainstream of mammalian development [29]. Shark relaxin inhibits guinea pig uterine muscle in vitro and also relaxes the pubic symphysis, as does porcine relaxin. However, a role for relaxin, if any, in the shark is unknown.

Studies on a variety of species, including humans, leave little doubt that the corpus luteum is the source of relaxin. The source of luteal relaxin may be the granules observed in the granulosa lutein cells. Relaxin may also be produced and stored within granulocytes localized to the endometrium of rhesus monkeys and adult human females. Relaxin concentrations in luteal and other tissues are highest during pregnancy (Fig. 19.4). In the human relaxin concentrations are four times higher in the ovarian vein draining the ovary, which contains the corpus luteum of pregnancy, than in either peripheral plasma or the contralateral ovarian vein. Immunoreactive relaxin is present in the serum as early as the fourth week of pregnancy; it is detectable throughout the course of gestation but is only rarely detected in the plasma of nonpregnant women [27]. Plasma levels of immunoreactive relaxin rise to a peak shortly before parturition in rodents and pigs, which is correlated with the increase in cervical dilatability and the formation of an interpublic ligament (Fig. 19.5). Plasma RIA relaxin is also markedly elevated in late pregnancy in the dog, rhesus and Java monkeys, and humans. Relaxin has also been found in the testes of

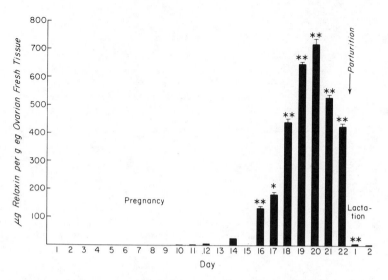

Figure 19.4 Mean relaxin immunoactivity levels (± S.E.) in ovarian extracts from pregnant and lactating rats. Ovaries obtained from two animals were pooled for each day shown. Multiple volumes of extract, containing 0.2 to 50 ngeq ovarian fresh tissue, were employed. Asterisks denote those mean relaxin concentrations which differ significantly from those of the preceding observation (*P < 0.05; **P < 0.01). (From Sherwood and Crnekovic, [34], with permission.)

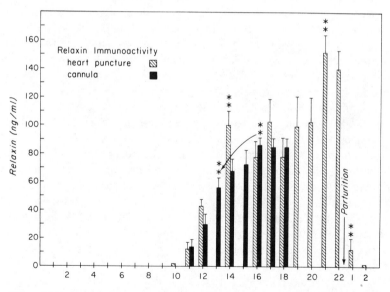

Figure 19.5 Relaxin immunoreactivity levels (± S.E.M.) in the peripheral sera of anesthetized (heart puncture) and unanesthetized (cannula) rats. Asterisks denote those mean values which differ significantly (*P < 0.05; **P < 0.01) from those using the same end point which precede or are indicated with an arrow. (From Sherwood et al., [36], with permission.)

armadillos and roosters but is undetectable in the testes and serum of a number of male mammals, including humans. The role, if any, of relaxin in the male is therefore unknown.

The biological effects of relaxin described are associated with pregnancy and parturition. Relaxin acts on the pubic symphysis to transform the connective tissues from a compact cartilaginous type to a more fluid, flexible structure. This results, in some species, in the formation of a ligament between the pubic bones. This increased flexibility and enlargement of the birth canal is important to successful parturition in a number of species. Although formation of an interpubic ligament may not occur, there is, nevertheless, a change in the ground substance of the connective tissue, which leads to increased flexibility of the public symphysis and attached bones.

Relaxin may be present within the endometrium of the uterus: In the rhesus monkey the peptide may function as a local hormone to control endothelioid cytomorphosis. This response involves hypertrophy and proliferation of the endothelial cells of the blood vessels just below the implanted embryo. This vascular response to relaxin could provide increased blood flow to the fetus. Relaxin also inhibits uterine motility by relaxing the myometrium. It has been speculated that because of its myometrium-inhibiting activity, relaxin may play a role in maintenance of pregnancy. Other effects of relaxin on the collagen framework and distensibility of the uterus, as well as similar effects on the uterine cervix, have been described. Relaxin and somatotropin may act synergistically in stimulating mammary gland growth. The evidence is rather convincing that relaxin subserves a multifunctional role in preparing the female for parturition and possibly other roles related to pregnancy.

Relaxin acts on the estrogen-primed uterus, but neither relaxin nor estrogen exerts its effects in hypophysectomized animals unless somatotropin is administered concomitantly with an estrogen and a relaxin. Estrogens may transform pubic symphysial chondrocytes and osteocytes to chrondroclasts and osteoclasts, respectively. The role of relaxin may be to release lysosomal hydrolases from these cells into the cartilage matrix. Relaxin increases the level of cAMP in the pubic symphyses of mice. The hormone does not increase the concentration of cAMP in nontarget tissues such as the liver; the increase in symphysial cAMP cannot be similarly elicited by insulin, a hormone of similar size and structure, or by glucagon, a known stimulator of liver cAMP production. The mechanism of action of relaxin on the pubic symphysis may therefore involve the intracellular messenger, cAMP [2]. Similarly, relaxin elevates cAMP levels in uterine strips taken from estrogen-primed female rats. The effects of relaxin on the uterus appear to be direct and not mediated through β-adrenoceptors whose activation also causes relaxation of the uterus.

Exogenous oxytocin increases relaxin levels in ovarian venous blood during late pregnancy in the pig. It is sugegsted that oxytocin may indirectly increase blood levels of relaxin via an oxytocic action on the uterine myometrium [20]. For example, oxytocin is known to stimulate $PGF_{2\alpha}$ production in the uterus and $PGF_{2\alpha}$ induces parturition in the pig, apparently through luteolytic action. Injections of $PGF_{2\alpha}$ sufficient to induce parturition in the pig increase prepartum levels of relaxin. Injection of the PG synthesis inhibitor, indomethacin, prior to parturition in the sow delays the relaxin surge for a number of days after termination of the drug [35]. In the human neither oxytocin nor $PGF_{2\alpha}$-induced labor, whether successful or not, is associated with significant elevations in serum relaxin levels. Labor in the human female therefore appears different from that of rodents and the pig where increased levels of the hormone are associated with parturition. This correlates with the observation that $PGF_{2\alpha}$, although luteolytic in many other mammals, does not have such an effect on the human corpus luteum of pregnancy.

Parturition in Humans

A model for the initiation of labor in the human [12] espouses that, as a result of the rising estrogen levels during gestation, the concentration of uterine oxytocin receptors increases. Rapid fetal growth near term increases uterine distension which may also contribute to the increase in uterine oxytocin receptors near term as shown in rats (Chapter 7). The increased numbers of oxytocin receptors probably lower the threshold of the uterus to a level where myometrial contractions are initiated. Oxytocin may bind to decidual receptors and stimulate prostaglandin biosynthesis. The coupling of oxytocin receptor activation and prostaglandin biosynthesis may be the crucial event in the initiation of labor. During spontaneous labor there is an increase in plasma oxytocin levels in the fetal umbilical artery compared to the umbilical vein, indicating a flow of oxytocin from the fetal toward the maternal compartment [5]. Oxytocin derived from the fetus may provide the stimulus for the increased production of prostaglandins at the onset of labor [12]. Hypothalamo-neurohypophysial maturation within the fetus, leading to fetal-adrenal activation and neurohypophysial hormone secretion, may provide the final essential directive for the induction of parturition.

LACTATION

In mammals two ectodermal ridges (so-called milk lines) appear on either side of the ventral midline early in fetal life. Localized thickenings become the mammary buds which in the female grow into the underlying dermis to form the primary mammary cords, the precursors of the duct systems. In the human male early mammary gland development is suppressed by gonadal androgens and, although there is an initial hypertrophy of the primary ducts and the secretion of a colostrumlike "witch's milk," caused by the maternal hormones of pregnancy, these glands soon become inactive. Further growth of the undeveloped mammae in the human female is not initiated until ovarian cycles begin. At puberty, further growth and branching of the ducts occurs and a lobular system is developed. Most of the increase in size of the mammary glands is due to interlobular fat deposition. Mammary growth and development at puberty is mainly in response to gonadal estrogens, but adrenal glucocorticoids and somatotropin may also be involved.

Proliferation of a lobular-alveolar system is initiated at pregnancy. Besides the requirement for estrogens and possibly glucocorticoids and somatotropin for continued duct growth, progesterone and prolactin are required for full development of the ductule system (Fig. 19.6). Placental lactogen may also be required for full development of the breasts in the pregnant human female. Milk production in the mature mammary gland occurs near parturition. The following hormones have been implicated as essential to mammary growth and lactogenesis in some species:

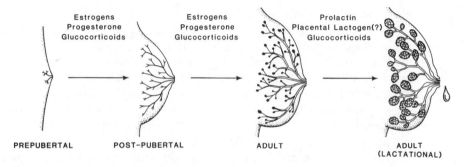

Figure 19.6 Hormonal regulation of mammary gland growth and development.

estrogens, progesterone, glucocorticoids, somatotropin, insulin, placental lactogen, and prolactin. The relative and temporal roles of these hormones for any one species remain to be clarified.

Although milk constituents begin to appear before parturition in most species, high rates of synthesis do not usually occur until after birth. Milk is synthesized within the cells lining the mammary gland alveoli. Milk is a complex nutrient consisting mainly of milk sugar, lactose, lipids, the milk proteins (casein and whey) as well as monovalent and divalent cations, and most interesting, immune antibodies. Glucose is converted to the milk sugar, lactose, by the enzyme, *lactose synthetase*, which is composed of two individual subunits. The catalytic subunit of the enzyme is galactosyltransferase, and α-lactalbumin is the regulatory subunit. In addition a number of major (e.g., casein) and minor milk proteins are synthesized. These products are released by macrovesicular exocytosis into the alveolar lumen where they are stored until ejected by the action of oxytocin on the myoepithelial cells covering the contraluminal surface of the alveolus (Fig. 7.4).

Milk secretion is regulated by PRL through an action on plasmalemmal receptors of mammary gland alveolar secretory cells [37]. In the rabbit an increase in PRL receptors, synchronous with the onset of lactation, occurs at the same time as the major rise in serum PRL levels at parturition. Estradiol stimulates the number of mammary gland PRL receptors, whereas progesterone suppresses this increase. PRL also induces the formation of its own receptors. The dramatic increase in lactogenesis that follows parturition can therefore be partly explained by the removal of the inhibitory action of progesterone on the mammary gland coupled to the positive actions of PRL on the stimulation of its own receptors. Suckling-induced PRL secretion is required for maintenance of postpartum lactogenesis in some animals, such as the human, but not in others such as the cow.

Prolactin, like other growth hormones, apparently does not exert its effects through the intermediary of cAMP. cAMP has anti-PRL-like action on the mammary gland. PRL stimulates cGMP production, but its role, if any, in lactogenesis is undetermined. An initial action of PRL at the level of the cell membrane is the stimulation of phospholipase A activity. This results in the conversion of phosphocholine to arachidonic acid which then serves as substrate for prostaglandin biosynthesis. Prostaglandins stimulate mRNA synthesis within mammary epithelial cells, mimicking the action of PRL, but it is unclear whether PG's affect membrane nucleotide cyclase activities or act in some way as cytoplasmic messengers. Plasma membranes from lactating rabbit mammary glands respond to PRL by releasing a factor capable of stimulating casein gene transcription by isolated mammary cell nuclei. Insulin and glucocorticoids appear to be absolutely essential for casein mRNA production by mouse mammary epithelial cells in response to PRL. Casein and α-lactalbumin synthesis is stimulated by PRL and can be blocked by concomitant administration of actinomycin D [30]. Prolactin also stimulates ornithine decarboxylase production through newly synthesized mRNA. This enzyme stimulates polyamine synthesis, and polymines (e.g., spermidine) themselves mimic the action of PRL suggesting that they may be obligate intracellular second messengers in the actions of PRL on milk synthesis. Stimulation of polyamine biosynthesis may be secondary to PRL stimulation of prostaglandin synthesis.

Fatty acids derived from dietary fat intake are converted within mammary gland epithelial cells to triglycerides (milk fats). These fatty acids are made available to mammary gland epithelial cells by activation of membrane bound lipoprotein lipase. The activity of this enzyme is negligible in nonlactating animals but is enhanced 2 to 3 days before parturition apparently in response to rising levels of PRL. Prolactin activation of lipoprotein lipase is blocked by simultaneous administration of actinomycin D, indicating that synthesis or activation of the enzyme requires mRNA-directed protein synthesis. Fatty acids are also synthesized within mammary gland epithelial cells in response to PRL.

In certain fishes PRL stimulates renal Na^+/K^+-activated ATPase and controls salt excretion by the nasal salt gland of some marine birds. Prolactin also activates the transport of Na^+ and K^+ in mammary tissue apparently through an action on a Na^+/K^+ pump which is localized almost exclusively to the basolateral membranes of mammary epithelial cells [9]. Control of transepithelial Na^+ transport may be the underlying and most basic action of PRL on mammary gland milk production [1, 17].

The secretion of PRL from the pituitary is under an inhibitory control by the hypothalamus (Chapter 6). A PRL release-inhibiting hormone, most probably dopamine, is released from hypothalamic dopaminergic neurons into the hypophysial portal system where the catecholamine is carried to the lactotrophs of the pars distalis. Inhibition of hypothalamic dopamine release or inhibition of dopamine interaction with lactotroph receptors (by ergot alkaloids; e.g., ergocryptine) results in PRL secretion.

The stimulus to PRL secretion is a neuroendocrine reflex involving neural afferents from the teats to the hypothalamus. A suckling-induced neuroendocrine reflex mechanism is also responsible for secretion of oxytocin from the neurohypophysis (Fig. 19.7). Blood concentrations of PRL increase progressively throughout pregnancy apparently due to the influence of increasing concentrations of placental steroids, particularly estrogens. Nevertheless, milk secretion is inhibited by a direct action of progesterone on the mammary glands. At parturition, blood levels of PRL are about 20 times greater than normal, but the level of the hormone remains elevated for only about a week postpartum in the absence of suckling. Blood concentrations of PRL remain high for the duration of lactation in breast-feeding women, and PRL is also released during each suckling episode in response to tactile stimulation of the nipple. Estrogens exert a profound action on pituitary mammotroph PRL production. The elevated plasma levels of estrogens just prior to parturition

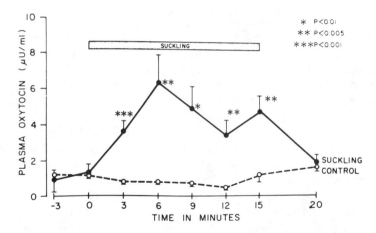

Figure 19.7   Mean (± S.E.M.) plasma oxytocin concentrations for six nursing and six control subjects. Asterisks indicate significance relative to control subjects (*P < 0.01; **P < 0.005; ***P < 0.001). (From Weitzman et al., [43], by permission.)

may, indeed, be important in stimulating lactogenesis through stimulation of PRL secretion. Estrogens appear to enhance mammotroph PRL secretion (at least in rats) by increasing the number of TRH receptors present in these cells, an action which is blocked by the estrogen receptor antagonist, tamoxifen (Fig. 19.8) [14]. TRH is stimulatory to pituitary PRL secretion in some mammals.

The placenta secretes large amounts of estrogens and progesterone, hormones inhibitory to FSH secretion during pregnancy. Therefore, plasma FSH levels are normally suppressed during pregnancy and at term are low or undetectable. Blood levels of FSH increase postpartum to normal follicular phase levels. Both pituitary and plasma levels of LH are also extremely low during pregnancy, apparently also due to a negative feedback inhibition by placental steroid hormones. Inhibition of

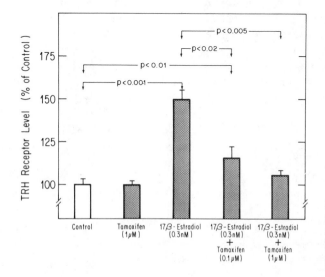

Figure 19.8   Effect of tamoxifen, an estrogen antagonist, on pituitary TRH receptor number. (From Gershengorn, Marcus-Samuels, and Geras, [14], with permission.)

pituitary gonadotropin production during pregnancy may provide an adaptive mechanism whereby further egg maturation and release is inhibited so that the nutritive needs of the nursing infant are sustained. In nonlactating women LH concentrations may remain low during the early puerperium (state of the woman after childbirth) but return to normal cyclic levels within 3 to 5 weeks when the PRL concentration returns to its normal low levels.

In lactating women blood estradiol concentrations are significantly lower than those of nonlactating women and no ovarian follicular development occurs during the period of lactation as long as PRL levels remain high. The mechanism and site of the inhibitory action of PRL on ovarian function is unknown. Plasma levels of LH and estradiol increase soon after weaning, concomitant with a drop in PRL secretion, indicating the resumption of ovarian activity. Because the return of menstruation and fertility is usually delayed in women who breast-feed, it has been suggested that breast-feeding acts as a natural birth spacer or "nature's own contraceptive" [38]. In those societies where breast-feeding is the sole source of nutrition for the baby, *lactational amenorrhea* (postpartum infertility) may last for 2 to 3 years [24]. The duration of the period between birth and the onset of a menstrual cycle in the mother is probably a function of the frequency and duration of suckling. Although breast-feeding usually delays conception, it cannot do so indefinitely and women can become pregnant before the breast-feeding infant is weaned.

HORMONAL CONTRACEPTION

The common contraceptive drugs in clinical use for women contain estrogens or progestogens, either singly or in a variety of combinations and concentrations [28]. The estrogens are usually synthetic derivatives of ethinyl estradiol (Fig. 19.9). The progestogens are usually 19-nortestosterone or 17-hydroxyprogesterone derivatives such as norethindrone (Fig. 19.9). The *combination contraceptive preparations* contain an estrogen and a progestogen and are often administered daily for 20 days and stopped for 5 days during which time withdrawal uterine bleeding (menses) occurs. Through a combined negative feedback to the hypothalamus (and pituitary?) LH and FSH secretions are suppressed. There is an absence of an LH-FSH surge, and the failure of a follicular phase rise in FSH secretion results in lack of ovarian follicular development. Endogenous blood levels of estradiol remain low due to suppression of LH and FSH secretion [6].

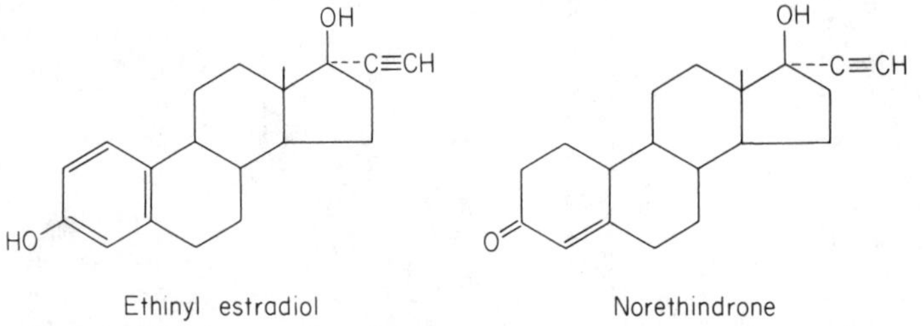

Ethinyl estradiol   Norethindrone

Figure 19.9 Examples of structures of two common contraceptive steroids, an estrogen, ethinyl estradiol, and a progestogen, norethindrone.

Progestogens administered alone have complex effects which relate to the dosage. Besides suppression of gonadotropin secretion and inhibition of follicular development, cervical mucus composition is modified, which may prevent sperm entry into the uterine cavity. In addition endometrial histology may be altered and thus interfere with implantation of the ovum should fertilization occur [28].

Some contraceptive steroid regimes consist of estrogens administered alone for a number of days (usually 15) followed by a progestogen for several days (usually 5). These *sequential contraceptive preparations* simulate to some degree the normal sequence of ovarian steroid secretion. A large dose of an estrogen has been used with some success as a postcoital contraceptive. Silastic steroid-impregnated devices that provide a slow delivery of a progestogen are being studied for possible use as contraceptive depot preparations. Even intrauterine devices (IUD's) impregnated with progestogens have been reported to provide significant contraceptive action.

Oral contraceptives increase the risk of venous thromboembolic disease apparently by increasing the size of the intravenous clots formed in response to endothelial injury or other stimuli that lead to thrombin formation. The estrogenic component of the oral contraceptives is responsible for the effect, apparently because it decreases antithrombin III activity. In addition to increasing the risk of venous thromboembolic disease oral contraceptives also increase the risks of myocardial infarction, thrombotic stroke, and hemorrhagic stroke. In women under age 35 the mortality rate ascribed to the use of oral contraceptives is about one-fourth or less that of the risk of death associated with complications of pregnancy among women using no method of contraception and is similar to the risk of death associated with the current use of other methods of contraception [39].

Superactive agonistic analogs of GnRH have been developed for potential use in hypogonadal men and women. These stimulatory analogs have been discovered to exert paradoxical inhibitory effects on pituitary-gonadal function in both sexes. Postovulatory administration of these stimulatory analogs may have a luteo-

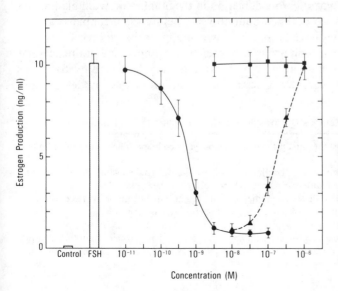

Figure 19.10 In vitro demonstration of GnRH hormone inhibition of estrogen production by rat granulosa cells. Increasing concentrations of GnRH (10^{-11}–10^{-7} M; ●—●) were inhibitory to estrogen production but this inhibition was reversed by increasing concentrations of a GnRH antagonist (D-pGlu^1, D-Phe^2, D-Trp^{3,6}]-GnRH; ▲---▲). The antagonist was without intrinsic activity on estrogen biosynthesis (■—■). (From Hsueh and Ling, [16], with permission.)

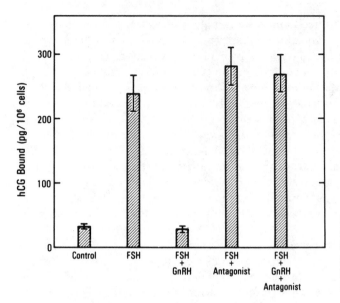

Figure 19.11 In vitro demonstration of FSH-induced LH/HCG receptor number in rat granulosa cells. The action of FSH is inhibited by GnRH an action antagonized by the GnRH antagonist. (From Hsueh and Ling, [16], with permission.)

lytic effect in women. The effects of these GnRH analogs may be mediated at the level of the pituitary, to cause a down regulation of gonadotropin GnRH receptors, and also at the level of the gonad through some unknown action (Figs. 19.10, 19.11). Other methods of hormonal contraception in the female are indicated in Table 19.1.

MENOPAUSE

The onset of menopause results from a loss in the cyclic activity of the ovary [7], which is believed to be caused by a failure at the level of the ovary to respond to gonadotropins. This is in part due to a depletion in the number of available follicles for growth. Fertility begins to decline about 10 years before the menopause and by age 50 most primary follicles have been lost. It would appear that germ cell atresia is determined by an intrinsic genetic program rather than by hormonal influences. As women approach menopause, there may be a striking increase in serum FSH levels relative to those of LH. Eventually, as estradiol secretion falls to low levels, both

TABLE 19.1 Theoretical Methods Of Nonsteroidal Contraception In The Female

Production of antibodies against the zona pellucida of the oocyte membrane which inhibit binding by spermatozoa.

Production of active immunization against chorionic gonadotropin. Antibodies against the N-terminus of the β subunit of hCG (which differs from the LH molecule) have been utilized with some success.

Production of agents that exert a direct luteolytic effect on the corpus luteum or interfere with the luteotropic action of the implanting blastocyst (e.g., competitive antagonist of hCG).

Production of antiprogestins to inhibit the progestational development of the endometrium.

Development of toxic drugs to act on the early human embryo. One plant protein, from the tuber of *Trichosanthes kiriloivii*, has a specific toxic effect on the syncytiotrophoblast of the human conceptus inducing a fall in hCG concentrations.

FSH and LH concentrations rise and remain elevated apparently due to the removal of the negative steroid feedback mechanism characteristic of active ovarian function. The premenopausal rise in FSH secretion may relate to the progressive loss of the putative ovarian hormone, inhibin, whose role is postulated to exert a negative feedback control of pituitary FSH secretion. Progressive loss of ovarian follicles and their maturation would be expected to reduce the production of inhibin.

In the absence of gonadal estrogens in the body during menopause it is not unexpected that a number of physiological changes take place. The uterus, an estrogen-dependent organ, becomes smaller and the endometrium atrophic. Atrophic vaginitis as well as vaginal dryness may occur but these changes can be reversed by exogenous estrogens given locally or systemically. There is an increased risk of coronary thrombosis in postmenopausal women, reaching a level of risk similar to that of men. After the menopause there is a reduction in the cortical thickness and the tensile strength of bones, resulting from an increase in loss of mineral content. *Postmenopausal osteoporosis* can be prevented by estrogen administration, but this depends on how soon after menopause estrogen replacement therapy begins.

During the *climacterium*, that period preceding termination of the reproductive period, some women experience episodic sensations of heat (menopausal flushes), usually involving the face and neck and upper part of the chest, which may be associated with profuse sweating. There is a close synchrony between these menopausal flushes and pulses of LH secretion. These flushes are not correlated with significant similar secretions of FSH, PRL, or catecholamines. The flushes are not caused by LH secretion per se as they occur in hypophysectomized women. Apparently a suprapituitary mechanism involving GnRH secretion is involved. It has been suggested that these flushes may be a manifestation of a classical withdrawal syndrome, mediated through changes in neurons sensitive to estrogens. A central adrenergic mechanism may be involved as α-adrenergic agonists provide some symptomatic relief [3].

There appears to be no relationship between the age of onset of menopause and the age of the onset of menarche. Also, the number of children born or the age at the time of birth of the first child does not appear to be related to the age of menopause [42]. The nutritional status of the individual may, however, influence the onset of menopause. The age of menopause varies in different countries: 49.8 for white North Americans; 51.4 in the Netherlands; 44 or younger in the Punjab, New Guinea, and Central Africa [15]. It appears that the age of menopause is increasing [11].

PATHOPHYSIOLOGY

Because of the complexity of the female reproductive system, the cyclic nature of ovarian hormone production and secretion, and the fact that the growth and development of a number of organs, in particular the uterus and mammary glands, are dependent on ovarian hormone secretion, it is not surprising that a large number of pathological states are attributable to endocrine dysfunctions. The pregnant state, dependent on a multitude of hormonal events unique to the female, is vulnerable to endocrine dysfunctions that can endanger the life of both the fetus and mother.

Endocrine Dysfunctions

Amenorrhea. This term designates a relatively common disturbance in the human female characterized by an absence of the monthly menstrual flow. The etiology relates to a deficiency in estrogen production and a failure therefore in the monthly proliferative growth of the endometrium and therefore an absence of monthly sloughing of the uterine lining. The failure of the menses to be initiated at puberty is referred to as *primary amenorrhea.* The etiology may relate to a genetic defect, resulting in a failure of gonadal maturation (or total gonadal dysgenesis), or more specifically to a defect in estrogen biosynthesis. *Secondary amenorrhea* refers to a failure to menstruate after regular menses have been initiated. Pregnancy and the menopause are, of course, examples of normal physiological bases for failure to resume the menses. Failure of pituitary gonadotropin secretion or hyperprolactinemia are defects that result in amenorrhea.

Isolated gonadotropin deficiency. This defect is characterized by a bihormonal deficiency of FSH and LH. In patients with isolated gonadotropin deficiency (IGD) administration of GnRH enhances FSH and LH secretion thus restoring normal gonadal function. It is likely that IGD may relate to a suprapituitary etiology involving an impaired synthesis and secretion of endogenous GnRH.

Polycystic ovarian disease. Women with this syndrome ovulate infrequently or not at all. The defect appears to relate to a failure of follicular maturation. Excess adrenal androgen production may be the etiological factor involved. Estrone levels are elevated relative to estradiol and may derive from excessive conversion of androstenedione to estrone. Elevated estrone may be inhibitory to pituitary FSH secretion but stimulatory to LH secretion thus leading to failure of follicular development and ovulation.

Hyperprolactinemia. The most common example of pituitary hypersecretion of a hormone involves prolactin. Not only does hyperprolactinemia lead to *galactorrhea* (excess milk production) but amenorrhea and anovulation are complicating sequelae of excessive PRL secretion. Breast engorgement due to excessive lactogenesis usually results from excessive PRL secretion from a pituitary adenoma (prolactinoma). The etiology of the prolactinoma is uncertain but could result from a failure of hypothalamic release of prolactin inhibiting factor thus leading to lactotroph hyperplasia and eventual adenoma formation. The onset of galactorrhea may date to a normal postpartum lactation that fails to be discontinued (Chiari-Frommel syndrome). Suckling of the breasts is the normal stimulus to PRL secretion. It appears that stimuli which increase afferent impulses in the neuroendocrine reflex pathway leading to PRL secretion, such as surgery, trauma, tight-fitting garments, or continued breast manipulation, may lead to galactorrhea (neurogenic galactorrhea-amenorrhea). The amenorrhea that accompanies the galactorrhea probably results from PRL inhibition of hypothalamic GnRH secretion and a subsequent block of the ovulatory surge of gonadotropins. In addition elevated plasma PRL levels are directly inhibitory to ovarian estrogen production, which may also be, in part, responsible for the accompanying amenorrhea. Women with increased PRL levels and a resulting decreased estrogen production may experience bone demineralization and associated incidence of clinical bone fractures [21]. Bromocryptine, a dopamine receptor agonist, is effective in establishing normal estrogen levels and ovulatory menstrual cycles in most hyperprolactinemic women.

Hirsutism and virilization. Hirsutism in the female may be due to a number of diverse causes. Enzymatic defects in adrenal cortisol metabolism that lead to excess androgen secretion (Chapter 15) or excess androgen production by an adrenal or ovarian tumor may cause hirsutism. Increased facial and body hair growth, increased muscle mass, and clitoral enlargement are manifestations of excessive adrenal (adult adrenogenital syndrome) or gonadal androgen production. Cyproterone acetate, an androgen antagonist, has been used successfully in the treatment of hirsutism and masculinization.

Hormones and breast cancer. The early observation that oophorectomy may effect a rapid remission of advanced breast cancer in some premenopausal women provided evidence that some human breast cancers may depend on sex steroids for their continued proliferation. Hypophysectomy and adrenalectomy are a means of hormone deprivation through endocrine ablation, but unfortunately not all women respond favorably to such radical treatment. This is because only 25% to 30% of human breast cancers are hormone dependent and therefore responsive to endocrine manipulation. Patients with hormone-dependent cancers may, however, be favorable candidates for endocrine therapy. It is important therefore to distinguish those women with such hormone-responsive cancers. It has been demonstrated that the quantitative determination of the estrogen receptor (estrophilin) content of an excised tumor specimen often provides useful information as the best type of therapy for the patient with advanced breast cancer. Tumors that contain low or negligible amounts of estrophilin rarely respond to endocrine ablation or other hormone therapy (e.g., antiestrogen administration), whereas patients with receptor-rich cancers often benefit from endocrine treatment [18].

REFERENCES

[1] BISBEE, C. A., T. E. MACHEN, and H. A. BERN. 1979. Mouse mammary epithelial cells on floating collagen gels: transepithelial ion transport and effects of prolactin. *Proc. Natl. Acad. Sci. USA* 76:536–40.

[2] BRADDON, S. A. 1978. Relaxin-dependent adenosine 3,5″-monophosphate concentration changes in the mouse public symphysis. *Endocrinology* 102:1292–99.

[3] CASPER, R. F., S. S. C. YEN, and M. M. WILKES. 1979. Menopausal flushes: a neuroendocrine link with pulsatile luteinizing hormone secretion. *Science* 205:823–25.

[4] CSAPO, A. I., E. F. CSAPO, E. FAYE, M. R. HANZL, and G. SALAU. 1973. The delay of spontaneous labor by naproxen in the rat model. *Prostaglandins* 3:827–37.

[5] DAWOOD, M. Y., O. YLIKORKALA, D. TRIVEDI, and F. FUCHS. 1979. Oxytocin in maternal circulation and amniotic fluid during pregnancy. *J. Clin. Endocrinol. Metab.* 49: 429–34.

[6] DROEGEMUELLER, W., and R. BRESSLER. 1980. Effectiveness and risks of contraception. *Ann. Rev. Physiol.* 31:329–43.

[7] ESKIN, B. A., ed. 1980. *The menopause*. New York: Masson Publ. Co.

[8] EVERETT, R. B., and P. C. MACDONALD. 1979. Endocrinology of the placenta. *Ann. Rev. Med.* 30:473–88.

[9] FALCONER, I. R. 1980. Aspects of the biochemistry, physiology and endocrinology of lactation. *Aust. J. Biol. Sci.* 33:71–84.

[10] FEVOLD, H., F. L. HISAW, and R. K. MEYER. 1930. The relaxative hormone of the corpus luteum. Its purification and concentration. *J. Am. Chem. Soc.* 52:3340–48.

[11] FLINT, M. 1978. Is there a secular trend in age of menopause? *Maturitas* 1:133–39.

[12] FUCHS, A., F. FUCHS, P. HUSSLEIN, M. SOLOFF, and M. J. SOLOFF. 1982. Oxytocin receptors and human parturition: a dual role for oxytocin in the initiation of labor. *Science* 215:1396–98.

[13] GARFIELD, R. E., S. SIMS, and E. E. DANIEL. 1977. Gap junctions: their presence and necessity in myometrium during parturition. *Science* 198:958–59.

[14] GERSHENGORN, M. C., B. E. MARCUS-SAMUELS, and E. GERAS. 1979. Estrogens increase the number of thyrotropin-releasing hormone receptors on mammotropic cells in culture. *Endocrinology* 105:171–76. © 1979 *The Endocrine Society*. Baltimore: The Williams & Wilkins Company.

[15] GRAY, R. H. 1976. The menopause—epidemiological and demographic considerations. In *The menopause*, ed. R. J. Beard, pp. 25–40. Lancaster, England: MTP Press Ltd.

[16] HSUEH, A. J. W., and N. C. LING. 1979. Effect of an antagonistic analog of gonadotropin releasing hormone upon ovarian granulosa cell function. *Life Sci.* 25:1223–30. © 1979, Pergamon Press, Ltd.

[17] JAFFE, R. B., ed. 1981. *Prolactin*. New York: Elsevier North-Holland, Inc.

[18] JENSEN, E. V., and E. R. DESOMBRE. 1977. The diagnostic implications of steroid binding in malignant tissues. *Advan. Clin. Chem.* 19:57–89.

[19] KEIRSE, M. J. N. C., A. B. M. ANDERSON, and J. B. GRAVENHORSE, eds. 1979. *Human parturition*. Leiden, the Netherlands: Leiden University Press.

[20] KERTILES, L. P., and L. L. ANDERSON. 1979. Effect of relaxin on cervical dilatation, parturition and lactation in the pig. *Biol. Reprod.* 21:57–68.

[21] KLIBANSKI, A., R. N. NEER, I. Z. BEITINS, E. C. RIDGWAY, N. T. ZERVAS, and J. W. McARTHUR. 1980. Decreased bone density in hyperprolactinemic women. *New Engl. J. Med.* 303:1511–14.

[22] LIGGINS, G. C., C. S. FORSTER, S. A. GRIEVES, and A. I. SCHWARTZ. 1977. Control of parturition in man. *Biol. Reprod.* 16:39–56.

[23] MARSHALL, J. M. 1981. Effects of ovarian steroids and pregnancy of adrenergic nerves of uterus and oviduct. *Am. J. Physiol.* 240:C165–C174.

[24] McNEILLY, A. S. 1979. Effects of lactation on fertility. *Brit. Med. Bull.* 35:151–54.

[25] NATHANIELSZ, P. W. 1978. Endocrine mechanisms of parturition. *Ann. Rev. Physiol.* 40:411–45.

[26] NIKITOVITCH-WINER, M. B., and J. W. EVERETT. 1959. Histologic changes in grafts of rat pituitary on the kidney and upon re-transplantation under the diencephalon. *Endocrinology* 65:357.

[27] O'BYRNE, E., B. T. CARRIERE, L. SORENSON, A. SEGALOFF, C. SCHWABE, and B. G. STEINETZ. 1978. Plasma immunoreactive relaxin levels in pregnant and nonpregnant women. *J. Clin. Endocrinol. & Metab.* 47:1106–10.

[28] ODELL, W. D., and M. E. MOLITCH. 1974. The pharmacology of contraceptive agents. *Ann. Rev. Pharmacol.* 14:413–34.

[29] REING, J. W., L. N. DANIEL, C. SCHWABE, L. K. GOWAN, B. G. STEINETZ, and E. M. O'BYRNE. 1981. Isolation and characterization of relaxin from the sand tiger shark (*Odontaspis taurus*). *Endocrinology* 109:537–43.

[30] ROSEN, J. M., R. J. MATUSIK, D. A. RICHARDS, P. GUPTA, and J. R. RODGERS. 1980. Multihormonal regulation of casein gene expression at the transcriptional and post-transcriptional levels in the mammary gland. *Rec. Prog. Horm. Res.* 36:157–93.

[31] ROTHCHILD, I. 1981. The regulation of the mammalian corpus luteum. *Rec. Prog. Horm. Res.* 37:183–298.

[32] SCHWABE, C., and J. C. MCDONALD. 1977. Relaxin: a disulfide homolog of insulin. *Science* 197:914–15.

[33] SCHWABE, C., B. STEINETZ, G. WEISS, A. SEGALOFF, J. K. MCDONALD, E. O'BYRNE, J. HOCKMAN, B. CARRIERE, and L. GOLDSMITH. 1978. Relaxin. *Rec. Proc. Horm. Res.* 34:123–211.

[34] SHERWOOD, O. D., and V. E. CRNEKOVIC. 1979. Development of a homologous radio-immunoassay for rat relaxin. *endocrinology* 104:893–97. © 1979 *The Endocrine Society*. Baltimore. The Williams & Wilkins Company.

[35] SHERWOOD, O. D., B. S. NARA, V. E. CRNEKOVIC, and N. L. FIRST. 1979. Relaxin concentrations in pig plasma after the administration of indomethacin and prostaglandin $F_{2\alpha}$ during late pregnancy. *Endocrinology* 104:1716–21.

[36] SHERWOOD, O. D., V. E. CRNEKOVIC, W. L. GORDON, and J. E. RUTHERFORD. 1980. Radioimmunoassay of relaxin throughout pregnancy and during parturition in the rat. Encorinology 107:691–98. © 1980 *The Endocrine Society*. Baltimore: The Williams & Wilkins Company.

[37] SHIU, R. P. C., and H. G. FRIESEN. 1980. Mechanism of action of prolactin in the control of mammary gland function. *Ann. Rev. Physiol.* 42:83–96.

[38] SHORT, R. V. 1976. Lactation—the central control of reproduction. In Ciba Foundation Symposium 45, *Breast-feeding and the mother*. Excerpta Medica pp. 73–86. Amsterdam: Elsevier North-Holland, Inc.

[39] STADEL, B. V. 1981. Oral contraceptives and cardiovascular disease. *New Engl. J. Med.* 305:612–18, 672–77.

[40] THORNBURN, G. D., and J. R. G. CHALLIS. 1979. Endocrine control of parturition. *Physiol. Rev.* 59:863–918.

[41] VAN TIENHOVEN, A. 1968. *Reproductive physiology*. Philadelphia: W. B. Saunders Company.

[42] WALSH, R. J. 1978. The age of menopause in Australian women. *Med. J. Aust.* 2:181–215.

[43] WEITZMAN, R. E., R. E. LEAKE, R. T. RUBIN, and D. A. FISHER. 1980. The effect of nursing on neurohypophyseal hormone and prolactin secretion in human subjects. *J. Clin. Endocrinol.* 51:836–39. © 1980. *The Endocrine Society*. Baltimore: The Williams & Wilkins Company.

20

Endocrine Role of the Pineal Gland

INTRODUCTION

The evidence is convincing that the pineal gland (epiphysis cerebri) is involved in the control of reproductive processes of certain mammals, possibly even humans. Clinical evidence reveals that children with parenchymal pinealomas may be delayed in their sexual development, whereas destructive (nonparenchymal) pinealomas are often associated with precocious puberty [24]. However, the detailed mechanisms by which the pineal affects reproductive processes are unclear. It is generally believed that the pineal secretes a hormone which has antigonadotropic properties. A vast amount of experimental data indicates *melatonin*, an indoleamine, as the pineal antigonadotropin [48], but other putative antigonadotropins have been espoused. This chapter summarizes the vast but sometimes conflicting literature on the role of the pineal in mammalian reproductive physiology. In addition the pineal as an endocrine organ controlling other physiological processes is also discussed. A number of monographs are available which provide further information on the anatomy, biochemistry, and physiology of this intriguing endocrine organ [33, 37, 38, 49].

PINEAL DEVELOPMENT AND MORPHOLOGY

The human pineal arises as a median evagination of the diencephalic roof of the embryonic brain. In most mammals the pineal gland moves away from the roof of the third ventricle and loses connection with the brain except for a thin stalk. The

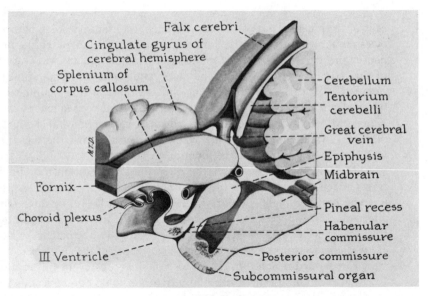

Figure 20.1 The human pineal gland (epiphysis) and its anatomical relation to the diencephalic roof. (From Wurtman, Axelrod, and Kelly, [48], with permission.)

adult human pineal (epiphysis) is a pine cone-shaped organ, a shape which suggested the organ's name (Fig. 20.1). The pineal is innervated by postganglionic fibers originating from the *superior cervical ganglia*; the pineal is therefore an effector organ of the autonomic nervous system [49]. The pineal parenchymal cells, pinealocytes, are derived from the ependymal lining of the epithalamus; both light and dark parenchymal cells can be distinguished in the mammalian pineal. The dark cells contain pigment granules of an unknown nature as well as glycogen deposits of undefined physiological significance. The dark pinealocytes are interconnected by tight junctions, suggesting that electrical signals may be communicated between the cells. Fibroblasts and glial cells make up the rest of the glandular mass which, in humans, is about 170 to 175 mg in average weight [46]. Calcification of the human pineal begins during the second decade of life and by 60 years 70% of all pineal glands may be at least partly calcified [37]. Nevertheless, there is no evidence that calcification signals a loss of function; on the contrary, biochemical studies indicate no change in biochemical activity of the pineal with age.

THE MELATONIN HYPOTHESIS

Historical Perspective

Early anatomists held various views on the physiological function of the pineal in the human. This unique unpaired structure that lies deeply recessed under the cerebral hemispheres of the brain drew their attention and speculation. The philosopher Descartes considered it the "seat of the soul." The possible physiological significance of the pineal was first recognized by Heubner who noted precocious sexual maturity in a young boy whose pineal was destroyed by a tumor. Holmgren noted that the

The Melatonin Hypothesis

cells of the pineal gland of an elasmobranch were sensorylike in nature: The pinealo-cytes resembled the sensory cells of the retina. Because some reptiles possess a prominent "third eye," the pineal of mammals including humans was considered a vestige of this primitive visual organ. The observation that the human pineal may become calcified at an early age further consolidated thought that the pineal was, indeed, a vestigial organ and therefore of little physiological consequence. A monograph by Kitay and Altschule [24] described, however, some remarkable clinical correlations of pineal dysfunction. The evidence clearly revealed that the pineal might in some way be related to reproductive function in humans.

McCord and Allen made the interesting observation that bovine pineal extracts added to the water in which tadpoles swam caused the larvae to blanch, that is, to become very light in color or even transparent [26]. This interesting pigmentary effect was duly appreciated by the dermatologist, Aaron Lerner, who was searching for a factor which might be responsible for vitiligo (white patches of skin) in humans. He was able to isolate and determine the structure of the substance, an indoleamine, which he named *melatonin*. This was a momentous event in the history of pineal research as this unique molecule of pineal origin could now be readily synthesized and made available for a variety of physiological studies. Melatonin, N-acetyl-5-methoxy-tryptamine (Fig. 20.2), proved to have potent effects on integumental pigmentation in some animals, but not humans, as will be discussed. Most importantly, however, this indoleamine was shown to have antigonadal effects on the mammalian reproductive system.

Profound changes in gonadal function are observed in many animals when exposed to continuous light or darkness. Maturation of the gonads of hamsters, for example, is delayed when these animals are maintained under conditions of continuous darkness. This effect can be prevented by pinealectomy (epiphysectomy). In contrast, continuous light leads to the early onset of sexual development and to a more rapid increase in gonadal weight; constant light also causes a reduction in size and function of the pineal gland. Pineal ablation in young rodents usually leads to accelerated gonadal maturation, and these developmental effects can be reduced by injections of pineal extracts. Melatonin, like pineal extracts, administered to young rodents also results in a delay of gonadal maturation. These observations are consistent with a hypothesis that photic cues received by an animal in some way affect pineal release of melatonin which then has an antigonadal action. The "melatonin hypothesis" has thus emerged [47]. Other evidence which further relates to this hypothesis will be examined.

Animal Studies

From studies on the hamster the role of the pineal in mammalian reproductive processes has been further elucidated [36, 37]. Changes in length of the daily photoperiod are especially important in controlling gonadal activity in the hamster, *Mesocricetus auratus*, which in its natural habitat breeds seasonally and hibernates. The repro-

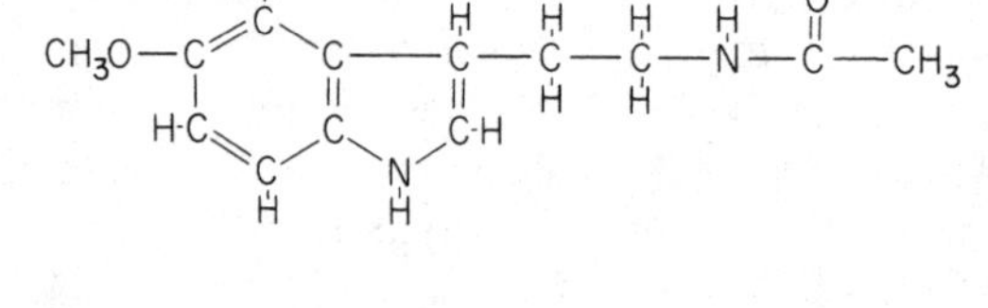

Figure 20.2 The structure of melatonin (N-acetyl-5-methoxytryptamine).

ductive organs of the hamster are extremely sensitive to the influence of environmental lighting and to the activity of the pineal gland. In the male short photoperiods or blinding lead to gonadal atrophy with complete loss of testicular spermatogenic activity. The gonads may be reduced to only 20% of their normal size. The accessory organs (seminal vesicles and coagulating glands) also atrophy, indicating a loss of support by gonadal androgens. These atrophic effects result from decreased secretion of FSH and LH from the pituitary. Pinealectomy prevents gonadal regression in hamsters maintained on nonstimulatory short days. In the female the data are less clear, but there is a decrease in uterine weight apparently due to decreased estrogen production in response to short photoperiods or blinding. Plasma gonadotropin levels of female golden hamsters on short days is decreased relative to that of females exposed to long days.

There is a daily rhythm of pineal melatonin synthesis in the hamster, a rhythm influenced by environmental lighting. Superior cervical ganglionectomy, however, abolishes the rhythm of pineal melatonin production. There is good evidence that melatonin is the hamster antigonadotropic hormone. The mechanism of antigonadotropic action has been determined through some ingenious experiments. There appears to be a short day-induced increase in the sensitivity of the hypothalamopituitary axis to the negative feedback effect of steroid hormones. Castrated male hamsters on short days are much more sensitive to the negative feedback effects of exogenous testosterone (as determined by measurements of serum gonadotropin levels) than are animals exposed to long days. This increased sensitivity is blocked or reduced by pinealectomy. Thus, the short day-induced increase in sensitivity of the hamster hypothalamo-hypophysial axis to testosterone feedback is mediated, at least in part, by the pineal gland [41].

Blinding does not cause permanent inhibition of testicular or ovarian function in the hamster. There is a spontaneous recrudescence of the gonads to the normal adult condition in hamsters that have been blinded for about 27 weeks. This could help explain what normally happens under hibernating conditions. Hamsters are reproductively competent when they emerge from their burrows in the spring. The spontaneous onset of the gonadal refractory condition appears to be a single occurrence, not a cyclical phenomenon, as the recrudesced gonads of blinded hamsters remain large indefinitely. In other species (ewe, starling), however, there is evidence for both a spontaneous onset and termination of reproductive activity which occur cyclically with a period of about a year (i.e., circannually) [15].

It is unclear why the gonads of blinded or hibernating hamsters spontaneously become activated. The hypothalamo-hypophysial-gonadal axis may become refractory to the pineal antigonadotropic hormone [18]. It has been shown that exogenous melatonin injections cause testicular regression in pinealectomized hamsters regardless of the photoperiod. Injections of melatonin during the early part of the day, however, are often ineffective in causing gonadal atrophy in intact hamsters. Also, in the presence of continuously elevated levels of melatonin (in animals carrying implants of melatonin) pinealectomized animals are rendered insensitive to daily injections of the hormone. Thus, the continuous exposure to melatonin possibly renders the target tissue relatively unresponsive to daily injections of melatonin. It may therefore be important that melatonin be released rhythmically from the pineal rather than continuously [10, 18, 37].

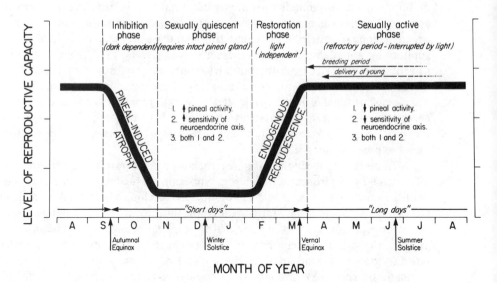

Figure 20.3 The role of the pineal in the annual reproduction cycle of a long-day breeder, the hamster. (From Reiter, [36], with permission.)

These observations leave little doubt that the pineal through the action of its antigonadotropic hormone, melatonin, is a key component in the control of reproductive processes in this mammal (Fig. 20.3). There is evidence that the pineal functions in a similar role in some other mammals and some nonmammalian species [17, 22].

Pineal Indoleamine Biosynthesis

The biochemistry of pineal indoleamine biosynthesis is well documented [33, 47]. Indoleamine biosynthesis involves utilization of the amino acid, tryptophan, which is converted to 5-hydroxytryptophan by the enzyme tryptophan hydroxylase (Fig. 20.4). The enzyme 5-hydroxytryptophan decarboxylase acts on 5-hydroxytryptophan to form 5-hydroxytryptamine (5-HT, *serotonin*) which is converted to *N*-acetylserotonin by the action of *N*-acetyltransferase. The *N*-acetylserotonin produced is O-methylated by hydroxyindole-O-methyltransferase (HIOMT) to form *N*-acetyl-5-methoxytryptamine (melatonin). It is believed that the increase in *N*-acetylserotonin concentration acts by a mass action effect to enhance the production of melatonin. Pineal melatonin biosynthesis is mainly controlled by *N*-acetyltransferase activity which may be the rate-limiting event in the production of this indoleamine. Others argue, however, that HIOMT activity may be of prime importance to melatonin biosynthesis. Melatonin is then metabolized in the liver to 6-hydroxymelatonin by melatonin hydroxylase and converted to a sulfate or to a glucuronide for urinary excretion.

Although acetylation to *N*-acetylserotonin is a necessary step in the biosynthesis of melatonin, deamination of serotonin by monoamine oxidase can also oc-

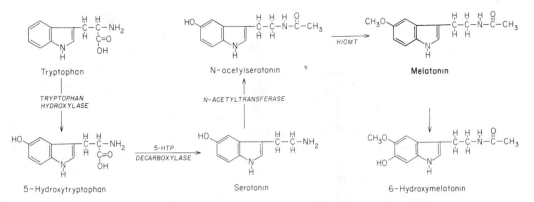

Figure 20.4 Pathway of melatonin biosynthesis and metabolism within the pineal gland.

cur in the pineal. The deaminated product may be either oxidized to 5-hydroxy-indoleacetic acid or reduced to 5-hydroxytryptophol. The latter compounds can then become O-methylated by HIOMT to give 5-methoxyindole acetic acid and 5-methoxytryptophol.

Effect of Light on Pineal Indoleamine Biosynthesis

Melatonin synthesis within the rat pineal is dramatically affected by photic cues received by the lateral eyes. At night there is an increase in the activity of N-acetyltransferase which is 10- to nearly 100-fold greater than values in the light. The concentration of N-acetylserotonin is subsequently increased to values ten to 30 times greater than observed under day conditions. HIOMT activity is also increased, which results in elevated levels of pineal melatonin. Pineal enzyme activities are rapidly depressed by light. Pineal serotonin levels reveal marked diurnal changes with highest levels noted during the daylight hours. Serotonin levels are depressed after darkness, probably because serotonin is the substrate for N-acetyltransferase action and is therefore converted to N-acetylserotonin. Reversal of external lighting conditions reverses the rhythm of pineal enzyme activity and indoleamine biosynthesis. Thus, a daily diurnal rhythm of pineal biosynthetic activity is observed and is controlled by the normal day-to-day changes in natural lighting. This diurnal fluctuation of pineal enzyme activity and melatonin synthesis is lost under conditions of continuous illumination. The rhythm is, however, maintained, though diminished, in animals kept in the dark. Some CNS site may be responsible for producing a cyclic signal which is responsible for the persistence of pineal rhythmicity. The daily rhythm of pineal indoleamine biosynthesis in the bird [7, 8] is depicted in Figure 20.5 and has also been carefully documented in the rat [25].

CNS Pathway in the Control of Pineal Indoleamine Biosynthesis

The role of the CNS in the control of pineal indoleamine biosynthesis in mammals has been determined by a variety of surgical techniques. Melatonin is synthesized in response to norepinephrine released from postganglionic neurons from the superior

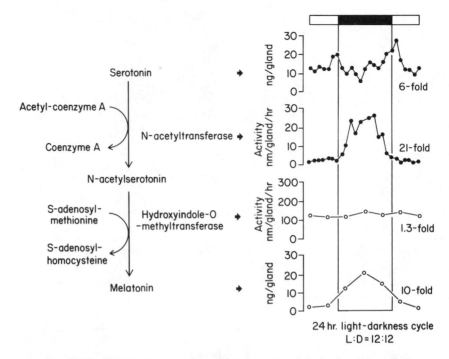

Serotonin   →

Acetyl-coenzyme A ⟍

Coenzyme A ↙   N-acetyltransferase →

N-acetylserotonin

S-adenosyl-
methionine   Hydroxyindole-O →
-methyltransferase

S-adenosyl- ↙
homocysteine

Melatonin   →

ng/gland   30 20 10 0   6-fold

Activity nm/gland/hr   30 20 10 0   21-fold

Activity nm/gland/hr   300 200 100 0   1.3-fold

ng/gland   30 20 10 0   10-fold

24 hr. light-darkness cycle
L:D = 12:12

Figure 20.5   Pathway for serotonin conversion to melatonin in the pineal gland. Daily measurements over a 24-hour period of serotonin content, *N*-acetyltransferase activity (NAT), hydroxyindole-O-methyltransferase activity (HIOMT), and melatonin content in chick pineals were made. The bar at the top of the graph represents the 24-hour lighting regimen in which the birds were held (L:D 12:12:12 hours of light in alternation with 12 hours of dark). The daily change in melatonin is believed to be a consequence of the daily change in NAT. The numbers (x-fold) on the graph are the ratio of peak to nadir values. (Modified from Binkley, [7], with permission.)

cervical ganglia. Thus, the pineal is considered to be a *neuroendocrine transducer*, like the adrenal chromaffin tissue, as neural input to these organs is converted into an endocrine output [48]. Postganglionic stimulation of pinealocytes depends on the absence of light activation of the retina of the lateral eyes. Light information perceived by the eyes is conveyed to the *suprachiasmatic nuclei* of the brain by way of a retinohypothalamic pathway [28].

  Neuronal circuits from the suprachiasmatic nuclei convey information via the medial forebrain bundle to the upper thoracic spinal cord and then out to the superior cervical ganglia. From these ganglia the postganglionic neurons proceed to innervate the pineal. Disruption of this neural pathway anywhere between the lateral eyes and the suprachiasmatic nuclei stimulates pineal indoleamine biosynthesis. Removal of the superior cervical ganglia (ganglionectomy) or decentralization of the ganglia, on the other hand, abolishes the rhythms of indoleamine biosynthesis. Lesions of the medial forebrain bundle also block pineal *N*-acetyltransferase rhythms as do lesions of the suprachiasmatic nuclei. A summary of the surgical procedures is provided (Fig. 20.6). These data suggest that the suprachiasmatic nuclei may be the CNS site responsible for generation of the nocturnal activity of pineal indoleamine

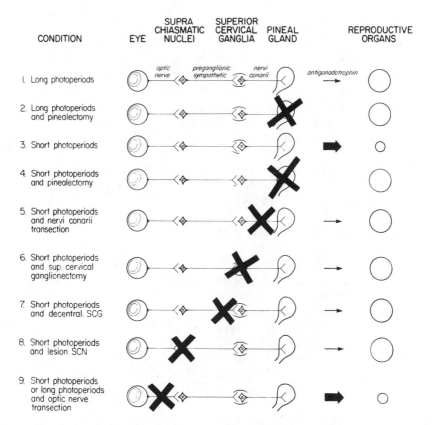

CONDITION	EYE	SUPRA CHIASMATIC NUCLEI	SUPERIOR CERVICAL GANGLIA	PINEAL GLAND	REPRODUCTIVE ORGANS
1. Long photoperiods		optic nerve	preganglionic sympathetic	nervi conarii	antigonadotrophin
2. Long photoperiods and pinealectomy					
3. Short photoperiods					
4. Short photoperiods and pinealectomy					
5. Short photoperiods and nervi conarii transection					
6. Short photoperiods and sup. cervical ganglionectomy					
7. Short photoperiods and decentral. SCG					
8. Short photoperiods and lesion SCN					
9. Short photoperiods or long photoperiods and optic nerve transection					

Figure 20.6 Surgical procedures which eliminate or exaggerate pineal antigonadotropic activity in mammals. The bold X's represent removal of the organ or surgical transection of a fiber tract. The thickness of the arrows indicates the antigonadotropic capability of the pineal gland. The phrase preganglionic sympathetic fibers refers to a multitude of neurons which intervene between the suprachiasmatic nuclei (SCN) and the superior cervical ganglia (SCG). Decentral. SCG (decentralization of the SCG) refers to separating the SCG from their connections with the central nervous system. (From Reiter, [36], with permission.)

biosynthesis in mammals. The circadian oscillatory activity of the cells of the suprachiasmatic nuclei may be entrained to the daily photoperiod [25].

Intracellular Control of Pineal Indoleamine Biosynthesis

Norepinephrine released from superior cervical postganglionic neurons interacts with pinealocyte β-adrenergic receptors, which leads to an increase in pineal cyclic AMP production. Elevation of this intracellular second messenger results in the conversion of tryptophan to serotonin and then serotonin to N-acetylserotonin. This response is mimicked by dibutyryl cyclic AMP or theophylline, a phosphodiesterase inhibitor, which elevates pineal cyclic AMP levels. Norepinephrine, but not dibutyryl cyclic AMP, increases uptake of tryptophan into pinealocytes. The neurotransmitter therefore has a twofold effect: It increases intracellular levels of the substrate, tryptophan, as well as cyclic AMP, whose action is to enhance enzymatic utilization of the substrate for melatonin biosynthesis. Injection of propranolol, a β-adrenergic receptor antagonist, just before the onset of darkness inhibits the nighttime rise in pineal N-acetyltransferase activity as does reserpine, a drug that depletes adrenergic neurons of catecholamines. A single dose of isoproterenol, a β-adrenergic receptor agonist, administered during the day causes an immediate increase in pineal N-acetyltransferase activity. Electrical stimulation of the superior cervical ganglia causes a rapid increase in the concentration of cyclic AMP in the pineal gland of rats [20]. These experimental manipulations clearly reveal the role of noradrenergic postganglionic neurons in the control of pineal biosynthetic activity [25, 49]. A summary depicting the CNS pathways and mechanisms controlling pineal function is given (Fig. 20.7).

Melatonin Secretion and Circulation

Melatonin is present in the plasma and urine of all animals studied, including humans, and pinealectomy reduces the circulating levels of the indoleamine in experimental animals. As for pineal melatonin, plasma levels of melatonin of humans and other animals (sheep, pig, rat, cow, donkey, camel, chicken, salmon, lizard) are highest at middark and lowest at midlight periods (Fig. 20.8) [43]. In addition to the daily melatonin rhythm in blood and urine of primates there is a diurnal melatonin rhythm in primate cerebrospinal fluid (CSF) [39]. Night peak values are two to 15 times higher than day values. This increase occurs soon after lights are turned off, and the decrease toward day values occurs rapidly after lights are turned on

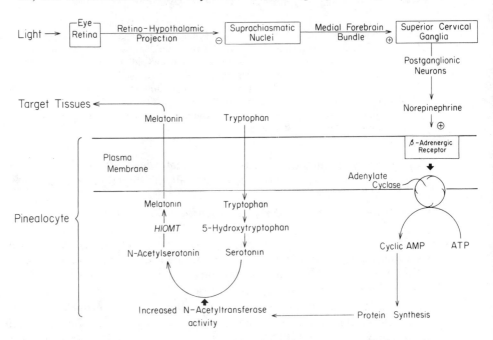

Figure 20.7 CNS pathway and mechanisms controlling pineal indole metabolism in mammals.

Endocrine Role of the Pineal Gland   Chap. 20

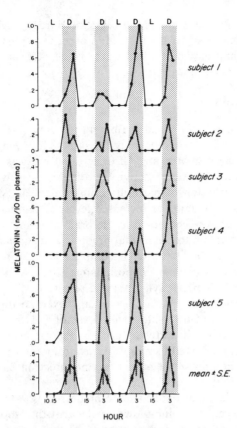

Figure 20.8 Diurnal plasma melatonin levels in humans. Note the nocturnal elevation during four consecutive cycles in five adult male subjects. (From Vaughan, Meyer, and Reiter, [44], *Journal of Clinical Endocrinology and Metabolism*, vol. 42, pp. 752–764. © 1976 Philadelphia: J. B. Lippincott Publishing Company, with permission.)

again (Fig. 20.9). The changes in CSF melatonin concentrations appear to reflect daily changes in plasma melatonin concentrations. It is not clear, however, whether melatonin is secreted into the CSF only, into the plasma only, or into both [43]. A 24-hour rhythm in the concentration of CSF melatonin suggests the possibility that the CSF may be an important route of communication between the pineal gland and other parts of the brain [49].

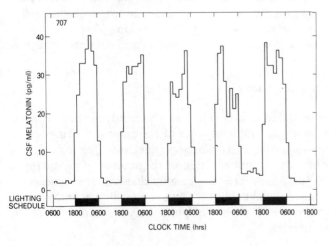

Figure 20.9 Diurnal pattern of CSF melatonin in the rhesus monkey. An individual animal was studied for 6 consecutive days and CSF was collected every 90 minutes. (From Reppert et al., [39], with permission.)

The Melatonin Hypothesis

HIOMT activity is present in some blood cells, the Harderian gland [11], and the retina, and melatonin may also be synthesized in other extrapineal sites such as the hypothalamus, retina, and gastrointestinal tract. These sites may assume some functional significance following pinealectomy.

Site of Action of Melatonin

There is evidence for brain, pituitary, and peripheral antigonadotropic actions of melatonin. The evidence for a CNS effect is derived from the following information. Pinealectomy leads to increased motor and EEG activity, whereas melatonin administration reduces spontaneous motor activity, promotes sleep with slow EEG activity, and prolongs the duration of barbiturate-induced sleep. Melatonin may modify CNS neurotransmitter function as increased levels of gamma aminobutyric acid (GABA) and serotonin have been noted in the brain after melatonin administration [49]. Melatonin implants into the medial preoptic and suprachiasmatic and retrochiasmatic areas of the mouse brain elicit complete gonadal regression [17]. It is suggested that melatonin mediates its hypothalamic effect by inhibition of gonadotropin-releasing hormone (GnRH) synthesis and secretion.

There is additional evidence that melatonin can also exert an antigonadotropic action directly on the pituitary. GnRH-induced release of LH from neonatal rat pituitaries in organ culture is significantly reduced in the presence of melatonin, but this effect cannot be demonstrated using pituitaries from adult rats or neonatal or adult hamsters [1]. In the human melatonin has no effect on basal or GnRH-stimulated LH secretion [37, 38].

There is also evidence that exogenous melatonin decreases testicular androgen synthesis and that the indoleamine is inhibitory to the growth response of the rat ventral prostate gland to exogenous testosterone. Melatonin also decreases the weight of both the testes and the ventral prostate gland of hypophysectomized rats receiving testosterone. Pinealectomy enhances the growth response of the seminal vesicles to testosterone in castrated rats and administration of the indoleamine prevents the response to the androgen. These results suggest that the inhibitory influence of systematically administered melatonin on the accessory sex organs may be due to its antagonistic effect at the level of the gonads. Melatonin excretion in normal males and females increases at puberty. Gonadal function may influence melatonin secretion during puberty, and melatonin may play a role in adrenarche (pubertal changes induced by adrenal androgens) by an action on adrenal steroidogenesis [32].

Pineal Rhythms and Biological Clocks

The pineal gland synthesizes melatonin in response to photic information received from the lateral eyes. Because of the rapid response of the epiphysial synthesizing machinery and the short half-life of the released product, melatonin, circulating levels of the indoleamine may be an accurate reflection of the amount of photic input to the lateral eyes. The pineal may therefore provide a mechanism for the measurement of the duration of the dark and light periods. Thus, in animals whose reproductive patterns fit into a specific seasonal scheme the pineal may play a pivotal role in the control of their gonadal function.

In mammals light information is first perceived by photoreceptor elements of the lateral eyes; this information is then relayed through a retinohypothalamic pathway to the suprachiasmatic nuclei (SCN) [40]. A rhythm of N-acetyltransferase activity is, however, maintained in blinded animals kept in constant lighting or in normal animals in continuous darkness. It is suggested that the signal generator is an oscillator (*biological clock*) with a period of about 24 hours that only transmits a signal to the pineal gland periodically. The pineal rhythm is truly circadian in nature. Biological clocks are synchronized or entrained by periodically recurring environmental stimuli. Although more than one mammalian circadian clock may exist, the SCN is considered the "master" oscillatory system [52].

OTHER PUTATIVE PINEAL HORMONES

Pineal substances other than melatonin are also reported to possess antigonadotropic activity. However, the evidence is not very convincing. A number of peptide hormones have, however, been localized to the pineal, but their physiological significance there remains to be clarified. The indoleamine 5-methoxytryptophol, which is synthesized from 5-hydroxytryptophol by the action of HIOMT, is reported to possess antigonadotropic activity. A variety of other unidentified indolic and peptide substances are also reported to possess antigonadal activity [6, 14].

It has been claimed that the mammalian pineal contains and synthesizes arginine vasotocin (AVT) and that oxytocin and arginine vasopressin may also be present in the mammalian epithalamus. AVT is said to inhibit compensatory ovarian hypertrophy and pituitary ACTH and LH release and to stimulate PRL secretion. AVT is also said to inhibit pineal N-acetyltransferase activity and to decrease norepinephrine-stimulated pineal indoleamine biosynthesis. It has been reported that melatonin injected intravenously or directly into the third ventricle releases AVT into the CSF. Thus, it is claimed that the antigonadotropic actions of melatonin are mediated indirectly through the actions of AVT. Exogenous melatonin, however, induces gonadal regression in pinealectomized hamsters thus providing evidence for a direct action of melatonin rather than an indirect action through the intermediary action of AVT. There is convincing evidence that AVT is not present in the mammalian brain [13]. There is no doubt that one or more neurohypophysiallike peptides are present within the epithalamus in substantial amounts. These peptides are, however, mainly confined to the ependymal portions of the pineal rather than to the pineal proper [5]. Thus, whatever their epithalamic significance, it may not necessarily be related to pineal function.

Immunocytochemical studies reveal that the rat pineal gland also contains an α-MSH-like compound which is similar but not identical to α-MSH. Further evidence suggests that this melanotropin may be related to the AVT-like peptide reported present in the pineal, as immunocytochemical studies localized these MSH-like and AVT-like substances to the same cells of the pineal. It is not known, however, whether these substances are the same peptide or are separate entities. A circadian rhythm of α-MSH concentration exists in the rat pineal gland which suggests a role for the melanotropin in the rhythmic activity of the pineal gland [29].

The pineal gland is reported to be a supplemental source of hypothalamic-releasing hormones. As measured by radioimmunoassay, both GnRH and TRH are present within ovine, bovine, and porcine pineal glands in rather high concentrations. There is a seasonal variation in GnRH content of rat pineals with a dramatic increase in pineal GnRH in the spring. Again, it is possible that these releasing-factor activities are not localized to the pineal per se but rather to the ependymal portions of the pineal. One must be cautious in assigning a pineal role to these epithalamic substances.

OTHER PROPOSED ROLES OF THE PINEAL

The pineal has been suggested to affect almost every endocrine gland in the body as well as many physiological activities. The pineal may, like its diencephalic hypothalamic counterpart the pituitary, function in the control of a large number of physiological processes. A few of the more recognized roles of the pineal will be described.

Prolactin and Somatotropin Secretion

There is evidence that the pineal affects the synthesis and secretion of pituitary prolactin [43]. The 24-hour pattern of plasma melatonin closely resembles that described for PRL which has a nocturnal rise also enhanced by sleeping. Blinding of female rats leads to depressed pituitary PRL stores, whereas plasma levels of PRL are usually elevated. These effects are reversed by pinealectomy, superior cervical ganglionectomy, or postganglionic transection of the nerves innervating the pineal. Melatonin has no direct effect on PRL secretion from the pituitary in vitro but, when injected into the third ventricle of rats, elevates plasma prolactin levels. It is suggested that the pineal is in some way inhibitory to hypothalamic PRL-inhibiting factor (PIF) release. Removal of the inhibitory PIF influence would, of course, lead to PRL secretion.

Somatotropin synthesis and secretion also appear to be impaired by the release of some pineal component [38]. Removal of the eyes of young rats results in lowered growth rate, an effect abolished by pinealectomy. Young rats placed in constant darkness also have lower pituitary and plasma STH levels and they grow more slowly. These effects, too, are abolished by pinealectomy. The mechanism responsible for these antigrowth effects of the pineal is undetermined.

Ocular Melatonin

Melatonin is present in the retina of many animals as are the enzymes N-acetyltransferase (NAT) and HIOMT, and serotonin is converted to melatonin in the eye in vitro [16]. Like the pineal, ocular NAT activity shows a daily light-dark cycle which can be modified by environmental lighting [9]. Ocular melatonin probably gets into the bloodstream as rhythms of circulating melatonin are often still present after pinealectomy.

Melatonin synthesis by the eye might serve some endocrine role or melatonin may act locally to regulate some ocular function. For example, the normal cyclic shedding of the outer retinal segment of the rat is blocked by reserpine treatment which also abolishes the circadian rhythm of indoleamine biosynthesis. Melatonin may therefore regulate the cyclic metabolism of photoreceptor cells [21]. In addition the photoreceptors of some poikilotherms are retracted during periods of bright illumination, an event facilitated by melatonin. Pigment migration within retinal melanocytes also occurs in response to photic cues in some species. Pinealectomy abolishes this response, whereas melatonin has the opposite effect. Melatonin may therefore play an important role in retinal light sensitivity and visual acuity in some vertebrates [31].

Adrenal Steroidogenesis

Ovariectomy of the rat results in increased adrenal secretion of the major metabolites of corticosterone (5 α-dihydrocorticosterone and 5 α-tetrahydrocorticosterone) with a proportionate fall in the production of corticosterone. Secretion of these metabolites declines after pinealectomy and corticosterone output is restored to normal levels. Melatonin administration in vivo reverses the effects of pinealectomy by stimulating adrenal 5 α-reductase activity thus leading to decreased corticosterone synthesis. Melatonin is equally effective in hypophysectomized and pinealectomized animals. Melatonin stimulation of adrenal 5 α-reductase activity contrasts with that of other hormones, such as ACTH, PRL, STH, testosterone, and estradiol, which inhibit activity of the enzyme. These observations suggest a direct inhibitory role of the pineal and melatonin on adrenal glucocorticoid synthesis [30]. Numerous other experiments implicate the pineal in the control of rhythms of adrenocortical steroid synthesis by an indirect action on the control of pituitary ACTH secretion. Other contrasting evidence supports a stimulatory role of pineal indoleamines on adrenocortical steroid synthesis.

Adrenal Catecholamines

Adrenal chromaffin cell dopamine-β-hydroxylase activity has a 24-hour rhythm which is increased with the onset of darkness [4]. The nocturnal rise in enzyme activity does not occur under conditions of constant light or if animals are pinealectomized. Conditions of stress, such as insulin-induced hypoglycemia, cause activation of pineal enzymes and melatonin synthesis. This pineal response is depressed by bilateral adrenalectomy and may depend on adrenal epinephrine for activation. Epinephrine could be expected to stimulate pineal melatonin biosynthesis by stimulation of pinealocyte β-adrenergic receptors. Thus, pineal melatonin and adrenal epinephrine each appear to have a reciprocal action on the synthesis of the other. Because of the effects of the pineal on adrenal steroidal and adrenal chromaffin function, melatonin might be considered a hormone of stress [49]. Numerous other functions for the pineal and melatonin have been suggested.

The Pineal and the Circadian System of Birds

In the bird, as in mammals, the activity of the enzymes responsible for melatonin synthesis (NAT and HIOMT) and the amount of melatonin in the pineal gland are enhanced in darkness and depressed in light. Serum levels of melatonin are increased during the dark in birds. Even after blinding, changes in pineal indoleamine biosynthesis occur in response to environmental lighting. The thin skull of birds may allow light to penetrate directly to the pineal. In addition a circadian rhythm of pineal melatonin synthesis occurs in isolated pineals maintained in organ culture in the absence of light; these isolated pineals are directly light sensitive [8, 12].

In the sparrow *Passer domesticus* the pineal gland is essential for persistence of the circadian locomotor rhythm under conditions of constant darkness. Removal of the pineal results in arrhythmic locomotor activity. Pinealectomized sparrows will nevertheless still entrain to light-dark cycles and reveal other signs that are partially indicative of a circadian system. The free-running rhythm of locomotor activity is not abolished by disruption of the neural input to the pineal or its neural output. Most interestingly, rhythmicity can be restored to pinealectomized birds by the implantation of a donor pineal to the anterior chamber of the eye. The transplanted pineal transfers the phase of the donor bird's rhythm to the host. The avian pineal therefore seems to be coupled to other components of the circadian system by an endocrine rather than a neural mechanism [27, 51].

It has been suggested that the avian pineal contains a self-sustained oscillator which produces a rhythmic hormonal output. Furthermore, it is believed that circadian fluctuations of this hormone entrain a damped oscillator located elsewhere in the body which in turn drives the locomotor activity. In this model each oscillator would have separate access to environmental light cycles. Locomotor and other behaviors of pinealectomized birds would be determined exclusively by the damped oscillator but would be unable to free run (in the absence of light cues) because the self-sustained oscillator is lacking. Restoration of the damped oscillator to its normal state can be reestablished by cyclic hormonal output from a transplanted pineal [27, 51].

The continuous administration of melatonin reduces the total amount of perch-hopping activity in sparrows, an effect reversed to normal after cessation of melatonin treatment. The evidence suggests that the pineal through its product melatonin may play a role in both the timing and the amount of activity expressed throughout the activity and resting cycle in birds. Pinealectomy abolishes the normal circadian rhythm of body temperature in constant darkness and also alters significantly the amplitude of body temperature rhythms entrained to light cycles. There is evidence that the pineal gland may influence thermoregulatory behavior and physiology in some reptiles and mammals [35, 42]. In some birds reproductive activity is clearly related to photoperiodic events, but the pineal gland and melatonin have not been implicated in the control of such activity [34].

Pineal-Melatonin Control of Chromatophores

The discovery of McCord and Allen [26] that bovine pineal glands contain a factor which causes tadpoles to lighten in color was ultimately responsible for the search and elucidation of the structure of melatonin. There is now good evidence that melatonin controls color change in certain poikilothermic vertebrates, at least at certain developmental stages. When amphibian larvae are placed in the dark they rapidly become lighter in color. This body-blanching response is eliminated by pinealectomy but is mimicked when melatonin is added to the water in which larvae swim [2]. Melatonin-induced lightening of amphibian larvae is due to the direct effect of the indoleamine on melanosome aggregation within dermal melanophores (Chapter 8).

There is strong experimental evidence that the body-blanching response of larval amphibians as well as that of cyclostomes to darkness is due to melatonin release from the pineal [3].

The normal background response of larval and adult amphibians to a light- or dark-colored background is controlled by the presence or absence of circulating levels of MSH and is not under the control of the pineal gland [3]. The control of chromatic responses by the pineal gland and melatonin in other vertebrates has not been studied in depth. Melanophores of certain species of fishes and reptiles do respond to melatonin but this need not necessarily imply that the indoleamine plays any normal role in the control of chromatic behavior in these vertebrates.

The fact that melatonin is extraordinarily effective in reversing the darkening (melanosome-dispersing) action of MSH is of broader significance than melatonin's immediate chromatic effect. Although there is strong evidence that melatonin is the mammalian pineal antigonadotropin, less information exists as to its locus of action. There is only meager information relative to the putative hypothalamic neurons, pituitary cells, or gonadal cells on which the indoleamine may mediate its actions [17]. Thus, because the cellular site of action is unknown, the mechanism of melatonin action has not been easily studied. The melanophores of some frogs, lizards, and fishes, however, provide model systems for deriving some information on melatonin mechanisms of action and have been used as a bioassay for the indoleamine. The cellular mechanisms by which chemical messengers work are generally similar between species. Therefore, it might be expected that studies of melatonin actions on integumental melanophores may be applicable to other cellular systems including those of humans. From a study of many structural analogs of melatonin, it was determined that a methoxy group on the fifth carbon atom of the indole nucleus is necessary for melanosome aggregation (skin lightening) within melanophores [19]. The N-acetyl group, on the other hand, is necessary for binding of melatonin to its receptor. This can be demonstrated by the use of N-acetyltryptamine which lacks intrinsic agonistic (lightening) activity but is competitively inhibitory to the actions of melatonin. The tryptamine nucleus and the 5-methoxy and N-acetyl groups are therefore essential for complete activity of melatonin. The proposed structural requirements of the melatonin receptor of frog skin melanophores in terms of binding site affinity and intrinsic agonistic activity are shown (Fig. 20.10). Because melanosome dispersion within melanophores is mediated by cyclic AMP, it might be conjectured that melanosome aggregation could be effected through the actions of cyclic GMP. Melatonin has been shown to enhance guanylate cyclase in a variety of tissues [45].

The Photosensitive Pineal of Poikilotherms

In the mammal light information is received through the lateral eyes and conveyed through the CNS to control pineal melatonin synthesis. As discussed at the outset of this chapter, cells of the pineal of certain poikilotherms might be sensory in nature. From elegant electron microscopic studies, the pinealocytes of amphibians, reptiles, and teleosts are sensory in structure and function (Fig. 20.11). The morphology of these cells resembles that of the retinal photoreceptors of the lateral eyes. In addition electrophysiological recordings indicate that these pineal sensory elements are directly photosensitive and are apparently activated in the absence of

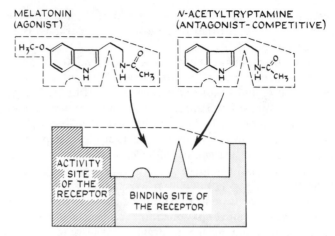

MELATONIN RECEPTOR

Figure 20.10 Schematic representation of the melatonin receptor based on structure-function studies of melatonin-related analogs. (Reprinted with permission from Heward and Hadley, *Life Sciences*, vol. 17, pp. 1167–1178. © 1975 Pergamon Press, Ltd.)

light to synthesize and release melatonin. As in mammals there is a diurnal rhythm of plasma melatonin in poikilotherms (fishes, lizards) which is totally or partially abolished by pinealectomy, but other sources of melatonin may exist [23, 35].

Infant rats do not require lateral eyes for the cyclic nocturnal fall in their pineal serotonin levels [53]. This drop in pineal serotonin can, however, be inhibited by continuous illumination. Thus, these young rodents appear to see even though their eyelids are closed. If, however, the heads of these animals are completely covered with black hoods, there is a decrease in pineal 5-HT levels. There is evidence that the pinealocytes of newborn rats contain photoreceptor organelles as in poikilothermic

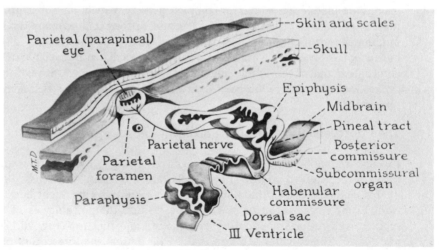

Figure 20.11 The lizard pineal gland and its anatomical relation to the diencephalic roof. (From Wurtman, Axelrod, and Kelly, [48], with permission.)

vertebrates [50]. Thus, in their ontogeny these cells recapitulate their phylogeny relative to the structure of these elements.

From a comparative evolutionary standpoint it is interesting that the earliest pineal systems (cyclostomes, elasmobranch and teleost fishes, amphibians, and reptiles and birds) are directly photosensitive. In all these vertebrates the pineal synthesizes and releases melatonin in the absence of light. There is also evidence that the pineals of these animals are not directly controlled by nervous input.

In adult mammals, on the other hand, the same biochemical events take place in the pineal cells in the absence of light, but the pinealocytes are regulated via photic cues received initially by the lateral eyes. Photostimulation of the lateral eyes results in neural information that is then conveyed to the pinealocytes. Even in their ontogeny the pinealocytes of both birds and mammals, at least in those few studied, possess photosensitive sensory cells. Thus there has been a gradual transformation from a directly photosensitive sensory system to an indirectly regulated system (in mammals) controlled through the nervous system by information received from the lateral eyes. Nevertheless, the evidence is clear that the pineal glands of all vertebrates, whether directly photoreceptive or not, are actively engaged in the biosynthesis of indoleamines.

PINEAL PATHOPHYSIOLOGY

Two contrasting types of pinealoma are associated with precocious or delayed sexual maturation. Parenchymal pinealomas, which consist of an enlarged mass of pinealocytes, are associated with delayed puberty. Destructive pinealomas, which consist of nonparenchymal (e.g., connective tissue) tissue, are associated with enhanced precocious development of sexual maturation. The interpretation of these clinical observations is as follows. An overactive pineal (parenchymal pinealoma) secretes an excess of a factor which is inhibitory to gonadal development. In the absence of this factor, because of destruction of the pineal, the antigonadotropin is absent and the individual experiences a precocious development of the gonads. Pineal tumors are rare in the female, but about one-third of all males below the age of sexual maturation who have pineal tumors undergo precocious puberty [24, 37].

CONCLUSIONS AND SPECULATIONS

There is a solid body of evidence supporting a role for the pineal in the control of reproductive function in certain mammals including humans. All the criteria have been met that should establish the mammalian pineal gland as an endocrine organ. An equal body of experimental data, which supports melatonin as the pineal antigonadotropin, is summarized.

1. Removal of the gland, pinealectomy, prevents the inhibitory effects ascribed to the pineal in the intact animal.
2. Extracts of the pineal (replacement therapy) in the pinealectomized animal mimic the inhibitory action of the pineal in the intact animal.

3. Enzyme activity within the pineal is most active under conditions (short photoperiods) where the pineal is known to be antigonadotropic.

4. Denervation of the pineal results in decreased pineal indoleamine biosynthesis.

5. Melatonin, an indoleamine with antigonadotropic activity, is synthesized within the pineal.

6. Melatonin synthesis and secretion is most active in darkness, a condition correlated with the antigonadotropic activity of the pineal.

7. There is a diurnal rhythm of plasma and CSF melatonin levels in mammals which is correlated with the rhythm of pineal indoleamine biosynthesis.

8. Melatonin is inhibitory to hypothalamic GnRH release and pituitary gonadotropin release which may account for its known antigonadotropic actions.

9. No other indoleamines or other hormones or putative chemical messengers are similarly related to pineal activity and reproductive function.

10. Clinical evidence in humans clearly equates pineal dysfunction with subsequent effects on gonadal development.

Because other hormones are present within the pineal gland, an argument need not exist against melatonin as the mammalian antigonadotropic hormone. The pineal gland might well function as the epithalamic equivalent of the hypothalamic pituitary gland. The pineal may, like the pituitary, control a diverse number of functions.

In certain poikilotherms the pineal and melatonin clearly function in the control of integumental chromatophore responses. Here, again, melatonin is released under conditions of darkness to induce a specialized chromatic behavior at certain developmental stages. This may be the most ancient functional role for this indoleamine.

The presence of other peptide hormones in the pineal and epithalamus is not unique as they are distributed throughout most of the CNS (Chapter 21). These so-called pineal peptides may not be major constituents of the pineal per se, but rather, they may be more prevalent in adjacent epithalamic areas. Thus, although these substances may be removed with the pineal, they may only be ependymal "contaminants" and therefore of no physiological relevance to pineal function. The ependyma of the epithalamus and other regions of the spinal cord may turn out, however, to be a rich source of chemical messengers which regulate other undetermined physiological functions.

REFERENCES

[1] BACON, A., C. SATTLER, and J. E. MARTIN. 1981. Melatonin effect on the hamster pituitary response to LHRH. *Biol. Reprod.* 24:993–99.

[2] BAGNARA, J. T. 1960. Pineal regulation of body lightening reaction in amphibian larvae. *Science* 132:1481–83.

[3] BAGNARA, J. T., and M. E. HADLEY. 1970. Endocrinology of the amphibian pineal. *Am. Zool.* 10:201–16.

[4] BANERJI, T. K., and W. B. QUAY. 1976. Adrenal dopamine-β-hydroxylase activity: 24-hour rhythmicity and evidence for pineal control. *Experientia* 32:253–54.

[5] BENSON, B., M. J. MATTHEWS, M. E. HADLEY, S. POWERS, and V. J. HRUBY. 1976. Differential localization of antigonadotropic and vasotocin activities in bovine and rat pineal. *Life Sci.* 19:747–54.

[6] BENSON, B., and I. EBELS. 1978. Pineal peptides. *J. Neural Trans. Suppl.* 13:157–73.

[7] BINKLEY, S. A. 1979. Pineal rhythms *in vivo* and *in vitro*. *Comp. Biochem. Physiol.* 64A: 201–206. Copyright © 1979, Pergamon Press, Ltd.

[8] BINKLEY, S. A., J. B. REIBMAN, and K. B. REILLY. 1978. The pineal gland: a biological clock in vitro. *Science* 202:1198–1201.

[9] BINKLEY, S. A., M. HRYSHCHYSHYN, and K. B. REILLY. 1979. *N*-acetyltransferase activity responds to environmental lighting in the eye as well as in the pineal gland. *Nature* 281: 479–81.

[10] BITTMAN, E. L. 1978. Hamster refractoriness: the role of insensitivity of pineal target tissues. *Science* 202:648–50.

[11] BUBENIK, G. A., G. M. BROWN, and L. J. TROTA. 1976. Immunohistochemical localization of melatonin in the rat Harderian gland. *J. Histochem. Cytochem.* 24:1173–77.

[12] DEGUCHI, T. 1979. Circadian rhythm of serotonin *N*-acetyltransferase activity in organ culture of chicken pineal gland. *Science* 203:1245–47.

[13] DOGTEROM, J., F. G. SNYDEWINT, P. PÉVET, and D. F. SWAAB. 1980. Studies on the presence of vasopressin, oxytocin and vasotocin in the pineal gland, subcommissural organ and fetal pituitary gland failure to demonstrate vasotocin in mammals. *J. Endocrinol.* 84:115–23.

[14] EBELS, I., and B. BENSON. 1978. A survey of the evidence that unidentified pineal substances affect the reproductive system in mammals. *Prog. Reprod. Biol.* 4:51–89.

[15] ELLIS, G. B., S. B. LOSEE, and F. W. TUREK. 1979. Prolonged exposure of castrated male hamsters to a nonstimulatory photoperiod: spontaneous change in sensitivity of the hypothalamo-pituitary axis to testosterone feedback. *Endocrinology* 104:631–35.

[16] GERN, W. A., and C. L. RALPH. 1979. Melatonin synthesis in the retina. *Science* 204: 183–84.

[17] GLASS, J. D., and G. R. LYNCH. 1981. Melatonin: identification of sites of antigonadal action in mouse brain. *Science* 214:821–23.

[18] GOLDMAN, B., V. HALL, C. HOLLISTER, P. ROYCHOUDHURY, and L. TAMARKIN. 1979. Effects of melatonin on the reproductive system in intact and pinealectomized male hamsters maintained under various photoperiods. *Endocrinology* 104:82–88.

[19] HEWARD, C. B., and M. E. HADLEY. 1975. Structure-activity relationships of melatonin and related indoleamines. *Life Sci.* 17:1167–78.

[20] HEYDORN, W. E., A. FRAZER, and B. WEISS. 1981. Electrical stimulation of sympathetic nerves increases the concentration of cyclic AMP in rat pineal gland. *Proc. Natl. Acad. Sci. USA* 78:7176–79.

[21] HOLLYFIELD, J. G., and S. F. BASINGER. 1978. Cyclic metabolism of photoreceptor cells. *Invest. Ophthalmol. Vis. Sci.* 17:88–89.

[22] JOHNSON, L. Y., and R. J. REITER. 1978. The pineal gland and its effects on mammalian reproduction. *Prog. Reprod. Biol.* 4:116–56.

[23] KENNAWAY, D. J., R. G. FRITH, G. PHILLIPOU, C. D. MATTHEWS, and R. F. SEAMARK. 1977. A specific radioimmunoassay for melatonin in biological tissue and fluids and its validation by gas chromatography-mass spectrometry. *Endocrinology* 101:119–27.

[24] KITAY, J. I., and M. D. ALTSCHULE. 1954. *The pineal gland*. Cambridge, Ma.: Harvard University Press.

[25] KLEIN, D. C., M. A. A. NAMBOODIRI, and D. A. AUERBACH. 1981. The melatonin rhythm generating system: developmental aspects. *Life Sci.* 28:1975–86.

[26] McCORD, C. P., and F. P. ALLEN. 1917. Evidence associating pineal gland function with alterations in pigmentation. *J. Exp. Zool.* 23:207–24.

[27] MENAKER, M., and N. ZIMMERMAN. 1976. Role of the pineal in the circadian system of birds. *Am. Zool.* 16:45–55.

[28] MOORE, R. Y. 1978. The innervation of the mammalian pineal gland. *Prog. Reprod. Biol.* 4:1–29.

[29] O'DONOHUE, T. L., R. L. MILLER, R. C. PENDLETON, and D. M. JACOBOWITZ. 1980. Demonstration of an exogenous circadian rhythm of α-melanocyte stimulating hormone in the rat pineal gland. *Brain Res.* 186:145–55.

[30] OGLE, T. F., and J. I. KITAY. 1978. *In vitro* effects of melatonin and serotonin on adrenal steroidogenesis. *Proc. Soc. Exp. Biol. Med.* 157:103–105.

[31] PANG, S. F., H. S. YU, and P. L. TANG. 1982. Regulation of melatonin in the retinae of guinea pigs: effect of environmental lighting. *J. Exp. Zool.* 222:11–15.

[32] PENNY, R. 1982. Melatonin excretion in normal males and females: increase during puberty. *Metabolism:* 31:816–23.

[33] QUAY, W. B. 1974. *Pineal chemistry.* Springfield, Ill.: Charles C. Thomas, Publisher.

[34] RALPH, C. L. 1978. Pineal control of reproduction: nonmammalian vertebrates. *Prog. Reprod. Biol.* 4:30–50.

[35] RALPH, C. L., T. FIRTH, W. A. GERN, and D. W. OWENS. 1979. The pineal gland and thermoregulation. *Biol. Rev.* 54:41–72.

[36] REITER, R. J. 1978. Interaction of photoperiod, pineal and seasonal reproduction as exemplified by findings in the hamster. *Prog. Reprod. Biol.* 4:169–90.

[37] REITER, R. J. (ed.). 1982. *The pineal and its hormones.* New York: Alan R. Liss.

[38] RELKIN, R. 1976. *The pineal.* Montreal: Eden Press.

[39] REPPERT, S. M., M. J. PERLOW, L. TAMARKIN, and D. C. KLEIN. 1979. A diurnal rhythm in primate cerebrospinal fluid. *Endocrinology* 104:295–301. © 1979 American Roentgen Ray Society. Williams & Wilkins Company.

[40] TAKAHASHI, J. S., and M. ZATZ. 1982. Regulation of circadian rhythmicity. *Science* 217:1104–1111.

[41] TUREK, F. W. 1979. Role of the pineal gland in photoperiod-induced changes in hypothalamic-pituitary sensitivity to testosterone feedback in castrated male hamsters. *Endocrinology* 104:636–40.

[42] UNDERWOOD, H. 1981. Effects of pinealectomy and melatonin on the photoperiodic gonadal response of the male lizard *Anolis carolinensis. J. Exp. Zool.* 217:417–22.

[43] VAUGHAN, M. K., and D. E. BLASK. 1978. Arginine vasotocin—a search for its function in mammals. *Prog. Reprod. Biol.* 4:90–115.

[44] VAUGHAN, G. M., G. G. MEYER, and R. J. REITER. 1978. Evidence for a pineal-gonad relationship in the human. *Prog. Reprod. Biol.* 4:191–223.

[45] VESELY, D. L. 1980. Melatonin enhances guanylate cyclase activity in a variety of tissues. *Mol. Cell. Biochem.* 35:55–58.

[46] WETTERBERG, L. 1978. Melatonin in humans: physiological and clinical studies. *J. Neural Trans. Suppl.* 13:289–310.

[47] WURTMAN, R. J., and J. AXELROD. 1965. The pineal gland. *Sci. Amer.* 213:50–60.

[48] WURTMAN, R. J., J. AXELROD, and D. E. KELLY. 1968. *The pineal.* New York: Academic Press, Inc.

[49] WURTMAN, R. J., and M. A. MOSKOWITZ. 1977. The pineal organ. *New Engl. J. Med.* 296:1329–33, 1383–86.

[50] ZIMMERMAN, B. L., and M. O. M. TSO. 1975. Morphologic evidence of photoreceptor differentiation of pinealocytes in the neonatal rat. *J. Cell Biol.* 66:60–75.

[51] ZIMMERMAN, N. H., and M. MENAKER. 1979. The pineal gland: a pacemaker within the circadian system of the house sparrow. *Proc. Natl. Acad. Sci. USA* 76:999–1003.

[52] ZUCKER, I. 1976. Light, behavior, and biologic rhythms. *Hosp. Prac.* 11(10):83–91.

[53] ZWEIG, M., S. H. SNYDER, and J. AXELROD. 1966. Evidence for a nonretinal pathway of light in the pineal gland of newborn rats. *Proc. Natl. Acad. Sci.* 56:515–20.

21

NEUROHORMONES

INTRODUCTION

Classically, the endocrine system was separated from the nervous system based on its supposed different physiological role. The brain, in particular the hypothalamus, however, can be considered an endocrine organ as it synthesizes and secretes a large number of chemical messengers. Most interesting has been the discovery that many and possibly all classical peptide hormones are now also found within the brain and other nervous tissues [23]. For example, the gastrointestinal peptides cholecystokinin and substance P are found in the brain, as are α-MSH and ACTH, hormones of the pituitary. A number of peptides isolated and characterized from mammalian brain and gastrointestinal tract (e.g., TRH, somatostatin, and substance P) have been found to be chemically similar, in some cases identical, to peptides present in amphibian skin. Possibly not surprising, certain peptides originally discovered in amphibian skin are present within mammalian tissues including the brain.

Pearse formulated a unifying concept, the APUD hypothesis, that postulates that neurons and endocrine cells producing peptide hormones share common cytochemical and ultrastructural features [41]. APUD, an acronym for Amine content and/or Precursor Uptake and Decarboxylation, describes common features of neuron and endocrine cells. It is believed that both these cell types share a common embryonic origin in that they are derived from the neuroectoderm. Therefore, the ability of a neuron, a pituitary cell, or a skin cell to produce a peptide hormone is because they are all derived from a "neuroendocrine-programmed" ectoblast [41]. This concept of a common cellular embryological origin may therefore provide a reasonable explanation for the observation that peptide hormones are common to both the CNS as well as the pituitary gland and to such peripheral organs as the GI tract and skin.

The diverse anatomical distribution of a particular peptide hormone implies that the hormone might regulate a variety of physiological functions. Within the nervous system peptide hormones function as neurotransmitters or neuromodulators or both, depending on their particular distribution within the tissue. To function as a neurotransmitter, a peptide hormone should fulfill certain criteria: (1) It should be synthesized within neurons and concentrated in presynaptic terminals; (2) it should be released by presynaptic stimulation; (3) it should have specific high-affinity, saturable, and reversible binding sites on postsynaptic membranes; (4) it should be metabolically degraded by nervous tissue; and (5) it should evoke a postsynaptic potential. Similar criteria would apply to neuromodulatory peptides of nervous system origin. This chapter summarizes present knowledge of the role of peptide hormones as neurotransmitters or neuromodulators.

THE ENDORPHINS

In 1965 Li discovered a peptide in the pituitary of cattle which he named β-lipotropin [30]. This so-called lipotropic peptide β-LPH, named for its action on adipose tissue, was considered for many years to be a hormone in search of a function. With the discovery in the brain of endogenous morphinelike peptides, β-LPH may at last have found a function. Opiate receptors have been discovered in the brain and have been pharmacologically characterized by their interaction with opiate agonists and antagonists such as morphine and naloxone, respectively (Fig. 21.1). Because it is reasonable to conclude that such highly specific receptors have not evolved to interact with exogenous opiate alkaloids, it was suggested that endogenous opiatelike substances might exist as natural ligands for the identified opiate receptors. Two compounds possess-

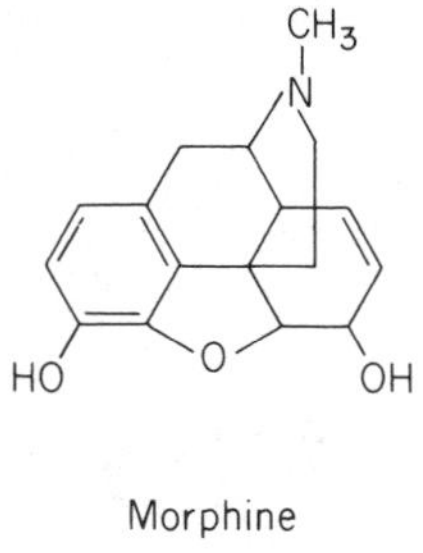

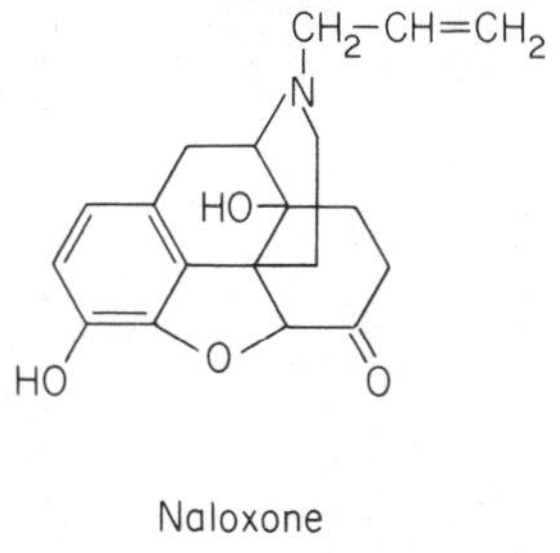

Figure 21.1 Structures of an opiate receptor agonist (morphine) and antagonist (naloxone).

Morphine   Naloxone

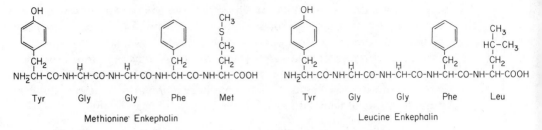

Figure 21.2   Structures of Met- and Leu-enkephalins.

ing opiatelike activity were isolated from bovine brain tissue as pentapeptides, differing only in their terminal amino acid sequence (Fig. 21.2) and possessing either leucine or methionine [48]. These peptides are referred to as *enkephalins*, and methionine enkephalin was recognized to be identical to an amino acid sequence of a larger peptide of the pituitary, β-LPH (Fig. 21.3) [30].

Endorphin is the name given to the class of substances isolated from the brain and pituitary gland that have such opiatelike activity [2, 20]. It was also discovered that the pituitary contains an endogenous opioid with a molecular weight greater than the enkephalins. This peptide was isolated, sequenced, and found to correspond to the 61–91 sequence of bovine β-LPH (Fig. 21.3). This β-endorphin as well as the enkephalins and more recently discovered endorphins are under intense study as possible candidates as the body's own antipain (analgesic) hormones [48]. If, indeed, these peptides prove to play such a role, β-LPH might be considered to function as a prohormone for the production of at least some of these endorphins.

Source, Synthesis, Chemistry, and Metabolism

Pituitary β-LPH is found in both the pars distalis and pars intermedia in association with ACTH. Corticotrophs and melanotrophs of the pars distalis and pars intermedia, respectively, of the pituitary produce a large molecular weight (31,000 daltons) protein which contains the sequence of β-LPH and ACTH. The term *pro-opiomelanocortin* was suggested for this protein that appears to be the common precursor for β-endorphin and corticotropin. Pro-opiomelanocortin is found within secretory granules of corticotrophs of the pars distalis and the granules of secretory cells of the melanotrophs

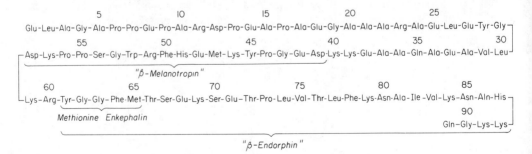

Figure 21.3   Structure of bovine β-lipotropin illustrating the sequences of Met-enkephalin, β-endorphin, and β-MSH.

of the pars intermedia. The precursor protein serves as a prohormone for ACTH production in the pars distalis; in the pars intermedia enzymatic activity results in cleavage of pro-opiomelanocortin to yield α-MSH (Fig. 8.4). The complete amino acid sequence of bovine pro-opiomelanocortin has been reported [37]. A high molecular weight protein containing β-endorphin as well as ACTH immunoreactivities has been isolated from the human placenta. This protein was identified as the heavy chain of the human immunoglobulin class lgG_1. This demonstrates that homologies in amino acid sequences exist between physiologically unrelated molecules.

The so-called lipotropic activity of β-LPH is a common property of β-LPH and other melanotropic peptides that possess structural similarities. There is no clear evidence, however, that any one of the peptides plays a normal physiological role in affecting adipose tissue lipolysis. It is unclear whether β-endorphin or its metabolic products present within corticotrophs or melanotrophs of the pituitary play any hormonal role or are only necessary byproducts of ACTH and α-MSH secretion. Although a so-called β-MSH has been localized to the pars intermedia, this peptide (Fig. 8.1), which is present within the structure of β-LPH (Fig. 21.3), appears to be an artifact of extraction. There is no evidence that β-MSH is secreted from the pars intermedia other than as a component of β-LPH (Chapter 8).

Although there is no evidence that β-endorphin of pituitary origin serves any physiologically relevant humoral role, another opioid peptide, dynorphin, has been isolated from the posterior pituitary. This heptadecapeptide contains Leu-enkephalin as its NH_2-terminal sequence (Fig. 21.4). The potency of this peptide is greater than that of any other known endogenous opiatelike peptide, but the peptide's physiological role is undetermined [20]. Cells that stain immunocytochemically for dynorphin are found within specific sites within the hypothalamus and myenteric plexus of the gut. Within the pituitary the peptide is specifically localized to the neurohypophysis. Dynorphin and vasopressin occur in the same hypothalamic magnocellular neurons of rats; their synthesis, however, appears to be under separate genetic control. Dynorphin is not present within oxytocin-containing neurons [60]. Also within the neurohypophysis are a number of large molecular weight (80,000 daltons) proteins that may not only serve as precursor proteins for neurophysins and neurohypophysial hormones but also contain within their structure sequences similar to corticotropin and β-endorphin. These composite prohormones have been referred to as neurohypophysial coenophorins; other regionally specific coenophorins may be localized to other regions of the brain [28].

A number of independent endorphin pathways in the brain have been delineated: a β-endorphin system with a single cell group in the hypothalamus and long axons innervating midbrain and limbic structures and two enkephalin systems with multiple cell groups throughout the spinal cord and brainstem which possess relatively short axons [1]. The immunocytochemical mapping of Leu- and Met-enkephalins suggests that the two pentapeptides occur in completely separate nerve cells in neural pathways that anatomically differ considerably. The relative proportions of Met- and Leu-enkephalin vary between different brain regions and also between different species,

Tyr-Gly-Gly-Phe-Leu-Arg-Arg-Ile-Arg-Pro-Lys-Leu-Lys-Trp-Asp-Asn-Gln

Figure 21.4 Primary structure of porcine dynorphin, a superpotent endorphin.

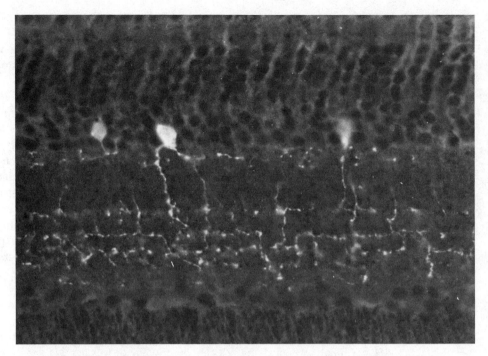

Figure 21.5 Immunocytochemical localization of Leu-enkephalin to an amacrine cell of the avian retina. (From Brecha, Karten, and Laverack, [5], with permission.)

further demonstrating the existence of separate populations of Met- and Leu-enkephalin nerves. Many areas of the brain that are rich in enkephalins correspond to areas closely associated with dopaminergic, noradrenergic, serotonergic, and substance P-containing neuronal systems. Many enkephalin-containing neurons appear to be short interneurons (Fig. 21.5).

Outside the CNS there is a rich enkephalinergic innervation of the gastrointestinal tract, and there is evidence that the enkephalins may also be contained in various autonomic nerves and ganglion cells and in mucosal cells of the stomach. Present evidence suggests that β-LPH, ACTH, and β-endorphin sequences occur within the same neurons within the brain and pro-opiomelanocortin may therefore also function as a prohormone for β-endorphin, α-MSH, or ACTH production within the CNS. The enkephalins, on the other hand, appear to be derived from different, unidentified precursors; "big" forms of both Met-enkephalin and Leu-enkephalin have been discovered. The amino acid sequence of these peptides differs from that of β-LPH suggesting separate precursors for β-endorphin and each of the enkephalins.

The enkephalins are labile to proteolytic enzymes, a property which would be consistent with a role for the enkephalins as neurotransmitters. Termination of enkephalin action is apparently the result of enzymatic degradation rather than uptake into neurons or glia as there appears no high affinity uptake system for enkephalins in synaptosomal preparations. The primary step in the very rapid degradation of the enkephalins involves N-terminal cleavage of tyrosine to yield the inactive tetrapeptides. β-Endorphin is far more stable that the enkephalins; its conformation apparently protects the N-terminal tyrosine from hydrolysis. Substitution of D-Ala in the 2 position of the enkephalins (e.g., [Tyr-D-Ala^2-Gly-Phe-Met]-enkephalin), greatly prolongs the analgesic actions of these peptides in vivo. These D-amino-substituted peptides are less susceptible to proteolytic degradation, which apparently accounts for their increased biological activity.

Physiological Roles

The physiological roles of the identified opioid systems are not fully elucidated. The endorphins are found in high concentrations in brain areas involved in pain transmission, respiration, motor activity, pituitary hormone secretion, and mood. The suggestion of a relationship between the endorphins and ACTH secretion is intriguing as behavioral studies indicate that stress increases the concentrations of endorphin in blood and brain, with parallel changes in pain threshold. Histochemical localization also suggests that the opioid substances may have potentially important relations to noradrenergic and dopaminergic systems. If the endorphins, indeed, are a component of the basic systems which modulate responses to pain and stress, they may be critical in behavioral and emotional responses to the environment [1, 27].

Analgesic function. The most clearly understood action of an endorphin is in the spinal cord where small enkephalin-containing neurons impinge on the terminals of peripheral sensory nerve cells that convey pain information to the spinal cord (Fig. 21.6). These primary afferent neurons contain (and release) another peptide known as substance P, and the application of an enkephalin (or an opiate) depresses the release of substance P [22, 48]. In this manner it is thought that pain stimuli can be suppressed at the very point where they enter the central nervous system. But enkephalin-containing neurons are also found at higher levels of the pain pathways and in brain areas thought to connect pain impulses with emotional responses to pain.

One fascinating finding suggests that endorphins and their receptors can affect acupuncture-induced analgesia. For example, the firing rate of cells in the spinal cord is greatly increased in response to painful stimuli. Acupuncture suppressed this increased electrical activity, but this effect of acupuncture was completely blocked by the specific opiate antagonist, naloxone. The acupuncture effect was slow in onset and it long outlasted the acupuncture stimulation, suggesting a hormonal rather than

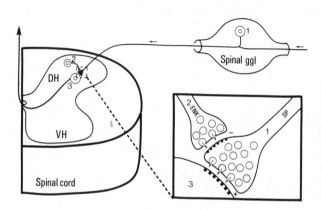

Figure 21.6 Schematic illustration of the hypothetical interaction between (1) substance P-containing (pain-conveying?) primary afferents and (2) enkephalin interneurons in the dorsal horn (DH). The third neuron represents a pathway ascending to higher centers. VH = ventral horn. (From Hökfelt et al., [22], with permission.)

The Endorphins

a direct neuronal response. It was reported that an opioidlike material present in rat blood (anodynin) disappears after hypophysectomy. It has also been shown that acupuncture analgesia in mice is blocked by naloxone and abolished by hypophysectomy. It was suggested, therefore, that the pituitary is the source of an endogenous opioid-like substance that is released in response to nervous stimulation.

Several studies have implicated an endogenous opiate system in human behavior specifically related to pain and psychiatric disorders. It was found that stimulation of the periaqueductal gray matter of the brain produces naloxone-reversible analgesia in patients suffering from intractable pain. This response was accompanied by an increase in ventricular endorphinlike activity. These data support the findings that basal levels of endogenous opioids in the CSF of patients with persistent pain are depressed. These observations suggest, as do the animal studies cited earlier, that analgesic brain stimulation may result in the release of an endogenous opiatelike substance. Preliminary trials have suggested that β-endorphin itself produces significant pain relief when administered to terminal cancer patients. These results offer the possibility that with further well-controlled clinical trials a more detailed understanding of the mechanisms of pain and pain relief may be achieved.

Endorphins as possible adrenomedullary hormones. Stressful stimuli often elicit marked neurogenic stimulation of the adrenal medulla. Many forms of stress also induce significant analgesia which can be partially blocked by naloxone. A large number of enkephalin-containing peptides are present in mammalian adrenal chromaffin tissue. They are stored within chromaffin vesicles and are cosecreted in response to the same stimuli that induce catecholamine secretion. Denervation of the rat adrenal increases the amounts of enkephalin and enkephalin-containing polypeptides in the gland. These peptides may all derive from a pro-enkephalin through proteolysis. One such peptide (peptide E) contains within its structure both the Met- and Leu-enkephalin sequences (Fig. 21.7). This peptide is 30 times more potent than [Met]-enkephalin. It is suggested that free enkephalins may not be the physiologically relevant end product derived from pro-enkephalin but, rather, that peptide E and other adrenal enkephalin-containing peptides may serve as unique physiological regulatory substances [24]. Specifically, it has been suggested that adrenomedullary enkephalins may contribute to the attenuation of pain during life-threatening stress [55].

Control of pituitary hormone secretion. There is evidence that opioid peptides may play a physiological role in controlling the release of pituitary hormones. For example, in the pig-tailed monkey the concentration of β-endorphin is more than 100 times greater in the hypophysial blood than in the peripheral plasma [58]. Intravenous injections of opioid peptides cause the release of PRL, STH, AVP, and MSH. These peptides are, however, inhibitory to FSH and LH secretion, and these effects of the endorphins on pituitary hormone release are reversed by naloxone. Opioid peptides and antagonists are without any effect on isolated pituitaries, suggesting that their

1		5			10			15			20			25

Tyr–Gly–Gly–Phe–Met–Arg–Arg–Val–Gly–Arg–Pro–Glu–Trp–Trp–Met–Asp–Tyr–Gln–Lys–Arg–Tyr–Gly–Gly–Phe–Leu

Figure 21.7 Primary structure of bovine peptide E derived from adrenal chromaffin tissue. The sequences of Met- and Leu-enkephalin within the peptide are indicated [24].

effects are mediated at the level of the hypothalamus. The simplest interpretation is that endogenous opioid peptides inhibit dopaminergic (or noradrenergic) pathways that normally control some pituitary hormone secretions. Prolactin secretion from the adenohypophysis is normally inhibited by a prolactin inhibiting factor which apparently is dopamine (Chapter 5). Endorphin inhibition of dopamine secretion would therefore result in PRL secretion. These results demonstrate that the release of prolactin under physiological conditions can be reduced by blockade of opiate receptors, which further suggests that endogenous endorphins participate tonically in the regulation of PRL hormone secretion. Likewise, β-endorphin inhibition of dopamine or norepinephrine secretion from median eminence catecholaminergic neurons (which is stimulatory to hypothalamic gonadotropin releasing hormone neurons) would account for the inhibition of FSH and LH secretion that follows central administration of an endorphin. Again, opiate receptor antagonists stimulate gonadotropin secretion suggesting that GnRH secretion is under tonic inhibition by an exogenous endorphin.

Role in reproductive physiology. A synthetic analog of Met-enkephalin that is resistant to enzymatic degradation inhibits copulatory behavior in sexually active male rats; its action is prevented by naloxone, a specific inhibitor of opioid receptors. Naloxone itself induces copulatory behavior in inactive male rats, which suggests that endorphins normally exert a tonic inhibition of copulatory behavior. These observations provide strong evidence that endorphins may be important in the regulation of sexual behavior [19]. Table 21.1 summarizes the evidence that endorphins may function as neurohormones.

Mechanisms of Action

Endorphins modify the excitability of a variety of neurons in the central nervous system. Microiontophoresis of Met-enkephalin onto single neurons in the rat brainstem shows that the endorphin's predominant action suppresses the firing rate of spontaneously active neurons. Similar effects are obtained with the narcotic agonists morphine and etorphine; their actions and those of Met-enkephalin are blocked by iontophoretically applied naloxone. Endorphins and opiate narcotics inhibit spon-

TABLE 21.1 Evidence That Endorphins Function as Neurohormones

Electrical stimulation of particular areas of the brain produces analgesia.
Opiate drugs bind stereospecifically to nervous tissues ("opiate receptors").
Binding of opiate drugs to receptors is blocked by opiate drug antagonists.
Opiate antagonists (e.g., naloxone) partially inhibit electrically induced analgesia.
Brain and pituitary extracts contain opiatelike activity.
Peptides (endorphins) that induce analgesia have been isolated and chemically characterized from nervous tissue.
Endorphins displace morphine and related analogs from opiate receptors.
Opiate antagonists inhibit binding of endorphins to opiate receptors.
Regional differences of endorphin levels within the CNS parallel the distribution of opiate receptors.
Endorphins and opiate receptors are localized to neuronal tracts recognized to be involved in pain transmission.
Endorphins are localized immunocytochemically to discrete neurons.
Endorphins are released from nervous tissue by K^+ (depolarizing action) in a Ca^{2+}-dependent manner.

taneously responsive cells in the cortex, brainstem, caudate nucleus, and thalamus. In the hippocampus, however, pyramidal cells are usually excited and are also naloxone sensitive. Opiate receptors are apparently localized presynaptically on some nerve fibers and endorphins may reduce the release of dopamine and other neurotransmitters by an action on these receptors. A major function of endorphins may therefore be to mediate presynaptic inhibition on a variety of neuronal systems in the central nervous system. The presynaptic effects of endorphins or opiate narcotics on neuronal activity would depress or excite neurons depending on whether the presynaptic neurons are excitatory or inhibitory to the neurons being monitored electrophysiologically. Thus, disinhibition of an active neuron that is inhibitory to a quiescent neuron would result in excitation of this latter neuron. Although opiate receptors mediate neuronal inhibition in most brain regions, the ultimate action of exogenous opiates on a given region may depend on the "local cytoarchitectonics" [63].

Endorphins interact with opiate receptors as shown by their ability to displace radiolabeled narcotic agonists and antagonists from the receptors. Opiate receptors fall into a number of distinct classes as characterized by pharmacological and biochemical methods. The specific anatomical localizations suggest that the different types of receptors mediate different physiological functions. The so-called mu receptors (μ) may mediate analgesic actions, whereas delta receptors (δ) may preferentially regulate emotional behavior [49]. The μ and δ receptors are regulated by Met- and Leu-enkephalins, respectively. Dynorphin appears to be a specific endogenous ligand for the kappa (κ) subclass of opioid receptor. Thus, the opiates, like adrenergic, cholinergic, and dopaminergic agonists, initiate their broad spectrum of diverse physiological actions by interaction with multiple receptor types. This provides some hope that opiate drugs might be developed that possess morphinelike analgesic actions but lack addictive effects [64].

Most peptide hormones work through effects on membrane cyclizing enzymes to elevate or lower intracellular cyclic nucleotide levels. Endorphins mediate their actions through inhibition of adenylate cyclase. In studies on a neuroblastoma hybrid cell line grown in tissue culture it was found that continuous exposure to opiates resulted initially in decreased cyclic AMP production. More of the opiate agonist was required to decrease cyclic AMP production to the original levels produced by the opiate; the cells had apparently become *tolerant* to the actions of the drug. It was found that the cells synthesized more adenylate cyclase and, upon removal of the opiate from the cells, cyclic AMP levels rose dramatically and responded excessively to other hormonal stimulation. This excessive production of cyclic AMP may represent the biochemical correlate of withdrawal symptoms noted in humans taken off opiate drugs [25]. There is evidence that opiate drugs and peptides also mediate their actions on nervous tissue through stimulation of cyclic GMP production.

Pathophysiology

Classical *tolerance* and *dependence* develop in rodents continuously infused with endorphins. The animals are also cross dependent on morphine and vice versa. This might be expected as the receptors for opiate drugs and peptides are identical. It has been suggested that heroin addicts at some stage in their addiction may suffer from an endorphin deficiency. Excess target tissue hormones (e.g., cortisol) are known to exert a negative feedback to hypothalamic production of releasing hormones (i.e., CRH). Possibly the production of brain or pituitary endorphins is shut off in a similar manner due to feedback inhibition by opiate drugs. Addicts then might be suffering from a true hormone (endorphin) deficiency.

According to the catecholamine theory of schizophrenia, psychosis results from the overproduction of dopamine and therefore overstimulation of dopaminergic receptors. There is good evidence that endorphins affect certain CNS dopaminergic pathways. The opiate antagonist, naloxone, alters some schizophrenic symptoms. This observation might support the hypothesis that endorphins may be involved in some schizophrenic symptomatology.

SUBSTANCE P

In 1931 von Euler discovered a substance in brain and intestinal mucosa that caused intestinal smooth muscle contraction and relaxed vascular smooth muscle. This active material was referred to as preparation P [56], but it was not until 1970 that by accident the chemical nature of substance P (SP) was elucidated. SP is a peptide with the following structure:

$$\text{Arg-Pro-Lys-Pro-Gln-Gln-Phe-Phe-Gly-Leu-Met-NH}_2$$

This undecapeptide has been immunocytochemically localized within nerve fibers of the peripheral and central nervous system. SP has fulfilled most criteria that establish it as a neurotransmitter, or at least a neuromodulator. For example, it is synthesized within the cell bodies of neurons and then transported axonally to nerve terminals where it is released by appropriate stimulation into a synapse. In addition synthetic SP mimics SP's putative actions. Electrophysiological studies on the actions of SP suggest that it may serve diverse functions in interneuronal communication [38, 54].

SP has been immunocytochemically localized to sensory pain fibers of the dorsal root ganglia. The higher concentration of SP in dorsal root neurons compared to ventral root nerves suggests that SP may be the neurotransmitter released by the central terminals of primary afferent sensory fibers. This suggestion is strengthened by the observation that SP is found in higher concentrations in the dorsal horn than in the ventral horn of the spinal cord. SP has an excitatory action on single neural units in the dorsal horn of the spinal cord. Further studies have shown that the units excited by SP are among those excited by noxious cutaneous stimulation; SP causes an enhancement of the responses of these nociceptive (pain-sensing) units to noxious stimulation.

Met-enkephalin blocks the release of SP from nerve terminals of sensory pain fibers, and the effect of the endorphin is antagonized by naloxone. The distribution of opiate receptors closely parallels that of SP neurons, and the SP neurons apparently contain binding sites (receptors) for the enkephalins. Thus, enkephalin-containing neurons within the dorsal horn may inhibit release of SP from dorsal root sensory neurons and thus inhibit pain transmission to the brain (Fig. 21.6). There is evidence that another major site of enkephalin modulation of the transfer of nociceptive information in the dorsal horn is on the projection neurons themselves [46]. The relationship between enkephalins and SP may be the physiological basis for the postulated "pain gate." This gate in the spinal cord lets pain impulses through to the brain. Prevention of SP release by enkephalin may be what closes the gate (Fig. 21.6).

The peripheral site of action of SP outside the CNS seems to be mainly on smooth muscle. SP lowers arterial blood pressure and is recognized as one of the most potent vasodilators. Almost all peripheral tissues contain SP-positive nerves, often in close association with blood vessels and secretory cells. The high potency of SP together with its presence in intrinsic nerves in the gut suggest that SP may function as a physiological modulator of smooth muscle activity in gut tissue (Chapter 10). Intestinal peristalsis changes from bidirectional to unidirectional shortly after birth, concomitant with the appearance in the myenteric plexa of peptidergic nerve fibers. A role for SP in the regulation of intestinal peristalsis has been suggested, and SP may be involved in the postnatal induction of propulsive motility (Chapter 10). Intraventricular injections of SP have a marked antidipsogenic effect without depressing food intake or producing other behavioral modification. It has been suggested that because SP is found in the brain, it may be a natural satiator of thirst.

All analogs of SP containing the C-terminal pentapeptide amine sequence possess potent biological activity. An analog of SP, [Tyr^8]-SP, is similar in activity to the native [Phe^8]-SP, which allows the tyrosine moiety to be iodinated for use in radioimmunoassay. Substance P stimulates adenylate cyclase activity in particulate preparations from rat and human brains. The peptide also increases cyclic AMP levels in cultured glioma cells and induces morphological differentiation in neuroblastoma and glioma cells. Substance P stimulates neurite outgrowth in cultured neuroblastoma cells and in chicken dorsal root ganglia. It is therefore speculated that SP may be important in the control of neuron growth in both central and peripheral nervous systems.

Substance P is structurally similar to certain peptides found in frog skin (Fig. 21.8). These substances are referred to as *tachykinins* (Greek: *takus*, fast) because of their rapid actions on smooth muscle. Physalaemin is found in the skin of the South American frog, *Physalaemus bigilonigerus*, and other species of this genus. The shorter peptide, phyllomedusin, is found in the skin of the Amazonian hylid frog, *Phyllomedusa bicolor*, and several related species. Eledosin, a peptide similar in structure to SP and other tachykinins, is found in the posterior salivary glands of the Mediterranean octopus of the genus *Eledone*. Because TRH, a brain hormone, is found in frog skin and bombesin, a peptide found in frog skin, is found in the brain, some

Substance P	Arg–	Pro	–Lys –	Pro	– Gln – Gln –	Phe	–Phe –	Gly – Leu – Met –NH$_2$
Physalaemin	pGlu– Ala – Asp–			Pro	– Asn – Lys –	Phe	– Tyr –	Gly – Leu – Met –NH$_2$
Phyllomedusin		pGlu – Asn –		Pro	– Asn – Arg –	Phe	– Ile –	Gly – Leu – Met –NH$_2$
Eledoisin	pGlu–	Pro	–Ser – Lys –		Asp – Ala –	Phe	– Ile –	Gly – Leu – Met –NH$_2$

Figure 21.8 Comparative primary structures of peptides related to substance P. Amino acid residues within the peptides located at identical positions to substance P are enclosed.

tachykinins may in time be discovered in the brain. On the other hand, SP and the other tachykinins may all be derived from a more primitive ancestral peptide whose structural gene has undergone a number of mutations in each of the species. Substance P immunoreactivity (IR-SP) has been localized to specific cells in the retina of the bullfrog and other vertebrate species. In the rat, monkey, and chicken, this IR-SP is apparently identical to authentic SP. Three distinct IR-SP substances are present in the frog and carp and appear to be different from SP and other SP-related peptides such as physalaemin and uperolein. It appears that the SP-like substances in the bull-frog and the carp represent novel peptide moieties [15].

SOMATOSTATIN

Somatostatin (SS), a tetradecapeptide, clearly functions as a hypophysiotropic factor regulating the release of somatotropin (Chapter 6). Immunoreactivity to SS is, however, found throughout the CNS; high concentrations are present in the preoptic regions, amygdala, circumventricular organs, CSF, spinal cord, and ganglion cells of various ganglia. The unique localization of SS in specific systems of neurons suggests that this peptide may be released as a neurotransmitter or neuroregulator. The release of SS from hypothalamic and other brain tissues by depolarizing stimuli is calcium dependent; these observations further support a neurohormonal role for somatostatin within the CNS.

Although the tetradecapeptide form of somatostatin (SS-14) is present in the brain, pancreas, GI tract, and thyroid gland of mammals, other forms of the peptide may also exist. A 28-amino acid peptide, somatostatin-28 (SS-28), has been isolated from the intestine and hypothalamus of several mammalian species. This peptide may represent the prosomatostatin form of SS-14 (Fig. 6.7). However, this peptide is about ten times more active than SS-14 inhibiting secretion from the pituitary, and it has been postulated that, on the basis of the selective actions of SS-28 compared to

TABLE 21.2 Known Effects of Somatostatin and Somatostatinlike Peptides on Physiological Processes

Site of action	Response[a]
Pituitary	↓ Somatotropin secretion
	↓ TSH secretion
Endocrine pancreas	↓ Insulin secretion
	↓ Glucagon secretion
Stomach	↓ Gastrin secretion
Exocrine pancreas	↓ CCK secretion
Toad bladder	Modulator of vasotocin-stimulated water permeability
Brain	↓ Adrenal epinephrine secretion
	↓ Bombesin-induced hypothermia
	↓ Gastric acid secretion
Rat colon	↓ VIP-stimulated fluid secretion
Elasmobranch rectal gland	↓ VIP-stimulated chloride secretion
Thyroid	↓ TSH-stimulated T_3 and T_4 release

[a]A decreased or inhibited response to somatostatin is indicated (↓).

SS-14, the longer peptide may serve as the physiologically relevant neuropeptide on some receptors and also as the prohormone substrate for SS-14 production. In the channel catfish (*Ictalurus punctatus*) at least two somatostatin mRNA species are present in the pancreas which code for hormones differing in both amino acid sequence and chain length. Again, it is suggested that processing of somatostatin precursors leads to additional peptide hormones that participate in the multiplicity of biological effects attributed to somatostatin [50].

Immunoreactive somatostatin has been localized to the urinary bladder of the toad where it may function locally as a regulator (modulator) of the cellular action of vasopressin on osmotic water flow through the bladder epithelium [18]. A summary of the known physiological roles or effects of the somatostatins is provided (Table 21.2).

HUMAN BOMBESIN AND NUTRIENT HOMEOSTASIS

Bombesin is a tetradecapeptide of the primary structure

pGlu-Glu-Arg-Leu-Gly-San-Gln-Trp-Ala-Val-Gly-His-Leu-Met-NH$_2$

which was originally isolated from the skin of the frog and is structurally related to other biologically active peptides found within the anuran integument (Table 21.3). Bombesinlike immunoactivity has been demonstrated by radioimmunoassay and immunocytochemical techniques to be present within mammalian brain, gastrointestinal tract, lung, and plasma [9]. The highest concentration of bombesinlike immunoreactivity is in the hypothalamus. A functional role for a mammalian bombesinlike ligand is further supported by the demonstration of high affinity receptors for bombesin in mammalian brain and exocrine pancreas. In the brain the material reacting within bombesin antibodies is chemically distinct from authentic bombesin [49]. A 27 amino acid peptide has been isolated from the porcine gut and termed gastrin releasing peptide (GRP). The C-terminal decapeptide fragment of GRP is almost identical to the C-terminal decapeptide of frog skin bombesin (Fig. 10.9). It is now believed that GRP is probably mammalian bombesin.

Bombesin acting within the CNS causes a lowering of body temperature and inhibits cold-induced pituitary TSH secretion, possibly by inhibiting TRH release from brain peptidergic neurons [8]. Thus, bombesin inhibits the thermogenic response of animals to cold acclimation. Bombesin-induced hypothermia is reversed by intracranial administration of TRH, prostaglandins (E-series), and naloxone. It has been suggested that bombesin or a related peptide and TRH may play dual roles in the control of body temperature. Microinjections of bombesin into various regions of the brain revealed that the neuroanatomic site of action of the peptide was the preoptic area of the hypothalamus.

Intracisternal injections of bombesin result in a complete suppression of gastric acid output. Intracranial injections of bombesin also promote the rapid development of hyperglycemia in rats, an effect apparently mediated through the CNS and involving adrenal release of catecholamines (Fig. 21.9) [8]. Somatostatin acting at the level of the brain reverses both the thermolytic and hyperglycemic actions of bombesin. Bombesin given intraperitoneally reduces feeding behavior in rodents. There is a post-

TABLE 21.3 Structures of Bombesin and Related Peptides Isolated from Amphibian Skin[a]

Peptide	Species	Sequence
Bombesin	*Bombina bombina*	(pyro)Glu-Gln-Arg-Leu-Gly-Asn-Gln-Trp-Ala-Val-Gly-His-Leu-Met-NH$_2$
Alytesin	*Alytes obstetricans*	(pyro)Glu-Gly-Arg-Leu-Gly-Thr-Gln-Trp-Ala-Val-Gly-His-Leu-Met-NH$_2$
Ranatensin	*Rana pipiens*	(pyro)Glu-Val-Pro-Gln-Trp-Ala-Val-Gly-His-Phe-Met-NH$_2$
Ranatensin R	*Rana rugosa*	Ser-Asp-Ala-Thr-Leu-Arg-Arg-Tyr-Asn-Gln-Trp-Ala-Thr-Gly-His-His-Phe-Met-NH$_2$
Ranatensin C	*Rana catesbiana*	(pyro)Glu-Thr-Pro-Gln-Trp-Ala-Thr-Gly-His-His-Phe-Met-NH$_2$
Litorin	*Litoria aurea*	(pyro)Glu-Gln-Trp-Ala-Val-Gly-His-Phe-Met-NH$_2$

[a]Modified from [14].

501

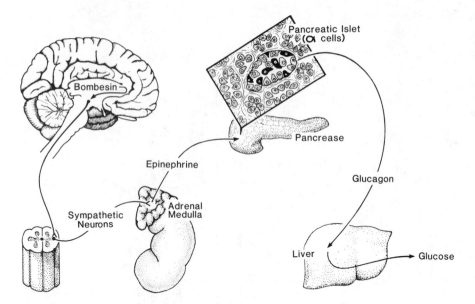

Figure 21.9 Hypothetical scheme for the role of bombesin, a neurohormone, in nutrient homeostasis. Although the human brain is depicted, experimental evidence linking bombesin to adrenomedullary epinephrine secretion is derived from studies on the rat brain. (Modified from Brown et al., [6], with permission.)

prandial rise in plasma bombesinlike immunoreactivity in dogs. Bombesin might affect appetite behavior indirectly by stimulating secretion of CCK, a peptide which is proposed to be a "satiety hormone." The various actions of bombesin may all be related to nutrient homeostasis as the common denominator of these effects is the behavioral and biochemical regulation of carbohydrate metabolism [6].

NEUROTENSIN

Neurotensin (NT), a tridecapeptide with the structure

pGlu-Leu-Tyr-Glu-Asn-Lys-Pro-Arg-Arg-Pro-Tyr-Ile-Leu,

was first isolated from the hypothalamus and gut of a number of mammals including humans. This peptide exhibits a wide spectrum of systemic actions which include hypotension, gut contraction, increased vascular permeability, hemoconcentration, hyperglycemia, and hyperglucagonemia. NT stimulates pituitary secretion of somatotropin and prolactin and, like bombesin, induces hypothermia in cold-exposed mice when administered intracisternally.

Neurotensin has been shown to bind stereospecifically to brain synaptosomes; the degree of binding of neurotensin and neurotensin analogs to cell membranes correlates closely with the known biological actions of the peptide. The hypothalamus contains the highest amount of NT-like immunoreactivity, and the distribution of synaptosomal receptors which specifically bind radiolabeled NT is generally similar to the regional distribution of NT-like peptide in the brain. The profiles of NT binding strongly suggest the presence of biologically important synaptic receptors for neurotensin. NT may therefore function as a neurohormone within the brain.

THYROTROPIN RELEASING HORMONE

The tripeptide pyroglutamyl-histidyl-proline amide (Fig. 1.3), thyrotropin releasing hormone (TRH), is the hypophysiotropic factor controlling pituitary thyrotropin (TSH) secretion. The widespread distribution of extrahypothalamic TRH along with its extrahypophysial effects suggests that this peptide may play a role in a number of CNS neuronal processes. It has even been suggested that although its name, TRH, may be useful for historical purposes, it is far too restrictive and may only describe a minor component of the tripeptide's physiological and pharmacological significance [44].

There is a widespread distribution of TRH immunoreactivity within the CNS of mammals including humans. Very high concentrations are also found in frog skin, and the peptide is even present within invertebrates [45]. Besides the hypothalamus, a TRH-like immunoreactive substance is present within the retina, pancreas, gastrointestinal tract, and numerous CNS sites including the spinal cord. TRH is present subcellularly in both hypothalamic and extrahypothalamic synaptosomes and saturable TRH binding to high affinity binding sites within the CNS can be demonstrated. The binding is highly tissue specific, and the receptor is specific for TRH and some of its analogs. Of many tissues examined, only the brain and pituitary display high affinity TRH binding. Thus, membrane receptors of the pituitary and brain interact selectively with sequence of amino acids characteristic of TRH.

These and other observations that TRH is catabolized by neuronal tissue, is released from CNS synaptosomal preparations by certain stimuli, and that selective changes in the regional brain content of TRH occur after various treatments are consistent with a functional role of TRH (besides its role in the control of pituitary hormone secretion). The demonstration that significant concentrations of the tripeptide are present within the medulla oblongata, particularly the nucleus tractus solitarius, the dorsal motor nucleus of the vagus, and nucleus ambiguus, suggests that TRH may be involved in the regulation of autonomic nervous system function [7].

TRH exerts unusual psychostimulant influences on the CNS independent of its role in endocrine function [62]. Most remarkable is its ability to counteract the depressant effects of drugs. TRH can antagonize the depressant effects of most classes of neuroleptics (substances that act on the nervous system), including general anesthetics, some tranquilizers, alcohol, and narcotics. Thus, TRH exhibits a general arousal action and will even arouse hibernating ground squirrels. TRH activates the EEG of rabbits and adult fowl, and, depending on the dose, the peptide induces such behavioral symptoms as hypermotility, muscle tremor, body shakes, lacrimation, hyperthermia, and piloerection. Many other actions of the peptide have been described.

Studies on the mechanism of action of TRH provide no unifying hypothesis concerning its mode of action. Thus, while the actions of TRH are antagonized by muscarinic cholinergic antagonists, TRH restoration of body temperature in cold acclimated rats is not affected. The peptide has a direct inhibitory effect on most hypothalamic neurons when applied iontophoretically. The multiplicity of actions of TRH suggests the widespread involvement of many neurotransmitter systems.

CHOLECYSTOKININ AND FEEDING BEHAVIOR

Most members of a species grow to an average weight characteristic of the group. It is proposed that certain brain centers control appetite behavior. Humoral and neural cues may interact with these neural centers to stimulate or inhibit feeding behavior. The relation of food intake to caloric needs is an example of one of the body's major homeostatic mechanisms [27].

Bilateral destruction of the ventral medial hypothalamus (VMH) produces a dramatic increase in food intake (hyperphagia). Destruction of the lateral hypothalamic nuclei, on the other hand, inhibits feeding (aphagia) which may lead to severe, long-lasting anorexia. Electrical stimulation of the VMH inhibits feeding behavior, whereas electrical stimulation of the LH initiates eating. During hunger and the onset of feeding electrical activity of the LH increases, whereas that of the VMH decreases. Norepinephrine infused into the medial or the lateral hypothalamus initiates or inhibits ingestive behavior. It was originally proposed that a *satiety center* (within the VMH) is tonically inhibitory (through noradrenergic neurons) to a *feeding center* (within the lateral hypothalamus) and that the presence or absence of humoral or local neural cues inhibitory or stimulatory to the satiety center would affect feeding-center activity. There is evidence that neural afferents deriving from both the VMH as well as the LH reciprocally affect the activity of the other area of the hypothalamus.

Cells within the VMH and LH may function as glucoreceptors by monitoring blood glucose levels to control food intake. Glucoreceptive neural units have been demonstrated by electrophysiological methods to be present in the VMH and LH. A nonmetabolizable glucose compound, 2-deoxy-D-glucose (2-DG), which blocks the intracellular utilization of glucose and therefore causes glucoprivation, stimulates feeding when injected intracisternally. The 2-DG-induced feeding response is blocked if animals are pretreated with the α-adrenoceptor antagonist phentolamine. These observations and other evidence suggest that central glucoreceptors may be noradrenergic neurons or that these glucostats mediate their actions indirectly through such neurons.

Other humoral or neural cues may also control the activity of the putative hypothalamic satiety and feeding centers. Partially digested food, chyme, released into the duodenum of the small intestine from the stomach, triggers the release of a number of GI hormones that regulate the release of pancreatic digestive enzymes and the motility of the digestive tract (Chapter 10). Specific metabolic substrates of the chyme, such as proteins, lipids, carbohydrates, or degradative products thereof, also interact with cellular receptors of the gut epithelium to activate specific GI hormone secretions. Besides local effects on gastrointestinal activity, these metabolic substrates or GI hormones may provide cues that inform the animal of its short-term metabolic status. The food intake of hungry rats, for example, is reduced if the rats' blood is mixed with blood from a recently fed rat, but not if too much time has elapsed between feeding and the blood transfusion.

Cholecystokinin (CCK) is released from the duodenum in response to certain factors present in the chyme from the stomach. CCK stimulates gallbladder contraction, secretion of pancreatic enzymes, and numerous other GI functions. There is now evidence that CCK may also function as a satiety signal [35]. Systemic injections of CCK inhibit food intake in the rat and the rhesus monkey in a dose-related manner [36]. In humans a consistent dose-response relationship has not been noted, although rapid intravenous injection of CCK does reduce food intake. CCK (synthetic octapeptide), in a dose-dependent manner, also prolongs the intermeal interval in the rat by considerably delaying the start of the next meal. This is important as a CCK-satiety hypothesis would suppose that elevation of CCK in the plasma as an animal eats would inhibit feeding; as long as the level of CCK in the blood remains high, food intake would be expected to be inhibited.

The C-terminal octapeptide of CCK is inhibitory to food intake (but not water intake), and some analogs of CCK are more potent than the native peptide on such CCK-mediated responses as gallbladder contraction and pancreatic enzyme secretion. These peptides are also more effective in reducing food intake; thus a common CCK receptor is implicated in the control of satiety and GI function. Caerulein, a decapeptide isolated from the skin of a frog, shares a very similar C-terminal sequence with CCK (Fig. 10.13) and it is also effective in altering food intake.

If CCK plays a role as a humoral factor controlling food intake, where is its site of action? The effects of systemically injected CCK are abolished by vagotomy (the gastric branch of the vagus nerve), suggesting that vagal afferents may provide important satiety cues to the hypothalamus. Nevertheless, there is convincing evidence for a central site of action of CCK or a structurally related peptide. Injections of CCK into the cerebral ventricles inhibit feeding in sheep. The relative lack of effect of systemically injected CCK compared to the satiety effects of the peptide at much lowered concentrations when administered intracerebroventricularly suggests that CCK acts on CNS structures involved in food intake [12]. This is further substantiated by the observation that injections of anti-CCK sera into the cerebral ventricles stimulate feeding in sheep. Rats with lesions in the VMH show reduced sensitivity to caerulein, whereas rats with lateral hypothalamic damage exhibit heightened sensitivity to the peptide. Microinjections of caerulein into the VMH, but not into the LH, limit feeding. In addition tritiated caerulein is selectively bound to tissue in the VMH. Systemic injections or local application of CCK-related peptides activate neural units within the LH; the particular response elicited is influenced by the nutritional state of the animal. A peptide immunologically closely related to CCK-octapeptide, the C-terminal eight amino acid sequence of CCK, is present within the brain where it is localized to specific neurons. A peptide similar to CCK-4 (the COOH-terminal tetrapeptide of CCK) has also been described as being localized to specific brain areas. Feeding responses elicited by hypothalamic infusions of norepinephrine are blocked by CCK administered either intraperitoneally or to NE-sensitive hypothalamic sites. In addition systemic administration of CCK releases NE within the hypothalamus. A tentative hypothesis is that CCK released by the gastrointestinal tract or afferent vagal neurons is stimulatory to noradrenergic neurons of the VMH which, through the release of norepinephrine, are inhibitory to the lateral hypothalamic feeding centers.

THE BRAIN RENIN-ANGIOTENSIN SYSTEM

Angiotensin II controls aldosterone secretion and elevates blood pressure by a direct vasoconstrictor action and by stimulation of adrenal aldosterone secretion. This octapeptide is produced by the action of renin, an enzyme released by the kidney, on the protein substrate angiotensinogen produced by the liver (Chapter 15). All components of the renin-angiotensin system have been found in the brain. Central as well as peripheral administration of angiotensin II stimulates drinking (dipsogenic) behavior and vasopressin secretion from the neurohypophysis. Both actions of the octapeptide lead to physiological responses important to water balance and the maintenance of blood pressure.

The organum vasculosum of the lateral terminalis (OVLT) and the subfornical organ (SFO) are *circumventricular organs* of the brain that lack a *blood-brain barrier*. They are uniquely suited as receptor sites for bloodborne electrolytes as well as biologically active substances normally excluded by the brain. The evidence for a role of these organs as well as a brain renin-angiotensin system in the control of thirst and water balance is outlined in Table 21.4. The production of angiotensin II in the brain may not, however, be limited solely to a role in water homeostasis but may subserve other functions as well.

BRAIN MELANOTROPINS AND BEHAVIOR

A number of peptide hormones are believed to act directly on the brain to affect learning or behavior. Some peptides are being tested clinically to determine their value in treating a number of conditions including Parkinson's disease, schizophrenia, de-

TABLE 21.4 Evidence for an Endogenous Brain Renin-Angiotensin System

Isorenin is present in the brain even after bilateral nephrectomy.

Brain isorenin converts angiotensin I to angiotensin II.

Angiotensinases are present in the brain which cleave angiotensin II into smaller (inactive?) fragments.

Angiotensin II has effects on blood pressure when injected in low doses (which are ineffective intravenously) into the brain ventricles. Ventricularly administered angiotensin II also causes copious drinking, whereas an intravenous infusion does not.

Microiontophoretic application of angiotensin II to the proposed receptive area of the brain, the organum vasculosum of the lamina terminalis (OVLT), induces neural excitation.

Lesions of the OVLT area produce a syndrome of transient adipsia and loss of responsiveness to ventricular angiotensin II injections.

In vitro radioreceptor assays reveal specific binding sites for angiotensin II in the OVLT which are increased in number in tissue taken from hypertensive rats.

Specific angiotensin II binding sites have been visualized in the brain by fluorescent microscopy using a biologically active fluorescent angiotensin II agonist.

Neurons in brain cell cultures specifically bind angiotensin II.

The subfornical organ (SFO) has efferent neural projections to sites within the brain (the OVLT and the supraoptic nuclei) known to be involved in drinking behavior and the secretion of vasopressin [32].

Lesions of the SFO eliminate the dipsogenic responses to physiologically relevant doses of angiotensin II.

pression, and learning disorders. The hormones that have attracted the most attention are MSH and ACTH which are partially similar in structure (Chapter 8). Two general types of conditioning experiments have been used in these studies. In *avoidance conditioning* the animal must learn to perform a specific task, such as running from one compartment of a shuttle box into the other, to avoid an unpleasant experience such as an electric shock. In *appetitive* or *approach conditioning*, which is considered to be unstressful, the animal must acquire the behavior in order to achieve a reward such as food or drink.

Injections of either MSH or ACTH are claimed to enhance the acquisition of avoidance responses in the rat [13]. These peptides are also said to increase the resistance to avoidance behavior extinction; that is, animals treated with the peptides persist in the task longer than untreated animals even after the shock is terminated for a period of time. The influence of ACTH is independent of its action on the adrenal cortex as it is active in adrenalectomized rats. Also, α-MSH and corticotropin fragments (ACTH$_{1-10}$ and ACTH$_{4-10}$) increase resistance to extinction of avoidance behavior, whereas ACTH$_{11-24}$, which is devoid of action on the adrenal, is without such an effect. The tetrapeptide ACTH$_{6-9}$ sequence is also said to be effective but less potent. This is the same minimal sequence believed required for melanotropic activity. Thus, the sequence affecting these behavioral responses appears to be localized to the central sequence -His-Phe-Arg-Trp- which is common to α-MSH, β-MSH, and ACTH (Fig. 8.1).

Data obtained from electrophysiological studies indicate that ACTH analogs have a CNS excitatory action. The locus of these effects was determined by lesion and implantation studies to be the thalamic area and the limbic forebrain structures of the brain. Apparently the thalamic reticular area is important in integrative behavior because all incoming information converges in this structure. Implantation of MSH and ACTH peptides in this region of the brain effectively alters extinction of conditioned behavior. MSH- and ACTH-like peptides may therefore modulate neuronal transmission at this nodal point in sensory integration [13].

Although most original studies were related to avoidance behavior, other investigators believe that MSH/ACTH peptides facilitate learning by improving the motivation or ability of an animal to pay attention to the task rather than by acting on memory processes per se. Although most studies using MSH/ACTH peptides have involved rodents, there is evidence that these peptides also influence memory processes in humans [3].

The pituitary is not believed to be the source of the MSH or ACTH that may regulate brain-mediated behavioral responses. Neurons are located within the arcuate nucleus which contains pro-opiomelanocortin and therefore intramolecular sequences for corticotropin and melanotropins. These neurons project to other parts of the brain, and it is possible that an MSH- and ACTH-like peptide may be released to function as a neurotransmitter or neuromodulator to affect behavioral processes related to learning and memory retention.

There is evidence that MSH- and ACTH-like peptides may function in a role opposite that of opioid peptides in controlling pain sensitivity. These peptides inhibit endorphin-induced analgesia without having any analgesic effect themselves. Injections of ACTH$_{1-24}$ into the lateral ventricles of the brain cause hyperalgesia in rats;

this increased sensitivity to pain is antagonized by morphine but increased by naloxone. In addition MSH/ACTH peptides are said to induce a withdrawal syndrome in morphine-dependent animals. It has been hypothesized, therefore, that MSH- and ACTH-like peptides may be considered endogenous antagonists of opiates and that they may cause hyperalgesia by displacing the endogenous opiates from their receptors [4]. Another body of conflicting data argues that the actions of MSH- and ACTH-like peptides on the brain are analgesic in nature [59].

Within the brain are neurons that synthesize more than one putative neurotransmitter. The opiomelanotropinergic neurons may release a number of neuropeptides, all derived from the precursor protein pro-opiomelanocortin within some neurons. Deacetylated α-MSH is an initial product derived from the precursor protein. The N-acetylated native form of α-MSH is much more potent than desacetyl-α-MSH in eliciting behavioral activity in the rat. β-Endorphin is also derived from pro-opiomelanocortin but in the acetylated form is less active than the nonacetylated endorphin. Within multineurotransmitter neurons, differential regulation of acetylating enzymes may alter the ratios of α-MSH and β-endorphin produced by these neurons [39]. Conceivably, therefore, behavior regulated by either α-MSH or β-endorphin might be determined by modulating neural inputs that effectively control the chemical nature of the secreted neuropeptides.

NEUROHYPOPHYSIAL HORMONES AND BEHAVIOR

The neurohypophysial hormones vasopressin and oxytocin are classical peptidergic neurohormones which play important regulatory roles in water homeostasis and reproductive processes, respectively. Although these neurosecretions are released into the systemic circulation to reach their target tissues, they are also released from other neurons within the brain where they appear to regulate a number of specific behaviors.

Vasopressin is claimed to be involved in the acquisition and maintenance of adaptive behavior [13]. Removal of the posterior lobe of the rat pituitary attenuates resistance to extinction of certain avoidance behavior. Administration of vasopressin restores the maintenance of avoidance behavior of posterior lobectomized rats. In intact rats vasopressin and related peptides increase resistance to extinction of active avoidance behavior. These peptides also facilitate passive avoidance behavior acquisition. Vasopressin and related peptides have a long-term effect on the maintenance of active and passive avoidance behavior which may be noted for a period of days to weeks depending on the dose administered. Intracerebroventricular administration of antisera to arginine vasopressin after a learning experience leads to a deficit in passive avoidance retention. These and other data suggest that these peptides, like the melanotropins, are involved in learning and memory processes.

The site of the behavioral effect of vasopressin and related peptides is in the midbrain limbic structures as concluded from lesion and microinjection studies. Structure-activity studies indicate that arginine vasopressin is more active than lysine vasopressin. Removal of the C-terminal glycinamide decreases the potency about 50%, but such peptides lack almost all other endocrine activities (e.g., antidiuresis). This indicates a dissociation between the endocrine and behavioral activities of the vasopressins. The physiological role of vasopressin in memory is said to be demonstrated in the Brattleboro rat with hereditary diabetes insipidus due to a lack of ADH secretion. Rats homozygous for this condition are said to be inferior in acquiring and maintaining active and passive avoidance behavior traits compared to heterozygous or normal rats. The abnormal EEG patterns characteristic of these rats are normalized by administration of vasopressin or related analogs.

A group of neurophysin-containing fibers from the paraventricular nucleus diverge from the ventrally arching fibers and pass dorsally toward the lateral ventricles where they appear to terminate within the choroid plexus. The response of the choroid plexus to exogenously administered vasopressin suggests a possible functional role for a vasopressin/neurophysin projection to the choroid plexus. Innervation of the choroid plexus by vasopressinergic fibers may serve to control fluid and electrolyte balance within the cerebrospinal fluid by acting on choroid receptors whose function may be similar to that of the distal convoluted tubules of the kidney. There is also evidence for the presence of vasopressin in the septal area of the brain, an observation which strengthens the proposed role of vasopressin in the control of certain aspects of behavior.

In the human the neurohypophysial hormone analog 1-desamino-8-D-arginine vasopressin (DDAVP) was shown to influence learning and memory. Cognitively unimpaired (alert) as well as cognitively impaired adults treated with this analog for several days learn certain types of information more effectively. DDAVP also appears to reverse partially the retrograde amnesia that follows electroconvulsive treatment [61].

There is evidence that neurohypophysial hormones may be released into the cerebral spinal fluid. Electrical stimulation of the paraventricular nucleus, for example, is followed by a significant rise of oxytocin in the CSF. It was hypothesized that during the time of increased synthesis and secretion of oxytocin at parturition oxytocin might be released into the CSF and affect subsequent behavior. Indeed, an intracerebroventricular injection of oxytocin into virgin female rats did induce maternal behavior, whereas vasopressin was without such an effect. However, maternal behavior was only manifested in females during the period of the cycle when estrogen levels were elevated. Oxytocin was without an effect on maternal behavior in ovariectomized females but did induce such behavior in ovariectomized females pretreated with estradiol [43]. These observations suggest that the characteristic maternal behavior exhibited by the rat at parturition may be activated by the interaction of estrogens and oxytocin within the brain.

THE CAUDAL NEUROSECRETORY SYSTEM (UROPHYSIS) AND THE UROTENSINS

Within the spinal cord of some teleost and cartilaginous fishes are groups of neurosecretory neurons which possess all the characteristics of a neuroendocrine system, anatomically analogous to the neurohypophysis [10]. This *caudal neurosecretory system* or *urophysis* contains two types of secretory cells based on staining reactions, granule morphology, and response to osmotic or electrophysiological stimuli. Two types of granules have been isolated and each is associated with its own hormonal-

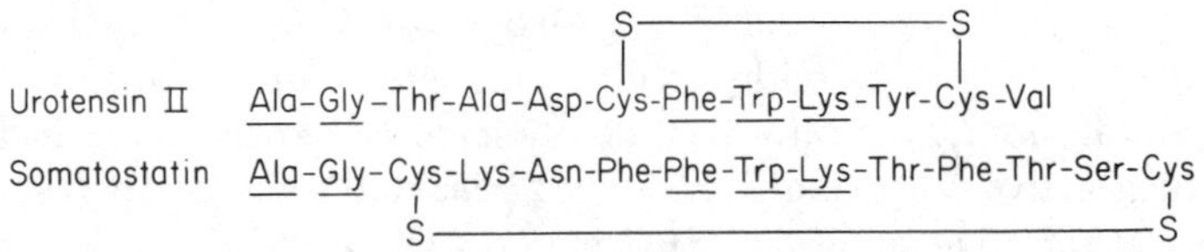

$$S\text{————}S$$

Urotensin II   Ala-Gly-Thr-Ala-Asp-Cys-Phe-Trp-Lys-Tyr-Cys-Val

Somatostatin   Ala-Gly-Cys-Lys-Asn-Phe-Phe-Trp-Lys-Thr-Phe-Thr-Ser-Cys

$$S\text{————————————}S$$

Figure 21.10 Comparative primary structures of urotensin II and somatostatin. (From Pearson et al., [42], with permission.)

like factor (urotensin I and II). Both aminergic and cholinergic inputs to urophysial secretion are implicated in some species of fishes. The *urotensins* are neuropeptides and, like the neurohypophysial hormones of the pars nervosa, are associated with two or more transport proteins, *urophysins*, which specifically bind either urotensin I or II.

Extracts of the urophysis are vasoactive in all vertebrate species studied. In general a vasopressor response is observed in poikilothermic vertebrates and a vasodepressor effect in homeotherms. There is evidence that these differential effects are produced by two distinct peptides: The vasodepressor factor is referred to as urotensin I, whereas urotensin II is the name given the vasopressor principle of the urophysis. Both urotensins are apparently present in all fish urophyses thus far examined, suggesting that they are indeed peptidergic hormones of this neurosecretory system. The presence of a third urotensin (III) is based solely on experimental data; urotensin IV appears to be arginine vasotocin (AVT).

Urophysectomy in several teleost species results in ionic imbalance, and exposure of euryhaline teleosts to different salinities results in marked histological and ultrastructural changes in the urophysial cells. In addition injections of urophysial extracts increase plasma ion levels in fishes. Experimental evidence strongly suggests that urotensin II may act directly on the ion-transporting cells of the urinary bladder involved in teleostean seawater osmoregulation [31].

Urotensin II, isolated from the urophysis of the teleostean fish *Gillichthys mirabilis* is reported [42] to be a dodecapeptide with an amino acid sequence somewhat similar to somatostatin (Fig. 21.10). The primary structure of urotensin I has also been determined (Fig. 21.11) and found to be strikingly similar to that of a putative corticotropin releasing hormone of sheep and to sauvagine, a peptide isolated and characterized from frog skin [29]. There is hope that with the elucidation of the structure of urotensin I synthetic analogs may be produced of pharmacological value in the clinical treatment of hypertension in humans.

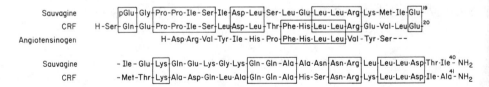

Figure 21.11 Comparative primary structures of: urotensin I (teleost), CRF (ovine), and sauvagine (frog). Amino acid residues of CRF and SVG located at identical positions to urotensin I are enclosed [52].

Further study may reveal that all the known classical hormonal peptides will also be found within the nervous system. Except for the gonadotropins, all pituitary hormones have been found by immunocytochemical methods to be present within the CNS. It has been argued that these peptides are of pituitary origin; however, these hormones are still present after hypophysectomy. Also, in some cases, nervous tissue has been shown to synthesize these peptides, and in addition immunocytochemical methods have localized the peptides to individual neurons. Thus, their specific anatomical localization to certain brain areas, their intraneuronal presence, and the fact that they are released from synaptosomes argue strongly for a CNS neurotransmitter or neuromodulatory role for these neuropeptides. The neuropeptides or related structures localized to the mammalian brain are schematically illustrated (front cover figure).

Corticotropin Releasing Hormone

The primary structure of a putative CRH has finally been determined (Fig. 6.10). Although CRH functions importantly in the control of pituitary corticotropin (ACTH) secretion, evidence suggests that it may also subserve other physiological functions. Intracerebroventricular injections of CRH elevate blood pressure, increase heart rate, and increase plasma levels of catecholamines and vasopressin [17]. These responses, characteristic of those usually induced by stressful stimuli, are mediated at an extra-pituitary site within the brain and are not secondary to ACTH secretion as they are induced in hypophysectomized animals. Because the hypothalamus is the primary site of CNS control of sympathetic outflow, it is possible that CRH acting within the brain as a neurohormone may activate, in concert with the pituitary-adrenal axis, the sympathetic nervous system during stress [17].

Within the primary structure of CRH are sequences homologous to those found in other peptides: angiotensinogen, sauvagine, and urotensin I (Fig. 21.11). It was suggested that the sequence, -Phe-His-Leu-Leu-, found in both CRH and angiotensinogen, may reflect a distant evolutionary relatedness between the two molecules, particularly as both polypeptides control different functions of the adrenal cortex [52]. Sauvagine is a peptide that has been isolated from the skin of the South American frog *Phyllomedusa sauvagei*. This is reminiscent of the observation that other brain and gut peptides, such as substance P, cholecystokinin, bombesin, bradykinin, and opiate peptides, are also found in the integument of the frog [33]. Sauvagine also shares a close structural similarity to urotensin I, a peptide isolated from the teleost urophysis.

Gonadotropin Releasing Hormone

Besides its well-established role in the control of pituitary gonadotropin secretion, GnRH may function as a neurotransmitter and a neuromodulator within the central and peripheral nervous systems. Injections of GnRH increase sexual behavior in estrogen-primed ovariectomized or hypophysectomized female rats and in androgen-primed castrated male rats. This is a specific action of the peptide as other hypophysiotropins are without such an action, and the effects on mating behavior are not duplicated by gonadal steroids in the absence of GnRH. GnRH has been localized by radioimmunoassay to specific sites within the brain. Intrahypothalamic (medial preoptic area, MPOA) injections of GnRH potentiate lordosis behavior. In contrast, infusions of antibodies to GnRH decrease lordosis behavior in steroid-primed animals. GnRH-responsive neurons have been monitored within the MPOA. GnRH has been identified within symptosomal preparations and has been localized to cell bodies and nerve terminals known to be involved in the initiation of specific CNS-dependent behaviors. There is interest in the possibility that GnRH or related analogs might be useful in the treatment of human sexual impotence.

Bradykinin

Bradykinin, a hypotensive peptide, is derived from a plasma kininogen through the enzymatic action of a kallikrein. A bradykininlike system appears to be also present within the brain. Immunocytochemical studies reveal that a substance identical or closely similar to the bradykinin nonapeptide is localized specifically within the hypothalamus, particularly to the periventricular and dorsomedial nuclei [11].

The presence of endogenous bradykininlike activity in hypothalamic extracts has been demonstrated through bioassays unique for demonstrating bradykinin activity. Injections of bradykinin into the lateral ventricles of the brain elevate systemic blood pressure, an effect abolished by lateral septal lesions. The fact that injections of bradykinin into the periaqueductal gray elicit analgesia is in harmony with data that this particular area of the brain is involved in analgesic phenomena.

Insulin

Insulin receptors are selectively localized to axons and axon terminals in the external median eminence and the hypothalamic arcuate nucleus of the rat as determined by autoradiography using $[^{125}I]$-insulin [53]. Insulin acts directly on cells of the medial basal hypothalamus and alters the electrical activity of ventral hypothalamic neurons. It stimulates the release of norepinephrine within certain hypothalamic areas and in hyperinsulinemic-hyperphagic rats catecholamine turnover in the median eminence is selectively increased. Thus it is possible that fluctuations in bloodborne insulin may modulate hypothalamic neurons and program feeding behavior, body weight, and glucose homeostasis [53].

Vasoactive Intestinal Peptide

Although originally discovered within the gastrointestinal tract, VIP is also present within both the peripheral and central nervous systems. VIP shares a structural similarity with glucagon, secretin, and gastric inhibitory peptide (Fig. 10.3). The peripheral effects of the peptide include lowering of blood pressure by causing vasodilation, suppression of gastric acid secretion, and stimulation of fluid secretion within the small intestine and colon (Chapter 10). Central effects of VIP include increased arousal

TABLE 21.5 Evidence for a CNS Neurotransmitter Role of Vasoactive Intestinal Peptide

VIP is particularly concentrated in the telencephalic areas of the brain.

VIP has a potent excitatory action on cortical neurons.

Peripheral VIP-containing neurons are present in certain autonomic ganglia and nerves.

The VIP-ergic neurons in the gut are mainly intrinsic with cell bodies localized in the submucosal and myenteric plexa.

VIP stimulates adenylate cyclase activity in brain tissue from areas known to contain VIP nerve terminals.

VIP exerts a direct action on smooth muscle cells.

A local release of VIP occurs from VIP-innervated target organs when the physiological response is provoked by nerve stimulation.

Radiolabeled VIP binds to rat brain membranes with high affinity. The binding is specific, saturable, and reversible.

Tissue VIP-stimulated adenylate cyclase activity parallels tissue VIP receptor density suggesting that both are linked.

Immunoreactive VIP is present in portal hypophysial blood in much higher concentrations than in systemic arterial blood.

VIP is selectively distributed in the brain, with highest concentrations in the neocortex, hypothalamus, corpus striatum, and amygdala.

VIP is concentrated in synaptosomal fractions of brain tissue homogenates.

VIP is released from synaptosomal preparations by depolarizing stimuli in the presence of Ca^{2+}.

VIP is demonstrable by immunofluorescence in nerve terminals and neurons.

---

and stimulation of secretion of a number of pituitary hormones. Table 21.5 summarizes evidence that VIP functions within the nervous system as a neurotransmitter or neuromodulator.

Somatotropin and Prolactin

Significant amounts of immunoreactive STH have been discovered in the amygdaloid nucleus of the limbic system. Immunohistochemical staining also reveals the presence of STH-like immunoreactivity in some other brain areas. Cells of the amygdala from both intact and hypophysectomized animals produce STH when placed in tissue culture. This observation argues for the synthesis of hormones in situ by this central nervous system structure of the brain. Extracts of the amygdala stimulate epiphysial cartilage growth as does pituitary STH [40].

Prolactin has also been shown by immunocytochemical studies to be present in nerve fibers in certain brain areas. PRL-responsive neurons are present within the dorsomedial and ventromedial nuclei in the rat brain. Intraventricular or systemic injections of PRL selectively increase the metabolic activity of tuberoinfundibular dopaminergic neurons. These neurons function in the inhibitory control of pituitary PRL secretion. PRL may regulate its own secretion by feedback effects on the tubero-infundibular neurons. Specific PRL binding sites have been demonstrated in the ependyma of the rat choroid plexus. PRL may regulate CSF ion composition through an initial action on receptor sites of the choroid plexus. On the other hand, the PRL binding sites may function in the uptake of PRL from the blood and delivery of the hormone to the CSF where PRL might then be delivered to other brain areas [57].

Brain Calcitonin

Calcitoninlike activity has been localized to the brain of a number of vertebrate species. Immunoreactive CT, indistinguishable from human CT, has also been identified in extracts of the hypothalamus (and pituitary) of humans [16]. Concentrations of the peptide are highest in the median eminence and the posterior hypothalamus with lesser amounts found in other parts of the brain. Specific binding of radiolabeled CT were highest in those brain areas associated with levels of endogenous CT. Intracerebroventricular injections induce prolactin secretion in rats. Other effects of central administration of the peptide were noted that could not be similarly evoked by systemic injections of the hormone. Whether CT functions as a neurotransmitter or neuromodulator within the brain remains to be determined.

EVOLUTION OF NEUROPEPTIDES

It is evident that peptides of identical or related primary structure are found in a wide variety of tissues. Originally, peptides, such as gastrointestinal hormones, were isolated from the gastrointestinal mucosa and their putative functions characterized. After determination of their primary structures, subsequent synthesis of these peptides allowed antibodies to be produced for radioimmunoassay and immunocytochemical studies. This then provided evidence for the localization of these peptides to the CNS and even to specific neurons within the brain and spinal cord. Thus, new functions are suggested for these peptides in addition to the original roles classically ascribed [21].

The discovery that peptides in the mammalian GI tract and brain are often found within amphibian skin and vice versa suggests that further elucidation of peptide structures from the tissues of nonmammalian vertebrates may provide important clues for the discovery of analogous peptides in mammalian tissues. Sauvagine, for example, may prove to be a prototype of a new family of peptides having structural counterparts in the brain and nervous system of mammals and other vertebrates [33].

New Theory of Hormones

While determining the presence of the vertebrate peptide hormones within more primitive organisms, the discovery was made that peptide hormones (or immunologically similar peptides) are, indeed, present within tissues of flies, worms, protozoa, and even bacteria [26]. It has been suggested that a primitive role of chemical messengers may have been as tissue growth factors. They may have been released initially as intracellular chemical messengers to regulate cellular growth processes. Subsequently their release into the extracellular environment may have provided a stimulus to their own growth or to other cells of the same cellular species. This point is well documented in the cellular slime mold.

The role of cyclic AMP as an intracellular messenger of hormone action in vertebrates is well established. This cyclic nucleotide is also an intermediate in the action of some insect hormones. Most interesting was the discovery that cyclic AMP is used in communication in cellular slime molds and in that capacity serves as the initial stimulus for amoeboid movement and subsequent morphogenesis. *Dictyostelium discoideum* is a cellular slime mold which passes through a number of distinctive stages in its life cycle. Initially, spores germinate to yield irregularly shaped, solitary, amoeboidlike cells that live on microorganisms usually available on the forest floor. During this stage the individual cells grow and divide by binary fission. When food sources are depleted, the starving amoebae mass together in response to periodic pulses of a chemical attractant and form multicellular aggregates. The cells initially begin moving in a pulsatile manner toward a central point and then form pulsating streams of aggregating cells. Aggregation is initiated by a small number of cells which release an attractant, originally known as *acrasin*. Eventually it was discovered that acrasin was identical to cyclic AMP. In response to cAMP cells move toward the cyclic nucleotide and in the process release their own pulse of cAMP. After releasing or responding to cAMP, the cells appear insensitive to the nucleotide for several minutes apparently because it is destroyed by a membrane cAMP phosphodiesterase. When a new pulse of cAMP arrives, the cells respond again; thus the amoebae migrate in pulsatile steps in response to alternations in sensitivity to the attractant [51].

Cyclic AMP apparently interacts with cellular receptors of the amoebae because slime molds that fail to respond to cAMP do not bind radiolabeled cAMP. The starvation stimulus apparently induces the formation of cAMP receptor proteins in the plasma membrane of amoebae which allows them to recognize the aggregation signal. The actual mechanism of perception of cAMP is not understood, but it is possible that the amoebae compute the difference in concentration of cAMP from the front to the back of the cells and thereby sense the presence of a gradient of the nucleotide. Other theories are equally attractive [34]. Movement, per se, involves activation of contractile proteins on the side of the cells that receives the signal to move. It is possible that cAMP may activate ion channels and elevate local intracellular levels of Ca^{2+}. Calmodulin or other intracellular Ca^{2+} receptors might then activate the contractile machinery required for amoeboid movement.

In its role as an extracellular chemical messenger cAMP functions in the classical sense as a pheromone. This might be considered a more primitive function of the cyclic nucleotide. Not all species of slime molds respond chemotactically to cAMP: Other chemical attractants, possibly small peptides, may be utilized. It is possible that a large number of chemically diverse "communicational molecules" may be employed by microorganisms [34]. Studies of these chemical messengers may provide important insights into the role of similar molecules that may be important in directing morphogenic movements in early development of invertebrate and vertebrate species.

Early in evolution, cell-cell communication in multicellular organisms may have been effected by local hormones. Although a paracrine mechanism of communication might be envisioned as operative in "simple" multicellular organisms (e.g., *Volvox*), more rapid delivery of a local hormone to a more distant site may have necessitated cellular elongation (dendritogenesis and axonal development). This would have resulted in the evolution of the first neurons whose original secretions may have been purely paracrine in nature (Fig. 10.5). Chemotactic orientation to a chemical gradient may have provided the initial stimulus to cellular elongation. Nerve growth factor, for example, provides the hormonal stimulus to directed growth of sympathetic neurons.

Evolution of Neuropeptides   **515**

The development of the complex structural element, the synapse, might be viewed as a later evolutionary acquisition. Release of a hormone into a synaptic cleft would have provided the mechanism for a more localized (efficient) delivery of the chemical messenger. Further evolution of the synapse may have involved localized membrane ion flow, rapid transmembrane electrical changes, and action potential transmission, features which characterize neurotransmitter mechanisms of action.

To mediate their actions hormones must be recognized by target cells. A version of the old "chicken-or-the-egg" argument—what came first, the hormone or the receptor—is raised. Both hormones and receptors most likely evolved simultaneously. Even the most primitive of cells needed to "sense" the environment. Change in salinity is known to stimulate morphological changes in some single-celled organisms. Some cellular receptor substance must therefore be able to interact with and subsequently respond to changes in Na^+ or Cl^- concentration. Even in mammals, chemoreceptors detect changes in Na^+ concentration of the blood. Calmodulin, the newly discovered intracellular Ca^{2+} receptor (Chapter 4), may well represent a reasonable example of such a chemoreceptive protein.

Peptide hormones probably evolved from cellular proteins that originally served other functions. Enzymatic hydrolysis, both intracellularly and extracellularly, may have then yielded smaller biologically active sequences that evolved a hormonal function. Point mutations of DNA bases would have provided new protein species necessary for the evolutionary selection process. It might be expected that selection would have favored enhanced hormone-receptor interaction. Through mutational changes in the DNA, the hormones and their receptors would have evolved together to provide sensitivity and selectivity characteristic of hormones and their receptors. Stability of peptide structures may have involved posttranslational modifications of the carboxy- and amino-terminal groups of some peptide hormones. Gene duplication followed by base mutations would have provided the means for variation of hormonal structure and subsequent evolution of the various families of hormones (Fig. 21.12).

With the development of diverse tissue types, other forms of hormones may have evolved. Mesodermal tissues, for example, are the specific source of steroid hormones. But the ability to synthesize steroid-like structures is not the sole provenance of animal tissues. Plants are able to produce vitamin D-like and estrogenic steroids. It is possible that their raison d'etre is to modify (adversely) physiological processes of animal tissues. For example, certain plant steroids may affect insect growth and development and cause egg maturation to occur at a seasonally inappropriate time.

In the vertebrate steroid hormones play important roles in modulating cellular responses to peptide hormones (Chapter 4). Many peptide hormones are virtually inactive in the absence of steroid hormones. The modulatory actions of steroid hormones on the brain are particularly important and through feedback mechanisms regulate the secretion of peptidergic hypophysiotropins (Chapter 6). Although the classical target tissues of vitamin D are the gut, kidney, and bone, the brain has been discovered to be a new site. Within the brain vitamin D may selectively affect specific neuronal populations causing changes in metabolism, neurite growth, and production and secretion of certain neurotransmitters, as has been demonstrated for other steroid hormone actions on the brain [47].

From an evolutionary perspective it appears that ancestral molecules supplied

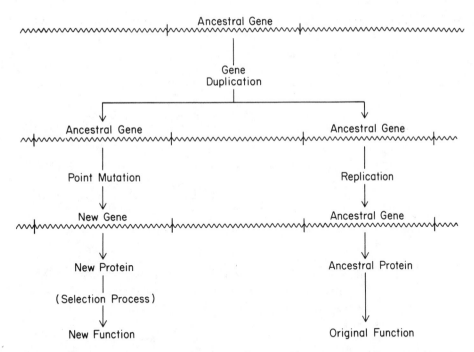

Figure 21.12 Scheme of peptide hormone evolution through gene duplication and base mutation.

the raw material on which evolutionary selective processes provided the present-day diversity of vertebrate hormones. Most importantly, these ancestral hormones often evolved to regulate species-specific physiological processes. The evolution of the terrestrial vertebrate from an aquatic habitat probably necessitated the need to put old hormones to new or additional uses or to evolve new hormones. Conservation of water and calcium may have become particularly important processes that required new hormonal control systems in the terrestrial habitat. The ancestral prolactin molecule antedated the evolutionary acquisition of mammary glands in the vertebrates. Melanotropins may have been particularly important hormones for certain species of animals where adaptative coloration was of survival value. In certain large groups of birds and many mammals MSH appears no longer to serve such a role. This is particularly evident in humans and birds where the source of MSH, the pars intermedia, is even lacking. However, in some mammals, including humans, MSH is present within the brain where it may function as a neurohormone to regulate other behavioral and physiological processes.

REFERENCES

[1] BARCHAS, J. D., H. AKIL, G. R. ELLIOTT, R. B. HOLMAN, and S. J. WATSON. 1978. Behavioral neurochemistry: neuroregulators and behavioral states. *Science* 200:964–73.

[2] BEAUMONT, A., and J. HUGHES. 1979. Biology of opioid peptides. *Ann. Rev. Pharmacol.* 19:245–67.

[3] BECKWITH, B. E., and C. A. SANDMAN. 1978. Behavioral influences of the neuropeptides ACTH and MSH: a methodological review. *Neurosci. Behav. Rev.* 2:311–38.

[4] BERTOLINI, A., and G. L. GESSA. 1981. Behavioral effects of ACTH and MSH peptides. *J. Endocrinol. Invest.* 4:241–51.

[5] BRECHA, N., H. J. KARTEN, and C. LAVERACK. 1979. Enkephalin-containing amacrine cells in the avian retina: immunohistochemical localization. *Proc. Natl. Acad. Sci. USA* 76: 3010–14.

[6] BROWN, M. 1981a. Neuropeptides: central nervous system effects on nutrient homeostasis. *Diabetologia* 20:299–304.

[7] ———. 1981b. Thyrotropin releasing factor: a putative CNS regulator of the autonomic nervous system. *Life Sci.* 28:1789–95.

[8] BROWN, M., J. RIVIER, and W. VALE. 1977. Bombesin: potent effects on thermoregulation in the rat. *Science* 196:998–1000.

[9] BROWN, M., R. ALLEN, J. VILLARREAL, J. RIVIER, and W. VALE. 1978. Bombesin-like activity: radioimmunologic assessment in biological tissues. *Life Sci.* 23:2721–28.

[10] CHAN, D. K. O., and H. A. BERN. 1976. The caudal neurosecretory system. *Cell Tiss. Res.* 174:339–54.

[11] CORRÊA, F. M. A., R. B. INNES, G. R. UHL, and S. H. SNYDER. 1979. Bradykinin-like immunoreactive neuronal systems localized histochemically in rat brain. *Proc. Nat. Acad. Sci. USA* 76:1489–93.

[12] DELLA-FERA, M. A., and C. A. BAILE. 1979. Cholecystokinin octapeptide: continuous picomole injections into the cerebral ventricles of sheep suppresses feeding. *Science* 206: 471–73.

[13] DE WIED, D. 1976. Hormonal influences on motivation, learning, and memory processes. *Hosp. Prac.* 11(1):123–31

[14] ERSPAMER, V. 1980. Peptides of the amphibian skin active on the gut II. Bombesin-like peptides isolation, structure, and basic functions. In *Gastrointestinal hormones*, ed. G. B. Glass, pp. 343–61. New York: Raven Press.

[15] ESKAY, R. L., J. F. FURNESS, and R. T. LONG. 1981. Substance P activity in the bullfrog retina: localization and identification in several vertebrate species. *Science* 212:1049–50.

[16] FISCHER, J. A., P. H. TOBLER, M. KAUFMANN, W. BORN, H. NENKE, P. E. COOPER, J. M. SAGAR, and J. B. MARTIN. 1981. Calcitonin: regional distribution of the hormone and its binding sites in the human brain and pituitary. *Proc. Natl. Acad. Sci.* 78:7801–7805.

[17] FISHER, L. A., W. VALE, J. SPIESS, C. RIVIER, and M. R. BROWN. 1982. Corticotropin-releasing factor alters mean arterial pressure, heart rate and plasma levels of catecholamines and vasopressin. *Proc. Natl. Acad. Sci. USA* 78:7801–7805.

[18] FORREST, J. N., JR., S. REICHLIN, and D. B. P. GOODMAN. 1980. Somatostatin: an endogenous peptide in the toad urinary bladder inhibits vasopressin-stimulated water flow. *Proc. Natl. Acad. Sci.* 77:4984–87.

[19] GESSA, G. L., E. PAGLIETTI, and B. PELLIGRINI QUARANTOTTI. 1979. Induction of copulatory behavior in sexually inactive rats by naloxone. *Science* 204:203–204.

[20] GOLDSTEIN, A., W. FISCHLI, L. I. LOWNEY, M. HUNKAPILLER, and L. HOOD. 1981. Porcine pituitary dynorphin: complete amino acid sequence of the biologically active heptadecapeptide. *Proc. Natl. Acad. Sci. USA* 78:7219–23.

[21] GUILLEMIN, R. 1977. The expanding significance of hypothalamic peptides, or, is endo-crinology a branch of neuroendocrinology? *Rec. Prog. Horm. Res.* 33:1–28.

[22] HÖKFELT, T., O. JOHANSSON, A. LJUNGDAHL, J. LUNDBERG, M. SCHULTZBERG, L. TERENIUS, M. GOLDSTEIN, R. ELDE, H. STEINBUSCH, and A. VERHOFSTAD. 1979. Histochemistry of transmitter interactions-neural coupling and coexistence of transmitters. In *Advances in pharmacology and therapeutics*, ed. S. Simon, pp. 131–42. © 1979 New York: Pergamon Press, Inc.

[23] IVERSEN, L. L. 1979. The chemistry of the brain. *Sci. Amer.* 241:134–49.

[24] KILPATRICK, D. L., T. TANIGUCHI, B. N. JONES, A. S. STERN, J. E. SHIVELY, J. HULLIHAN, S. KIMURA, S. STEIN, and S. UNDENFRIEND. 1981. A highly potent 3200-dalton adrenal opioid peptide that contains both a [Met]- and [Leu]-enkephalin sequence. *Proc. Natl. Acad. Sci. USA* 78:3265–68.

[25] KLEE, W. A. 1979. Molecular mechanisms of opioid action in neuroblastoma × glioma cells. In *Mechanisms of pain and analgesic compounds*, eds. R. F. Beirs, Jr. and E. G. Bassett, pp. 361–72. New York: Raven Press.

[26] KOLATA, G. 1982. New theory of hormones proposed. *Science* 215:1383–84.

[27] KRIEGER, D. T., and J. B. MARTIN. 1981. Brain peptides. *New Engl. J. Med.* 304:876–85, 944–50.

[28] LAUBER, M., P. NICOLAS, H. BOUSSETTA, C. FAHY, P. BÉGUIN, M. COMIER, H. VAUDRY, and P. COHEN. 1981. The M 80,000 common forms of neurophysin and vasopressin from bovine neurohypophyses have corticotropin- and β-endorphin-like sequences and liberate by proteolysis biologically active corticotropin. *Proc. Natl. Acad. Sci. USA* 78:6086–90.

[29] LEDERIS, K., A. LETTER, D. MCMASTER and G. MOORE. 1982. Complete amino acid se-quence of urotensin I, a hypotensive and corticotropin-releasing neuropeptide from *Catostomus. Science* 128:162–64.

[30] LI, C. H. 1978. β-Endorphin: a new biologically active peptide from pituitary glands. In *Hormonal proteins and peptides*, ed. C. H. Li, pp. 35–73. New York: Academic Press, Inc.

[31] LORETZ, C. A., and H. A. BERN. 1981. Stimulation of sodium transport across the teleost urinary bladder by urotensin II. *Gen. Comp. Endocrinol.* 43:325–30.

[32] MISELIS, R. R., R. E. SHAPIRO, and P. J. HAND. 1979. Subfornical organ efferents to neural systems for control of body water. *Science* 205:1022–25.

[33] MONTECUCCHI, P. C., and A. HENSCHEN. 1981. Amino acid composition and sequence analysis of sauvagine, a new active peptide from the skin of *Phyllomedusa sauvagei. Int. J. Peptide Res.* 18:113–20.

[34] NEWELL, P. C. 1977. How cells communicate: the system used by slime molds. *Endeavor* 1:63–68.

[35] MUELLER, K., and S. HSIAO. 1978. Current status of cholecystokinin as a short-term satiety hormone. *Neurosci. Behav. Rev.* 2:79–87.

[36] MYERS, R. D., and M. L. MCCALEB. 1981. Feeding: satiety signal from intestine triggers brain's noradrenergic mechanism. *Science* 209:1035–37.

[37] NAKANISHI, S., A. INOUE, T. KITA, M. NAKAMURA, A. C. Y. CHANG, S. N. COHEN, and S. NUMA. 1979. Nucleotide sequence of cloned cDNA for bovine corticotropin-β-lipotropin precursor. *Nature* 278:423–27.

[38] NICOLL, R. A., C. SCHENKER, and S. E. LEEMAN. 1980. Substance P as a transmitter can-didate. *Ann. Rev. Neurosci.* 3:227–68.

[39] O'Donohue, T. L., and D. M. Dorsa. 1982. The opiomelanotropinergic neuronal and endocrine systems. *Peptides* 3:353-95.

[40] Pacold, S. T., L. Kirsteins, S. Hojvat, and A. M. Lawrence. 1978. Biologically active pituitary hormones in the rat brain amygdaloid nucleus. *Science* 199:804-805.

[41] Pearse, A. G. E. 1981. The diffuse neuroendocrine system: falsification and verification of a concept. In: *Cellular basis of chemical messengers in the digestive system*, eds. M. I. Grossman, M. A. B. Brazier & J. Lechago, pp. 13-19. New York: Academic Press, Inc.

[42] Pearson, D., J. E. Shively, B. R. Clark, I. I. Geschwind, M. Barkley, R. Nishioka, and H. A. Bern. 1980. Urotensin II: a somatostatin-like peptide in the caudal neurosecretory system of fishes. *Proc. Natl. Acad. Sci.* 77:5021-24.

[43] Pedersen, C. A., J. A. Ascher, Y. L. Monroe, and A. J. Prange, Jr. 1982. Oxytocin induces maternal behavior in virgin female rats. *Science* 216:648-50.

[44] Reichlin, S. 1980. Peptides in neuroendocrine regulation. In *Peptides: integrators of cell and tissue function*, ed. F. E. Bloom, pp. 235-50. New York: Raven Press.

[45] Reichlin, S., R. Siperstein, I. M. D. Jackson, A. E. Boyd, and Y. Petel. 1976. Hypothalamic hormones. *Ann. Rev. Physiol.* 38:389-424.

[46] Ruda, M. A. 1982. Opiates and pain pathways: demonstration of enkephalin synapses on dorsal horn projection neurons. *Science* 215: 1523-25.

[47] Stumpf, W. E., M. Sar, and S. A. Clark. 1982. Brain target sites for 1,25-dihydroxyvitamin D_2. *Science* 215:1403-1405.

[48] Snyder, S. H. 1977. Opiate receptors and internal opiates. *Sci. Amer.* 236:44-56.

[49] _____. 1980. Brain peptides as neurotransmitters. *Science* 209:976-83.

[50] Taylor, W. L., K. J. Collier, R. J. Deschenes, H. L. Weith, and J. E. Dixon. 1981. Sequence analysis of a cDNA coding for a pancreatic precursor to somatostatin. *Proc. Natl. Acad. Sci.* 78:6694-98.

[51] Tomchik, K. J., and P. N. Devreotes. 1981. Adenosine 3',5'-monophosphate waves in *Dictyostelium discoideum*: a demonstration by isotope dilution-fluorography. *Science* 212:443-46.

[52] Vale, W., J. Spiess, C. Rivier, and J. Rivier. 1981. Characterization of a 41-residue bovine hypothalamic peptide that stimulates secretion of corticotropin and β-endorphin. *Science* 213:1394-97.

[53] Van Houten, M., B. I. Posner, B. M. Kopriwa, and J. R. Brawer. 1980. Insulin binding sites localized to nerve terminals in rat median eminence and arcuate nucleus. *Science* 207:1081-83.

[54] Vincent, J. D., and J. L. Barker. 1979. Substance P: evidence for diverse roles in neuronal function from cultured mouse spinal neurons. *Science* 205:1409-11.

[55] Viveros, O. H., E. J. Diliberto, Jr., E. Hazum, and K. J. Chang. 1980. Enkephalins as possible adrenomedullary hormones: storage, secretion, and regulation of synthesis. In *Neural peptides and neuronal communication*, eds. E. Costa and M. Trabucchi, pp. 191-204. New York: Raven Press.

[56] von Euler, U. S., and B. Pernow, eds. 1977. *Substance P*. New York: Raven Press.

[57] Walsh, R. J., B. I. Posner, B. M. Kopriwa, and J. R. Brown. 1978. Prolactin binding sites in the rat brain. *Science* 201:1041-42.

[58] Wardlow, S. L., W. B. Wehrenberg, M. Ferin, P. W. Carmel, and A. G. Frantz. 1980. High levels of β-endorphin in hypophyseal portal blood. *Endocrinology* 106:1323-26.

[59] Watson, S. J., H. Akil, and J. M. Walker. 1980. Anatomical and biochemical studies of the opioid peptides and related substances in the brain. *Peptides 1* (Suppl. 1):11-20.

[60] WATSON, S. J., H. AKIL, W. FISCHLI, A. GOLDSTEIN, E. ZIMMERMAN, G. NILAVER, and T. B. VAN WIMERSMA GREIDANUS. 1982. Dynorphin and vasopressin: common localization in magnocellular neurons. *Science* 216:85–87.

[61] WEINGARTNER, H., P. GOLD, J. C. BALLENGER, S. A. SMALLBERG, R. SUMMERS, D. R. RUBINOW, R. M. POST, and F. K. GOODWIN. 1981. Effects of vasopressin on human memory functions. *Science* 211:601–603.

[62] YARBROUGH, G. G. 1979. On the neuropharmacology of thyrotropin releasing hormone (TRH). *Prog. Neurobiol.* 12:291–312.

[63] ZIEGLGANSBERGER, W. 1980. Peptides in the regulation of neuronal function. In *Integrators of cell and tissue function*, ed. F. E. Bloom, pp. 219–33. New York: Raven Press.

[64] ZUKIN, S., and S. R. ZUKIN. 1981. Multiple opiate receptors: emerging concepts. *Life Sci.* 29:2681–90.

Appendix

SOME COMMON ENDOCRINE ABBREVIATIONS AND TERMINOLOGY

ACTH	Adrenocorticotropic hormone (corticotropin)
ADH	Antidiuretic hormone
AMP	Adenosine 3,5′-monophosphate
ANS	Autonomic nervous system
APUD	Amine precursor uptake and decarboxylation
AVP	Arginine vasopressin
AVT	Arginine vasotocin
cAMP	Cyclic adenosine monophosphate
CaBP	Calcium binding protein
CBG	(corticosteroid binding globulin, transcortin)
CCK	Cholecystokinin
cGMP	Cyclic guanosine monophosphate
CNS	Central nervous system
COMT	Catechol-O-methyltransferase
CRH	Corticotropin releasing hormone
CSF	Cerebral spinal fluid
CT	Calcitonin
DBH	(dopamine β-hydroxylase)

DHT	Dihydrotestosterone
DIT	Diiodotyrosine
DOPA	(dihydroxyphenylalanine)
EGF	Epidermal growth factor
FGF	Fibroblast growth factor
FSH	Follicle stimulating hormone (follitropin)
GH	Growth hormone (somatotropin, STH)
GHRH	(growth hormone releasing hormone, somatocrinin)
GIP	Gastric inhibitory peptide
GnRH	Gonadotropin releasing hormone (LH/FSH-RH)
GTP	Guanosine triphosphate
HCG	Human chorionic gonadotropin (choriogonadotropin)
HCS	Human chorionic somatomammotropin
HIOMT	Hydroxyindole-O-methyltransferase
HPL	Human placental lactogen
5-HT	5-Hydroxytryptamine (serotonin)
IGF	Insulinlike growth factors (I and II)
LATS	Long-acting thyroid stimulator (thyroid stimulating antibody, TSAb)
LH	Luteinizing hormone (lutropin)
β-LPH	β-Lipotropin
LVP	Lysine vasopressin
MAO	Monoamine oxidase
MIF	MSH release inhibiting factor (melanostatin)
MIT	Monoiodotyrosine
MRF	Müllerian regression factor
mRNA	Messenger ribonucleic acid
α-MSH	α-Melanocyte (or melanophore) stimulating hormone (α-melanotropin)
NSILA	Nonsuppressible insulinlike activity
PBI	Protein bound iodine
PDGF	Platelet-derived growth factor
PGE$_2$	Prostaglandin E$_2$
PGF$_{2\alpha}$	Prostaglandin F$_{2\alpha}$
PIF	Prolactin inhibiting factor
PMS	Pregnant mare serum
PNMT	Phenylethanolamine-N-methyltransferase
PRL	Prolactin
PTH	Parathormone
rT$_3$	(reverse T$_3$)
STH	Somatotropin (growth hormone, GH)
T$_3$	Triiodothyronine
T$_4$	Thyroxine (tetraiodothyronine)
TBG	Thyroxine binding globulin
tRNA	Transfer ribonucleic acid
TRH	Thyrotropin releasing hormone
TSH	Thyroid stimulating hormone (thyrotropin)
VIP	Vasoactive intestinal peptide
VMA	Vanillylmandelic acid

Some Common Endocrine Abbreviations and Terminology

VERTEBRATE HORMONES

Hormone	Molecular Weight	
Acetylcholine	147	
Aldosterone	360	
Angiotensin II	1046	
Arginine vasopressin (AVP)	1084	
Bombesin	1620	(f)[a]
Bradykinin	1060	
Caerulein	1353	(f)
Calcitonin (thyrocalcitonin)	3418	
Cholecystokinin (CCK)		
Chymodenin[b]		
Corticosterone	346	
Corticotropin, adrenocorticotropin (ACTH)		
Corticotropin releasing hormone (CRH)		
Cortisol	363	
Cortisone	361	
Dihydrotestosterone	366	
Dopamine	153	
β-Endorphin	3465	
Epidermal growth factor (EGF)		
Epinephrine	183	
Erythropoietin; erythrocyte stimulating factor (ESF)[b]		
Estradiol	262	
Fibroblast growth factor (FGF)[b]		
Follicle stimulating hormone (FSH); follitropin		
Gamma aminobutyric acid (GABA)	103	
Gastric inhibitory peptide (GIP)	5104	(p)
Gastrin (1–17)	2098	
Glucagon		
Gonadotropin releasing hormone (GnRH); gonadoliberin	1182	
Histamine	111	
Human chorionic gonadotropin (choriogonadotropin, hCG)		
Human placental lactogen (hPL); chorionic somatomammotropin		
Inhibin[b]		
Insulin		
Insulinlike growth factor I (IGF-I)		
Insulinlike growth factor II (IGF-II)		
Leucine enkephalin (Leu-enkephalin)		
Leukotrienes, LTE_4		
Luteinizing hormone (lutropin, LH)		
Lysine vasopressin (LVP)	1056	
Lyslbradykinin	1188	
α-Melanocyte stimulating hormone (α-MSH); α-melanotropin	1665	
Melatonin (N-acetyl-5-methoxytryptamine)	232	
Mesotocin	1007	
Methionine enkephalin (Met-enkephalin)	574	
Motilin	2699	(p)
MSH release inhibiting factor (MIF)		
Müllerian regression factor (MRF)[b]		
Nerve growth factor (NGF)		
Neurotensin (NT)	1673	
Norepinephrine (NE)	103	

Oxytocin	1007	
Pancreatic polypeptide (PP)	4221	(b)
Parathormone (PTH)		
Platelet-derived growth factor (PDGF)[b]		
Progesterone	314	
Prolactin inhibiting factor (PIF)		
Prostacyclin I_2 (PGI$_2$)		
Prostaglandin E_2 (PGE$_2$)	353	
Prostaglandin $F_{2\alpha}$ (PGF$_{2\alpha}$)	355	
Relaxin		
Secretin	3055	(p)
Serotonin (5-hydroxytryptamine, 5-HT)	176	
Serum thymic factor (STF)	876	
Somatomedin A[b]		
Somatomedin B		
Somatomedin C[b]		
Somatostatin (SS); somatotropin release inhibiting hormone (SRIH)	1639	
Somatotropin (STH)		
Substance P (SP)	1347	(b)
Testosterone	288	
Thromboxane A_2 (TXA$_2$)		
Thymopoietin		
Thymosin$_{\alpha 1}$		
Thymosin$_{\alpha 4}$		
Thyrotropin; thyroid stimulating hormone (TSH)		
Thyrotropin releasing hormone (TRH)	362	
Thyroxine (T$_4$)	777	
Triiodothyronine (T$_3$)	651	
Urogastrone[c]		
Vasoactive intestinal peptide (VIP)	3326	(p)
Vasotocin	1050	
Vitamin D (1,25-dihydroxycholecalciferol)(1,25-(OH)$_2$D$_3$) (calcitriol)	417	

[a]All hormones are of human origin unless otherwise noted (p, porcine; b, bovine; f, frog). The molecular weights (MW) are derived from the constituent amino acids of the peptides. It should be noted that commercially available or synthetically prepared peptides may contain a number of counter ions (e.g., acetate, Na$^+$, etc.) depending on the final purification and isolation procedures. This should be carefully considered when using the dry weight of the lyophilized powder to prepare molar concentrations of the peptides.

[b]Structure undetermined.

[c]Probably identical to epidermal growth factor (EGF).

Bibliography

BOOKS AND MONOGRAPHS

BARRINGTON, E. J. W. 1964. *Hormones and evolution*. London: The English Universities Press, Ltd.

——. 1975. *An introduction to general and comparative endocrinology*. 2nd ed. London: Oxford University Press, Inc.

BENTLEY, P. J. 1982. *Comparative vertebrate endocrinology*, 2nd ed. Cambridge, England: Cambridge University Press.

DEGROOT, L. J., G. F. CAHILL, JR., L. MARTINI, D. H. NELSON, W. D. ODELL, J. T. POTTS, JR., E. STEINBERGER, and A. I. WINEGRAD, eds. 1979. *Endocrinology*, vols. 1–3. New York: Grune & Stratton, Inc.

FRIEDEN, E. H. 1976. *Chemical endocrinology*. New York: Academic Press, Inc.

FRIEDEN, E. H., and H. LIPNER. 1971. *Biochemical endocrinology of the vertebrates*. Englewood Cliffs, N.J.: Prentice Hall Publishing Co., Inc.

FRYE, B. E. 1967. *Hormonal control in vertebrates*. New York: Macmillan, Inc.

GANONG, W. F. 1981. *Review of medical physiology*. 10th ed. Los Altos, Ca.: Lange Med. Publ.

GORBMAN, A., W. W. DICKHOFF, S. R. VIGNA, N. B. CLARK and C. L. RALPH. 1983. *Comparative endocrinology*. New York: John Wiley & Sons, Inc.

KRIEGER, D. T., and J. C. HUGHES. 1980. *Neuroendocrinology. A hospital practice book*. Sunderland, Ma.: Sinauer Associates.

LEE, J. and J. LAYCOCK. 1978. *Essential endocrinology*. New York: Oxford University Press.

LI, C. H., *ed.* 1973–1981. *Hormonal proteins and peptides*, vols. 1–10. New York: Academic Press, Inc.

MARTIN, C. R. 1976. *Textbook of endocrine physiology*. Baltimore: The Williams & Wilkins Company.

Norris, D. O. 1980. *Vertebrate endocrinology*. Philadelphia: Lea & Febiger.

Sawin, C. T. 1969. *The hormones*. Boston: Little, Brown & Company.

Tepperman, J. 1980. *Metabolic and endocrine physiology*. 4th ed. Chicago: Year Book Medical Publishers, Inc.

Turner, C. D., and J. T. Bagnara. 1976. *General endocrinology*. 6th ed. Philadelphia: W. B. Saunders Company.

Williams, R. H. 1981. *Textbook of endocrinology*. 6th ed. Philadelphia: W. B. Saunders Company.

MAJOR ENDOCRINOLOGY JOURNALS

Acta Endocrinologica (Acta Endocrinol.)
Advances In Cyclic Nucleotide Research (Advan. Cyclic Nucl. Res.)
Annales d'Endocrinologie (Ann. d'Endocrinol.)
Clinical Endocrinology (Clin. Endocrinol.)
Endocrine Research Communications (Endoc. Res. Commun.)
Endocrinologica Japonica (Endocrinol. Jap.)
Endocrinology
Endokrinologie
General and Comparative Endocrinology (Gen. Comp. Endocrinol.)
Hormone and Metabolic Research (Horm. Met. Res.)
Hormones and Behavior (Hormone Behav.)
Journal of Clinical Endocrinology And Metabolism (J. Clin. Endocrinol. Metab.)
Journal of Endocrinology (J. Endocrinol.)
Molecular and Cellular Endocrinology (Mol. Cell. Endocrinol.)
Neuroendocrinology

ENDOCRINOLOGY-RELATED JOURNALS

Advances In Prostaglandin and Thromboxane Research
Advances In Steroid Biochemistry and Pharmacology
American Journal of Physiology (Am. J. Physiol.)
Cell and Tissue Research (Cell Tissue Res.)
Clinical Investigation (Clin. Invest.)
Diabetes
FEBS Letters
Federation Proceedings (Fed. Proc.)
Journal of Biological Chemistry (J. Biol. Chem.)
Journal of Clinical Investigation (J. Clin. Invest.)
Journal of Cyclic Nucleotide Research
Journal of Experimental Zoology (J. Exp. Zool.)
Journal of General Physiology (J. Gen. Physiol.)
Journal of Neurophysiology
Journal of Physiology (J. Physiol.)
Laboratory Investigation (Lab. Invest.)
Life Sciences (Life Sci.)

Nature
Neuroscience Letters (Neurosci. Lett.)
New England Journal of Medicine (New Eng. J. Med.)
Peptides
Proceedings of the National Academy of Sciences, USA (PNAS USA)
Prostaglandins
Receptors
Regulatory Peptides
Science
Steroids

SERIAL PUBLICATIONS

Annual Review of Biochemistry (Ann. Rev. Biochem.)
Annual Review of Medicine (Ann. Rev. Med.)
Annual Review of Neuroscience (Ann. Rev. Neurosci.)
Annual Review of Pharmacology and Toxicology (Ann. Rev. Pharmacol. Toxicol.)
Annual Review of Physiology (Ann. Rev. Physiol.)
Contemporary Endocrinology (formerly *The Year In Endocrinology*)
Frontiers In Neuroendocrinology (Front. Neuroendocrinol.)
Physiological Reviews (Physiol. Rev.)
Recent Progress In Hormone Research (Rec. Prog. Horm. Res.)
Vitamins and Hormones (Vit. Horm.)

Index

C

Cabbage goiter, 298
Caffeine, 51
Calciferin-binding protein (*See* Transcalciferin)
Calciferol (*See* Ergocalciferol)
Calcitonin, 21, 104, *187–207*
  brain, 5, 14
  feeding behavior and, 190
  source (thyroid), 297
Calcitriol (1, 25-(OH)$_2$-D$_3$) (*See* Vitamin D)
Calcium:
  calmodulin and, 76
  dependent regulatory protein, 76
  homeostasis, 78, *182–207*
  hormonal control of, 182
  hormone action and, 75
  ionophores, 53
  metabolism of, 183
  receptor, 76
  role in hormone action, 76
  stimulus-response coupling and, 75
Calciuria, 186
Calmodulin, 75, 333
Calorigenesis:
  thyroid hormones and, 303, 314
cAMP (*See* Cyclic AMP)
Cancer, 266
  estrogens and breast cancer, 463
Cannabinoids:
  male reproductive function and, 417
Cannon, Walter, 4, 9, 319
Carbacol, 52
Carbimazole:
  antithyroid action of, 309
Carbohydrate metabolism:
  catecholamine effects on, 337
  general considerations, 239
  glucocorticoid effects on, 360
  thyroid hormone effects on, 304
Carboxypeptidase, 33
Carbutamide, 298
Cardiac glycosides, 41
Carotenemia, 310
Carotenes, 310
Carotid sinus:
  vasopressin secretion and, 152
Carpopedal spasms:
  hypocalcemia and, 203
Carrier-mediated process, 304
Cartilage, 266, 285
Cascade phenomenon:
  in glycogenolysis, 65
Casein synthesis, 455
Castration, 1, 402

Catalytic subunit:
  of cAMP dependent protein kinase, 64, 79
Catecholamine(s), 318–43
  biosynthesis, 326
  catabolism, 327
  reversal, 329
Catecholamine-0-methyltransferase (COMT), 34
Catecholestrogens, 434
Catechol-0-methyltransferase (COMT), 377
Caudal neurosecretory system, 507
CBG (*See* Corticosteroid-binding globulin)
CCK (*See* Cholecystokinin)
CCK-octapeptide, 505
C (clear) cells:
  source of calcitonin, 187
Cell cycle, 265
Cerebral spinal fluid (CSF), 499
  melatonin and, 475
  neurohypophysial hormones and, 145, 508
Cerulein (caerulein), 231
Cervix (of the uterus), 147, 423
  cervical mucus, 437, 459
cGMP (*See* Cyclic GMP)
Chalones, 22, 23, 26, 283
Chemical messengers, 23
Chemoreceptors, 12
Chief cells:
  parathyroid glands, 184
  stomach, 217
Chlorpromazine:
  dopamine receptors and, 52, 53, 124, 165
  melanotropin secretion and, 165
  prolactin secretion and, 52
Chlorpropamide, 253
Cholecalciferol (Vitamin D$_3$), 191
Cholecystokinin (CCK), 21, 211, 218
  calcitonin secretion and, 190
  gall bladder contraction and, 68
  -pancreozymin and, (CCK-PZ),
  satiety and, 504
Cholera toxin, 81
Cholesterol:
  ester hydrolase, 353
  steroid hormone biosynthesis, 348, 351
Cholinergic:
  agonists, 328
  antagonists, 328
  receptors, 328
Cholinomimetic agents, 328
Chondrocytes, 285
Choriogonadotropin (*See* Chorionic
      gonadotropin)
Chorionic gonadotropin (choriogonadotropin),
      93, 99, 446
  growth effects of, 270

Morphological color change, 167
Mosaicism, 395
Motilin, 21, 210, 214, 215
MRF (*See* Müllerian regression factor)
MSA (*See* Multiplication stimulating activity)
α-MSH (*See* Melanotropins, α-melanotropin)
MSH release inhibiting factor (MIF)
    (melanostatin), 125
Müllerian ducts, 384
Müllerian regression factor (MRF), 384
Multiple endocrine adenomas (MEA's), 258
Multiplication stimulating activity (MSA),
    268
Muscarinic receptors, 329
Muscle:
  hormone action on
    catecholamines, 335, 449
    glucocorticoids, 362, 411
    neurohypophysial hormones, 149
    prostaglandins, 335
Musk, 413
Myasthenia gravis:
  cholinergic receptors and, 81
Myelinogenesis:
  thyroid hormones and, 303
Myenteric plexus of Auerbach, 209
Myoepithelial cells, 147, 149, 455
Myometrium, 73, 423, 426
  catecholamines and, 335
  parturition and, 447, 450
  prostaglandins and, 449
Myxedema, 37, 108, 308, 310, 336

N

N-Acetyl-5-methoxytroptamine (*See* Melatonin)
N-Acetylserotonin, 470, 473
N-Acetyltransferase (NAT), 470
Na$^+$,-K$^+$-ATPase (*See* Sodium-potassium pump),
    50
  aldosterone and, 365
  prolactin and, 456
  thyroid hormones and, 305, 306
Naloxone, 489
Nasal salt glands:
  glucocorticoid affects on, 373
Negative:
  feedback, 9, 61
  nitrogen balance, 258
  receptor cooperativity, 62
Nephrectomy, 278
Nephrogenic diabetes insipidus, 155
Nerve growth factor (NGF), 61, *271*, 303, 325,
    413

Nervous system:
  glucocorticoid effects on, 353, 362
  gonadal steroid effects on, 388, 391
  thyroid hormone effects on, 303, 308
Neural crest, 322
Neuraminidase, 279
Neuroblastoma, 340
Neuroblasts, 325, 340
Neurocrine secretion, 32
Neuroectoderm, 87, 325
Neuroendocrine:
  reflex, 301, 456
  transducer, 472
Neuroendocrinology, 7, 12, 142
Neurogenic:
  diabetes insipidus, 155
  hyperprolactinemia, 462
Neuroglial cells, 141
Neurohemal organ, 142
Neurohormones, 4, 23, 488
Neurohypophysial hormone(s), 92, *106*, *140–59*
  behavior and, 508
Neurohypophysis (pars nervosa), 141, 144, 161
Neurointermediate lobe, 87, 160
Neuromodulator(s), 19, 23
Neuropeptide(s), 5, 23, 30, 117
Neuropharmacology, 132
Neurophysin(s), 144, 491
Neuroregulators, 22, 23
Neurosecretion, 18, 141
Neurosecretory:
  granule, 141
  neurons, 114, 141
Neurotensin, 12, 211, 214, 215, 226, 502
Neurotransduction, 472
Neurotransmitter(s), 18, 23, 25, 29, *489*
Neurovascular hypothesis, 113
Neutral sex, 382
Nicotinic receptors, 328
Nociceptive stimuli, 498
Nonhistone (chromatin) proteins, 305, 432
Nonshivering (metabolic) thermogenesis, 315
Nonsteroidal estrogens, 433
Nonsuppressible insulin-like activity (NSILA-I,
    NSILA-II), 267
Noradrenaline (*See* Norepinephrine)
Norepinephrine (noradrenaline), 4, 18, 126, 320
Norethindrone:
  a contraceptive steroid, 458
Normetanephrine, 377
19-Nortestosterone, 458
Nuptial pads, 413
Nuptial plumage, 411
Nutrient homeostasis:
  bombesin and, 500

O

Oligomycin:
  a metabolic inhibitor, 51, 53
Oligosaccharides (of glycoprotein hormones), 99
Oocyte, 423
  maturation factor, 435
  maturation inhibitor (OMI), 435
Oogenesis, 382
Oophorectomy, 463
Opiate(s):
  endorphins and, 489
  (-like) peptides, 169, 489
  receptors, 489
Opiomelanotropinergic neurons, 508
Opportunistic breeders, 441
Oral ectoderm, 87
Orchidectomy:
  male castration, 44, 49, 405
Organizational effects:
  of steroid hormones, 388
Organs of Zuckerlandl, 324
Organum vasculosum (of the lateral terminalis, OVLT), 506
Ornithine decarboxylase (ODC), 273, 275, 307, 456
Oscillator (biological clock):
  pineal and, 477, 480
Osmoreceptors, 12
  aldosterone secretion and, 355
  vasopressin secretion and, 150
Osmoregulation (electrolyte balance), 13, 150, 355
Osteoblasts, 183, 199
Osteoclasts, 183, 199
Osteocytes, 182
Osteomalacia: 191, 203
  vitamin D-resistant, 204
  vitamin D-responsive, 204
Osteoporosis:
  postmenopausal, 204
Ouabain:
  Na^+-K^+ pump inhibitor), 50
Ovalbumin:
  estrogens and, 431
Ovarian:
  cycle, 424, 436
  regulatory (growth) factors, 435, 436
Ovariectomy, 44, 421, 449
  breast cancer and, 463
Ovaries, 422
Oviducts, 422, 431
Oviparity, 444
Oviposition, 196
Ovotestis:
  true hermaphroditism, 396
Ovoviparity, 444

Ovulation, 422, 438
  induced, 439, 440
  reflex, 439, 440
Oxidative coupling (in thyroid hormone biosynthesis), 295
Oxidative phosphorylation:
  thyroid hormone effects on: 303, 306
  uncouplers of, 51
Oxyntic cells (*See* Chief cells, stomach)
Oxyphil cells:
  parathyroid gland and, 184
Oxyphysin, 106, 144
Oxytocin, 18, 19, 22, 59, 92, 106, 107, 125, 130, *140–59*, 430
  coitus and, 147, 150
  estradiol and, 148
  parturition and, 450, 454
  progesterone and, 149
  receptors, 148
  reflex stimulation of, 144
  uterine contraction and, 154
Oxytocinase, 153
Oxytocinergic neurons, 144

P

Paget's disease, 204
Pain:
  gate, 493
  hormones, 169, 489
Palkovits punch, 117
Pancreas, 235
Pancreatic:
  amylase, 237
  cholera, 229
  enzymes, 210, 229
  hormones, 235, 263
  islet cell tumors, 258
  islets, 3
  lipase, 210
  polypeptide (PP), 211, 250
Pancreozymin (PZ), 218 (*See also* Cholecystokinin)
Panhypopituitarism, 95, 107
Para-aortic bodies (*See* Paraganglia)
Parabiosis, 44, 277
Paracrine;
  mechanism of secretion, 21, 216, 222, 237, 515
Parafollicular (C) cells, 21, 188
Paraganglia (para-aortic bodies), 324
Paragangliomas, 340
Paraphysis, 482
Parapineal organ, 482
Parasympathetic nervous system, 321
Parathormone, 21, 59, *183–87*
Parathyroidectomy, 184, 186
Parathyroid glands, 21, 183
Parathyroid hormone (*See* Parathormone)